S0-BEC-317

EXTRACRANIAL CEREBROVASCULAR DISEASE

EXTRACRANIAL CEREBROVASCULAR DISEASE

Diagnosis and Management

Edited by

Francis Robicsek, M.D.

Chairman, Department of Thoracic and
Cardiovascular Surgery,
Charlotte Memorial Hospital and
Medical Center,
Charlotte, North Carolina

and

Clinical Professor of Surgery
University of North Carolina at Chapel Hill,
Chapel Hill, North Carolina

Macmillan Publishing Company
NEW YORK

Collier Macmillan Canada, Inc.
TORONTO

Collier Macmillan Publishers
LONDON

Printed in the United States of America

Macmillan Publishing Company
866 Third Avenue, New York, New York, 10022

Collier Macmillan Canada, Inc.
Collier Macmillan Publishers · London

Library of Congress Cataloging-in-Publication Data

Extracranial cerebrovascular disease.

Includes index.
1. Cerebrovascular diseases. I. Robicsek, Francis.
[DNLM: 1. Cerebrovascular Disorders—diagnosis.
2. Cerebrovascular Disorders—therapy. WL 355 E96]
RC388.5.E98 1986 616.8′1 86-2835
ISBN 0-02-402540-2

Printing: 1 2 3 4 5 6 7 8 Year: 6 7 8 9 0 1 2 3 4

This book is dedicated to my family — Lilly, Steven,
Suzanne, John-Christopher, Frances,
and
The Charlotte Memorial Hospital

Foreword

Only 35 years ago, a patient diagnosed as suffering from a cerebral thrombosis was considered to have an intracranial arterial occlusion and great care was taken to diagnose which intracranial vessel was involved, the middle cerebral, the posterior cerebral, or the anterior cerebral. Today it is known that in at least 60 percent of such patients an extracranial arterial lesion is the cause of this problem, and in most of these patients the intracranial arteries are not occluded. This knowledge has changed, in a most significant way, the medical profession's management of such patients. The key to modern therapy is to study the extracranial cerebral arteries—the innominate, carotid, subclavian, and the vertebral—in every patient considered having a transient attack of cerebral ischemia or stroke caused by arterial thrombosis or embolus. Treatment is then based upon the concept that these common extracranial arterial lesions, when discovered, can be treated either medically or surgically and that in many patients the occurrence of stroke can be prevented.

Thousands of operations are done each year for atheromatous plaque or stenosis at the bifurcation of the common carotid arteries, and many more are performed for problems involving the subclavian-vertebral circulation. In addition the innominate and external carotid arteries are reconstructed, the latter when the ipsilateral internal carotid artery is totally occluded. During this period a newly recognized disease, fibromuscular hyperplasia of the internal carotid, has been described, and the management of old problems, such as arterial injuries, carotid body tumors, and aneurysms of the extracranial cerebral arteries, has been modernized to such a degree that the diagnosis and treatment of extracranial arterial disease are now an important part of medical practice.

In 1954, the American College of Surgeons held a sectional meeting in London, England. We at Saint Mary's Hospital, London, were asked to stage a clinical demonstration of such conditions and presented a patient who was suffering from transient attacks of cerebral ischemia caused by severe stenosis of the internal carotid artery. We presented her case to Edwin J. Wiley, who was there in military uniform. When the management of the patient was discussed, he stated that a thromboendarterectomy should be a satisfactory procedure, and this was the operation that we planned to do. The patient was also seen by M. E. DeBakey, Frank L. A. Gerbode, and George R. Dunlop, who later became president of the American College of Surgeons. All of them watched us operate. Since the lesion was very short and localized, it was resected and the artery was reconstructed by an end-to-end anastomosis between the common and internal carotid arteries. The external carotid artery was divided between ligatures. The patient lived symptom free for many years after the operation.

In our view the most important contribution of this early period was the realization that the best time to restore a normal flow through an extracranial artery is during the stage of stenosis, before the artery became completely occluded. Today the management of patients with transient attacks of cerebral ischemia owing to a plaque or an atheroma at the origin of the internal carotid artery may be either surgical or medical. Such a plaque or atheroma may cause many problems, two of which are of special importance: microembolization, often from an ulcerated plaque, and the reduction of blood flow by a hemodynamically significant arterial stenosis. Such a stricture is a clear indication for surgical correction. In the case of microembolization from a plaque or atheroma, the debate is between treatment with antiplatelet drugs and by surgical removal of the plaque. In experienced hands, surgery can be performed with a combined mortality and morbidity risk of less than 2 percent, and it has been proven effective in preventing strokes.

The place of surgery in the management of total occlusion of the internal carotid artery has been discussed by many authors. The key to success in such a patient is to obtain a good backflow from the internal carotid artery. This is essential. If satisfactory backflow cannot be obtained, reconstruction of an external carotid stenosis may benefit the patient. Our position in 1986 can be summarized as follows: A patient with a total occlusion of the internal carotid artery should not have the artery explored surgically if there is an acute profound neurological deficit, if the patient is asymptomatic, or if it is suspected that the thrombosis has originated in the intracranial carotid circulation. On the other hand, patients who may benefit from carotid thromboendarterectomy for total internal carotid occlusion include mentally intact patients with fixed neurological deficits, patients with crescendo transient ischemic attacks, and some patients with a stroke in evolution.

In 1986, after 30 years' experience with reconstruction of the extracranial cerebral arteries, it can be stated that (1) the best indication for operation is a patient suffering from transient ischemic attacks owing to an arterial stenosis or a plaque which is a source of microemboli, (2) a patient with a total occlusion of an extracranial cerebral artery may benefit from arterial reconstruction when conditions are suitable, and (3) the best and most frequently used procedure is thromboendarterectomy with or without patch-graft angioplasty.

Francis Robicsek, chairman of the Department of Thoracic and Cardiovascular Surgery in Charlotte Memorial Hospital and Medical Center, Charlotte, North Carolina, together with a number of colleagues, the contributors to this book, have been pioneers in the development of cardiovascular surgery and especially of the treatment of patients with extracranial arterial disease. This authoritative work will, I am sure, be widely read and quoted. It is an honor to be asked to write this Foreword, because I have been interested in this problem from the onset of the modern era of patient care.

Charles G. Rob, M.D.

Preface

This book was written in anticipation of continued rapid expansion of the number of clinically recognized cases of extracranial cerebrovascular disease that undoubtedly has been brought about by improvements and more extensive application of noninvasive methods of diagnosis. It represents a consolidated effort of multidisciplinary approach to the management of extracranial cerebrovascular disease.

During the processes of writing and editing this book, we encountered several difficulties that appeared to be particular to the subject. As it often has been said, progress in medical science has become so rapid that it virtually outruns the slower process of writing, printing, and editing so that from the time a problem is presented an appropriate solution may have already been found. Somehow in the case of a comprehensive book on extracranial vascular disease this postulate seems to be working in reverse: for by the time the solution of a clinical problem has been presented in print it has already come under heavy fire and thus the process of problem-solving has to begin anew. A typical example of this "problem-solving in reverse" is the changing view on extracranial-intracranial bypass procedures. They were regarded as probably the most important advance in cerebrovascular surgery at the time of this authorship but fell in somewhat disrepute during the twelve months of editing and publication. Another problem that heavily hinders production of a comprehensive book on extracranial cerebrovascular surgery is the dubious results of clinical evaluations made by advocates of different therapeutic methods who staunchly and unwaveringly defend opposing views. Because of the lack of convincing proof, expression of different views on some subjects was allowed in consecutive chapters, thus the burden is put on the reader to decide the method and evaluation he finds more convincing. Multiple authorship also required us to take occasional editorial liberties to avoid unnecessary repetition of identical data or similar views. However, the reader will discern that some occasional overlap has been permitted wherever it was deemed necessary not to interrupt a train of thought or the development of a concept.

The contents of the book are divided into four units:

Unit I examines basic considerations including the history of recognition and the development of treatment modalities applied in extracranial cerebrovascular disease, the anatomy of vessels, the characteristics of the regulation of blood flow through them, and their pathological alterations.

Unit II is dedicated to the clinical picture and angiographic and noninvasive diagnosis with a separate chapter devoted to ophthalmological considerations.

Unit III, the major section of this textbook, encompasses the different treatment modalities of extracranial carotid artery disease, both acute and chronic, caused by a variety of pathological entities. Different chapters deal in depth with the clinical background: indications for surgery, anesthetic and surgical techniques in various occlusive aneurysmatic and neoplastic entities, as well as the carotid sinus hypersensitive syndrome. In the description of various techniques of arterial reconstruction not only standard techniques are described in detail but also proper attention is given to different variants, to their specific indications, inherent advantages, and potential complications.

Finally, *Unit IV* discusses the pathology and treatment of occlusive brachiocephalic disease with a primary emphasis on its influence on cerebral blood flow.

This book has been written with the primary aim to enlarge and to enrich the scope and understanding of the clinician, surgeon, and nonsurgeon alike.

Francis Robicsek

Acknowledgments

Presenting this book to the reader, I am using the opportunity to express my gratitude to those who made its completion a reality. First of all I want to thank Dr. Charles Rob, pioneer in carotid surgery, for honoring us by writing a Foreword to this volume, and to the line of illustrious authors, all renowned experts in their field, who participated in the assembly of this monograph. Without the cooperation of this panel of medical experts—anatomists, pharmacologists, physiologists, neurologists, neuroradiologists, neurovascular surgeons and neurosurgeons—it would not have been possible to present the crucial problems of extracranial cerebrovascular surgery from the broad view of a true multidisciplinary approach but only from the narrow angle of a subspecialist. For their most significant contribution I will remain grateful.

I also want to thank my associate of twenty years, Ms. Nell Franklin, and Mr. William Poveromo for the valuable assistance I received in the editorial work, Ms. Patricia Johnson for her medical illustrations of the highest quality, and my family for their support and tolerance in creating the atmosphere from which this book was born.

Last, but not least, I want to thank Alys von Lehmden-Maslin, Senior Editor Medicine Macmillan Publishing Company, for her guidance and encouragement throughout the preparation of this volume.

Contributors

Evelyn M. Anderson, M.D. Assistant Professor of Thoracic Cardiovascular Surgery, University of Illinois at Chicago, and Luthern General Hospital, Chicago, Illinois

Giorgio M. Aru, M.D. Clinica Chirurgica dell Universita, Padova, Italy

Gustav V. R. Born, M.D. Professor of Pharmacology, Department of Pharmacology, University of London at King's College, London, England

Andrew L. Carney, M.D. Assistant Professor of Thoracic and Cardiovascular Surgery, University of Illinois at Chicago, and Luthern General Hospital, Chicago, Illinois

John E. Connolly, M.D. Professor of Surgery, University of California at Irvine, Chief of Vascular Surgery, University of California Irvine Medical Center, Irvine, California

Joseph W. Cook, M.D. Department of Thoracic and Cardiovascular Surgery, Charlotte Memorial Hospital and Medical Center, Charlotte, North Carolina

Joseph M. Craver, M.D. Associate Professor of Cardiovascular Surgery, Emory University School of Medicine, Atlanta, Georgia

Ivan K. Crosby, M.D. Baylor University Medical Center, Clinical Associate Professor, Department of Surgery, University of Texas Health Sciences Center, Southwestern Medical School, Dallas, Texas. Former Professor of Surgery, Division of Thoracic and Cardiovascular Surgery, University of Virginia School of Medicine, Charlottesville, Virginia

C. Stephen Ford, M.D. Instructor, Department of Neurology, Bowman Gray School of Medicine, Winston-Salem, North Carolina

Anthony J. Furlan, M.D. Director, Cerebrovascular Program, Head, Adult Clinical Neurology, Cleveland Clinic, Cleveland, Ohio

Vincenzo Gallucci, M.D. Professor of Thoracic Surgery, Clinica Chirurgica dell Universita, Padova, Italy

Michael T. Gillette, M.D. Associate Chairman, Department of Anesthesiology, Charlotte Memorial Hospital and Medical Center, Charlotte, North Carolina

George R. Hanna, M.D. Professor of Neurology, University of Virginia School of Medicine, Charlottesville, Virginia

Charles R. Hatcher, M.D. Chief, Department of Cardiovascular Surgery, Emory University School of Medicine, Atlanta, Georgia

E. Ralph Heinz, M.D. Professor of Radiology (Neuroradiology), Duke University Medical Center, Durham, North Carolina. Former Chairman of the Department of Radiology, University of Pittsburgh, Pennsylvania

Edward Gray Hill, Jr., M.D. Department of Neurology, Bowman Gray School of Medicine, Winston-Salem, North Carolina

Kaichiro Ishikawa, M.D. Lecturer, Faculty of Medicine, Kyoto University, Kyoto, Japan

Ellis L. Jones, M.D. Professor of Thoracic and Cardiovascular Surgery, Emory University School of Medicine, Atlanta, Georgia

John M. Keshishian, M.D. Clinical Professor of Surgery, The George Washington University Medical Center, Clinical Professor of Surgery, Uniformed Services University of the Health Sciences. Chief of Vascular Surgery, Washington Hospital Center. Senior Attending in Thoracic and Vascular Surgery, The George Washington University Hospital, Washington, D.C.

Martin J. Kreshon, M.D. Charlotte Eye, Ear, Nose, and Throat Hospital, Charlotte, North Carolina. Assistant Clinical Professor, Duke University, Durham, North Carolina

Richard A. Michalik, M.D. Instructor in Surgery, Emory University School of Medicine, Atlanta, Georgia

Arl V. Moore, Jr., M.D. Charlotte Memorial Hospital and Medical Center, Charlotte, North Carolina. Clinical Associate Professor, Radiology Department, Duke University Medical Center, Durham, North Carolina

R. Gregory Parsons, M.D. Neuroradiology Section Chief, Charlotte Memorial Hospital and Medical Center, Charlotte, North Carolina

Philip Polido, M.D. Department of Surgery, Harbor/UCLA Medical Center, Torrance, California

Jeffrey K. Raines, Ph.D. Research Director and Director, Vascular Laboratory, Miami Heart Institute, Miami, Florida

Norman M. Rich, M.D. Professor and Chairman, Department of Surgery, Uniformed Services University of the Health Sciences, Bethesda, Maryland

Charles G. Rob, M.D. Professor of Surgery, Uniformed Services University of the Health Sciences, F. Edward Hebert School of Medicine, Bethesda, Maryland

Francis Robicsek, M.D. Chairman, Department of Thoracic and Cardiovascular Surgery, Charlotte Memorial Hospital and Medical Center, Charlotte, North Carolina. Clinical Professor of Surgery, University of North Carolina, Chapel Hill, North Carolina

Duke S. Samson, M.D. Professor and Chairman, Department of Surgery, Division of Neurological Surgery, University of Texas Health Science Center at Dallas, Dallas, Texas

Stewart M. Scott, M.D. Chief, Surgical Service, V. A. Medical Center, Asheville, North Carolina. Clinical Professor of Surgery, Duke University Medical Center, Durham, North Carolina

James F. Toole, M.D. Chairman, Department of Neurology, Bowman Gray School of Medicine, Winston-Salem, North Carolina

Christopher G. Ullrich, M.D. Department of Radiology, Charlotte Memorial Hospital and Medical Center, Charlotte, North Carolina. Assistant Professor of Radiology, Johns Hopkins University School of Medicine, Baltimore, Maryland

Frederick Walburn, Ph.D. Miami Heart Institute, Assistant Professor of Bioengineering, University of Miami, Miami, Florida

Samuel E. Wilson, M.D. Professor and Chairman, Department of Surgery, Harbor/UCLA Medical Center, Torrance, California

Contents

EXTRACRANIAL CEREBROVASCULAR DISEASE

UNIT I

General Considerations

1

Introduction

FRANCIS ROBICSEK

This apoplexy is, as I take it, a kind of lethargy, . . . a kind of sleeping in the blood.
—William Shakespeare, *King Henry IV, Part 2*

Considering that stroke today ranks as the third leading cause of death in the United States and that in about 50 percent of the patients the occlusive lesion responsible is situated in the thoracic or cervical segments of the cerebral circulation, one may expect that in this modern day and age of medicine all or most problems of extracranial cerebrovascular surgery have been solved. This, however, is far from being the case.

Despite advances in the management of extracranial cerebrovascular disease during the past century, especially during the last few decades, there is still room for progress in this area. Although the amount of published clinical material regarding medical and surgical therapy of extracranial cerebrovascular disease is enormous, the number of continuing controversies on the treatment of the disease is notable. Sometimes it appears to be increasing. Even the mechanism of transient ischemic attack, the principal symptom of cerebrovascular disease, is poorly understood. It has been suggested that systemic hypotension caused by acute redistribution of blood volume acting in the presence of extracranial occlusions may be the cause of fleeting focal cerebral ischemia. Follow-up studies of this theory indeed found such precipitating factors, but in only a few cases. Similarly, attempts at trying to induce transient ischemic attacks by creating a hypotensive state also uniformly failed. These findings redirected attention toward the theory that transient ischemic attack may be caused by repeated embolization, which certainly gives anyone who has read Chiari's article, written in 1905, a sense of *dėja vu.* We also still fail to understand why a carotid plaque develops, why it develops in that location, why some plaques grow and others regress, and why some ulcerate and others calcify.

Other controversies involve indications for noninvasive studies. Very few clinicians would debate their general value in the study of the asymptomatic patient suspected of having extracranial occlusive disease or as the tool of choice in the follow-up study of a patient who has already undergone operation. But should the clinician be assured on the basis of noninvasive techniques alone if the tests turn out to be negative in the patient with typical symptoms? Or would the clinician be willing to establish the operative indication exclusively on the basis of positive noninvasive studies?

What constitutes the indication for arteriography? Has digital subtraction angiography replaced the direct approach? How far should the angiographer go in the visualization of blood vessels?

If a lesion is found, what constitutes an indication for surgery? Should asymptomatic stenosis be operated upon? Nonstenotic ulcers? Buckles and kinks? Is there a place for balloon angioplasty in the management of carotid occlusive disease? What should we do about "strokes in development?" What is the significance of an asymptomatic subclavian steal? Has carotid artery surgery been proved beneficial in global ischemia? Should completely occluded internal carotid arteries be explored? Will a successful endarterectomy improve mental status?

If surgery is decided upon, what is the best method of protecting the brain while the carotid is operated upon? Should indwelling shunts be used always, never, or selectively? If selectively, then what are the criteria for use? Does the routine use of patch arterioplasty prevent recurrence? Does simultaneous bilateral carotid surgery increase or diminish the total surgical risk? In internal carotid artery occlusion and ipsilateral external carotid artery stricture is it proper to restrict the operation to external carotid arterioplasty, or should the initial procedure include extra- and intracranial anastomoses as well? Are the risks of "extraanatomic" technique really lower and the results truly equal to those of "anatomic" operations? What are the true "late results" of carotid endarterectomy?

To recommend the "optimal" technique for carotid endarterectomy is an impossible task. Although some aspects of this operation, such as the desirability of optical magnification and fine sutures, are well established, others, such as the "best" means of cerebral protection, are still undecided and, it now appears, may remain so for years to come. The reason for the indecision is the multiplicity of variables which may exist in different clinical reports, e.g., a surgeon with superb technique and a less-than-ideal method of cerebral protection may obtain similar or better results than a surgeon with less technical ability but more physiological insight. Local or general anesthesia, shunt or no shunt, patch or no patch, every possible combination has its supporters who back their position with reports of good results. These questions, still unanswered after several decades of in-depth experimental research and extensive clinical experience, dozens of specialty and interspecialty meetings, and several national and international cooperative studies, are now joined by the newly emerging problems of interspecialty competition and professional qualification procedures.

In the preparation of this volume, besides being the Editor, my activity as author concerns the chapters on history and on the surgical aspects of carotid and brachiocephalic disease, where I present the views and the surgical philosophy my associates and I practice at the Department of Thoracic and Cardiovascular Surgery of the Charlotte Memorial Hospital and Medical Center. With the panel of authors who have contributed to this volume we have addressed these questions, perhaps answered some, and raised others. This book is intended to be not the definitive statement on the management of extracranial cerebrovascular disease but the reflection of our knowledge in the year 1986.

Francis Robicsek

2

The Medical History of Extracranial Cerebrovascular Disease

FRANCIS ROBICSEK

If I have seen farther, it is by standing on the shoulders of giants.

—Sir Isaac Newton

CLINICAL BACKGROUND

The Dawn of Understanding

As one can discern from the words of the Old Testament, the devastating clinical effects of stroke were known in ancient times. An accurate description of hemiplegia is found in Psalm 137:506: ". . . let my right hand wither! Let my tongue cleave to the roof of my mouth."

Some of the basic terms for carotid disease come from the ancient Greek medical literature. Hippocrates, about the turn of the fourth century B.C., not only used the term "apoplexy" ("to strike down") but also gave a faithful and accurate description of strokes, prodromal symptoms, and transient ischemic attacks (Adams, 1886) and knew that lesions of the carotid artery resulted in contralateral hemiplegia (Dandy, 1945).

According to Rufus of Ephesus, who lived about 100 A.D., the term *carotid* was derived from the Greek word meaning "to stun, stupefy, or fall into deep sleep." The reason for so naming the artery was that compressing it caused loss of consciousness—"sleep." This was also described by Ambroise Paré: ". . . the arteries which they call *carotides* or *soporales,* the arteries for sleep" (Paré, 1968).

Recognition in the Middle Ages

The first meaningful description of the cerebral vessels, including the vertebral-basilar system, was given by the noted Swiss physician Johann Jakob Wepfer. In his *Treatise de Apoplexiae,* printed in Schaffhausen in 1658, he described the hemispheric supply of the brain by the carotid arteries, "which proceed intact and not divided," and made the first known reference to the association of pathological changes in the cerebral vessels and symptoms of cerebral ischemia. (Wepfer, 1704).

That the seventeenth-century anatomists fully appreciated the significance of collateral circulation is also apparent from a letter written by the English physician Richard Lower in 1668: "The carotidal and vertebral arteries have so many anastomoses so divinely contrived inside the dura mater, before they go up the brain . . . that if three arteries were quite obstructed, the fourth would convey blood into all parts of the brain and cerebellum, sufficient for life and motion" (Gurdjian, 1979).

They also recognized that differences in the quality of pulses and blood pressure in the upper extremities may also be caused by conditions such as brachiocephalic stenosis, aortic arch aneurysms, and congenital arch anomalies. In 1828, in the *De Motu Cordis,* Harvey (1941) described a case in which "the pulse in the corresponding arm was small in consequence of the greater portion of the blood being diverted into the tumor [aneurysm] and so intercepted." William Hunter (1757) mentioned a similar case in which a large arch aneurysm blocked the pulse to the left arm and temple.

Understanding Brachiocephalic Disease

In 1761, Giovan Battista Morgagni, of Padua, who was himself to die of cerebrovascular occlusive disease, described what was probably the first case of "pulseless disease," a 40-year-old woman who died of "spasmodic asthma" and whose "radial pulse was never perceived." At autopsy, Morgagni found that the aorta above the valves became "thicker and harder, while its internal layers, which in many places had become yellow, showed many signs of change into bone tissue, as could be noted at the outset of one of the subclavian arteries" (di Giacomo, 1984).

In 1839, John Davy reported the case of a 55-year-old army officer with absent arterial pulses in his arms who had symptoms of cerebrovascular insufficiency. This appears to be the first report of the so-called "aortic arch syndrome." The patient died from a ruptured syphilitic aneurysm of the aorta, which turned out to be the cause of obstruction of the arch branches (Davy, 1839). A few years later, R.B. Todd (1844) described a patient who had a stroke caused by innominate artery dissection.

In 1856, W.S. Savory reported the now famous case of "Anna Maria W., 22," who had various neurological symptoms attributable to cerebral ischemia and who finally died from infection. Autopsy revealed that she had extensive extracranial occlusive disease which today would be diagnosed as arteritis. The left carotid and both subclavian arteries were found to be occluded and their walls thickened (Savory, 1856).

The importance of reversal of the vertebral flow was first recognized by A.W. Smythe (1869), who observed a patient who underwent ligation of the innominate and carotid arteries because of a subclavian aneurysm. The patient later had multiple attacks of syncope, which were relieved by ligation of the ipsilateral vertebral artery.

W.H. Broadbent, in a lecture given on May 14, 1875 at the Clinical Society of London, described the autopsy findings of a more advanced example of the aortic arch syndrome of atherosclerotic origin occurring in a middle-aged man. His interest in the case was primarily that of explaining the bilateral absence of radial artery pulsations. Cerebral symptoms were not referred to.

In 1908, Takayasu, a Japanese ophthalmologist, without mentioning any changes in the arterial pulses of the neck or arm, reported the occurrence of "peculiar changes in the central blood vessels of the retina" thought to be due to ischemia in the eyes of a young woman patient, probably a victim of aortic arch syndrome. The disease was later named for him, despite the fact that it was not he but two of his colleagues, Onishi and Kagoshima (Judge *et al.*, 1962) who correlated such ocular changes with absent arm pulses. The Japanese physician Shimizu (Shimizu and Sana, 1951) enlarged upon the description, and at approximately the same time Frövig reported that a number of different disease processes could cause the same symptoms. It was then that he first used the term "aortic arch syndrome" (Frövig and Loken, 1951). Takayasu's disease was thought to be limited to Japanese women until Harbitz and Raeder (1926) gave a somewhat sketchy description of the microscopic features of the disease in a non-Oriental patient. The first detailed clinicopathological description of the condition was rendered by Martorell-Otzet in 1944.

Retrograde basilar-vertebral flow was first shown angiographically by Contorni in 1960. The connection between this reversed flow owing to subclavian "siphonage" and symptoms of cerebral ischemia was established a year later in the report of Reivich and associates. They reported their observations obtained in two patients in whom an "anatomic lesion producing a reverse blood flow was a stenosis of the left subclavian artery proximal to the origin of the vertebral artery. The cause of reversed flow (through the vertebral) in these circumstances can be attributed to a fall of pressure distal to the stenosis below that of the vertebral-basilar junction, so that the pressure created in the vertebral artery is reversed" (Reivich *et al.*, 1961). Their clinical observations were supplemented by animal experiments in which they were able to reverse vertebral blood flow by ligating the proximal subclavian artery. Fisher (1961) named the syndrome "subclavian steal." This term became accepted by the profession, and the postulate served as a model for a number of other "steal" syndromes.

The Diseased Carotid Bifurcation

In 1809, the noted British surgeon Sir Ashley Cooper recognized and discussed the possibility of stroke after carotid ligation (Cooper,

1809). Almost 20 years later, Abercrombie drew an analogy between cerebral ischemia and gangrene of the legs (Abercrombie, 1828). The relationship between extracranial cerebrovascular disease and stroke was noted by Gull in 1855 (Thompson, 1983). A year later, Virchow (1856) described carotid thrombosis with ipsilateral blindness. In 1875, Gowers discussed the case of a 30-year-old man with blindness of the left eye, right-sided hemiplegia, and aphasia. Ophthalmoscopy revealed embolic material in the left retinal arteries. The patient eventually died from rheumatic heart disease. At autopsy, the left middle cerebral artery was found to be completely occluded by a blood clot, probably an embolus from the heart (Gowers, 1875). This is probably the first description of simultaneous cerebral and ophthalmic embolization from the heart.

The first report proving the existence of anastomosis between the internal and external carotid arteries was written by Elschnig in Germany in 1893. He demonstrated that dye injected into the maxillary artery of a cadaver easily passes into the opthalmic arteries of both sides. The first suggestion to restore blood supply to the brain was made by Gluck in his treatise "Die moderne Chirurgie des circulations Apparates," published in Germany in 1898. He was also the first to replace a segment of the common carotid artery with a vein graft in experimental animals.

Although the clinical picture of internal carotid thrombosis was fairly accurately described as early as 1881 by Penzoldt, the syndrome consisting of temporary hemiparesis, aphasia, and transient loss of consciousness was first tied conclusively to occlusive disease of the carotid arteries by Chiari, in Prague, in 1905. He observed the case of a 45-year-old woman who died from right-sided hemiplegia and cerebral hemorrhage. At autopsy, he found "embolic occlusion 1 cm long at the distal end of the left internal carotid artery." Searching for the origin of the embolus, he "detected the source of the emboli in the form of a parietal thrombosis situated in the left wall of the final centimeter of the common carotid and reaching 1⅓ cm into the internal carotid." Chiari also found thrombus deposited on atherosclerotic plaques in an additional seven of 400 consecutive autopsies and concluded that "there is a common occurrence of endarteritis chronic deformans, and resulting thrombosis in the areas of carotid bifurcation, and . . . thrombus may embolize from this area to the cerebral arteries" (Chiari, 1905). The postulate that emboli may break away from ulcerated carotid plaques and cause symptoms of cerebral ischemia forwarded by Chiari still constitutes the basis of one of the two most generally accepted theories of transient ischemic attacks. Chiari also emphasized the need for investigation of the cervical carotid vessels in all cases of apoplexia, but his advice was largely disregarded by his contemporaries.

One of the most important individuals in the development of an understanding of extracranial occlusive carotid disease was J. Ramsey Hunt, who in 1914 described in detail the clinical syndrome of spherical hemiplegia and contralateral amaurosis fugax owing to cervical carotid disease and emphasized that the latter is a common cause of "brain softening" and stroke. He presented a strong case connecting extracranial cerebrovascular disease with stroke, and also urged that "in all cases presenting with cerebral symptoms of vascular origin the main arteries of the neck should be carefully examined for a possible diminution or absence of pulsation."

He further stated that he "would advocate the same attitude toward this group of cases as toward intermittent claudication, gangrene and other vascular symptoms of the extremities" (Hunt, 1914).

Also in 1914, Matas described his compression test, which challenged the efficiency of collateral circulation. Bailliart in 1917 investigated the behavior of the arterial pressure in the retinal arteries. His studies were the precursors of modern ophthalmodynamometry (Bailliart, 1917).

The first report on cerebral angiography was presented by Egas Moniz, of Lisbon, at the July 7, 1927 session of the Société de Neurologie (Moniz, 1927) in Paris. He presented satisfactory angiograms in five patients using intracarotid injection of strontium bromide and sodium iodide. Babinski (1927), the doyen of French neurology, congratulated Moniz, saying that the radiograms presented by Moniz were "remarkable."

A carotid occlusion (presumably a thrombosed aneurysm) was first diagnosed by angiography by Sjöqvist in 1936. One year later, Moniz presented four patients in whom the diagnosis of internal carotid artery occlusion was made by angiography and concluded that whenever the clinical symptoms suggest internal carotid artery occlusion, "cerebral angiography will always provide diagnostic certainty" (Moniz *et al.*, 1937). Hultquist in 1942 published an extensive monograph on the pathogenesis and propagation of carotid occlusive disease. His study was based on 3,500 consecutive autopsies in which cervical carotid occlusion was found in 91 instances (Hultquist and Jena, 1951).

From 1946 to 1948, it gradually became clear that the symptoms of carotid disease may be caused not only by complete occlusion but also in a rather sizable group of patients by stenosis of the vessel at one or several points.

In 1944, Krayenbuhl recommended that determination of the retinal artery pressure described by Bailliart (1917) should be applied in the diagnosis of internal carotid artery occlusion. In 1950, Milletti noted that systolic retinal pressure decreases 50 percent on compression of the carotid on the patent side but that no change occurs on the occluded side.

During the 1950s, arteriosclerotic occlusion emerged as a frequently occurring and clinically recognizable entity.

In 1955, Millikan and associates described the syndrome of "intermittent insufficiency of the carotid arterial system," whose characteristics were similar to the "cerebral intermittent claudication" described by Hunt in 1914. They emphasized the relationship of these attacks to the state of the collateral circulation and to changes in blood pressure. This was also demonstrated in the clinical observations of Meyer and associates (1956), who were able to reproduce the attacks in patients with carotid artery disease by changing their position on a tilt table.

During the fourth and fifth decades of our century, Carl Fisher, along with Ramsey Hunt, made what were probably the most important advances in clarifying and defining the clinical picture of carotid stenosis. In a study published in 1943, Fisher revived Chiari's theory that ulcerative plaques of the carotid bifurcation may cause cerebral embolism. Fisher wrote: "During our study of brain embolism, in many cases no source for the embolus could be found in the conventional locations—the pulmonary veins, the left auricle, the left ventricle or the ascending aorta. . . . Methodical search for disease of the internal carotid artery at autopsy was therefore undertaken and has been surprisingly rewarding" (Fisher and Adams, 1951). Fisher also called attention to the bifurcation atheroma as a frequent cause of contralateral transient and permanent motor dysfunction, and went so far as to predict that "vascular surgery will find a way to bypass the occluded portion of the artery during the period of ominous fleeting symptoms" (Fisher and Adams, 1951). In 1954, Fisher published clinical histories of eight patients with internal carotid occlusions verified at autopsy and furnished important clues to the mechanism of many heretofore puzzling cerebral symptoms, such as transient episodes of blindness, aphasia, paresthesia, and paralysis, as well as headache and dizziness. While bruits over the orbit were already known in the early nineteenth century, it was not until 1954 that Fisher, and Shapiro and Peyton described the carotid bruit as an important physical sign of occlusive disease (Fisher, 1954; Shapiro and Peyton, 1954).

The effectiveness of collateral channels from the external to the internal carotid artery was emphasized by Hutchinson and Yates (1957), who showed that these collaterals are even more effective than those of the vertebral artery.

Fibromuscular dysplasia of the internal carotid artery was first described by Palubinskas and Ripley in 1964. A year later, Connett and Lansche (1965) reported the case history of a patient with this disease who developed occlusion of the internal carotid artery and hemiparesis.

MILESTONES IN GENERAL VASCULAR SURGERY

Naturally, surgery of the extracranial cerebral vessels developed not as an isolated technique but as an integral part of vascular surgery as a whole. Some of the most important events in vascular surgery, which strongly influenced the development of extracranial cerebrovascular surgery are summarized below.

The technique of vascular suture developed in the second half of the nineteenth and the very early part of the twentieth centuries. The first repair of an injured vessel was credited to Hallowell (1909), who tied the suture around a pin stuck through the edges of the torn artery. In 1879, vascular anastomosis was first applied in a systematic and successful manner by Nikolai Eck, the creator of the portal-caval anastomosis (Child, 1953). Although individual reports of successful vascular surgery—primarily repair of injured vessels but also replacement with autogenous veins—appeared sporadically in the literature (Goyanes, 1906; Murphy, 1897), it was left to investigators of the early twentieth century (Jáboulay, 1902; Carrel and Guthrie, 1906) to firmly establish the technique of vascular repair and replacement. A most important contribution to the development of vascular surgery was that of Dorfler (1899), who demonstrated that penetration of the intima by silk sutures does not necessarily induce thrombosis.

The first operation to restore blood flow in an intrinsically occluded artery was credited to Labey (1911), who in 1911 performed the first successful arterial embolectomy. Important "nonsurgical" events that profoundly influenced cerebrovascular surgery were the identification of heparin in 1916 by McLean (1916) and the development of angiography. The first description of microvascular surgery was probably by Carrel and Guthrie in their classic monograph on anastomosis of small vessels (1906).

The 1930s and 1940s saw the development of a school of vascular surgeons headed by René Leriche, who had among his assistants Michael DeBakey, F. Cid dos Santos, and Jean Kunlin, and who maintained close contact with leading American surgeons of his time, such as Matas and Halsted.

Most important events of the fourth and fifth decades of this century were the invention and broad application of arterial substitutes and suture materials, the arterial homograft of Gross (1951), and the synthetic vascular prosthesis of Voorhees and associates (1952), which was brought to clinical popularity by DeBakey and associates (1958) and others.

The reverse saphenous vein as a bypass graft was introduced by Kunlin (1949) and later popularized by Linton (1955), Dale and associates (1959), and others. Undoubtedly, some of the most important unsung heroes of vascular surgery were the biomedical engineers, to whom we are all indebted for the development of the atraumatic and synthetic suture materials.

The technique of endarterectomy for the treatment of occlusive arteriosclerosis was introduced into the armamentarium of the vascular surgeon by Reboul, Loubry, and dos Santos; as dos Santos later said, it proved to be "the end of the myth of the need for intact intima" (dos Santos, 1976).

The modern principles of carotid endarterectomy were based on the work of Wylie on the iliac and femoral vessels. Compared with the early 1960s, few surgeons now perform endarterectomy except for the shortest arterial lesions. It has remained, however, a standard procedure for desobliteration of the carotid bifurcation.

In 1952, Freeman and Leeds introduced the principle of extraanatomical bypass, and in 1966, Mical and associates first used the temporary indwelling shunt. Another milestone in vascular surgery was the application of the operative microscope by Jacobson and Suarez (1960), which led to the development of extraintracranial bypass procedures.

NONRECONSTRUCTIVE CAROTID SURGERY

The first operations on the carotid artery were limited to ligation of the vessel. According to Cutter (1920), it was Jean Louis Petit who first noted that occlusion of the carotid artery is a condition compatible with life. He made his observation in a patient with an aneurysm of the common carotid artery whom he had followed for seven years and who at autopsy proved to have the lumen of the vessel completely occluded by thrombi.

The first report of operative ligation of the common carotid artery was that of Amroise Paré in 1552. His patient, however, developed aphasia and hemiplegia. Elective ligation of the common carotid artery with survival was performed by Hebenstreit and reported in 1793 (Hamby, 1952). The first case published in the English literature was that of John Abernathy (1811, 1815). Abernathy was a pupil of John Hunter, who operated on a man whose carotid artery was gored by the horns of a cow. The patient survived the operation without any undue immediate consequences but suffered hemiplegia and died the following day. While the procedure is believed to have taken place in 1798, it was not reported until 1804. Twitchell in 1843 reported carotid artery ligation for penetrating trauma with survival.

The first operations for carotid aneurysms consisted primarily of proximal but occasionally also of distal ligations. Such procedures were performed by Cogswell in 1803 (Cogswell, 1824) and by Sir Ashley Paston Cooper in 1809. Cooper's first patient died of hemorrhage; his second, of infection. On June 22, 1809, Cooper repeated the operation, this time successfully, and the patient lived 13 years thereafter (Cooper, 1836).

Ligation remained the treatment of choice for the management of carotid artery aneurysms until the middle of this century. The first carotid ligation for carotid corpus cavernosum fistula was performed by Benjamin Travers in 1809, and the first for intracranial aneurysm by Victor Horsley in 1885 (Dandy, 1942). Ligation was performed with increasing frequency, not only for aneurysms and injury but also for tumorous involvement, arteriovenous communications, etc., until the dangers of the procedure became generally known.

In 1902, Jáboulay suggested to Carrel that carotid-to-jugular-vein anastomosis might help revascularize the brain when there is sufficient blood supply owing to thrombosis. In 1911, Matas modified the technique of proximal carotid ligation for aneurysms by applying metal bands in lieu of ligatures.

In the later 1930s, the operation most frequently performed for carotid artery occlusion was excision of the occluded segment according to the principles of Leriche (Leriche, 1931). The first such intervention was performed by Chao and associates (1938) at the Medical College of Peking in 1935 on a 48-year-old Russian who "seemed to be constantly worried" and "appeared to be emotional with rather frequent exhibitions of tears." Their second patient was a 27-year-old student, the only patient recorded in the annals of carotid surgery who after having collapsed "was taken by rickshaw to his residence." To the surprise of the surgeons, the mental conditions of both patients improved after the operation and they concluded that in such cases "excision of the thrombosed artery should be carried out."

Throughout the 1940s, the treatment of choice for cervical internal carotid occlusion remained excision and ligation to "prevent the propagation of the clot and release vasospasm" (Gurdjian and Webster, 1958). In a few cases in which the symptoms seemingly improved, the beneficial effect may have been the cessation of repeated embolization from the occluded site.

Other early attempts to treat occlusive carotid disease with equally dubious results included procaine block of the cervical sympathetic ganglia, cervical sympathectomy, and brain revascularization using a muscle pedicle introduced by Henschen (1950).

To present a complete history of the development of extracranial carotid surgery, the procedure introduced by Sciaroni (1948) must be mentioned; he named it "reversal of the circulation of the brain." It consisted of creating side-to-side anastomosis between the common carotid artery and the internal jugular vein. The resulting arteriovenous fistula was expected to increase cerebral blood flow, alleviate symptoms of paralysis and epileptic seizures, and cure hypertension. Sciaroni's example was soon followed by others describing excellent results. Because of such enthusiastic reports, the operation was performed for several years before it fell into disrepute.

THE AGE OF RECONSTRUCTIVE CAROTID SURGERY

The feasibility of restoring flow through the interrupted carotid artery by anastomosis and vein grafts was proven experimentally by Gluck in Germany (1898), by Jáboulay in France (1902), and by Carrel in the United States (1902, 1908).

Nonocclusive Carotid Disease

The earliest successful carotid reconstructions were performed in patients with aneurysms long before similar operations were performed for occlusive disease. The reason for this is simple: surgeons who operated on aneurysms were able to do so because of the ease of diagnosis of the lesion. They did not have to wait for the development of angiography, without which the presence of carotid occlusion or stenosis can hardly be established.

The first surgeon to restore carotid continuity after resection for aneurysm, or, as a matter of fact, for any kind of carotid lesion, was von Parczewski, who in 1916 resected an arteriovenous aneurysm of the common carotid artery and restored continuity by performing an end-to-end anastomosis. His example was soon followed by von Haberer, who in 1918 successfully applied resection and lateral suture as well as resection and end-to-end anastomosis in soldiers of the German army wounded in World War I. In the same year Lexer and Denck also gave reports of successful resection of the common carotid with end-to-end anastomosis for war-inflicted aneurysms (Sloan, 1921).

It is not generally recognized what an important role surgical oncologists played in the development of carotid artery surgery. Their involvement with surgical restoration of the carotid artery stems from the frequent involvement of the carotid artery during radical neck dissections for malignancy. Similarly, breakdown of the common carotid artery sometimes occurs after intensive radiation treatment of the neck. Complete excision of the tumor may also necessitate the resection of the invaded vessel. While initially such cases were handled by ligation, it was soon realized that ligation of the carotid artery bears an unacceptable mortality and stroke rate.

Surgical oncologists, unlike their colleagues operating on carotid aneurysms, were not hampered by a lack of sophisticated technology in establishing the diagnosis. This gave them a considerable edge over those involved in the treatment of occlusive disease. The latter were for the most part general surgeons caught in desperate situations that called for bold responses. And some of them did indeed respond with measures that were far ahead of their time. The first report (Sloan, 1921) of carotid reconstruction in English is that of Harry G. Sloan, who in July 1920 operated on a patient with recurrent carcinoma of the lip with cervical metastases. He wrote: "We nicked the common carotid as it lay in a mass of scar tissue. . . . Before the bleeding was controlled by finger compression above and below the bleeding, the vessel wall was badly damaged by hemostats for about three-fourths of a centimeter. . . . We decided to excise the damaged area of the vessel and make an end-to-end anastomosis. Using a mosquito hemostat for a needle holder, we succeeded in placing the sutures. We employed Carrel's original method of suture, i.e., three guy sutures through all the coats of the vessel." Sloan's patient fully recovered without neurological deficit and was noted to have good temporal pulses after the operation. Enderlen, in an article on carotid body tumors published in 1938, described a similar case in which he had operated 20 years previously. A most important but not very well known figure in carotid surgery is John J. Conley, who practiced at Saint Vincent's Hospital in New York City in the early 1950s. Conley's special expertise was oncological surgery of the neck, in the course of which he often removed portions of the internal and common carotid arteries. Realizing the "gravity of sudden impairment of blood supply to the brain" and "in the hope of salvaging some patients who would otherwise die of cancer and fatal carotid hemorrhage," Conley designed an appropriate operation. It consisted of end-to-end anastomosis between the distal stumps of the internal and external carotid arteries which permitted the blood to flow through the anastomotic connections of the external carotid artery from the contralateral side into the external carotid artery. In describing this ingenious technique in 1952, Conley mentioned that vascular transplants of autogenous veins would be even more advantageous to maintain adequate blood supply to the brain. A year later, he reported for the first time in the surgical literature, a case in whom a portion of the common carotid artery which had ruptured owing to irradiation was replaced with a segment of autogenous saphenous vein.

In the same report, Conley published a series of case histories describing the clinical course of patients operated upon for tumors of the carotid body or for extensive cancerous invasion of the neck in whom carotid artery excision had become a necessity. With a technique and planning that would withstand the scrutiny of modern times, Conley successfully replaced the common and/or internal carotid arteries in 11 patients. He operated on his first patient in March 1951 and corrected the deficiency in the internal and common carotid arteries by the "immediate anastomosis of a segment of the great saphenous vein into this area" (Conley and Pack, 1952). With his impressive series of patients, Conley proved to be a surgeon far ahead of his time.

Occlusive Carotid Disease

Like many other surgical advances, surgery for carotid occlusion has developed over an unnecessarily long period of time from its conception to its wide general application today. This is especially true when we consider that sophisticated operations on the carotid artery, including resection and end-to-end anastomosis as well as replacement with autogenous vein grafts for tumors and aneurysms, were performed 30 years before the first such operation was done for carotid occlusion. In seeking to chart an accurate history of surgery for occlusive carotid disease, difficulties are encountered in establishing the chronology of the first interventions. For example, the first carotid reconstruction by resection and anastomosis was performed in 1951 but was not reported until 1954. Similarly, the first successful carotid endarterectomy was performed in 1953 but was not fully described until 19 years later. Moreover, in trying to identify the priority of surgical procedures and those who performed the initial operations to restore blood flow through the interrupted cervical carotid, several factors must be considered: the type of pathology, the type of procedure, the outcome of the operation, and the date of surgery versus the date of publication.

Surgery to restore patency in occlusive carotid disease began in the early 1950s with somewhat desperate attempts to salvage patients with acute strokes. As diagnostic methods, primarily angiography, evolved and became refined, a plethora of methods of restoring carotid flow were developed but later gave way to endarterectomy with or without patch arterioplasty as the procedure of choice for most cases of occlusive carotid artery disease. This development was slow, however, and the confused state of the art in 1953 is clearly reflected in the summary of Gurdjian and Webster (1958):

> Following diagnosis, the management may include, first, bilateral stellate block; second, excision of the cervical sympathetic on one or both sides; third, the use of anticoagulants; fourth, excision of the freshly formed clot to reestablish circulation through the thrombosed area; fifth, carotid artery ligation and excision of a portion of the thrombosed vessel; sixth, ligation of the carotid siphon intracranially.

Gordon Murray, in Toronto, performed what was probably the first successful operation to restore blood flow in an occluded common carotid artery in 1950 (Ross and McKussick, 1953). The first reconstruction of an occluded internal carotid artery was performed in Buenos Aires in 1951 on a 41-year-old man who has been admitted to the Instituto de Medicina Experimental with symptoms of convulsions, loss of consciousness, aphasia, blindness in the left eye, and right hemiparesis. Percutaneous left carotid angiography revealed a severe stricture of the internal carotid just above the bifurcation. The patient was operated upon by Carrea, Molins, and Murphy. During the course of the operation, "the internal carotid artery was cut about 5 mm above the abnormal area, the external carotid was also cut at the same level and the proximal carotid was anastomosed end-to-end to the distal portion of the internal carotid." The patient fully recovered from the hemiparesis and aphasia; however, he remained blind in the left eye. The patency of the vessel was confirmed by angiography. The case was reported four years later (Carrea *et al.,* 1955).

Although the technique of endarterectomy was introduced into the treatment of atherosclerotic occlusion of the aortoiliac system as early as 1947 by dos Santos, 15 years elapsed before it was first applied in carotid disease by Strully, Hurwitt, and Blankenberg on January 28, 1953 at the Montefiore Hospital in New York City. Their patient, a 52-year-old man; had a completely occluded internal carotid artery owing to arteriosclerotic stricture with superimposed thrombosis. During the operation, "a piece of clot with adherent intima was removed . . . but retrograde flow of blood could not be obtained." The procedure was finally terminated by resection of the carotid artery, but the continuity of the carotid circulation was not restored. The authors concluded that "if the diagnosis in this case had been made earlier it might have been possible to remove the clot completely" (Hurwitt *et al.,* 1960).

The first successful carotid endarterectomy was performed by DeBakey on August 7, 1953, in a 53-year-old man with transient ischemic attacks. The diagnosis was made without the benefit of angiography on the basis that "published reports had indicated that such lesions may be well localized at the bifurcation of the common carotid artery." The left carotid bifurcation was explored, and a "well-localized atheromatous plaque [which] produced severe stenosis at the origin of the internal, as well as the external carotid artery" and a "partially organized fresh clot partially filling the lumen of the common carotid artery" were removed (DeBakey *et al.,* 1959; DeBakey, 1975).

The operation which gave great impetus to the early development of surgery for carotid occlusion was that performed by Eastcott, Pickering, and Rob on May 19, 1954 and reported in the November issue of the *Lancet* in the same year. Their patient was a woman with transient ischemic attacks whose left carotid bifurcation was severely narrowed by an arteriosclerotic plaque. In the course of surgery, which was performed in moderate total-body-immersion hypothermia, the external carotid artery was divided and ligated, and the carotid bifurcation containing the occlusive atheroma was resected. The continuity of the carotid circulation was restored by direct anastomosis between the common carotid artery and the stump of the internal carotid artery. The patient fully recovered from the operation, and had no further attacks of cerebral ischemia (Eastcott *et al.,* 1954). In the following years,

DeBakey, Eastcott, Rob, Thompson, Moore, Baker, and Wylie exerted the primary influence on the development of carotid artery surgery.

On July 7, 1954, Denman, Ehni, and Duty performed an operation that included carotid artery resection and replacement of the removed segments with lyophilized homografts. Their case is noteworthy not only because the procedure was staged bilaterally but also because, while on one side the circulation to the internal carotid could not be restored, "the external carotid was patent and an arterial graft was inserted between it at the common carotid. Restoration of the external carotid circulation was considered desirable primarily because of its communication through the ophthalmic artery with the circle of Willis" (Denman *et al.,* 1955).

In 1956, Lin, Javid, and Doyle, at the Madigan Army Hospital in Tacoma, Washington, used an autogenous saphenous vein graft to restore continuity after resection of a segment of the internal carotid for occlusion (Lin *et al.,* 1956).

The earliest report in the literature of a successful carotid endarterectomy is that of Cooley, Al-Naaman, and Carton on March 4, 1956 at the Methodist Hospital in Houston. "A polyvinyl shunt with needle points at both ends was used to bypass the carotid circulation during the period of occlusion. With the external carotid temporarily occluded, internal carotid flow was maintained by means of the shunt while the atheromatous plaque was removed from the vessel" (Cooley *et al.,* 1956). Their report was also the first record of the application of a temporary shunt during carotid endarterectomy.

In August 1956, Lyons and Galbraith used the method of subclavian-to-common carotid graft to bypass a proximal common carotid occlusion employing a vascular prosthesis manufactured of nylon (Lyons and Galbraith, 1957). Side-to-side anastomosis between the external and internal carotid arteries to relieve occlusion of blood flow was performed by Wagner in 1958. In the same year, replacement of the carotid was performed with Dacron by Fields, Crawford, and DeBakey (Fields *et al.,* 1958) and with homograft by Roberts and associates (1958) and by Van Allen and associates (1958). In 1959, Bahnson performed the first bypass operation from the aortic arch to the carotid artery using homologous aorta as a graft (Bahnson *et al.,* 1959). Transposition of the subclavian to the common carotid artery was described by Parrott in 1964.

The carotid artery "back pressure" (the pressure measured in the internal carotid artery after proximal crossclamping) as a hemodynamic indicator of collateral cerebral blood flow was described by Crawford and associates in 1960 and used by Mical of Prague, Czechoslovakia (Mical *et al.,* 1966) and by Moore and associates (1969) of San Francisco to predict the tolerance of the brain to carotid crossclamping.

Indwelling temporary bypass shunting was first applied during carotid reconstruction by Mical, Hejnal, Heinol, and First at the Institute for Experimental Surgery, in Prague, in 1966. They used small plastic tubes inserted through the arteriotomy incision into the inside of the artery and, just as done earlier by Cooley (Cooley *et al.,* 1956), they applied external shunts armed on both ends with large-bore needles to maintain blood flow during surgery, not only on the carotid artery but also on the innominate and renal vessels and the descending thoracic aorta.

In the early 1960s, elective application of temporary shunting was advocated by Thompson and associates (1970). Selective application of the shunt on the basis of the measurement of the stump pressure was recommended by Moore and associates (1969) and on the basis of electrocardiographic monitoring by Callow (1980).

The concept of extraintracranial surgery can be traced to the clinical experiments of Henschen (1950), who attached a pedicle of the temporalis muscle to the surface of the brain to fashion a unique source of collateral circulation. The results were unconvincing. Woringer and Kunlin in 1963 first attempted extraintracranial bypass from the common to the internal carotid intracranially, but the patient died. In the same year, the same authors successfully performed common carotid-to-intracranial carotid artery bypass by bridging the defect with autogenous saphenous vein graft. Pool and Potts (1965) used a prosthetic graft to establish a bypass from the superficial temporal to the left anterior cerebral artery.

Extraintracranial surgery received further impetus from the introduction of microvascular techniques which allowed the performance of direct anastomosis between branches of the external and internal carotid arteries. This procedure had been suggested in 1951 by

Fisher, who said: "Anastomosis of the external carotid artery or one of its branches with the internal carotid about the area of narrowing should be feasible" (Fisher, 1951).

Using microsurgical techniques, Donaghy (1967) and Yasargil (1969) presented the feasibility, first experimentally and then clinically, of anastomosing the superficial temporal artery to the cortical branch of the middle cerebral artery, thus creating a well-functioning collateral between extra- and intracranial vessels suitable in cases in which patency of the cervical internal carotid arteries cannot be restored by direct surgery.

Since 1970, the scope of extraintracranial bypass procedures has been considerably broadened by the utilization of other arteries, such as the occipital and the auricular vessels (Ausman *et al.,* 1978; Sundt, 1974), as well as various arterial substitutes, primarily the saphenous vein.

VERTEBRAL ARTERY SURGERY

The first operation on the vertebral artery was performed in 1853 by Maisonneuve and Savrot (French and Haines, 1950), who ligated the first portion of the vertebral artery for trauma. Unfortunately, the patient died 17 days after surgery of septicemia and embolism. As mentioned previously, in 1864, Smythe ligated the vertebral artery in a 32-year-old patient with subclavian artery aneurysm. In 1888, Rudolph Matas successfully excised an aneurysm of the vertebral artery between the occiput and the atlas. Reports on vertebral artery ligation and its complications have been forwarded by Dandy (1944), Fisher (1961), and French (1950).

In 1946, Elkin and Harris published a report of ten successful operations for arteriovenous communications of the vertebral artery. In 1958, Crawford inserted a bypass graft from the subclavian to the distal vertebral artery, and in the same year, Crawford, DeBakey, and Fields reported reconstruction of vertebral flow using both the technique of subclavian-to-vertebral bypass graft and direct vertebral endarterectomy (Crawford *et al.,* 1958). In the late 1950s Imparato performed a patch angioplasty of the cervical vertebral artery (Imparato, 1967). In 1970, Wylie and Ehrenfeld described anastomosis of the proximal segment of the vertebral to the common carotid artery. In 1975, Carney and Emanuele (1977) performed side-to-end subclavian-proximal vertebral anastomosis in the neck and the first segmental resection and primary anastomosis of the vertebral artery at the level of C1 – C2. In 1976, Berguer and Bauer described the vein bypass from the subclavian to the proximal vertebral artery.

In 1966, Clark and Perry mobilized the vertebral artery above the level to C1 to gain length and to perform an external carotid vertebral anastomosis in 1977. Corkill and associates in 1977 reported direct anastomosis of the external carotid to the midvertebral artery. Subsequently, numerous reports have appeared utilizing modifications of this technique.

In August 1977, Carney performed the first vein bypass from the common carotid to the distal vertebral artery at the base of the skull. In 1979, George and Laurian performed an anatomical study of the skull base in 20 specimens and reported a case of subclavian-distal vertebral artery bypass.

In 1982, Carney reported an experience of 45 procedures at the skull base and noted the variety of pathologic features encountered. The surgical procedures performed were highly varied, but the end-to-side technique for the distal anastomosis was recommended with preservation of the native vessel. Extraintracranial bypass techniques were introduced into the management of cervical vertebral artery disease by Ausman (1978) and Sundt (1978).

SURGERY FOR OCCLUSIVE DISEASE OF THE BRACHIOCEPHALIC VESSELS

The first endarterectomy to restore blood flow through the innominate artery was carried out in March 1954 by Davis, Grove, and Julian (Davis *et al.,* 1956). The patient, who also had atherosclerotic occlusive disease of the innominate artery, presented with dizziness, blurring of vision, poor memory, and frequent syncope. After innominate endarterectomy, a strong pulse appeared on the right carotid, and the patient's condition improved significantly.

The first operation to relieve occlusive subclavian artery disease was carried out by Cate and Scott at Vanderbilt University, Nashville, Tennessee, on September 7, 1957 (Cate and Scott, 1959). The procedure was performed by splitting the upper half of the sternum and removing an atherosclerotic plug from the origin of the left subclavian and the left vertebral using a partly occluding clamp on the aorta. Their case was presented at the Twelfth Annual Meeting of the Society for Vascular Surgery, San Francisco, California, on June 22, 1958. At the same meeting, DeBakey gave a report of a similar operation performed by Crawford (DeBakey *et al.,* 1959).

In the development of grafting procedures on the brachiocephalic arteries, the same phenomenon can be observed that is seen in carotid artery disease: grafts for nonocclusive disease were performed years before those performed for occlusive disease. In 1954, Mahorner and Spencer published a report on a bypass graft after resection of an innominate artery aneurysm. The first graft for proximal occlusion of the brachiocephalic vessels was performed by DeBakey and associates four years later, when they utilized an aortic bifurcation graft to bypass the obstruction of the innominate and carotid arteries (DeBakey *et al.,* 1958).

Carotid-to-subclavian bypass went through several phases with repeated "backtracks" to procedures seldom utilized today. In 1953, the Baylor group in Houston (Dietrich *et al.,* 1967) advocated the performance of carotid-subclavian bypass using a Dacron vascular prosthesis anastomosed end-to-side to both vessels. Good results with carotid-subclavian bypass grafts were soon reported by several other authors. In 1964, Parrott recommended the creation of carotid-to-subclavian anastomosis by direct end-to-side implantation of the latter into the midsection of the common carotid artery. In 1965, DeBakey and associates reported a number of bypass operations from the carotid to the subclavian artery. In 1969, one-stage surgical correction of both carotid bifurcation stenosis and subclavian artery occlusion was carried out by Najafi, Dye, and Javid (Najafi *et al.,* 1969).

Ehrenfeld and associates (1968) first applied the transcervical crossover graft using saphenous vein between the two subclavian arteries in a patient with underlying cardiac disease and previous mediastinal surgery for innominate artery stenosis. The method of axillary-to-axillary bypass graft was reported by Myers and associates in 1971. In October 1970, Sproul (1971) used femoro-axillary bypass graft to correct cerebral ischemia in a patient with innominate artery stenosis as well as left carotid and subclavian occlusion. The same procedure was also used to relieve arm ischemia (Moseley and Porter, 1973). In 1976, Berguer, Andaya, and Bauer (Berguer *et al.,* 1976) reported subclavian-to-vertebral artery autogenous vein grafts. Carotid-to-vertebral anastomosis was carried out by Clark and Perry in 1966.

Only the most important highlights in the medical history of extracranial cerebrovascular disease have been touched upon here. It is not something that only happened in the distant past. It is very much alive, is still occurring, and will undoubtedly continue tomorrow. The road traveled is long but the end of the story still lies beyond the far horizon. Newer modalities in diagnosis and treatment and especially in prevention will certainly be found; they will exceed but not excell the work of those pioneers whose imagination, courage, and endeavor have taken us where we are today.

REFERENCES

Abercrombie, J.: *Pathological and Practical Researches on Diseases of Brain and Cord.* Waugh and Innes, Edinburgh, 1828.

Abernathy, J.: *Surgical Observations on Injuries of the Head.* Dobson, Philadelphia, **2**:72, 1811.

Abernathy, J.: *Surgical Works.* Vol. 2. Longman, London, 1815.

Adams, F.: *The Genuine Works of Hippocrates.* William Wood, New York, 1886.

Ausman, J.I.; Lindsay, W.; Ramsay, R.C., and Chou, S.N.: Ipsilateral subclavian to external carotid and STA-MGA bypasses for retinal ischemia. *Surg. Neurol.,* **9**:5–8, 1978.

Babinski, M.: Discussion of Moniz, E.: L'encéphalographie arterielle: son importance dans la localisation des tumeurs cérébrales. *Rev. Neurol. (Paris),* **2**:72–90, 1927.

Bahnson, H.T.; Spencer, F.C.; and Quattlebaum, J.K, Jr.: Surgical treatment of occlusive disease of the carotid artery. *Ann. Surg.,* **149**:711–20, 1959.

Bailliart, P.: Circulation artérielle rétinienne: essais de la determination de la tension artérielle dans les branches de l'artère centrale de la rétine. *Ann. Ocul.,* **154**:257–71, 1917.

Berguer, R.; Andaya, L.V.; and Bauer, R.B.: Vertebral artery bypass. *Arch. Surg.,* **111**:976–79, 1976.

Berguer, R., and Bauer, R.B.: Subclavian artery to external carotid artery bypass graft: improvement of cerebral blood supply. *Arch. Surg.,* **111**:893–96, 1976.

Broadbent, W.H.: Absence of pulsation in both radial arteries, vessels being full of blood. *Trans. Clin. Soc. London.,* **8**:165–68, 1875.

Callow, A.D.: David M. Hume memorial lecture. An overview of the stroke problem in the carotid territory. *Am. J. Surg.,* **140**:181–91, 1980.

Carney, A.L.; Emanuele, R., and Anderson, E.M.: *Surgery of the Vertebral Artery.* Medicom A-V Production, Chicago, 1977.

Carney, A.L., and Anderson, E.M.: The system approach to brain blood flow. In *Advances in Neurology. Diagnosis and Treatment of Brain Ischemia.* Raven Press, New York, 1982, pp. 1-30.

Carney, A.L.; Emanuele, R.; and Anderson, E.M.: *Carotid Distal Vertebral Artery Bypass.* Medicom A-V Productions, Chicago, 1977.

Carrea, R.; Molina, M.; and Murphy, G.: Surgery on spontaneous thrombosis of the internal carotid in the neck; carotido-carotid anastomosis: case report and analysis of the literature on surgical cases. *Medicine,* **15**:29-39, 1955.

Carrel, A.: Results of transplantation of blood vessels, organs, and limbs. *J.A.M.A.,* **51**:1662-67, 1908.

Carrel, A., and Guthrie, C.C.: Uniterminal and biterminal venous transplantations. *Surg. Gynecol. Obstet.,* **2**:266, 1906.

Carrel, A., and Morel, B.: Anastomose bout à bout de la jugulaire et de la jugulaire et de la carotide primitive. *Lyon. Med.,* **99**:114-16, 1902.

Cate, W.R., and Scott, H.W., Jr.: Cerebral ischemia of central origin: relief by subclavian-vertebral artery thromboendarterectomy. *Surgery,* **45**:19-31, 1959.

Chao, W.H.; Kwan, S.T.; Lyman, R.S.; and Loucks, H.H.: Thrombosis of the left internal carotid artery. *Arch. Surg.,* **37**:100-11, 1938.

Chiari, H.: Über das Verhalten des Teilungswinkels der Carotis bei der Endarteritis chronica deformans. *Verh. Dtsch. Pathol. Ges.,* 1905.

Child, C.G.: Eck's fistula. *Surg. Gynecol. Obstet.,* **96**:375-76, 1953.

Clark, K., and Perry, M.O.: Carotid-vertebral anastomosis: an alternate technique for surgical repair of subclavian steal syndrome. *Ann. Surg.,* **163**:414-16, 1966.

Cogswell, M.F.: Account of an operation for the extirpation of a tumour, in which a ligature was applied to the carotid artery. *N. Engl. J. Med. Surg.,* **13**:357-60, 1824.

Conley, J.J., and Pack, G.T.: Surgical procedure for lessening the hazard of carotid bulb excision. *Surgery,* **31**:845-58, 1952.

Connett, M.C., and Lansche, J.M.: Fibromuscular hyperplasia of the internal carotid artery: report of a case. *Ann. Surg.,* **162**:59-62, 1965.

Contorni, L.: The vertebro-vertebral collateral circulation in the subclavian artery at its origin. *Minerva Chir.,* **15**:268-71, 1960.

Cooley, D.A.; Al-Naaman, Y.D.; and Carton, C.A.: Surgical treatment of arteriosclerotic occlusion of common carotid artery. *J. Neurosurg.,* **13**:500-506, 1956.

Cooper, A.: Account of the first successful operation performed on the common carotid artery for aneurysm in the year 1808, with post-mortem examination in 1821. *Guy's Hosp. Rep.,* **1**:53-59, 1836.

Cooper, A.: Second case of carotid aneurysm. *Med. Chir. Trans.,* **1**:222-33, 1809.

Corkill, G.; French, B.N.; Michas, C.; Cobb, C.A.; and Mims, T.J.: External carotid-vertebral artery anastomosis for vertebrobasilar insufficiency. *Surg. Neurol.* **7**:109-15, 1977.

Crawford, E.S.; DeBakey, M.E.; Blaisdell, F.W.; Morris, G.C., Jr.; and Fields, W.S.: Hemodynamic alterations in patients with cerebral arterial insufficiency before and after operation. *Surgery,* **48**:76-94, 1960.

Crawford, E.S.; DeBakey, M.E.; and Fields, W.S.: Roentgenographic diagnosis and surgical treatment of basilar artery insufficiency. *J.A.M.A.,* **168**:509-14, 1958.

Cutter, I.S.: Ligation of the common carotid artery: Amos Twitchell. *Surg. Gynecol. Obstet. (Internat. Obstet. Surg.),* **48**:1-3, 1920.

Dale, W.A.; DeWeese, J.A.; and Scott, W.J.M.: Autogenous venous shunt grafts. *Surgery,* **46**:145-63, 1959.

Dandy, W.E.: Results following ligation of the internal carotid artery. *Arch. Surg.,* **45**:521-33, 1942.

Dandy, W.E.: *Intracranial Arterial Aneurysms.* Comstock Publishing Co., Ithaca, New York, 1944.

Dandy W.E.: *Surgery of the Brain.* W.F. Prior, Hagerstown, Pennsylvania, 1945.

Davis, J.B.; Grove, W.J.; and Julian, O.C.: Thrombic occlusion of the branches of the aortic arch. Martorell's syndrome: report of a case treated surgically. *Ann. Surg.,* **144**:124-26, 1956.

Davy, J.: *Researches, Physiological and Anatomic.* Smith, Elder, London, **1**:426, 1839.

DeBakey, M.E.: Successful carotid endarterectomy for cerebrovascular insufficiency: nineteen-year follow-up. *J.A.M.A.,* **233**:1083-85, 1975.

DeBakey, M.E.; Cooley, D.A.; Crawford, E.S.; and Morris, G.C., Jr.: The clinical application of a new flexible knitted Dacron arterial substitute. *Ann. Surg.,* **24**:862-69, 1958.

DeBakey, M.E.; Crawford, E.S.; Cooley, D.A., and Morris, G.C., Jr.: Surgical considerations of occlusive disease of innominate, carotid, subclavian, and vertebral arteries. *Ann. Surg.,* **149**:690-710, 1959.

DeBakey, M.E.; Crawford, E.S.; Cooley, D.A.; Morris, G.C., Jr.; Garrett, H.E., and Fields, W.S.: Cerebral arterial insufficiency: one to 11-year results following arterial reconstructive operation. *Ann. Surg.,* **161**:921-45, 1965.

Denman, F.R.; Ehni, G.; and Duty, W.S.: Insidious thrombotic occlusion of cervical carotid arteries treated by arterial graft: a case report. *Surgery,* **38**:569-77, 1955.

Diethrich, E.B.; Garrett, H.E.; Ameriso, J.; Crawford, E.S.; El-Bayar, M.; and DeBakey, M.E.: Occlusive disease of the common carotid and subclavian arteries treated by carotid-subclavian bypass: analysis of 125 cases. *Am. J. Surg.,* **114**:800-8, 1967.

di Giacomo, V.: A case of Takayasu's disease occurred over two hundred years ago. *Angiology,* **35**:750-54, 1984.

Donaghy, R.M.P.: Patch and bypass in microangional surgery. In Donaghy, R.M.P., and Yasargil, M.G. (eds.): *Micro-Vascular Surgery.* Mosby, Saint Louis, Missouri, 75-86, 1967.

Dorfler, J.: Über Arteriennaht. *Beitr. Chir.,* 25:781, 1899.

dos Santos, J.C.: Leriche memorial lecture. From embolectomy to endarterectomy or the fall of a myth. *J. Cardiovasc. Surg.,* **17**:113-28, 1976.

dos Santos, J.C.: Sur la desobstruction des thromboses artérielles anciennes. *Mem. Acad. Chir.,* **73**:409-11, 1947.

Eastcott, H.H.G.; Pickering, G.W.; and Rob, C.G.: Reconstruction of internal carotid artery in a patient with intermittent attacks of hemiplegia. *Lancet,* v.267, v.2: 994-96, 1954.

Ehrenfeld, W.K.; Levin, S.M.; and Wylie, E.J.: Venous crossover bypass grafts for arterial insufficiency. *Ann. Surg.,* **167**:287-91, 1968.

Elkin, D.C., Harris, M.H.: Arteriovenous aneurysm of the vertebral vessels. Report of ten cases. *Ann. Surg.,* **124**:934-51, 1946.

Elschnig, A.: Über den Einfluss des Verschlusses der Arteria Ophthalmica und der Carotis auf das Sehorgan. *Albrecht Von Graefes Arch. Klin. Exp. Ophthalmol.,* **39**:151, 1893.

Enderlen, E.: Surgery of carotid body tumors. *Zentralbl. Chir.,* **46**:2530-31, 1938.

Fields, W.S.; Crawford, E.S.; and DeBakey, M.E.: Surgical considerations in cerebral arterial insufficiency. *Neurology,* **8**:801–8, 1958.

Fisher, C.M.: Clinical syndromes in cerebral arterial occlusion. In Fields, W.S. (ed.): *Pathogenesis and Treatment of Cerebrovascular Disease.* Charles C. Thomas, Springfield, Illinois, 151, 1961.

Fischer, M.: Occlusion of the carotid arteries: further experiences. *Arch. Neurol. Psychiatry,* **72**:187–204, 1954.

Fisher, C.M.; Gore, I.; Okabe, N.; and White, P.D.: Atherosclerosis of the carotid and vertebral arteries: extracranial and intracranial. *J. Neuropathol. Exp. Neurol.,* **24**:455–76, 1965.

Fisher, C.M., and Adams, R.D.: Observations on brain embolism with special reference to the mechanism of hemorrhagic infarction [abstr.]. *J. Neuropathol. Exp. Neurol.,* **10**:92–3, 1951.

Freeman, N.E., and Leeds, F.H.: Operations on large arteries: application of recent advances. *Calif. Med.,* **77**:229–33, 1952.

French, L.A., and Haines, G.L.: Unilateral vertebral artery ligation: report of a case ending fatally with thrombosis of the basilar artery. *Neurosurgery,* **7**:156–58, 1950.

Frövig, A.G., and Loken, A.C.: The syndrome of obliteration of the arterial branches of the aortic arch, due to arteritis: postmortem angiographic and pathological study. *Acta. Psychiatr. Neurol. Scand.,* **25**:313–37, 1951.

George, B., and Laurian, C.: Surgical possibilities in the third portion of the vertebral artery. *Acta Neurochir.* [Suppl.], **28,** 263–69, 1979.

Gluck, T.: Die moderne Chirurgie des circulations Apparates. *Berl. Klin.,* **129**:1–29, 1898.

Gowers, W.R.: Simultaneous embolism of central retinal and middle cerebral arteries. *Lancet,* **2**:794–96, 1875.

Goyanes, J.: Nuevos trabajos de chirurgia vascular, substitución plástica de los arterias por las venas o arterioplástica venosa: applicada como neuvo método al tratamiento de los aneurismas. *El Siglo. Med.,* **53**:446–51, 1906.

Gross, R.E.: Treatment of certain aortic coarctations by homologous grafts: a report of nineteen cases. *Ann. Surg.,* **134**:753–68, 1951.

Gurdjian, E.S.: History of occlusive cerebrovascular disease. 1. From Wepfler to Moniz. *Arch. Neurol.,* **36**:340–43, 1979.

Gurdjian, E.S., and Webster, J.E.: Thrombo-endarterectomy of the carotid bifurcation and the internal carotid artery. *Surg. Gynecol. Obstet.,* **106**:421–26, 1958.

Gurdjian, E.S., and Webster, J.E.: Thrombosis of the internal carotid artery in the neck and in the cranial cavity: symptoms and signs, diagnosis and treatment. *Trans. Am. Neurol.,* **241**:242–54, 1951.

Hallowell: In Lambert: Medical observations and inquiries. Vol. II, 1762. Cited by E.A. Smith, E.A.: *Suture of Arteries: An Experimental Research.* Oxford University Press, London, 1909.

Hamby, W.B.: *Intracranial Aneurysms.* Charles C Thomas, Springfield, Illinois, 1952.

Harbitz, F., and Raeder, J.G.: *Nord. Med. (Laegevisdensk),* **87**:529, 1926.

Harvey, W.: *De motu cordis* (1628). C. Leak. (Trans.). Charles C. Thomas, Springfield, Illinois, 1941.

Henschen, C.: Operative Revaskularisation des zirkulatorisch geschadigten Gehirns durch Auflage gestielter Muskellappen (Encephalomyosynangiose.). *Langenbecks Arch. Klin. Chir.,* **264**:392–401, 1950.

Hultquist, G.T., and Jena, G.F.: Quoted in Fisher, M., and Adams, R.D.: Observations on brain embolism with special reference to the mechanism of hemorrhagic infarction [abstr.]. *J. Neuropathol. Exp. Neurol.,* **10**:92–3, 1951.

Hunt, J.R.: The role of the carotid arteries in the causation of vascular lesions of the brain, with remarks on certain special features of the symptomatology. *Am. J. Med. Sci.,* **147**:704–13, 1914.

Hunter, W.: The history of an aneurysm of the aorta with some remarks on aneurysms in general in medical observations and injuries. In Sotheby, P. (ed.): *Medical Observations and Inquiries.* London. **1**:323–57, 1757.

Hurwitt, E.S.; Carton, C.A.; Fell, S.C.; Kessler, L.A.; Seidenberg, B., and Shapiro, J.H.: Critical evaluation and surgical correction of obstructions in the branches of the aortic arch. *Ann. Surg.,* **152**:472–84, 1960.

Hutchinson, E.C., and Yates, P.O.: Cortico-vertebral stenosis. *Lancet,* **1**:2–8, 1957.

Imparato, A.M., and Pen-Tze Lin, J.: Vertebral artery reconstruction, internal plication and vein patch angioplasty. *Ann. Surg.,* **166**:213–21, 1967.

Jáboulay, M.: Chirurgie des artères, ses applications à quelques lesions de l'artère fémoral. *Sem. Med.,* **22**:405–406, 1902.

Jacobson, J.H., and Suarez, E.L.: Microsurgery in anastomosis of small vessels. *Surg. Forum,* **11**:243–5, 1960.

Judge, R.D.; Currier, R.D.; Gracie, W.A.; and Figley, M.M.: Takayasu's arteritis and the aortic arch syndrome. *Am. J. Med.,* **32**:379–92, 1962.

Krayenbuhl, H., and Weber, G.: Die Thrombose der Arteria Carotid Interna und ihre Beziehung zur Endarteritis obliterans v. Winiwarter-Buerger. *Helv. Med. Acta,* **11**:289–33, 1944.

Kunlin, J.: Le traitement de l'artérite obliterante par la greffe veineuse. *Arch. Mal. Coeur,* **42**:371–72, 1949.

Labey: In Mosny, E., and Dumont, J.: Embolie femorale au cours d'un restrecissement mitral pur. Arteriotomie Guerison. *Bull. Acad. Med. (Paris),* **66**:358, 1911.

Leriche, R.: Arterectomy in the treatment of localized arterial obliteration. *Am. J. Surg.,* **14**:55–67, 1931.

Lin, P.M.; Javid, H.; and Doyle, E.J.: Partial internal carotid artery occlusion treated by primary resection and vein graft. *J. Neurosurg.,* **13**:650–55, 1956.

Linton, R.R.: Some practical considerations in the surgery of blood vessel grafts. *Surgery,* **38**:817–34, 1955.

Lyons, C., and Galbraith, G.: Surgical treatment of atherosclerotic occlusion of the internal carotid artery. *Ann. Surg.,* **146**:487–98, 1957.

McLean, J.: The thromboplastic action of cephalin. *Am. J. Physiol.,* **41**:250–51, 1916.

Mahorner, H., and Spencer, R.: Shunt grafts. *Ann. Surg.,* **139**:439–46, 1954.

Martorell-Otzet, F., and Fabré, T.J.: El sindrome de obliteraction de los truncos supraaórticos. *Med. Clin. (Barcelona),* **3**:26–30, 1944.

Matas, R.: Testing the efficiency of the collateral circulation as a preliminary to the occlusion of the great surgical arteries. *J.A.M.A.,* **63**:1441–47, 1914.

Matas, R.: Traumatic aneurysm of the left brachial artery. *Med. News,* **53**:462, 1888.

Matas, R.: Aneurysms and wounds of the vertebral arteries. *Ann. Surg.,* **18**:477–516, 1893.

Meyer, J.S.; Leiderman, H.; and Denny-Brown, D.: Electroencephalographic study of insufficiency of the basilar and carotid arteries in man. *Neurology,* **6**:455–77, 1956.

Mical, V.V.; Hejhal, J.; Hejhal, L.; and Firt, P.: Zeitweilige Shunts in der vaskularen Chirurgie. *Thoraxchirurgie,* **14**:35, 1966.

Milletti, M.: Does a clinical syndrome of primary thrombosis of the internal carotid artery exist? *Acta Neurochir.*, **1**:196–231, 1950.

Millikan, C.H.; Siekert, R.G.; and Whisnant, J.P. *Cerebral Vascular Diseases.* Grune & Stratton, New York, 1955.

Moniz, E.: L'encéphalographie artérielle: son importancé dans la localization des tumeurs cérébrales. *Rev. Neurol.*, **2**:72–90, 1927.

Moniz, E.; Lima, A.; and De Lacerda, R.: Hemiplegies par thrombose de la carotide interne. *Press. Med.*, **45**:977–80, 1937.

Moore, O.S.; Karlan, M.; and Sigler, L.: Factors influencing the safety of carotid ligation. *Am. J. Surg.*, **118**:666–68, 1969.

Morgagni, G.B.: De sedibus et causes morborum per anatemen indignatis. Quoted in di Giacomo, V.: A case of Takayasu's disease occurred over two hundred years ago. *Angiology*, **35**:750–54, 1984.

Moseley, H.S., and Porter, J.M.: Femoral-axillary artery bypass for arm ischemia. *Arch. Surg.*, **106**:347–48, 1973.

Murphy, J.B.: Resection of arteries and veins injured in continuity: end-to-end suture: experimental and clinical research. *Med. Record*, **51**:73, 1897.

Myers, W.O.; Lawton, B.R.; and Sautter, R.D.: Axillo-axillary bypass graft. *J.A.M.A.*, **217**:826–34, 1971.

Najafi, H.; Dye, W.D.; Javid, H.; Hunter, J.A.; Ostermiller, W.E.; and Julian O.C.: Carotid bifurcation stenosis and ipsilateral subclavian steal. *Arch. Surg.*, **99**:289–92, 1969.

Palubinskas, A.J., and Ripley, H.R.: Fibromuscular hyperplasia in extrarenal arteries. *Radiology*, **82**:451–55, 1964.

Parczewski, S. von: Resection and anastomosis of the common carotid. *Münch. Med. Wochenschr.*, **63**(46):1646, 1916.

Paré, A.: *The workes of that famous chirurgion Ambrose Parey, Translated out of Latine and compared with the French by Thomas Johnson: From the first English Edition, London, 1634.* Milford House, New York, 1968.

Parrott, J.C.: The subclavian steal syndrome. *Arch. Surg.*, **88**:661–65, 1964.

Penzoldt, F.: Über Thrombose (autochtone oder embolische) der Carotis. *Dtsch. Arch. Klin. Med.*, **28**:80–93, 1881.

Pool, J.L., and Potts, D.G.: *Aneurysms and Arteriovenous Anomalies of the Brain: Diagnosis and Treatment.* Harper & Row, New York, 417, 1965.

Reivich, M.; Holling, H.E.; Roberts, B.; and Toole, J.F.: Reversal of blood flow through the vertebral artery and its effect on cerebral circulation. *N. Engl. J. Med.*, **265**:878–85, 1961.

Rob, C.: Technique of surgical therapy. In Millikan, C.H.; Siekert, R.G., and Whisnant, J.P. (eds.): *Cerebral Vascular Diseases.* Grune & Stratton, New York, 1961, p. 112.

Roberts, B.; Peskin, G.W.; and Wood, F.A.: Internal carotid artery thrombosis. *Arch. Surg.*, **76**:483–91, 1958.

Ross, R.S., and McKusick, V.A.: Aortic arch syndromes: diminished or absent pulses in arteries arising from the aortic arch. *Arch. Intern. Med.*, **92**:701–40, 1953.

Savory, W.S.: Case of a young woman in whom the main arteries of both upper extremities and of the left side of the neck were throughout completely obliterated. *Med. Chir. Trans.*, **39**:205–19, 1856.

Sciaroni, G.H.: Reversal of circulation of the brain. *Am. J. Surg.*, **76**:150–64, 1948.

Shapiro, S.K., and Peyton, W.T.: Spontaneous thrombosis of the carotid arteries. *Neurology*, **4**:83–100, 1954.

Shimizu, K., and Sana, K.: Pulseless disease. *J. Neuropathol. Clin. Neurol.*, **1**:37–47, 1951.

Sjöqvist, O.: Über intrakranielle Aneurysmen der Arteria Carotis und deren Beziehung zur ophthalmoplegischen Migraine. *Nervenarzt*, **9**:233–41, 1936.

Sloan, H.G.: Successful end-to-end suture of the common carotid artery in man. *Surg. Gynecol. Obstet.*, **33**:62–64, 1921.

Smythe, A.W.: A case of successful ligature of the innominate artery. *New Orleans J. Med.*, **22**:464–69, 1869.

Sproul, G.: Femoral-axillary bypass for cerebral vascular insufficiency. *Arch. Surg.*, **103**:746–47, 1971.

Strully, K.J.; Hurwitt, E.S.; and Blankenberg, H.W.: Thromboendarterectomy for thrombosis of the internal carotid artery in the neck. *J. Neurosurg.*, **10**:474–82, 1953.

Sundt, T.M., Jr.: Surgical therapy of occlusive vascular diseases of the brain. *Surg. Annu.*, **6**:393–411, 1974.

Sundt, T.M., Jr.; Smith, H.C.; Campbell, J.K.; Vlietstra, R.E.; Cucchiara, R.F.; and Stanson, A.W.: Transluminal angioplasty for basilar artery stenosis. *Mayo. Clin. Proc.*, **55**:673–680, 1980.

Sundt, T.M., Jr., and Tiepgras, C.: Occipital artery-middle cerebral anastomoses for cerebral artery occlusive disease. *J. Neurosurg.* **48**:916–28, 1978.

Takayasu, M.: A case with peculiar changes of the central retinal vessels. *Acta Soc. Ophthalmol. Jpn.*, **12**:554, 1908.

Thompson, J.E.: The development of carotid artery surgery. *Arch. Surg.*, **107**:643–48, 1973.

Thompson, J.E.; Austin, D.J.; and Patman, R.D.: Carotid endarterectomy for cerebrovascular insufficiency: long-term results in 592 patients followed up to thirteen years. *Ann. Surg.*, **172**:663–79, 1970.

Thompson, J.E.; Austin, D.J.; and Patman, R.D.: Endarterectomy of the totally occluded carotid artery for stroke. *Arch. Surg.*, **95**:791–801, 1967.

Todd, R.B.: Account of a case of a dissecting aneurysm of the aorta, innominate and right carotid arteries giving rise to suppression of the brain. *Med. Chir. Trans.*, 2nd ser., **27**:301–24, 1844.

Twitchell, A.: Gunshot wound of the face and neck treated by ligation of the carotid artery. *N. Engl. Q. J. Med. Surg.*, **1**:188–93, 1843.

Van Allen, M.W.; Blodi, F.L.; and Brintnall, E.S.: Retinal artery blood pressure measurements in diagnosis and surgery of spontaneous carotid occlusions. *J. Neurosurg.*, **15**:19–29, 1958.

Virchow, R.: *Thrombose und Embolie: Gefässen Zündung und septische Infektion in gesammelte Abhandlungen zur wissenschaftlichen Medicin.* A.M. Meidinger, Frankfurt, 219–732, 1856.

Voorhees, A.B., Jr.; Jaretski, A., III; and Blakemore, A.H.: The use of tubes constructed from Vinyon "N" cloth in bridging arterial defects. *Ann. Surg.*, **135**:332–36, 1952.

Wepfer, J.: *Observatio Anatomica.* Zurich, 1704.

Woringer, E., and Kunlin, J.: Anastomose entre la carotide primitive et la carotide intracranielle ou la Sylvienne par greffon selon la technique de la suture suspendue. *Neurochirurgie*, **9**:181–88, 1963.

Wylie, E.J., and Ehrenfeld, W.K.: *Extracranial Occlusive Cerebrovascular Disease. Diagnosis and Management.* W. B. Saunders, Philadelphia, 1970.

Yasargil, M.G.: Anastomosis between the superficial temporal artery and a branch of the middle cerebral artery. In Yasargil, M.G. (ed.): *Microsurgery Applied to Neurosurgery.* George Thieme Verlag, Stuttgart, 1969.

3

Surgical Anatomy of the Extracranial Vessels

EDWARD GRAY HILL, JR.

Pertinent discussion of extracranial arterial anatomy should begin with the aortic arch and terminate with the branches of the external carotid arteries. An adequate understanding of this anatomy also requires a knowledge of embryology, variants, and collateral flow.

EMBRYOLOGY OF THE EXTRACRANIAL CEREBRAL ARTERIES

Embryologically, the first four of the six aortic arches give rise to the extracranial cerebral vessels. During development, these aortic arches connect the dorsal aorta to the aortic sac, which is the most distal part of the truncus arteriosus. The six arches are not present simultaneously but develop in a craniocaudal sequence over time (see Figure 3–1). Eventual orientation and distribution of the extracranial cerebral arteries that arise from these arches depend upon the order of development of the central nervous system tissue which they are destined to nourish.

The first aortic arches serve as channels supplying the primitive internal carotid arteries. The second arches evolve into the hyoid and stapedial arteries, which in turn give rise to branches of the external carotid artery. After regression of portions of the dorsal aorta between the third and fourth aortic arches, the third aortic arches remain to form the common carotid and the proximal internal carotid artery. The right fourth aortic arch, with a portion of the right dorsal aorta, forms the initial portion of the right subclavian artery. The left fourth aortic arch takes part in the formation of the definitive aortic arch and the left subclavian artery. Both subclavian arteries also receive a contribution from the intersegmental arteries of the embryonic vertebral column.

Initially, the main sources of blood flow to the anterior, middle, and posterior cerebral arteries consist of the internal carotid arteries because neural tissue supplied by the posterior cerebral arteries lies more anteriorly. As development continues, the arteries migrate posteriorly with the tissue they serve, and eventually the posterior cerebral arterial blood flow is provided through the vertebral-basilar circulation. Generally in the course of embryologic development, the extracranial cerebral arterial branches obtain their blood supply from the source that is nearest at a particular stage of development.

Paired dorsal aortal and the cervical intersegmental arteries anastomose longitudinally to develop the vertebral arteries. The seventh intersegmental arteries form the junction between the subclavian and vertebral arteries. The thoracic and lumbar intersegmental arteries persist. The basilar artery develops from the fusion of the two vertebral arteries. This is an example of economy of distribution, another principle that governs the development of the extracranial cerebral vasculature.

Embryological development makes persistence of eight carotid-vertebral communications possible, although only the posterior communicating artery is the anastomosis nor-

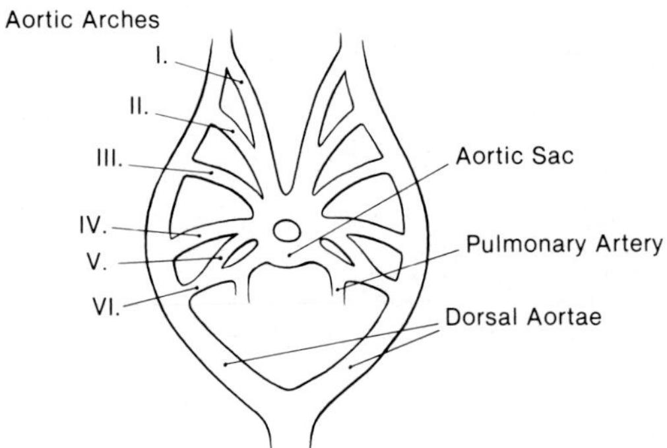

Figure 3–1. The six embryologic aortic arches develop in a craniocaudal sequence over time. They are not present simultaneously.

mally remaining. The next-most-common persistent anastomoses are the primitive trigeminal artery and the primitive hypoglossal artery. Detailed understanding of the embryological development of the extracranial vasculature facilitates a fuller appreciation and even anticipation of anatomical variations and the understanding of collateral pathways.

ANATOMY OF THE EXTRACRANIAL CEREBRAL VESSELS

The Aortic Arch

The three primary branches of the aortic arch are the innominate, the left common carotid, and the left subclavian arteries. The innominate artery is approximately 4 to 5 cm long. As it leaves the aortic arch, it passes superiorly and posteriorly until it reaches the approximate level of the right sternoclavicular junction. At this point, it divides into the right common carotid and the subclavian arteries. The left common carotid artery originates left of the innominate trunk from the highest portion of the aortic arch. It ascends through the superior mediastinum, and it stays ventral to the trachea, the esophagus, the left recurrent nerve, and the thoracic duct. On the left side of the thoracic carotid are the left vagus and phrenic nerves. The left carotid artery enters the neck above the left sternoclavicular joint. The left subclavian artery rises from the aortic arch just distal to the left common carotid (see Figure 3–2).

Variations in the origin of the brachiocephalic arteries are frequent (approximately 35 percent) and clinically important. The most common variant (16 percent) is the left common carotid rising from the arch of the aorta at a point closer than usual to the innominate artery. The left common carotid may actually originate from the innominate artery (8 percent). In 6 percent of cases, the left vertebral artery rises from the arch of the aorta, instead of originating from the left subclavian artery. The right subclavian may arise directly from the aortic arch (4 percent) but left of all other vessels. In 1 percent of cases, the right carotid artery begins at the arch. In less than 1 percent of cases, there is a left innominate artery from which the left common carotid artery arises.

Common Carotid Arteries

The right common carotid, a branch of the innominate artery, and the left common carotid, which arises from the aortic arch, are the principal arteries supplying the head and the neck. The right common carotid artery begins dorsal to the sternoclavicular joint. As noted in Figure 3–3, in rare cases the right carotid arises from the aortic arch.

The left common carotid originates left of the innominate trunk from the highest portion of the aortic arch. The course of the thoracic portion of this artery is discussed in the previous section. The left common carotid artery enters the neck dorsal to the left sternoclavicular joint. In the lower neck, the two common carotid arteries are separated only by the trachea. At the level of the thyroid gland, the larynx and the pharynx project ventrally between the two carotid arteries. The caudal portions of the cervical carotid arteries are covered by the sternocleidomastoid, sternohyoid, sternothyroid, and omohyoid muscles. As the common carotid arteries continue cranially, they are more superficial and are covered only by the cervical fascia and the platysma muscle.

The common carotid arteries are enclosed in a sheath which is derived from the deep cervical fascia. This sheath also contains the internal jugular vein and the vagus nerve. The jugular vein is lateral to the common carotid artery. The vagus nerve lies between the artery and vein and on a plane dorsal to both (see Figure 21–1).

The common carotid arteries are situated in the anterior cervical triangle, the margins of which are composed of the stylohyoid and the posterior belly of the digastric muscle in the superior aspect, the superior belly of the omo-

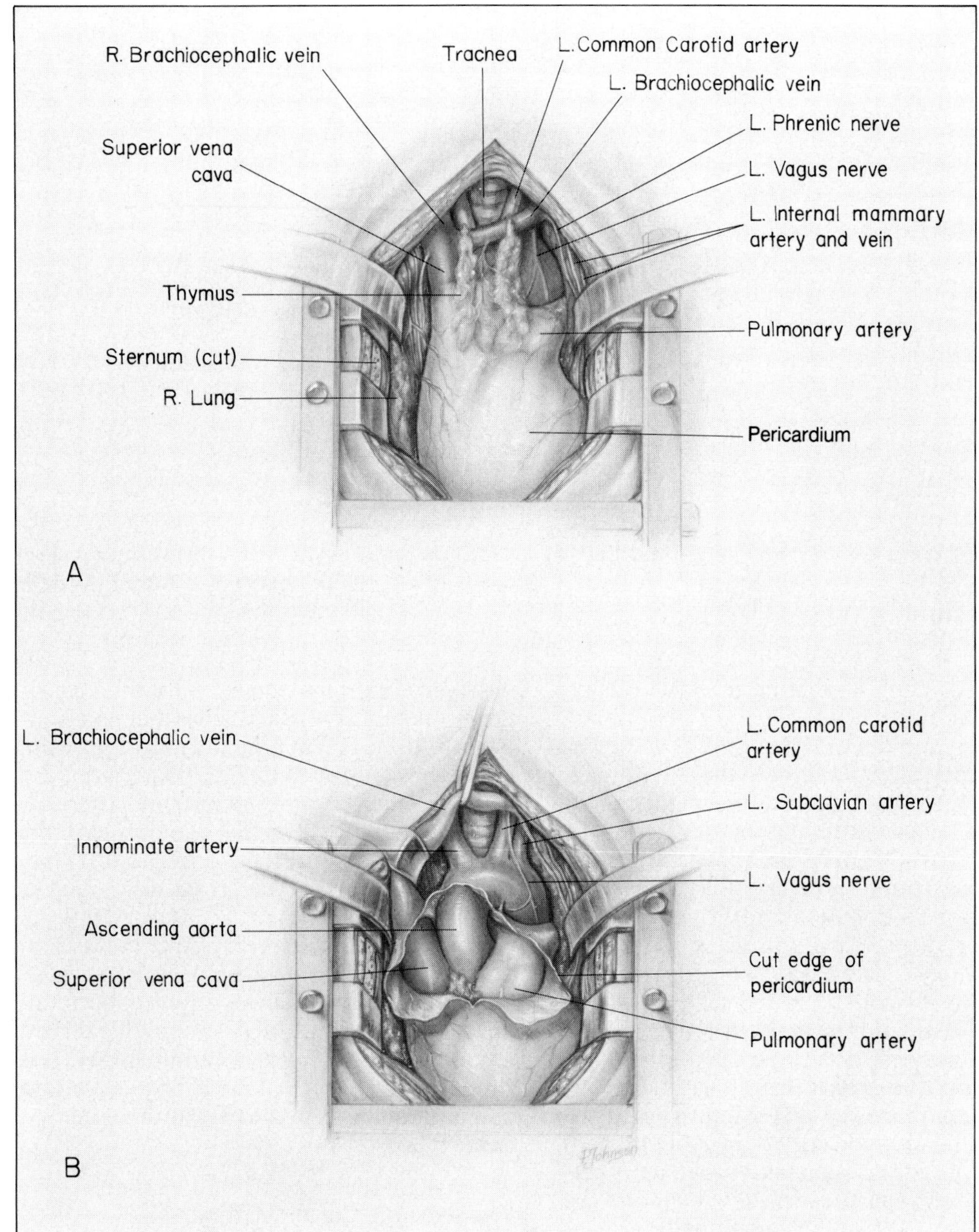

Figure 3–2. Anatomy of the arch of the aorta as seen through a median sternotomy incision: Midline incision through skin and subcutaneous tissues, with the pectoralis muscles exposed (*A*). The sternum is split and retracted, and the pericardial sac is exposed. Note the location of the vagus and phrenic nerves on the left (*B*).

hyoid at the medial aspect, and the sternocleidomastoid muscle at the lateral aspect.

The anterior cervical triangle constitutes an important surgical window within which the common carotid artery is crossed ventrally in an oblique medial-to-lateral direction by the sternocleidomastoid branch of the superior thyroidal artery. The superior and middle thyroidal veins usually follow a path superficial to the carotid sheath, but pierce it to drain into the internal jugular vein. Occasionally, the carotid sheath also encloses the descending hypoglossal and the ascending cervical nerves, as well as their thin connecting loop, the ansa

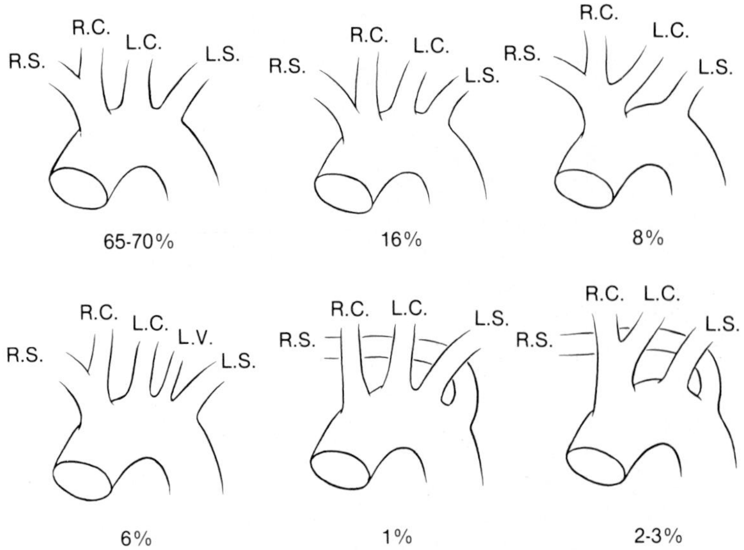

Figure 3–3. Variations in the anatomy of the branches of the aortic arch. First illustrated is the "normal" configuration, which occurs in 65 to 70 percent of cases. Other variations are shown in order of decreasing frequency. RS-right subclavian, RC-right common carotid, LC-left common carotid, LS-left subclavian, LV-left vertebral.

cervicalis, which is superifical to the carotid artery (see Figure 3–4).

The middle thyroid vein crosses the common carotid artery inferior to the anterior cervical triangle at or below the level of the cricoid cartilage. The anterior jugular vein crosses the common carotid artery just above the clavicle but is considerably more superficial, being separated from the common carotid by the sternothyroid and sternohyoid muscles. The recurrent laryngeal nerve passes obliquely dorsal to and at the caudal end of the cervical carotid artery. The inferior thyroid artery (a branch of the thyrocervical trunk) crosses dorsal to the inferior portion of the common carotid artery. The common carotid artery bifurcates at the level of the thyroid cartilage in more than 70 percent of cases. In an additional 15 to 20 percent, it bifurcates between this point and the hyoid bone. Most of the remaining 10 percent bifurcate higher, between the hyoid bone and the angle of the mandible. The low bifurcation, which is situated caudal to the superior border of the thyroid cartilage, is rare. A very rare anomaly is the completely absent common carotid, with the internal and external carotid arteries originating directly from the innominate artery or from the aortic arch.

The common carotid artery usually has no branches. However, a common variant (in some studies almost 45 percent) is the superior thyroidal artery arising from the distal common carotid artery usually within 2.5 cm of the bifurcation. Other branches that occasionally rise from the common carotid artery are the laryngeal, the ascending pharyngeal, the inferior thyroidal, and the vertebral artery.

The carotid body is small, often ovoid, and 2 to 5 mm in diameter. It lies dorsal to the bifurcation of the common carotid artery and is supplied by branches of the vagus nerve. Its chemoreceptor endings are part of the visceral afferent system of the body.

The term "carotid sinus" refers to the terminal common carotid artery and the dilated first centimeter of the internal carotid artery. It is supplied by a branch of the hypoglossal nerve and it participates in the regulation of the systemic blood pressure.

The External Carotid Artery

The common carotid artery divides into the internal and the external carotid arteries. The main trunk of the external carotid artery curves behind the angle of the mandible, where it branches into the maxillary and superficial temporal arteries. As a rule, the external carotid artery is slightly smaller than the internal carotid artery (see Figure 3–4C and D).

Generally, the main trunk of the external carotid artery is covered by the anterior or medial margin of the sternocleidomastoid muscle and is crossed by the hypoglossal nerve. The

Table 3–1. Nerves Relating to the Extracranial Vasculature in the Neck

Superficial Exposure (Sternocleidomastoid Muscle Intact)

- Facial nerve: deep to the platysma muscle; a cervical branch of which anastomoses with transverse cervical at anterior border of sternocleidomastoid muscle (communicating nerve)
- Great auricular nerve: crosses obliquely over sternocleidomastoid muscle toward angle of mandible and postauricular area
- Lesser occipital nerve: crosses over posterior attachment of sternocleidomastoid muscle to mastoid and occipital areas
- Spinal accessory nerve: passes at posterior aspect of sternocleidomastoid muscle across posterior triangle to disappear under trapezius muscle
- Transverse cervical nerve: crosses midbelly of sternocleidomastoid muscle to innervate anterior neck

Exposure Deep to Sternocleidomastoid Muscle

- Ansa cervicalis
  - Inferior root: from ventral rami of second and third cervical nerves; runs dorsal to internal jugular vein, then crosses superficial to it to join superior root
  - Superior root: descends from hypoglossal nerve and runs lateral to internal and common carotid arteries; connects with inferior root after inferior root passes over internal jugular vein
- Second cervical nerve (ventral ramus): dorsal to internal jugular vein
- Third cervical nerve (ventral ramus): dorsal to internal jugular vein
- Fourth cervical nerve (ventral ramus): dorsal to internal jugular vein
- Brachial plexus: in base of neck, arising dorsal to scalenus anterior muscle
- Phrenic nerve: arises from ventral ramus of fourth cervical nerve, runs dorsal to internal jugular vein, and laterally flanks brachiocephalic artery (on right)
- Superior laryngeal nerve: courses medially and dorsally to external carotid artery
- Vagus nerve: runs dorsolateral to carotid artery
- Hypoglossal nerve: loops inferior to posterior belly of digastric muscle and superficial to external carotid and disappears under stylohyoid muscle

Exposure Deep to Carotid Artery and Jugular Vein

- Cervical sympathetic trunk, including superior cervical ganglion, accessory cervical ganglion, and middle cervical ganglion: lies deep to carotid artery
- Superior cardiac branch of vagus nerve: between vagus and sympathetic trunk
- Superior cervical cardiac nerve: branches from sympathetic trunk
- Recurrent laryngeal nerve: deep to common carotid artery and thyroid gland
- Middle cervical cardiac nerve: branches from sympathetic trunk low in neck

superior laryngeal nerve courses medially and dorsally to the external carotid artery and is crossed by the lingual, common facial, and superior thyroid veins, as well as by the digastric and stylohyoid muscles. Beyond the angle of the mandible, the external carotid artery penetrates into the substance of the parotid gland, deep to the facial nerve.

The superior thyroid artery is the first branch to rise from the external carotid artery. It usually originates at the level of the hyoid bone and supplies the thyroid gland to which it gives two main branches. Other branches of the superior thyroid artery include the infrahyoid, sternocleidomastoid, superior laryngeal, and cricothyroid arteries. Variations in the origin of this vessel have been previously discussed (see Figure 14–17).

The second, and usually the smallest, branch of the external carotid is the ascending pharyngeal artery. It rises from the posterior aspect of the external carotid soon after the origin of that vessel and ascends vertically to the base of the skull. Its branches include the pharyngeal, palatine, prevertebral, inferior tympanic, and posterior meningeal arteries.

The third branch of the external carotid is the lingual artery which arises near the hyoid bone. This artery first courses cranially and then curves caudally and ventrally, forming a loop crossed by the hypoglossal nerve.

The facial artery is the fourth branch of the external carotid and originates in the anterior cervical triangle very close to the angle of the mandible. It then curves around the inferior border of the mandible and crosses it onto the face at the anterior edge of the masseter muscle (see Figure 3–5). Frequently, the facial and lingual arteries arise from a common vessel, the linguofacial trunk. The facial artery may vary in size and in the extent to which it supplies the face.

The occipital artery arises opposite the facial artery from the posterior aspect of the external carotid artery. It begins near the posterior belly of the digastric muscle and ends in the posterior part of the scalp. In its course, it passes between the transverse process of the atlas and the mastoid process of the temporal bone. Later, this artery changes its direction and runs more vertically in a somewhat tortuous course in the superficial fascia of the scalp, then divides into numerous branches that supply the vertex of the skull and anastomose with the posterior auricular and temporal arteries.

The descending branch of the occipital artery is the largest and supplies the major muscles of the posterior neck, including the trapezius, semispinalis capitis, and cervicis muscles. This branch anastomoses with the ascending branch of the transverse cervical, the vertebral,

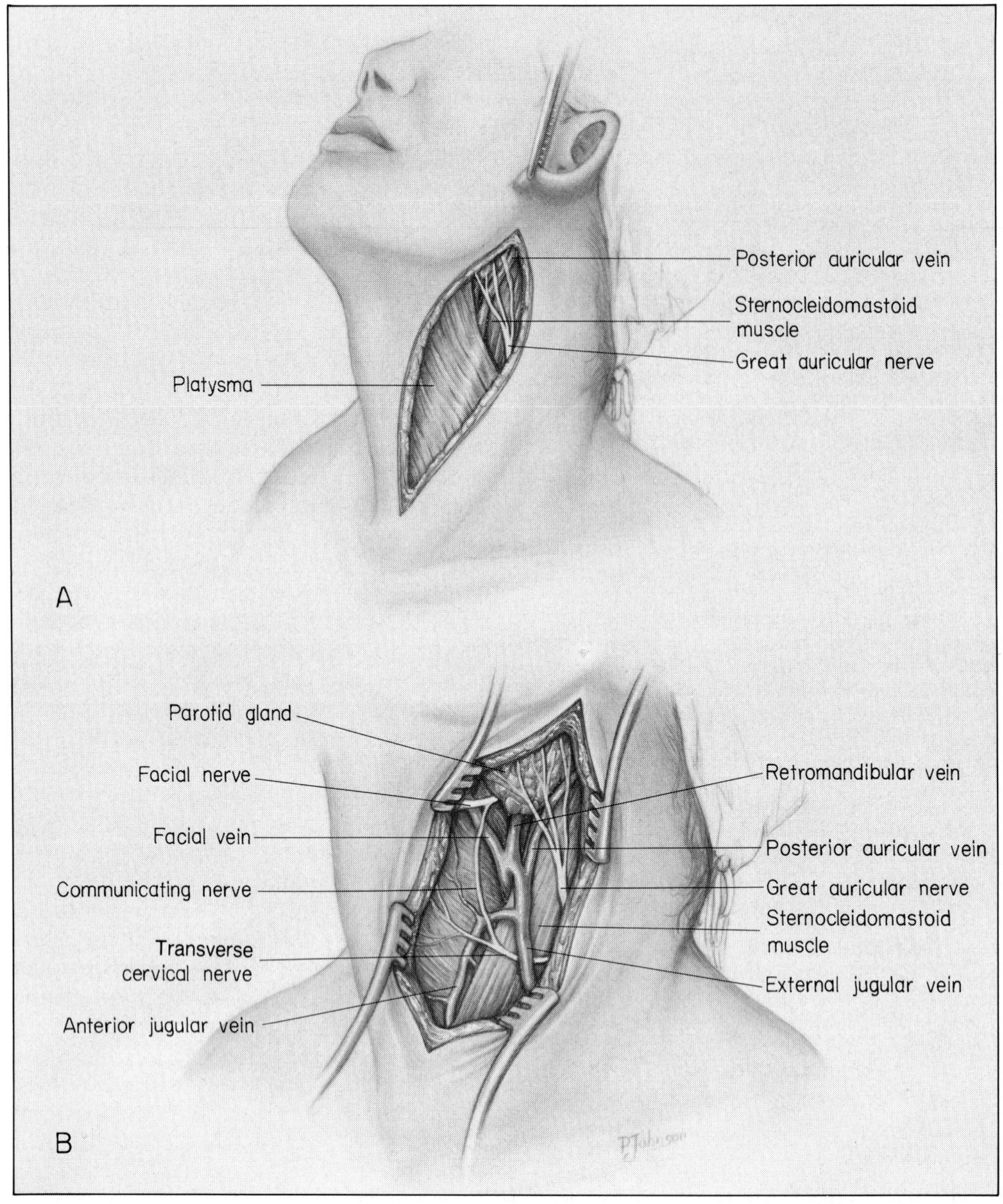

Figure 3–4. Anatomy of the neck as seen through an anterior cervical incision: subcutaneous incision with platysma superficial to the sternocleidomastoid muscle. The great auricular nerve is encountered at this level (*A*). Deeper dissection illustrates the venous drainage superficial to the carotid artery. The facial and transverse cervical nerves are visualized at this level (*B*). View of the carotid artery bifurcation and adjacent internal jugular vein, which is slightly posterior and superficial to the artery. The external jugular vein has been divided and ligated. Note the sternocleidomastoid branch of the occipital artery crossing over the hypoglossal nerve.

and the deep cervical, a branch of the costocervical trunk. These anastomoses are very important in establishing collateral circulation after occlusion of the common carotid or the subclavian artery.

The posterior auricular artery is a small branch of the external carotid artery arising near the styloid process. Its branches include the stylomastoid, auricular, and occipital arteries.

The superficial temporal artery is one of the two terminal branches of the external carotid. It begins within the parotid gland, courses over the zygomatic process, and eventually divides

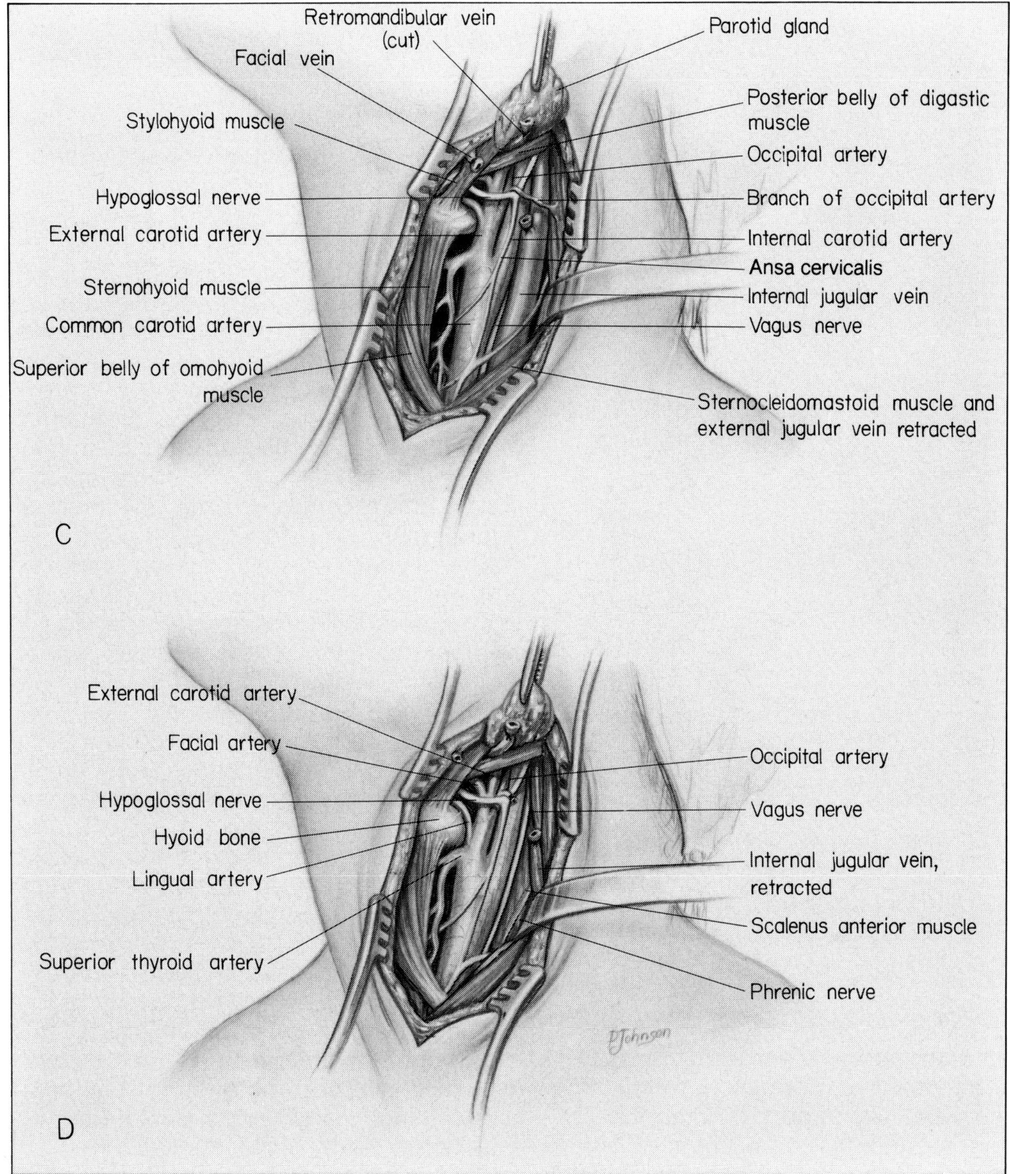

Figure 3–4 (continued). Anatomy of the neck as seen through an arterior cervical incision. The ansa cervicalis and vagus nerve are visualized (*C*). The internal jugular vein has been retracted to expose the carotid artery. Note the phrenic nerve coursing over the scalenus anterior muscle. The first three anterior branches of the external carotid artery are also seen (*D*).

into the frontal and parietal branches. In its course, it is crossed by the temporal and zygomatic branches of the facial nerve and is accompanied by the auriculotemporal nerve.

The maxillary artery is the larger of the terminal branches of the external carotid artery. It arises in the substance of the parotid gland, passes over the ramus of the mandible in an anterior direction, and then runs either superficial or deep to the lateral pterygoid muscle and ends in the pterygopalatine fossa. It supplies the deep structures of the face and divides into the mandibular, pterygoid, and pterygopalatine arteries.

The middle meningeal is one of five branches of the mandibular portion of the maxillary artery. It is the largest and most constant artery supplying the dura mater. Other branches of the mandibular artery include the deep auricular, anterior tympanic, inferior alveolar, and accessory meningeal vessels. The accessory meningeal artery supplies the tri-

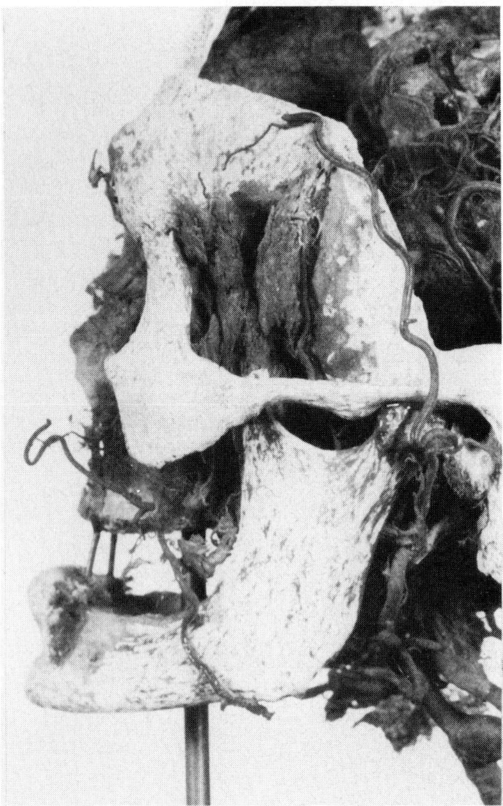

Figure 3-5. Resin cast of the vascular system of the upper neck and face shown against the bony anatomy. The facial artery courses in a tortuous manner toward the intermedial orbit. The superficial temporal artery traverses the zygomatic process to reach the temporal fossa.

geminal ganglion and the dura mater. Branches of the pterygoid portion of the maxillary artery are the deep temporal, pterygoid, mesenteric, and buccal arteries. Branches of the pterygopalatine portion of the maxillary artery include the posterior superior alveolar, infraorbital, and greater palatine arteries; the artery of the pterygoid canal; the pharyngeal, and sphenopalatine arteries. The proximal portion of the external carotid is usually located slightly anterior and medial to the internal carotid artery. During its embryological development, the external carotid migrates around the internal carotid. If the normal migratory route continues uninterrupted, the external carotid will lie lateral and posterior to the internal carotid artery. This has been referred to as the Prendes anomaly. It occurs in approximately 5 percent of the patients.

Rarely, the external carotid artery is absent; in this case the branches which would have originated from it arise from the internal carotid artery.

Internal Carotid Artery

The internal carotid artery begins at the bifurcation of the common carotid artery. Initially, it runs ventral to the transverse processes of the first three cervical vertebrae. In the petrous portion of the temporal bone, it crosses the foramen lacerum, passes through the carotid canal, and enters the middle cranial fossa of the skull where it is suspended in two layers of dura mater, which form the cavernous sinus. Within the cavernous sinus, the internal carotid makes a double curvature or siphon, passes between the optic and oculomotor nerves, and eventually reaches the circle of Willis (see Figure 3-6).

Its branchless proximal portion is usually posterior and lateral to the external carotid artery and somewhat overlapped by the sternocleidomastoid muscle. It then passes deep to the parotid gland, where it is crossed by the hypoglossal nerve, the digastric and stylohyoid muscles, the occipital and posterior auricular arteries. Dorsal to the internal carotid lie the superior cervical ganglion of the sympathetic trunk and the superior laryngeal nerve. Dorsolaterally to the internal carotid courses the vagus nerve, laterally the internal jugular vein, and medially the ascending pharyngeal artery. As the internal carotid reaches the base of the skull, the vagus, glossopharyngeal, accessory, and hypoglossal nerves lie between the artery and the internal jugular vein (which at this level is dorsal to the artery). The accompanying sympathetic fibers innervate the pupillodilator and superior tarsal muscles of the ipsilateral eye (see Figure 3-6).

The first branch of the internal carotid and the caroticotympanic artery rise in the petrous portion of the temporal bone. This can be an important collateral route via its anastomoses with external carotid branches in the event of internal carotid artery occlusion. The pterygoid artery (vidian artery) anastomoses in the pterygoid canal with a branch of the internal maxillary artery.

After the internal carotid artery emerges from the canal through the foramen lacerum and enters the cavernous sinus, it first ascends toward the posterior clinoid process, and then runs anteriorly and horizontally for about 2 cms. The vessel then takes an upward turn, passing on the medial aspect of the anterior

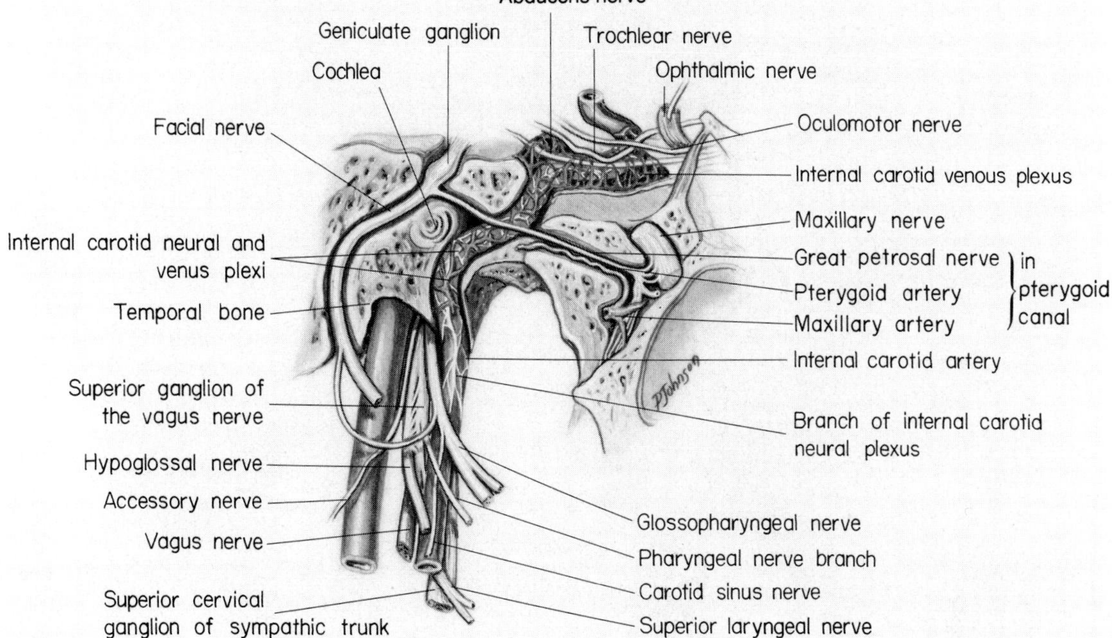

Figure 3–6. Lateral view of the carotid siphon.

clinoid process, and pierces the dural roof of the cavernous sinus to enter the subarachnoid space.

Several branches of the carotid artery arise in the cavernous sinus. The largest, most consistent, and most proximal branch is the meningohypophyseal trunk. It gives rise to the tentorial, inferior hypophyseal, and dorsal meningeal arteries. Other branches are the artery of the inferior cavernous sinus and McConnel's capsular artery. Cranial nerves II to VI and sympathetic fibers also pass through the cavernous sinus.

After entering the subarachnoid space on the medial side of the anterior clinoid process, the internal carotid artery lies posteriorly and superiorly to the lateral side of the optic chiasm. It gives rise to the ophthalmic artery, which passes through the optic canal below the optic nerve. The internal carotid, by dividing into the anterior and middle cerebral arteries, becomes part of the circle of Willis.

Vertebral and Basilar Arteries

The vertebral artery is the first branch of the subclavian artery. Initially, it courses between the longus colli and the scalenus anterior muscles, then angles dorsally to the transverse process of the sixth cervical vertebra and continues in a cranial direction through the foramina of the transverse processes of the upper six cervical vertebrae to the skull. After passing through the foramen of the atlas, the vertebral artery bends abruptly in a medial direction around the superior articular process. It then lies in a groove on the cranial surface of the posterior arch of the atlas and enters the cranial vault through the foramen magnum (see Figure 3–7).

As the vertebral artery passes through the foramina of the transverse processes, it is surrounded by branches from the inferior cervical sympathetic ganglion and by a plexus of veins that eventually unite in the lower neck to form the vertebral vein.

There are both cervical and cranial branches of the vertebral artery. The cervical branches are further divided into spinal and muscular categories. The spinal branches enter the vertebral canal through the intervertebral foramina and each divides into two tributaries. One branch supplies the spinal cord and its membrane, while the other branch divides into an ascending and descending portion which communicate with similar branches both cranially and caudally. The cranial branches include the meningeal, posterior and anterior spinal, posterior inferior cerebellar, and the medullary arteries. The meningeal branches arise from

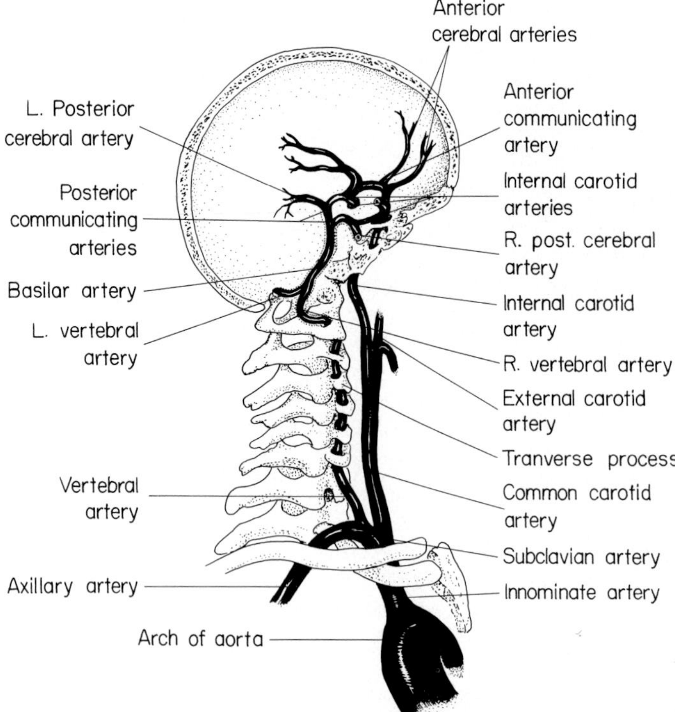

Figure 3–7. The relationship of the vertebral and carotid systems.

the horizontal segment between the atlas and the foramen magnum.

The vertebral arteries ascend to the ventral pontomedullary junction, where they unite to form the basilar artery. The anterior spinal rami arise from this distal segment of the vertebral artery and eventually unite to form the anterior spinal artery. The posterior inferior cerebellar arteries arise from the vertebral arteries at the level of the lower olive. Branches of the posterior inferior cerebellar artery supply the posterolateral medulla, the inferior posterior surface of the cerebellum, and the posterior part of the spinal cord (see Figure 3–8).

The basilar artery terminates in the premesenteric cistern. During its course, it gives off numerous small pontine branches. Its major branches include the labryinthine, the anterior inferior cerebellar, the superior cerebellar, and the posterior cerebral arteries. Shortly after the posterior cerebral arteries originate, they are joined by the posterior communicating arteries.

Variations of the vertebral arteries are frequent but usually of no clinical significance. Often one vertebral artery is larger than the other. In approximately 67 percent of the cases, it is the left vertebral artery that is dominant. One of the vertebral arteries, usually the left one, may arise from the aortic arch. In rare cases, the vertebral artery may arise from the common carotid artery in association with an anomalous subclavian artery. This represents persistence of the embryologic cervical intersegmental artery. More frequently, the innominate artery trifurcates, giving rise to the common carotid, vertebral, and subclavian arteries at once. Nearly 90 percent of the vertebral arteries enter the transverse processes at the sixth cervical vertebra. However, 8 percent enter at a higher level, and approximately 2 percent enter at the seventh cervical vertebra. When the vertebral artery is hypoplastic, which occurs more frequently on the right side, it may terminate in the posterior inferior cerebellar artery. In very rare cases, the vertebral artery (one or both) may fail to form between the first and second cervical vertebrae. If this anomaly is bilateral, collateral channels usually allow reconstitution of flow in the intracranial vertebrals, which continue as usual to form the basilar artery.

The most frequent variations of the basilar artery include partial duplication or island formation. The terminal branches of the basilar artery—the posterior cerebral arteries—arise phylogenetically from the internal carotid artery. In 22 percent of cases, the posterior cere-

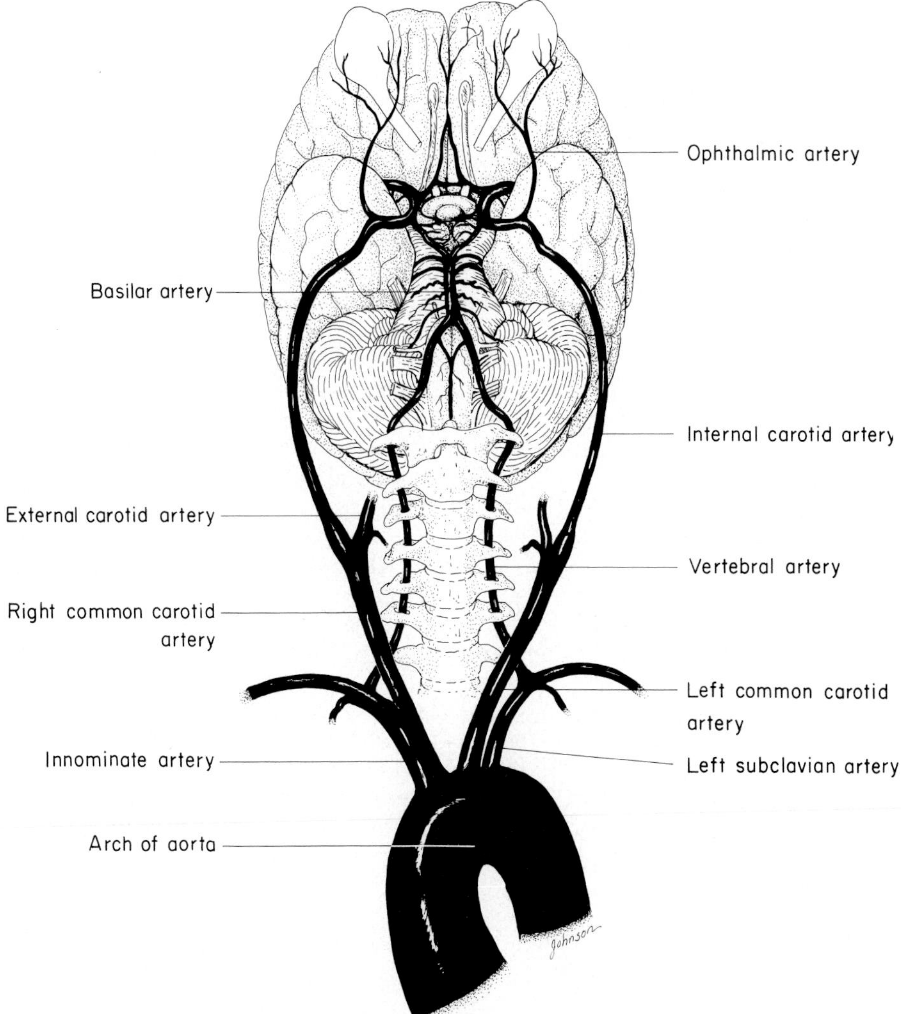

Figure 3–8. Inferior view of the brain illustrating the vertebral and basilar arteries (posterior circulation) and the circle of Willis.

bral artery remains a major internal carotid branch.

Circle of Willis

The circle of Willis is a polygonal-shaped arterial ring in the subarachnoid space which surrounds the infundibular stalk on the inferior surface of the brain. It is composed of the basilar artery (posterior circulation) and its terminal branches, the posterior cerebral arteries, the internal carotid artery (anterior circulation) and its terminal branches, and the middle and anterior cerebral arteries. The posterior cerebral and internal carotid arteries anastomose via the posterior communicating arteries, and the two anterior cerebral arteries anastomose through the anterior communicating artery, completing the polygon of the circle of Willis.

This anatomical situation occurs in only about 50 percent of cases. Variations include those in which the polygonal anastomotic integrity is maintained, but the components vary in their size or configuration. In other varieties, the anastomotic integrity is also lost. Because dye injected in the course of angiography into either the anterior or posterior circulation does not pass into the other arterial network, one has to conclude that the circle of Willis does not usually function as a distributor or equalizer of flow. This is probably fortunate, for its frequent variations render it somewhat unreliable in providing collateral circulation.

The variations that are functionally most significant include hypoplasia or agenesis of the communicating arteries. The most common variant is the posterior cerebral artery originating from the internal carotid siphon. Hypoplasia or agenesis of the anterior cerebral artery between the internal carotid artery and the anterior communicating arteries is more common than hypoplasia or agenesis of the communicating arteries.

Other Branches of the Subclavian Artery

Immediately beyond the origin of the vertebral artery, close to the medial border of the scalenus anterior muscle, the thyrocervical trunk rises from the subclavian artery. It divides into three branches: the inferior thyroid, the suprascapular, and the transverse cervical arteries. The inferior thyroid artery courses cranially, ventral to the vertebral artery, and reaches the longus colli muscle. The middle cervical ganglion often rests on this vessel. The inferior thyroid artery anastomoses with the superior thyroid artery. A prominent branch of the inferior thyroid is the ascending cervical artery, which arises between the scalenus anterior and the longus capitis, supplies muscles of the neck, and anastomoses with branches of the vertebral artery (see Figure 3–9).

As it passes in a lateral direction across the scalenus anterior and the phrenic nerve, the suprascapular artery is covered by the sternocleidomastoid muscle. It supplies branches to the sternocleidomastoid and supraspinatus muscles and terminates at the superior border of the scapula.

The transverse cervical artery has two equally frequent variants. When it arises as a common source, it gives rise to a superficial branch, which is the major blood supply to the trapezius muscle, and a deep branch, which feeds the levator scapulae and neighboring deep cervical muscles. If the deep branch comes from the subclavian artery instead of the thyrocervical trunk, it is called the descending scapular artery, and the superficial branch of the transverse cervical artery is called the superficial cervical artery.

The internal thoracic artery arises from the subclavian artery opposite the thyrocervical trunk. It descends just lateral to the sternal border on the inner surface of the anterior chest wall.

The costocervical trunk arises on the dorsal aspect of the subclavian artery opposite the thyrocervical trunk, deep to the scalenus anterior muscle on the right and medial to that muscle on the left. As the highest intercostal artery, it passes dorsally and superiorly, and

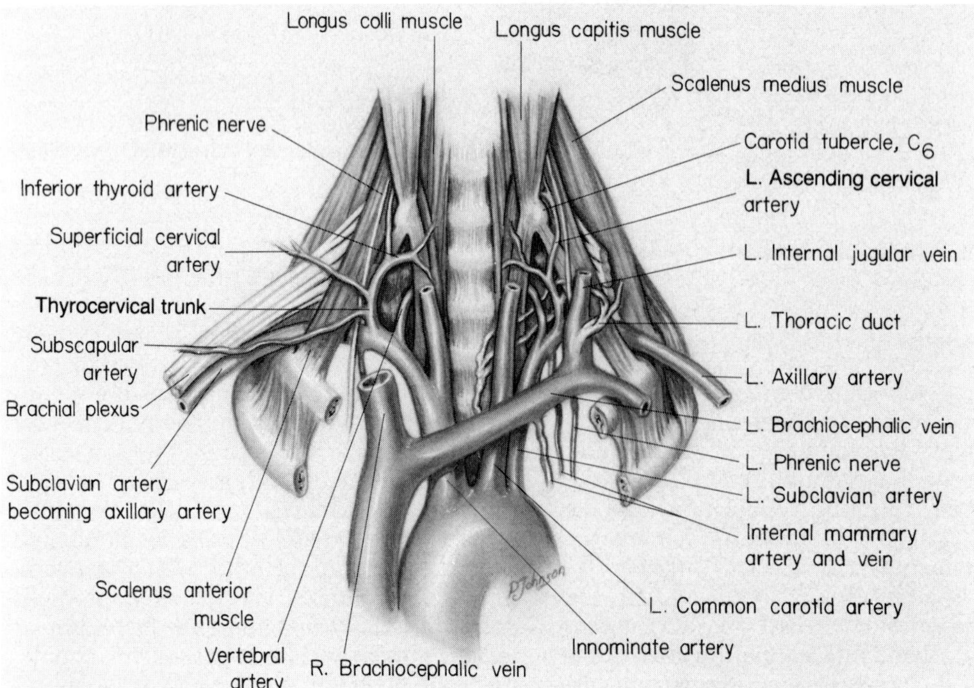

Figure 3–9. Anterior view of the extracranial vascular anatomy from the aortic arch and the supraclavicular area.

reaches the pleura ventral to the necks of the first and second ribs, where it anastomoses with the first aortic intercostal artery. The deep cervical artery usually arises from the costocervical trunk. Passing above the eighth cervical nerve and between the transverse process of the seventh cervical vertebra and the neck of the first rib, it ascends the dorsal neck between the semispinalis capitis and cervicis muscles. Occasionally, rather than arising from the costocervical trunk, it occurs as a separate branch from the subclavian artery (see Figure 3–10).

COLLATERAL FLOW

Atherosclerosis of the extracranial arteries has sites of predilection, including the innominate artery, the proximal subclavian arteries (often proximal to the origin of the vertebral artery), the proximal vertebral arteries, the proximal common carotid arteries, the carotid artery bifurcations, the proximal internal carotid arteries, the carotid artery siphons, the terminal vertebral arteries, and the basilar artery. When thrombosis occurs as a superimposed process on gradually developing atherosclerosis, it results in occlusion which usually does not extend beyond the next point of branching. Collateral flow may reenter the thrombosed vessel at the level of this branching.

Knowledge of these sites of atherosclerotic predilection, and of the preexisting collaterals available when atherosclerotic stenosis or occlusion occur, improves medical and surgical understanding and facilitates treatment. Extracranial anastomoses for collateral flow exist between the internal and external carotid arteries in the orbit, the external carotid and vertebral arteries, branches of the vertebral and subclavian arteries, and the subclavian and external carotid arteries. When the collaterals are adequate, they alleviate neurological deficits caused by stenosis or occlusion.

If there is an occlusion of the innominate artery, collateral flow may occur through four main channels. Forward flow through the left vertebral with reversal of flow through the right vertebral artery is a primary source of collateral flow. Branches of the left external carotid and left subclavian arteries anastomose with their counterparts on the right side providing collateral flow. Costocervical branches of the right subclavian artery anastomose with the first aortic intercostal arteries, supplying blood directly to the right subclavian artery. Communications between the intercostal arteries and branches of the axillary and internal mammary arteries allow retrograde flow into the right subclavian artery.

Occlusion of the proximal right and left subclavian arteries gives rise to collateral flow from five sources. Again, as in the description of collateral flow in innominate artery occlusion, forward flow in the contralateral vertebral artery with reversed flow in the ipsilateral vertebral artery provides an important collateral channel (see Figures 28–2 and 28–3). Descending branches of the occipital artery (branch of the external carotid artery) can anastomose with muscular branches of the vertebral artery, again providing retrograde flow through the vertebral artery to supply the area beyond the occlusion. Ipsilateral to the occlusion, branches of the external carotid which interconnect with branches of the thyrocervical trunk and branches of the costocervical trunk provide two further sources of collateral flow. The fifth source of collateral flow is through connections of the ascending and superficial cervical branches of the thyrocervical trunk with the deep cervical branch of the costocervical trunk.

When the common carotid artery is occluded proximally, there are five major sources of collateral flow into the ipsilateral internal and external carotid artery. When the proximal common carotid artery is occluded, anastomosis of the contralateral external carotid artery with the ipsilateral external carotid artery allows retrograde flow through the ipsilateral external and forward flow through the ipsilateral internal carotid artery. Branches of the thyrocervical and costocervical trunks of the subclavian artery anastomose with the branches of the ipsilateral external carotid artery. Muscular branches of the vertebral artery connect with the branches of the occipital artery, allowing further collateral flow. The inferior thyroid artery communicates with the superior thyroid artery, the first branch of the external carotid artery. The ascending cervical artery, which is a branch of the inferior thyroid, anastomoses with the occipital artery. When the carotid bifurcation is occluded, collateral flow for the internal and external carotid arteries must be considered separately. The five collaterals described for proximal carotid occlusion would still supply the external carotid artery.

In the case of proximal occlusion of the in-

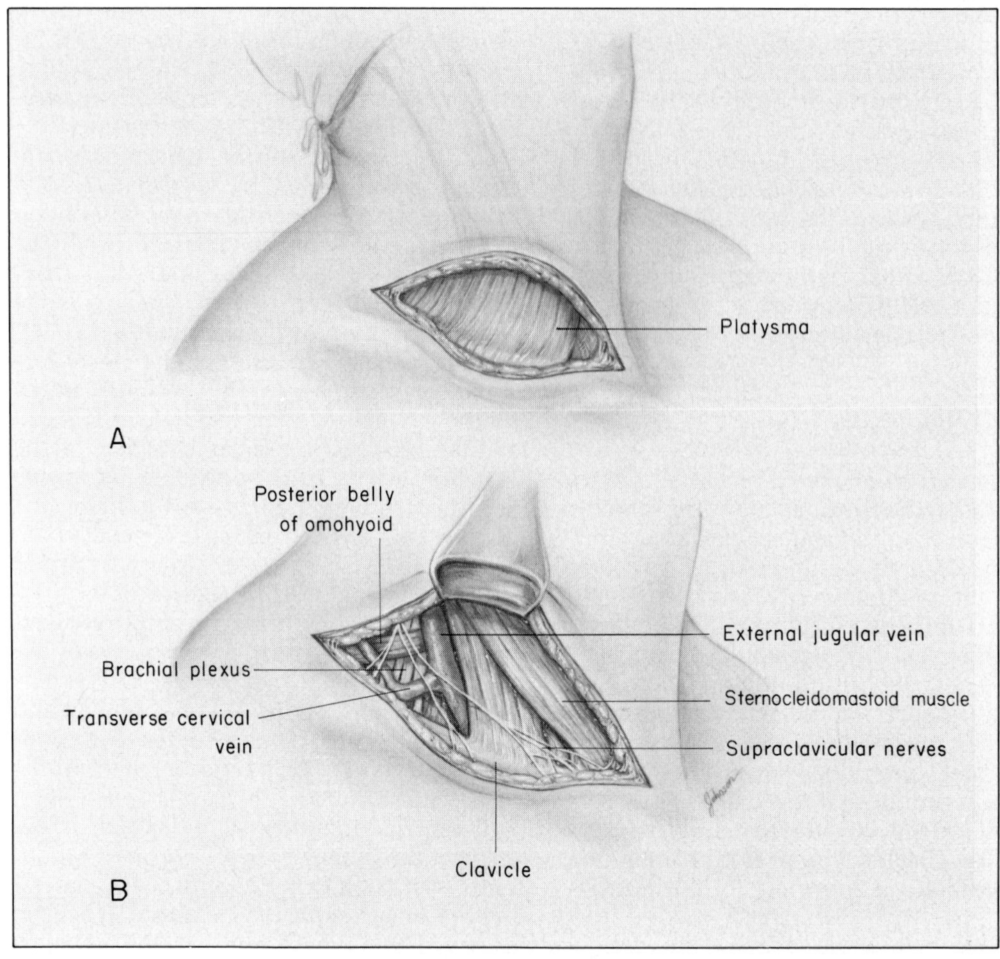

Figure 3-10. The anatomy of the lower neck seen through a supraclavicular incision. Superficial incision with platysma muscle exposed (*A*). The platysma divided and retracted with the sternocleidomastoid and omohyoid muscles. The external jugular and trasverse cervical veins are exposed. Nerves encountered at this level are listed (*B*).

ternal carotid artery, flow is maintained by four collaterals. The circle of Willis is one of the important collaterals through two pathways: (1) Cross-filling through the anterior communicating and anterior cerebral arteries to the internal carotid allows retrograde filling. (2) The basilar artery via the posterior communicating artery may supply retrograde internal carotid artery filling. The ophthalmic artery anastomoses with ipsilateral and contralateral branches of the middle meningeal artery, branches of the pterygopalatine portion of the maxillary artery, supraorbital and supratrochlear branches of the frontal division of the superficial temporal artery, and terminal branches of the angular artery. These provide important collateral flow. The caroticotympanic artery, the first branch of the internal carotid artery, anastomoses with the stylomastoid branch of the posterior auricular artery and the anterior tympanic branch of the internal maxillary artery.

If the internal carotid artery is occluded at the siphon, the possibility of collateral flow through the caroticotympanic artery no longer exists. The two collateral flow channels are still available, however, via the circle of Willis and the important collateral route through the ophthalmic artery.

In cases of vertebral artery occlusions, collateral flow at any level is possible through anastomoses of the segmental spinal branches of the vertebral arteries communicating with branches of the anterior spinal artery and the segmental branches of the cervical arteries. Basilar artery anastomoses are extensive. The

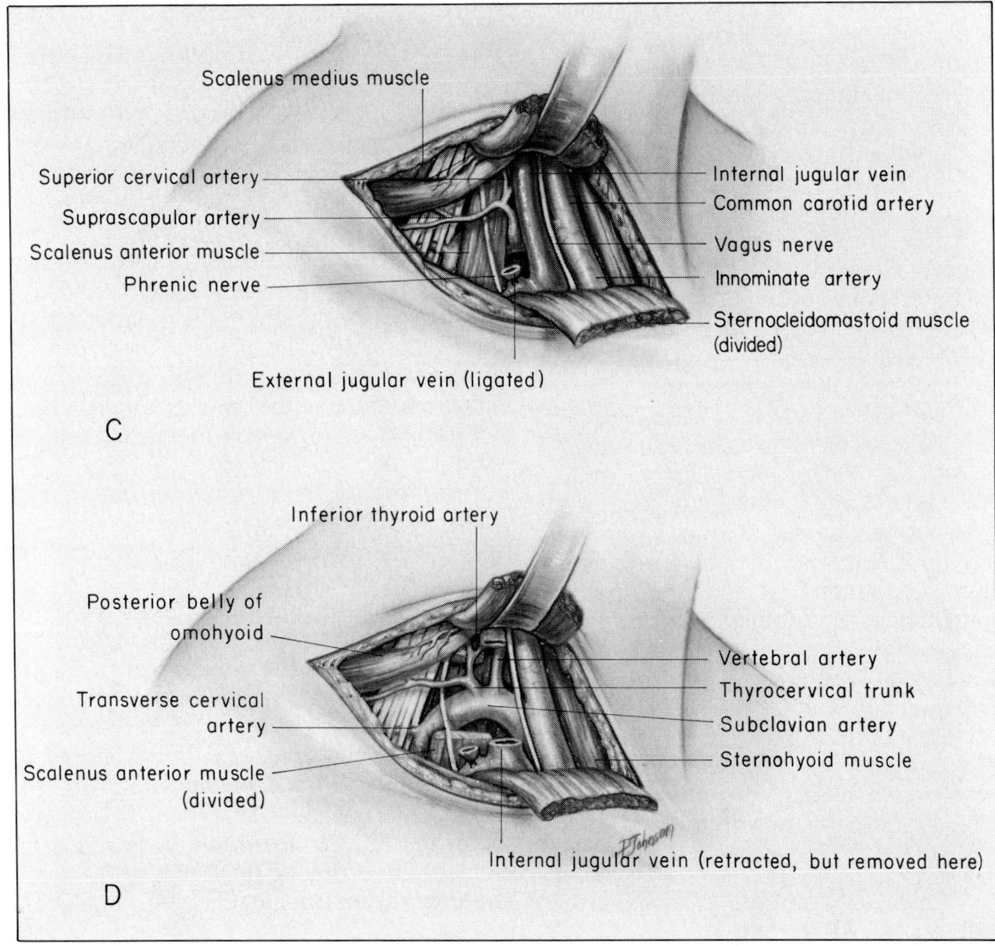

Figure 3–10 (continued). The anatomy of the neck seen through a supraclavicular incision. The sternocleidomastoid muscle is transected and the external jugular vein divided and ligated, with the internal jugular vein clearly visualized slightly superficial to the common carotid artery. The phrenic and vagus nerves are encountered at this level (*C*). The internal jugular vein is usually retracted but here has been removed to visualize underlying structures, including branches of the innominate and subclavian arteries (*D*).

anterior inferior cerebellar artery connects with the posterior inferior cerebellar and superior cerebellar arteries. The internal auditory and pontine arteries anastomose with the basilar artery. The superior cerebellar artery anastomoses not only with the anterior inferior cerebellar, but also with the posterior inferior cerebellar and posterior communicating arteries. The posterior cerebral artery interfaces with the middle and anterior cerebral arteries. These anastomoses are very important in cases of basilar artery stenosis or occlusion.

As previously discussed, the circle of Willis is frequently malformed and therefore is not always reliable in providing collateral circulation. Even when intact, the circle of Willis is not usually an equalizer of flow. However, if the demand for collateral flow develops, as in cases of carotid or basilar artery occlusion, the circle of Willis may provide essential communication between the two cerebral hemispheres and between the anterior and posterior arterial circuits.

Embryology predicts the possible persistence of eight carotid-vertebrobasilar anastomoses. Of these eight the posterior communicating artery is the only one that usually persists. Of the remaining seven possible persistent channels the most common are the trigeminal and the primitive hypoglossal arteries. They may become important as sources of collateral flow if they do remain. The trigeminal artery is seen on 0.1 to 0.2 percent of all angiograms. It arises from the internal carotid artery as it leaves the carotid canal in the petrous bone. When it is large, it may become the principal supplier to the basilar artery, and the vertebral arteries and inferior portion of the basilar may be correspondingly small. When the trigeminal artery is small, it contributes little to the vertebral-basilar circulation.

The next most frequent anomalous carotid–vertebral-basilar anastomosis is the primitive hypoglossal artery. It begins near the origin of the internal carotid artery, follows a tortuous course, and enters the posterior cranial fossa through the anterior condyloid foramen, terminating in the inferior basilar artery. When this anomaly occurs, the posterior communicating arteries are not visualized on angiography and the vertebral arteries are quite small. Whenever there is simultaneous filling of the vertebrobasilar circuit during carotid angiography, it usually occurs through these anomalous connections.

Leptomeningeal anastomoses occur over the surface of the cerebral and cerebellar hemispheres between the anterior and middle cerebral and between the middle cerebral and posterior cerebral arteries. These are called "watershed" areas and are thought to be especially sensitive to blood-flow reduction (see also Chapter 5 on blood flow to the brain).

THE VENOUS SYSTEM

Veins of the Cranium

The veins of the brain are tributaries of the internal jugular vein. There are two groups—cerebral and cerebellar veins. The cerebral veins are divided into superficial or external and deep or internal veins. While the superficial veins collect blood from the cortex and surrounding white matter, the deep veins drain the more central structures of the cerebrum. Both of these systems drain primarily into the dural sinuses which in turn empty into the internal jugular veins. The internal jugular veins exit the calvarium through the jugular foramina and course through the neck within the carotid sheaths.

An accessory route which drains blood from the brain is provided by the emissary and diploic veins, which connect the dural sinuses to the superficial veins of the scalp. These veins drain into the external jugular veins, which in turn empty into the subclavian veins.

Veins of the Face and Scalp

These veins can be divided into superficial and deep groups. The superficial veins include the facial, superficial temporal, posterior auricular, occipital, and retromandibular veins. The retromandibular vein joins the posterior auricular vein to form the external jugular vein.

The external jugular vein receives much of the drainage from the cranial exterior and deep face. It begins within the parotid gland near the angle of the mandible. It crosses the sternocleidomastoid obliquely and ends in the subclavian vein, lateral to the scalenus anterior muscle. Initially, it runs with the great auricular nerve.

Tributaries to the external jugular vein include the posterior external jugular, the anterior jugular, the transverse cervical, and the suprascapular veins.

The internal jugular vein drains the brain, face, and the neck. It is continuous with the transverse sinus and descends through the jugular foramen. It runs posterior and then lateral to the internal carotid artery and then lateral to the common carotid artery. At the base of the neck, it unites with the subclavian vein to form the brachiocephalic vein. At its origin, it is somewhat dilated; this dilation is called the jugular bulb. A second dilation near the termination of the internal jugular vein is called the inferior bulb.

At the base of the neck, the right internal jugular vein is a slight distance from the common carotid artery and crosses the first portion of the right subclavian artery. On the left side, the internal jugular vein often overlaps the common carotid artery. The left internal jugular vein is usually smaller than the right.

Important tributaries to the internal jugular vein include the inferior petrosal sinus; the facial, lingual, pharyngeal, superior, and middle thyroid; and the occipital veins. On the right side, the lymphatic duct enters at the point of union of the internal jugular and subclavian veins. On the left side, the thoracic duct enters at the same point of union.

The vertebral vein is formed from many small tributaries that converge in the suboccipital triangle to form a dense plexus around the vertebral artery, which ends in a single trunk emerging from the transverse foramen at the sixth or seventh cervical vertebra. Important tributaries include the anterior vertebral, accessory vertebral, and deep cervical veins. The vertebral vein occasionally communicates with the transverse sinus by a vein which courses through the condyloid canal. The vertebral vein may also receive some drainage from the occipital vein.

REFERENCES

Clemente, C.D.: *Anatomy: A Regional Atlas of the Human Body.* Lea and Febiger, Philadelphia, Pennsylvania, 1975.

Corliss, C.E.: *Patten's Human Embryology: Elements of Clinical Development.* McGraw-Hill, New York, 392–93, 1976.

Countee, R.W., and Vijayanathan, T.: External carotid artery in internal carotid artery occlusion: angiographic, therapeutic, and prognostic considerations. *Stroke,* **10**:450–60, 1979.

Day, A.L.: Anatomy of the extracranial vessels. In Smith, R.R. (ed.): *Stroke and the Extracranial Vessels.* Raven Press, New York, 1984.

Djindjian, R., and Merland, J.J.: *Super-Selective Arteriography of the External Carotid Artery.* Springer-Verlag, New York, 1978.

Grant, J.C.B.: *Grant's Atlas of Anatomy,* 6th ed. Williams & Wilkins, Baltimore, Maryland, 1972.

Gray, H., and Goss, C.M. (ed.): *Gray's Anatomy,* 29th American ed. Lea & Febiger, Philadelphia, Pennsylvania, 1975.

Hamilton, W.J., and Mossman, H.W.: *Human Embryology: Prenatal Development of Form and Function,* 4th ed. Williams & Wilkins, Baltimore, Maryland, 264–72, 1972.

Hershey, F.B., and Calman, C.H.: *Atlas of Vascular Surgery,* 3rd ed. Mosby, St. Louis, Missouri, 1973.

Hill, E.G., and McKinney, W.M.: Vascular anatomy and pathology of the head and neck: method of corrosion casting. In Carney, A.L., and Anderson, E.M. (eds.): *Advances in Neurology.* Vol. 30. *Diagnosis and Treatment of Brain Ischemia.* Raven Press, New York, 1981.

Langman, J.: *Medical Embryology,* 4th ed. Williams & Wilkins, Baltimore, Maryland, 184–202, 1981.

McHenry, L.C.: *Cerebral Circulation and Stroke.* Warren H. Green, Saint Louis, Missouri, 1978.

McVay, C.B.: *Surgical Anatomy,* 6th ed. W.B. Saunders, Philadelphia, Pennsylvania, 3–47, 248–91, 1984.

Palmer, F.J.: Origin of the right vertebral artery from the right common carotid artery: angiographic demonstration of three cases. *Br. J. Radiol.,* **50**:185–87, 1977.

Quattlebaum, J.L., Jr.; Wade, J.S.; and Wheddon, C.M.: Stroke associated with elongation and kinking of the carotid artery: long-term follow-up. *Ann. Surg.,* **1977**:572–79, 1973.

Ross-Russell, R.W. (ed.): *Cerebral Arterial Disease.* Churchill Livingstone, New York, 1976.

Schmidek, H.H., and Sweet, W.H. (eds.): *Operative Neurosurgical Techniques, Indications, and Results.* Grune & Stratton, New York, 671–828, 1982.

Toole, J.F.: *Cerebrovascular Disorders,* 3rd ed. Raven Press, New York, 1984.

Youmans, J.R. (ed.): *Neurological Surgery.* Vol. 3, 2nd ed. W.B. Saunders, Philadelphia, Pennsylvania, 1511–1626, 1982.

4

The Carotid Plaque

GUSTAV V.R. BORN

As long ago as 1905, carotid artery thrombosis was proposed as the only possible source of an embolus occluding the ipsilateral middle cerebral artery and causing contralateral hemiplegia. Some years later, it was recognized that carotid thromboembolism has a more general role in the causation of cerebrovascular disorders (Chiari, 1905; Hunt, 1914). Considerably later, it was again suggested that such thromboembolic processes could also account for transient monocular disturbances of vision associated with hemiparesis (Fisher, 1952). This postulate was soon supported by direct evidence (Fisher, 1959; Hollenhorst, 1961; Julian *et al.,* 1963; Gunning *et al.,* 1964; Millikan, 1965).

More recently, numerous clinical observations have contributed to the conclusion that embolization from atheromatous lesions at the carotid bifurcation is the most common cause of transient cerebral ischemia and one of the most frequent causes of stroke (Whisnant, 1976). This provided a satisfactory anatomic explanation for the frequency of contralateral hemiplegia, because the middle cerebral artery, which supplies the internal capsule, is the straightest continuation among the branches of the internal carotid and therefore the most susceptible to embolic obstruction.

To understand the basis for the surgical treatment of extracranial cardiovascular disease, it is necessary to consider the pathologic features of atheromatous plaques in the carotids, the pathogenesis of atherosclerosis both in general and in the particular setting of the carotid arteries, the complications of carotid plaques which give rise to their clinical manifestations, and the relations of the symptoms to the lesions that produce them.

PATHOLOGICAL FEATURES OF ATHEROMATOUS PLAQUES IN THE CAROTIDS

By far the most common site for atheromatous plaques in the extracranial circulation is the carotid bifurcation. This location is remarkably constant from case to case, being independent of racial and national origin as well as of sex and age (Solberg and Eggen, 1971). The first indication of the lesion is an intimal accumulation of lipids which raises the endothelial cover into a smooth bulge situated usually on the posterolateral wall of the carotid sinus. Subsequently, the lesion extends proximally into the common carotid and into the origins of the internal and external carotids as small patches which later become confluent. The confidence with which this almost invariable development can be described is due to recent, rigorously quantitative investigations (Grottum *et al.,* 1983) which are described later.

The fully developed fibro-fatty plaque covers the inside of the bifurcation, including part or all of the sinus. The length of the plaque varies from less than 1 cm to more than 3 cm. It is usually sharply defined distally but less so proximally, where it tends to merge into the diffusely thickened wall of the common carotid. A well-defined upper margin in the internal carotid permits comparatively clean surgical removal.

Underlying the plaque, the wall of the carotid bifurcation has different planes of cleavage along which dissection can be carried out. One such plane is between the intima and the media, the other between the media and the adventitia. The surgical availability of the cleavage planes depends on the extent to which the atheromatous process has affected the outer coats. Atheromatous infiltration and degeneration of the medial smooth muscle frequently require removal of most of the media (French and Rewcastle, 1974).

ATHEROGENESIS

The initial lesion of atherosclerosis manifests itself as patchy accumulations of fatty materials in the arterial wall; these are generally referred to as *fatty streaks.* Older lesions are described as *fibrous plaques,* which can become very hard and calcified. Whether there is a continuous progression from fatty streak to fibrous plaque is not yet completely certain.

Recent developments with computerized postmortem mapping of atherosclerotic lesions in human coronary and carotid arteries have shown close similarities in distribution of the earliest patches of accumulated lipids and fatty fibrous plaques (Fox *et al.,* 1982; Grottum *et al.,* 1983). This can be taken either as evidence for a pathogenetic association of the two types of lesions or as a proof of their independent development but with a common determinant such as blood flow.

Another possible precursor of the fibrous plaque is a gelatinous lesion containing smooth-muscle cells, fibroblasts, and collagen as well as high concentrations of plasma macromolecules, particularly low-density lipoproteins (LDLs) and fibrinogen (Smith and Smith, 1978). In the center of these lesions are extracellular accumulations of cholesterol esters, which, from their fatty-acid pattern, appear to be derived from LDLs. Thus, both varieties of early atherosclerotic lesions are characterized by the accumulation of lipids, mainly LDLs, from the circulating blood.

The accumulation of lipid is far from uniform; it affects some arteries, e.g., aorta, coronaries, and carotids, much more frequently and extensively than others, e.g., subclavian, brachial, and mesenteric vessels (Woolf, 1982). Lipid deposit in the involved arteries is not uniform but patchy, so that lipids tend to accumulate earliest and most frequently where arteries bend or branch, as, for example, at the bifurcation of the carotid.

At one time it was thought that atherosclerotic lesions consisted of fatty-acid "hyaline" products, such as collagen and elastin, resulting from the "degeneration" of normal constituents of arterial walls. There is evidence indeed for such degenerative processes in old human plaques, and epidemiological proof has established aging as a major risk factor in the clinical manifestations of atherosclerosis (Assmann and Schulte, 1982). Atherosclerosis, however, commonly begins in childhood or adolescence, long before any "degenerative" processes would be expected to start. There is no evidence of degenerative changes in the cells of affected arteries other than those associated with the accumulation of lipids from the plasma.

Attempts to explain the pathogenesis of atherosclerosis have led to three current hypotheses which merit consideration: i.e. that the atherogenic process is initiated by (1) thrombosis, (2) platelets, or (3) insudation of plasma lipids. These hypotheses and the evidence relating to them are considered later.

The Thrombogenic Hypothesis

The idea that atherogenesis is a consequence of intravascular thrombosis was already mentioned by von Rokitansky in 1852. This theory is based upon the observation of frequent association of thrombi with atheromatous plaques and on the demonstration that sections of advanced plaques often show layers reminiscent of the growth rings of trees, suggesting episodic deposition of thrombotic material (Duguid, 1946).

Despite the venerable history of the thrombogenic hypothesis, it is still uncertain to what extent, if at all, thrombosis contributes to atherosclerosis. Thrombi are, indeed, frequently found on advanced plaques, but usually as a complication of chronic ulceration or acute fissures (Davies and Thomas, 1981); thus, this cannot be taken as evidence that thrombi are part of the atheromatous process.

In relation to the thrombogenic hypothesis, it is essential to distinguish between venous and arterial thrombosis because of differences in pathogenesis. Venous thrombosis results from the clotting of blood in which soluble plasma fibrinogen is turned into insoluble fibrin. This reaction is greatly accelerated by platelets, which do not, however, contribute significantly to the thrombotic mass. Arterial thrombosis, in contrast, is initiated by the aggregation of platelets into cellular masses which may themselves become large enough to cause significant if not total obstruction of the blood flow.

Arterial as well as venous thrombosis depends on fibrinogen because it is an essential cofactor for platelet aggregation (Born and Cross, 1964; Cross, 1964). Both fibrinogen and fibrin have been unequivocally demonstrated in plaques by specific immunohistological techniques (Smith and Staples, 1982a,b). This, however, represents evidence not necessarily for the contribution of coagulation thrombosis to the formation of plaques, but more probably for the insudation of fibrinogen together with LDLs (see later) from the plasma into the arterial wall (Smith, 1983).

The proposition that atherogenesis depends on coagulation thrombosis is also incompatible with other evidence. Large veins are often afflicted by coagulation thrombosis, but atherosclerosis does not occur in them, not even in patients with advanced atherosclerosis of the arteries. Experimentally, the injection of emboli derived from blood clots into the pulmonary circulation gives rise to fibrous lesions that do not resemble those of atherosclerosis (Wartman *et al.,* 1951; Thomas *et al.,* 1956). Again, if plaque formation depended on coagulation thrombosis, it might be expected that patients with severe coagulation defects would have an exceptionally low incidence of clinical manifestations of atherosclerosis, such as myocardial infarction, and very little atherosclerosis demonstrable postmortem. This expectation is not supported by evidence, because the occurrence of atherosclerosis in patients with hemophilia A (Boivin, 1954), hemophilia B, or von Willebrand's disease (Silwer *et al.,* 1966) is similar to that of the general population.

The Platelet Hypothesis

The platelet hypothesis is a version of the thrombogenic theory which proposes that platelet aggregates rather than plasma clots persist as mural thrombi that later become organized into intimal thickenings (Mustard and Packham, 1975). This proposition is not supported by any directly relevant evidence, either experimental or pathological. The transformation of platelet aggregates into anything resembling atheromatous lesions has never been observed. Similarly, immunohistological examination of early plaques has failed to demonstrate the presence of intrinsic platelet antigens (Carstairs, 1965). Moreover, the lipids in early atheromatous lesions are so different from those of platelets as to make them a very unlikely source (Smith, 1970).

In recent years, other propositions for an essential role of platelets in atherogenesis have been presented. Platelets do not adhere to normal endothelium in arteries or any other vessels, but only where endothelium is damaged or absent, usually due to vascular injury. To associate platelets with atherogenesis, therefore, involves the assumption that the process begins with endothelial damage or injury (Ross and Harker, 1976). Atherogenesis is thus supposed to begin with some form of "injury" to the endothelium followed by the release of one or more platelet factors into the subendothelium that induce migration of medial smooth-muscle cells into the intima and their proliferation; the synthesis by the smooth-muscle cells of collagen, elastic fiber proteins, and proteoglycans; and the intra- and extracellular accumulation of lipid. "The concept of endothelial injury is central to current theories of atherogenesis" (Harker *et al.,* 1983). Most of the evidence collected in support of this hypothesis depends on experiments in which arterial endothelium is artificially damaged (Moore, 1981; Mustard *et al.,* 1984). Such endothelial damage has been brought about by various techniques, e.g., by introducing into the large artery of an experimental animal a catheter tipped with an inflatable balloon which removes the endothelium when withdrawn. "Too a considerable extent the response-to-injury hypothesis is based on the observation that removal of the endothelium by the balloon catheter technique leads to a characteristic intimal accumulation of smooth muscles" (Harker *et al.,* 1983). There is no clinical or pathological evidence to suggest that anything remotely similar to such gross endothelial damage occurs in man, except in the rare condition of homocystinemia, in which evidence of defective vascular endothelium is associated with the clinical manifestations of premature atherosclerosis (Harker *et al.,* 1974).

The Insudative Hypothesis

The proposition that the lipids in atherosclerotic lesions come from the blood plasma by "insudation" into the walls of susceptible arteries is also of respectable age (Virchow, 1862). The first experimental evidence for it (Anitschkow, 1933) was that the addition of one particular lipid, cholesterol, to the diet of experimental animals produced hypercholesterolemia and arterial lesions which resembled those occurring in humans. Because cholesterol and its esters are major components of plaques, they became a center of experimental and clinical attention during a long period in which the mechanism was elucidated by which insoluble lipids like cholesterol are rendered soluble in association with specific plasma proteins (Assmann, 1982).

If Virchow's proposition is restated in terms not of the influx of free lipids but of lipoproteins and fibrinogen into the arterial wall, the bulk of modern evidence indeed supports the insudative hypothesis. It has been established that the predominant lipids in developing atheromatous lesions are plasma LDLs and that the other major component is fibrinogen. Conclusive evidence of this was obtained using immunological techniques in which postmortem material from normal and atheromatous arteries with plaques at all stages of development was examined histologically by immunofluorescence with specific antiserums against plasma proteins and platelet antigens. In all plaques there was immunofluorescence, specific for LDLs. Their distribution corresponded closely with that of extracellular sudanophilic lipid dispersed diffusely in the ground substance of fatty streaks and with sudanophilic droplets along collagen and elastic fibers in later lesions. Many plaques were also fluorescent for fibrinogen. No lesion gave evidence of the presence of other plasma proteins, i.e., high-density lipoproteins, gammaglobulins, or albumin, or of platelet-specific antigens. Another technique elutes soluble proteins from sectioned lesions for subsequent immunological identification and quantification (Smith and Staples, 1980).

Much research on atherosclerosis is concerned with the questions of how these macromolecular components of the plasma accumulate in arterial walls, why some arteries are more susceptible to this than others, why in susceptible vessels the accumulation is patchy rather than uniform, and how this process is connected with the subsequent cellular and other changes characteristic of established plaques (Assman, 1982).

"The Endothelial Barrier"

Only recently has convincing evidence appeared on how LDLs move from blood into arterial walls through the continuous layer of endothelial cells covering the luminal surface. It has been widely assumed that the endothelial layer constitutes a barrier preventing these lipoproteins from penetrating into vessel walls. Evidence *against* such a barrier function (Smith and Slater, 1972; Smith and Staples, 1982a,b) is that the concentration of macromolecules in the arterial intima is directly related to their concentrations in the plasma and to their molecular weights, and particularly that the concentration of LDLs is higher in the normal intima than in the plasma and still higher in the early fibrous lesions of atherosclerosis. There is no evidence for a complex of a component of the intima with LDLs which might account for their high concentrations there (Smith and Staples, 1982b).

Until recently, evidence for a barrier function of endothelium was only inferred from the difficulty of conceiving how very large plasma proteins such as LDLs, with a mean molecular weight of about 2.5 times 10^6 daltons, can pass through what in a normal artery is an unbroken layer of viable cells apparently tightly joined (Florey, 1970).

For this reason, the "endothelial injury" hypothesis has been advanced to account also for the ability of plasma lipoproteins to pass from blood into arterial walls (Moore, 1981). Because various experimental injuries to endothelium may be followed by lipid infiltration, this hypothesis is at present much in favor. However, as already explained, such experiments produce artificial conditions of a kind very unlikely to be relevant to the pathogenesis of the actual human disease. Indeed, arterial walls denuded of endothelium contained fewer LDLs than did neighboring areas where the endothelium had regenerated (Falcone *et al.*, 1984). Furthermore, diet-induced hypercholesterolemia can bring about typical arterial lesions without loss of endothelium at any time up to at least one year (Joris *et al.*, 1983). In such experiments, the only consistent abnormality was an increase in the number of large mononuclear cells adhering to the intact endothelium, mainly at the openings of branches. These mononuclear cells emigrated and became lipid-laden "foam cells," characteristic of atheromatous lesions. "How the lipid reaches the macroplaques across an intact endothelium is not clear, possibly by transcytosis" (Joris *et al.*, 1983).

Indeed, there is now increasing evidence that atherogenic plasma proteins penetrate arterial walls by transcytosis through intact, normal endothelium. In experiments performed on rabbits, a continuous transfer of LDLs from blood into aortic walls with normal endothelium was observed (Stender and Zilversmith, 1980). Conversely, after loading aortas of rabbits with labeled plasma proteins, their clearance into the blood was found proportional to the logarithm of molecular size (Stender and Zilversmith, 1980). These observations are compatible with the movement of plasma proteins across endothelium by a diffusion-limited process which could take place either through interendothelial junctions or by transcellular transport (Stein and Stein, 1973).

Recent experiments with rat arteries in situ have demonstrated that LDLs traverse intact endothelial cells by two routes (Vasile *et al.*, 1983). One route utilizes a receptor-mediated mechanism involving coated pits on the cell surface. Binding to coated pits is part of the mechanism whereby LDLs are taken up into different types of cells, including endothelium, smooth-muscle, and fibroblast, on their way to metabolic breakdown and the control of cellular cholesterol concentrations (Goldstein and Brown, 1976). The other route is by a receptor-independent process in which LDL particles enter the vesicles or caveola characteristic of endothelium. The latter route, whereby LDLs are transported across the endothelial cells and delivered to the subendothelial tissues, accounts for over 90 percent of the total LDL uptake. Thus, it appears indeed that arterial endothelium interacts with circulating LDLs by their specific binding to high-affinity receptors which ensures the endothelial cells' own requirement for cholesterol, and also through another route in which low-affinity nonsaturable uptake by transcytotic vesicles makes cholesterol available to other cells of the arterial walls. It is the latter process which these observations suggest to be responsible for the atherogenic accumulation of plasma proteins.

The rates of uptake of LDLs by both mechanisms must depend on the concentration of LDLs in the plasma and on the efficiency of binding to the endothelial receptors. Regarding the former, this up-to-date version of the insudation hypothesis satisfactorily accounts for the well-established association of various hyperlipidemias with premature clinical manifestations of advanced atherosclerosis such as myocardial infarction (Assmann, 1982). Regarding the latter, there is evidence that binding efficiency of atherogenic proteins to endothelium depends on specific surface components. Thus, the uptake of LDLs is accelerated greatly and that of fibrinogen moderately after removal of sialic acids from the endothelium in living arteries (Görög and Born, 1982). This acceleration is not shared by plasma albumin, which, unlike LDLs and fibrinogen, is not a sialic protein. These observations suggest that the accumulation of atherogenic plasma proteins in arterial walls is limited, at least to some extent, by repulsive electrostatic interactions. This raises the pathological possibility that minor deficiencies of sialic acids on endothelium and/or on LDLs or fibrinogen could be associated with accelerated atherogenesis and the therapeutic possibility that a procedure capable of increasing acidic residues on arterial endothelium might diminish atherosclerosis.

LOCALIZATION OF ATHEROSCLEROTIC LESIONS

Beside the atherogenic process itself, the most important fact to be accounted for is the characteristic distribution of atherosclerotic plaques. These lesions, from the earliest to the fully developed, are most prevalent where large arteries bend or branch, for example, at the carotid bifurcation. This was first recognized at the beginning of this century (Chiari, 1905), but conclusive evidence had to await methods for measuring atheromatous lesions in major arteries such as the carotids (Samuel, 1956; Schwartz and Mitchell, 1961). For this purpose, arteries were opened longitudinally and stained with Sudan III or IV with measurements of stained areas on standardized segments (Svindland, 1984). This technique demonstrated the axial distribution of lesions at the carotid bifurcation (Solberg and Eggen, 1971). Only in the 1970s were techniques developed for complete mapping of the spatial distribution of lesions around bifurcations and branch orifices, first by reproducing the lesions on a coordinate grid (Cornhill and Roach, 1974) and most recently by computerized contour mapping of appropriately stained lesions (Kjaernes *et al.,* 1981). The results have confirmed that atherosclerotic lesions are concentrated in arterial curvatures and at branches and bifurcations.

A general explanation for this distribution assumes its dependence on changes in blood flow produced by curves and branchings. Hemodynamic effects could promote localized lesions by accelerating the influx or decelerating the efflux of atherogenic plasma proteins or by increasing retention by the arterial wall.

Blood flow in arteries occurs under high pressure; it is rapid, pulsatile, and asymmetric in velocity distributions as well as complicated in secondary motions and flow separations. Thus, the hemodynamic factors concerned are *pressure, wall shear stress,* and *flow separation,* with the formation of vortices, commonly known as *turbulent flow.*

That *pressure* is involved is implied by the restriction of atherosclerosis to the larger elastic and muscular arteries of the systemic circulation in which blood pressure is highest. The conclusion that blood pressure is a determinant of the disease is supported by the high incidence of clinical manifestations of the disease in patients with hypertension, an established "risk factor" (Assmann, 1982); by the association of pulmonary artery atherosclerosis with pulmonary hypertension (Moore *et al.,* 1982); and by the atherosclerotic thickening of veins subjected to arterial pressure in coronary bypass. The mechanism, however, whereby high blood pressure promotes atherosclerosis is still unknown.

Whether and to what extent atherosclerosis depends on the *shear stress* exerted on arterial walls by the flowing blood was until recently subject to controversy. This superficially plausible hypothesis maintains that the site of these lesions corresponds to localized flow regions of high shear stress (Fry, 1972, 1976), the proposed connecting link being "endothelial injury" (Moore, 1981; Mustard and Packham, 1975). These notions have been disproved by quantitative analysis of the distribution of atherosclerotic lesions in coronary, carotid, and other susceptible arteries (Fox and Seed, 1981; Svindland, 1984) which failed to establish association of atherosclerosis with high wall shear stress. At arterial bifurcations, the inner walls are exposed to high shear stress and the outer walls to low shear stress (Batten and Nerem, 1982). It is along the outer walls that the lesions begin and advance. Wall shear stress is low along the distal parts of the inner wall of arterial curvatures, which are again most affected by atherosclerosis. Therefore, the localization of atherosclerotic lesions is associated not with high but with low shear stress. The reason for this is unknown. One possible explanation (Caro, 1971) assumes a continuous diffusion of atherogenic lipid from the vessel wall into the bloodstream with a quantitative dependence of this transport on wall shear, so that low shear flow would favor retention of atherogenic lipids.

Flow separation describes the divergence of streamlines associated with changes in vessel geometry, commonly with the establishment of vortices. Flow separation occurs along the inner curvature of bends and along the outer walls of bifurcations. Although the latter predominates in the localization of atherosclerotic changes, it is by no means established that this association depends upon flow separation and the effects that accompany it. The blood flow is grossly and continuously turbulent in the ventricular chambers of the heart in which it is also under high pressure, without either "injury" to the endocardium or its general thickening through atherosclerotic deposits.

Correlation of Lesions with Hemodynamics in the Carotids

Rigorous correlations between the dynamics of blood flow through the carotid arteries and the distribution of early atherosclerotic lesions in them have been demonstrated in autopsies of young persons who died from noncardiovascular causes (Grottum *et al.,* 1983). Outlines of sudanophilic lesions in the arterial walls were computerized, scaled to a standardized size and shape, and added together; this provided contour lines connecting points occurring with equal frequency. The results (see Figures 4–1 and 4–2) revealed a definite pattern: the lesions begin on the outer walls of the bifurcation, while both the lateral and inner walls downstream from the flow divider remain free of lesions. Experiments with flow through casts of the carotid arteries have shown that flow velocities and shear stress are low along the outer walls of the bifurcation, whereas the shear stress is much higher along the flow divider (Zarins *et al.,* 1983), and confirm for the carotids the postulate of a relation between le-

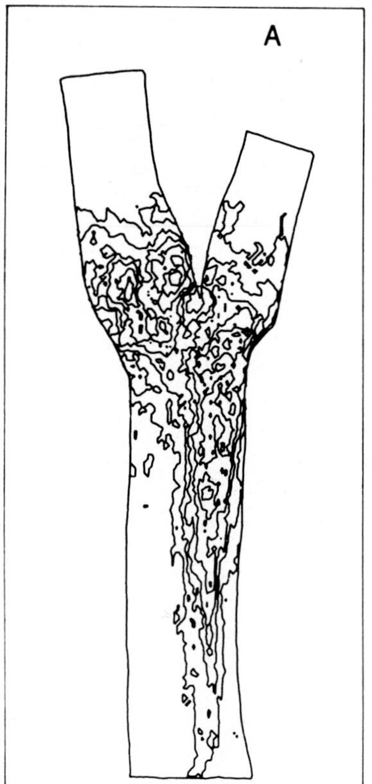

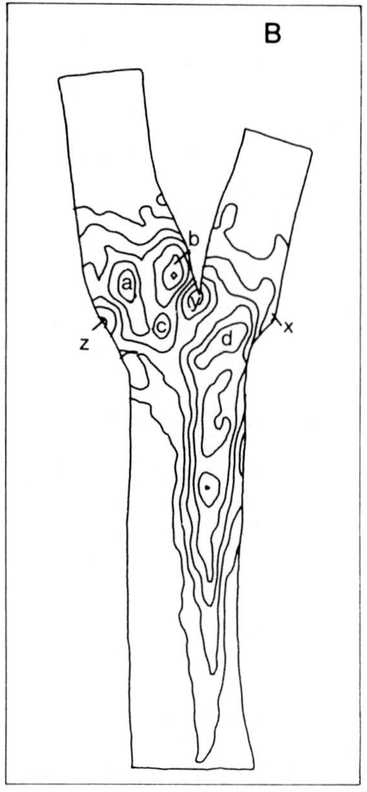

Figure 4-1. Frequency distribution of lesions in 37 carotid bifurcations. The results are displayed as contour lines connecting points with equal frequency of lesions. *(A)* The vertical distance between the contour lines is 10 percent of the theoretical maximum value: 37/10 = 3.7 arteries. *(B)* Frequency distribution of lesions as in *A*, after smoothing the distribution by replacing each number in the grid with a weighted average of the values within a small surrounding area. (From Grottum, P.; Svindland, A.; and Walle, L.: Localization of early atherosclerotic lesions in the right carotid bifurcation in humans. *Acta Pathol. Microbiol. Immunol. Scand.* (A), **91**:65–70, 1983, with permission.)

sions and blood-flow properties. This concept is further supported by the observation in the carotid sinus. In the proximal part of the internal carotid, the flow velocity is low and even reversed, with low shear stress at the wall; it is there that atheromatous lesions almost always appear first and advance the furthest. The carotid sinus is also subject to a blood-pressure peak, consistent with the atherogenic effect of high pressure.

The intimal coat of the carotids is thickest where the wall shear stress is low. On the assumption that intimal thickening represents atherosclerotic changes, this too indicates that the disease develops primarily in regions of comparatively low shear stress.

The proximal part of the common carotid usually remains unaffected by atherosclerosis except for the appearance of small plaques around its origin from the aorta and for an atheromatous ridge continuous with and extending proximally from the plaque in the bifurcation (Javid, 1979). Local vortices may be responsible for the plaques at the carotid origin, but the presence of the ridge is not readily accounted for by hemodynamic effects.

As remarkable as the constancy of plaque at the carotid bifurcation is the relative rarity of atheromatous lesions in the internal carotid artery beyond the bifurcation as far as the base of the skull. This segment of the artery is almost straight and without branches, so that the flow in it is comparatively smooth and laminar; the absence of atherosclerosis is, therefore, also consistent with the absence of turbulent flow.

In both internal and external carotids the flow of blood, although without gross disturbances, is helical with two counterrotating parallel vortices. This is of interest because of evidence for the helical disposition of lipid lesions in coronary arteries (Fox and Seed, 1981).

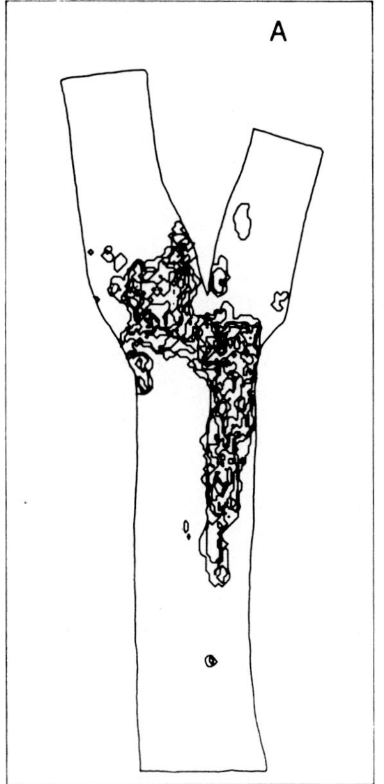

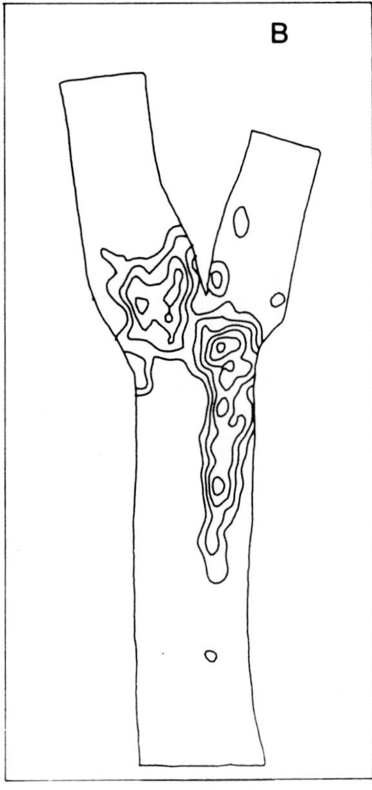

Figure 4–2. *(A)* Frequency distribution for the 12 least affected bifurcations as in Figure 4–1, but with vertical distance. 12/10 = 1.2 arteries. *(B)* Similar to *A*, but smoothed. (From Grottum, P.; Svindland, A.; and Walle, L.: Localization of early atherosclerotic lesions in the right carotid bifurcation in humans. *Acta Pathol. Microbiol. Immunol. Scand.* (A), **91**:65–70, 1983, with permission.)

This, however, has not yet been demonstrated in the carotid arteries.

COMPLICATIONS OF CAROTID PLAQUES

Asymptomatic carotid plaques can be present for many years. The appearance of symptoms is almost invariably associated with secondary changes which therefore assume predominant clinical importance. These secondary changes include (1) degeneration of the underlying arterial wall, (2) calcification, (3) ulceration, and (4) intraplaque hemorrhage.

Wall Degeneration

At the carotid bifurcation, the medial layer of smooth muscle is comparatively thick, and it usually contains several elastic laminae. Beneath atheromatous plaques, the smooth muscle tends to necrotize, and the elastic layers degenerate and disappear. These changes diminish the contractile and elastic resilience of the walls to blood pressure so that the plaque may come to lie in an aneurysmal dilatation. The cause of the medial degeneration is uncertain but presumably due to one or both of two effects: deposition of atheromatous lipids between and within smooth-muscle cells and impedance by the overlying plaque to the diffusion of nutrients and oxygen from the carotid blood.

Calcification

Plaques in the carotid bifurcation, as elsewhere, are subject to increasing calcification. How the accumulation of calcium depends on other components of plaque, particularly phospholipids, is still uncertain. Recent evidence indicates the presence of calcium-binding proteins in which high-affinity sites for calcium are vitamin K-dependent gamma-carboxy glutamate residues, like those of the calcium-binding proteins in the coagulation cascade (Keeley and Sitarz, 1983; P.M. Esnouf, personal communication). Calcification contributes to the diminished elasticity of the carotid wall and thereby to its susceptibility to aneurysmal dilatation.

Calcified plaques are hard and brittle; therefore, as a further complication, they tend to crack with the appearance of fissures or fractures. The exact mechanism responsible for this is unknown. Additional forces may be exerted on plaques by whatever smooth muscles remain viable around and beneath them.

Fissures or fractures are of great clinical significance because they are associated with hemorrhage into the plaque, which, together with the disruption of the surface, is the cause of mural thrombosis and embolization.

Ulceration

The relative thickness of the intimal deposit of lipids and the overlying fibrous cap varies greatly from one plaque to another. Thin fibrous caps tend to break apart at one or more sites. The resulting ulcers, on one hand, provide access of blood into the core of the plaque, which becomes distended by hemorrhage. On the other hand, plaque lipids may be forced out through the ulcer and embolize into the cerebral circulation. With the occurrence of hemorrhage and the exposure of collagen and microfibrils by ulceration, the conditions are established for the formation of mural thrombi of platelets (Born, 1978); it is the distal embolization of these thrombi that is responsible for most transient ischemic attacks and strokes (see Figures 16–1 and 16–2). Thus, in a series of 50 carotid endarterectomies small ulcers were present on 16 and large ulcers on 22 of the lesions, so that overall three out of four plaques were ulcerated (Blaisdell *et al.,* 1974).

Hemorrhage

Careful correlations of clinical with pathological evidence have established hemorrhage as the most frequent and most significant complication affecting plaques in the carotid bifurcation (Imparato *et al.,* 1979; Lusby *et al.,* 1982; Persson *et al.,* 1983). These correlations became known through the general introduction of carotid arteriography and through the study of atheromatous lesions removed surgically from the carotids. A significant association between fresh plaque hemorrhage and the onset of symptoms of cerebral ischemia has been demonstrated (Lusby *et al.,* 1983). It has already been emphasized that fissures or breaks in the surface of plaque are necessarily associated with hemorrhagic extravasation of blood into the plaque core. There is additional evidence that intraplaque hemorrhage may also result from the rupture of small vasa vasorum, many of which are demonstrable on histological sections through plaques (Fleming *et al.,* 1984).

In a typical series of patients undergoing carotid endarterectomy, recent intraplaque hemorrhage had occurred in 49 of 53 patients who also had symptoms of cerebral ischemia. By contrast, only seven of 26 asymptomatic patients (Lusby *et al.,* 1983) had intraplaque bleeding. Of the 53 patients with symptoms, many of whom had several attacks of cerebral ischemia, 43 (81 percent) had evidence of multiple hemorrhages. In 46 (86 percent), the lesions had reduced the carotid diameter by more than half. These multiple hemorrhages had occurred over long periods of time.

Thus, hemorrhage into plaques can be responsible for cerebral ischemic disease in three ways: (1) distention of plaque or with mural thrombosis causing local impedance to blood flow, (2) mural thrombosis with embolization, or (3) disruption and embolizing extrusion of lipid material from the plaque.

RELATION OF SYMPTOMS TO LESIONS

From the foregoing, it is evident that clinical manifestions of cerebral vascular insufficiency are consequences of carotid atheromata and their common complications. There is no regular, predictable association between the size, shape, or degree of stenosis of the primary lesion at the carotid bifurcation and the incidence of neurological symptoms. It has been known for many years that carotid stenosis may remain asymptomatic (Schwartz and Mitchell, 1961); only after the cross-sectional area of the carotid is reduced to less than 10 percent does blood flow decrease significantly (Spencer and Reid, 1979). Therefore, the relation between the properties of the lesion demonstrable angiographically in individual patients and their cerebrovascular symptoms is by no means straightforward.

Finally, it is of some interest that atherosclerosis of the carotid bifurcation may also be involved in an entirely different symptom complex, i.e., that produced by hypertension

(Angell-James, 1974). This possibility arises out of experiments in which atherosclerosis was induced in rabbits by the addition of cholesterol and sunflower-seed oil to the diet. After more than a year, the rabbits' mean blood pressure increased from 85 to 114 mm Hg. This was accompanied by highly significant decrease in sensitivity of the aortic baroreceptors and in the distensibility of the baroreceptor region, which was thickened by atheromatous deposits. In man, baroreceptors are situated in the carotid sinus; it is possible, therefore, that atherosclerosis affecting the sinus contributes to the blood-pressure abnormalities common in atherosclerotic patients. Such a mechanism could indeed contribute to the explanation of the role of hypertension in the disease.

REFERENCES

Angell-James, E.: Arterial baroreceptor activity in rabbits with experimental atherosclerosis. *Circ. Res.*, **34**:27–39, 1974.

Anitschkow, N.: Experimental arteriosclerosis in animals. In Cowdry, E.V. (ed.): *Arteriosclerosis.* Macmillan, New York, 1933.

Assmann, G.: *Lipid Metabolism and Atherosclerosis.* Schattauer, New York, 1982.

Assman, G., and Schulte, H.: Prediction and early detection of coronary heart disease. In Hauss, W.H. (ed.): *Second Münster International Symposium.* Westdeutscher Verlag, Opladen, 1982.

Batten, J.R., and Nerem, R.M.: Model study of flow in curved and planar arterial bifurcations. *Cardiovasc. Res.*, **16**:178–86, 1982.

Blaisdell, F.W.; Glickman, M.; and Trunkey, D.D.: Ulcerated atheroma of the carotid artery. *Arch. Surg.*, **108**:491–96, 1974.

Boivin, J.M.: Infarctus du myocarde chez un hemophile. *Arch. Mal Coeur.*, **47**:351–54, 1954.

Born, G.V.R.: Arterial thrombosis and its prevention. In Hayase, S., and Murao, S.J. (eds.): *Proceedings of the Eighth World Congress of Cardiology.* Excerpta Medica, Amsterdam, 1978.

Born, G.V.R., and Cross, M.J.: Effects of inorganic ions and of plasma proteins on the aggregation of blood platelets by adenosine diphosphate. *J. Physiol. (Lond.)*, **170**:397–414, 1964.

Caro, C.G.; Fitz-Gerald, J.M.; and Schroter, R.C.: Atheroma and arterial wall shear: observation, correlation and proposal of a shear dependent mass transfer mechanism of atherogenesis. *Proc. R. Soc. Lond. (Biol.)*, **177**:109–59, 1971.

Carstairs, K.C.: The identification of platelets and platelet antigen in histological sections. *J. Pathol. Bacteriol.*, **90**:225–31, 1965.

Chiari, H.: Über das Verhalten des Teilungswinkels der Carotis Communis bei der Endarteritis Chronica Deformans. *Verh. Dtsch. Ges. Pathol.*, **9**:326, 1905.

Cross, M.J.: Effect of fibrinogen in the aggregation of platelets by adenosine diphosphate. *Thromb. Diath. Hemorrh.*, **12**:524–27, 1964.

Cornhill, J.F., and Roach, M.R.: Quantitative method for the evaluation of atherosclerotic lesions. *Atherosclerosis*, **20**:131–36, 1974.

Davies, M.J., and Thomas, T.: The pathological basis and microanatomy of occlusive thrombus formation in human coronary arteries. *Phil. Trans. Soc. Lond.*, **294**:225–29, 1981.

Duguid, J.B.: Thrombosis as a factor in the pathogenesis of coronary atherosclerosis. *J. Pathol. Bacteriol.*, **58**:207–12, 1946.

Falcone, D.J.; Hajjar, D.P.; and Minick, C.R.: Lipoprotein and albumin in de-endothelialized and re-endothelialized aorta. *Am. J. Pathol.*, **114**:112–20, 1984.

Fisher, C.M.: Transient monocular blindness associated with hemiplegia. *Arch. Ophthalmol.*, **47**:167, 1952.

Fisher, C.M.: Observations of the fundus oculi in transient monocular blindness. *Neurology*, **9**:333–47, 1959.

Fleming, J.F.R.; Deck, J.H.N.; and Gotlieb, A.I.: Pathology of atherosclerotic plaques. In Smith, R.R. (ed.): *Stroke and the Extracranial Vessels.* Raven Press, New York, 1984.

Florey, H.W.: *General Pathology*, 4th ed. Lloyd-Luke, London, 1970.

Fox, B.J., and Seed, W.A.: Location of early atheroma in the human coronary arteries. *J. Biomech. Eng.*, **103**:208–12, 1981.

Fox, B.J.; Morgan B.; and Seed, W.A.: Distribution of fatty and fibrous plaques in young human coronary arteries. *Atherosclerosis*, **41**:337–47, 1982.

French, B.B., and Rewcastle, N.B.: Sequential morphological changes at the site of carotid endarterectomy. *J. Neurosurg.*, **41**:745–54, 1974.

Fry, D.L.: Localizing factors in arteriosclerosis and localizing factors in experimental atherosclerosis. In Likoff, W.; Segal, B.L.; Insull, W.; and Moyer, J.A. (eds.): *Atherosclerosis and Coronary Heart Disease.* Grune & Stratton, New York, 1972.

Fry, D.L.: Haemodynamic forces in atherogenesis. In Scheinberg, P. (ed.): *Cerebrovascular Diseases.* Raven Press, New York, 1976, pp. 77–95.

Goldstein, J.L., and Brown M.S.: Atherosclerosis: the low-density lipoprotein receptor hypothesis. *Metabolism*, **26**:1257–75, 1976.

Görög, P., and Born, G.V.R.: Increased uptake of circulating low-density lipoproteins and fibrinogen by arterial walls after removal of sialic acids from their endothelial surface. *Br. J. Exp. Pathol.*, **63**:447–51, 1982.

Grottum, P.; Svindland, A.; and Walle, L.: Localization of early atherosclerotic lesions in the right carotid bifurcation in humans. *Acta Pathol. Microbiol. Immunol. Scand. (A)*, **91**:65–70, 1983.

Gunning, A.J.; Pickering, G.W.; Robb-Smith, A.H.T.; and Russell, R.R.: Mural thrombosis of the internal carotid artery and subsequent embolization. *Q. J. Med.*, **33**:155–95, 1964.

Harker, L.A.; Slichter, S.J.; Scott, C.R.; and Ross, R.: Homocystinaemia vascular injury and arterial thrombosis. *N. Engl. J. Med.*, **291**:537–43, 1974.

Harker, L.A.; Schwartz, S.M.; and Ross, R.: Endothelial injury and repair. In Hauss, W.H. (ed.): *Second Münster International Arteriosclerosis Symposium.* Westdeutscher Verlag, Opladen, 1983.

Hollenhorst, R.W.: Significance of bright plaques in the retinal arterioles. *J.A.M.A.*, **178**:23–29, 1961.

Hunt, J.R.: The role of carotid arteries in the causation of vascular lesions of the brain, with remarks on certain features of symptomology. *Am. J. Med. Sci.*, **147**:704, 1914.

Imparato, A.M.; Riles, T.S.; and Gorstein, F.: The carotid bifurcation plaque: pathologic findings associated with cerebral ischemia. *Stroke,* **10**:238–45, 1979.

Javid, H.: Development of carotid plaque. *Am. J. Surg.,* **138**:224–27, 1979.

Joris, I.; Zand, T.; Nunnari, J.J.; Krolikowsky, F.J.; and Majno, G.: Studies on the pathogenesis of atherosclerosis 1. Adhesions and emigration of mononuclear cells in the aorta of hypercholesterolaemic rats. *Am. J. Pathol.,* **113**:341–58, 1983.

Julian, O.C.; Dye, W.S.; Javid, H.; and Hunter, J.A.: Ulcerative lesions of the carotid artery bifurcation. *Arch. Surg.,* **86**:803–09, 1963.

Keeley, F.W., and Sitarz, E.E.: Characterization of proteins from the calcified matrix of atherosclerotic human aorta. *Atherosclerosis,* **46**:29–40, 1983.

Kjaernes, M.; Svindland, A.; Walle, L.; and Wille, S.: Localization of early atherosclerotic lesions in an arterial bifurcation in humans. *Acta Pathol. Microbiol. Immunol. Scand.* (A), **89**:35–40, 1981.

Lusby, R.J.; Ferrell, L.D.; and Wylie, E.J.: The significance of intraplaque hemorrhage in the pathogenesis of carotid atherosclerosis. In Bergan, J.J., and Yao, J.S.T. (eds.): *Cerebrovascular Insufficiency.* Grune & Stratton, New York, 1983.

Lusby, R.J.; Ferrell, L.D.; Ehrenfeld, W.K.; Stoney, R.J.; and Wylie, E.J.: Carotid plaque hemorrhage: its role in production of cerebral ischemia. *Arch. Surg.,* **117**:1479–88, 1982.

Millikan, C.H.: The pathogenesis of transient focal cerebral ischemia. *Circulation,* **32**:438–50, 1965.

Moore, G.W.; Smith, R.L.R.; and Hutchins, G.M.: Pulmonary artery atherosclerosis. *Arch. Pathol. Lab. Med.,* **106**:378–80, 1982.

Moore, S.: Injury mechanisms in atherogenesis. In Moore, S. (ed.): *Vascular Injury and Atherosclerosis.* Marcel Dekker, New York, 1981.

Mustard, J.F.; Kinlough-Rathbone, R.L.; and Packham, M.A.: Platelet aggregation, vascular wall and ischemic heart disease. In Donato, L., and L'Abbale, A. (eds.): *Frontiers in Cardiology for the Eighties.* Academic Press, London, 1984.

Mustard, J.F., and Packham, M.A.: The role of blood and platelets in atherosclerosis and the complications of atherosclerosis. *Thromb. Diath. Haemorrh.,* **33**:444–56, 1975.

Persson, A.V.; Robichaux, W.T.; and Silverman, M.: The natural history of carotid plaque development. *Arch. Surg.,* **118**:1048–52, 1983.

Ross, R., and Harker, L.: Hyperlipidaemia and atherosclerosis: chronic hyperlipidaemia initiates and maintains lesions by endothelial cell desquamation and lipid accumulation. *Science,* **193**:1094–1100, 1976.

Samuel, K.C.: Atherosclerosis and occlusion of the internal carotid artery. *J. Pathol. Bacteriol.,* 381–401, 1956.

Schwartz, C.J., and Mitchell, J.R.A.: Atheroma of the carotid and vertebral arterial systems. *Br. Med. J.,* **2**:1057–63, 1961.

Silwer, J.; Cronberg, S.; and Nilsson, I.M.: Occurrence of arteriosclerosis in von Willebrand's disease. *Acta Med. Scand.,* **180**:475–84, 1966.

Smith, E.B.: Discussion. In Jones, R.J. (ed.): *Atherosclerosis: Proceedings of the Second International Symposium.* Springer-Verlag, Berlin, 1970.

Smith, E.B.: Endothelium and lipoprotein permeability. In Woolf, N. (ed.): *Biology and Pathology of the Vessel Wall.* Praeger, New York, 1983.

Smith, E.B., and Slater, R.H.: Relationship between low density lipoprotein in aortic intima and serum lipid levels. *Lancet,* **1**:463–69, 1972.

Smith, E.B., and Smith, R.H.: Early change in aortic intima. *Atheroscler. Rev.,* **1**:119–36, 1978.

Smith, E.B., and Staples, E.M.: Distribution of plasma proteins across the human aortic wall: barrier functions of endothelium and internal elastic lamina. *Atherosclerosis,* **37**:579–90, 1980.

Smith, E.B., and Staples, E.M.: Intimal and medial plasma protein concentrations and endothelial function. *Atherosclerosis,* **41**:295–308, 1982a.

Smith, E.B., and Staples, E.M.: Plasma protein concentrations in interstitial fluid from human aortas. *Proc. R. Soc. Lond. (Biol.),* **217**:59–75, 1982b.

Solberg, L.A., and Eggen, D.A.: Localization and sequence of development of atherosclerotic lesions in the carotid and vertebral arteries. *Circulation,* **43**:711–24, 1971.

Spencer, M.W., and Reid, J.M.: Quantitation of carotid stenosis with continuous wave (c-w) Doppler ultrasound. *Stroke,* **10**:326–30, 1979.

Stein, Y., and Stein, O.: Lipid synthesis and degradation and lipoprotein transport in mammalian aorta. In Porters, R., and Knight, J. (eds.): *Atherogenesis: Initiating Factors.* Ciba Foundation Symposium 12. Associated Scientific Publishers, Amsterdam, 1973.

Stender, S., and Zilversmith, D.B.: Mathematical models for the simultaneous measurement of arterial influx of esterified and free cholesterol from two lipoprotein fractions and *in vivo* hydrolysis of arterial cholesteryl ester. *Atherosclerosis,* **1**:38–49, 1980.

Svindland, A.: *Localization of Atherosclerotic Lesions in Human Arterial Bifurcations.* University Press, Oslo, 1984.

Thomas, W.A.; O'Neal, R.M.; and Lee, K.T.: Thromboembolism, pulmonary arteriosclerosis and fatty meals. *Arch. Pathol.,* **61**:380–89, 1956.

Vasile, E.; Simionescu, M.; and Simionescu, N.: Visualization of the binding, endocytosis, and transcytosis of low-density lipoprotein in the arterial endothelium *in situ. J. Cell. Biol.,* **96**:1677–89, 1983.

Virchow, R. von: Phlogose und Thrombose im Gefässystem. *Gesammelte Abhandlungen zur wissenschaftlichen Medizin.* Max Hirsch, Berlin, 1862.

von Rokitansky, C.: *A Manual of Pathological Anatomy.* Vol. 4 (trans. G.E. Day). Sydenham Society, London, 1852.

Wartman, W.; Jennings, R.B.; and Hudson, B.: Experimental arterial disease: the reaction of the pulmonary artery to minute emboli of blood clot. *Circulation,* **4**:747–55, 1951.

Whisnant, J.P.: A population study of stroke and TIA: Rochester, Minnesota. In Gillingham, F.J., and Williams, A.E. (eds.): *Stroke.* Churchill Livingstone, New York, 1976.

Woolf, N.: *The Pathology of Atherosclerosis,* Butterworth, London, 1982.

Zarins, C.K.; Giddens, D.D.; Bharadavaj, A.K.; Sottiurae, V.S.; Mabon, R.F.; and Glagov, S.: Carotid bifurcation atherosclerosis: quantitative correlation of plaque localization with flow velocity profiles and wall shear stress. *Circ. Res.,* **53**:502–14, 1983.

UNIT II

Diagnostic Considerations

5

Blood Flow to the Brain: The Direction of Change

ANDREW L. CARNEY and EVELYN M. ANDERSON

BASIC CONCEPTS OF CEREBRAL FLOW

Advancing technology has brought dramatic change to neurovascular surgery. Diagnostic methods now reveal detailed information never before available. Surgical techniques make procedures unheard of a decade ago readily applicable. The most dramatic changes, however, are conceptual; our ideas are changing. The clinical designations *stroke* and *transient ischemic attack* will probably be generally replaced by the more precise terms *infarction* and *regional ischemia* with specifications of location and qualification. Attention is being directed not only to the precise gross and microscopic pathology of the carotid bifurcation, but also to the circulation of the brain as a whole. This new terminology reflects a new precision in information. In many respects, these changes are reminiscent of those that occurred in cardiology and cardiac surgery more than a decade ago. *"Myocardial infarction"* has replaced *"heart attack"* just as *"brain infarction"* is now replacing *"stroke."*

The ischemic insult produces a three-dimensional lesion. The precise location, the structural composition, and the surrounding zones of ischemia constitute a spatial moeity that can be projected into the gross architecture of the brain. The position of such lesions often indicates the pathological mechanism, the clinical hazard, and the arterial branches involved. Angiography is necessary to identify precisely the blood supply to these branches. This is especially true of the posterior circulation, where the vascular tree is highly variable.

The spatial resolution attainable with the new generation of instruments, e.g., computed tomography (CT) and nuclear magnetic resonance (NMR) scanners, permits the identification of structural lesions and the quantitation of ischemia in the posterior fossa in a manner not previously possible. The advances in microvascular and vertebral artery surgery rest on such precise anatomical and hemodynamic data.

Access to the posterior fossa constitutes entry into the new world of sensation and perception. The sense organs, the cranial nerves, and the brain that integrates these components are also seats of new problems. First, sense-organ dysfunction must be distinguished from brain ischemia. Second, each medical specialty dealing with these problems has its own instrumentation, its own language, and its own perspective. Finally, the common language of brain hemodynamics and brain flow has not yet come into general usage.

There is increasing awareness of brain hemodynamics—the relationship of one vascular bed to another, of vessel flow in the neck to brain perfusion, and of system flow to brain function. The dynamic nature of blood flow to the brain and its alteration by mechanical and physiological factors make testing under static conditions or at only one site, e.g., the carotid bifurcation, incomplete. The progressive incorporation of stress into the neurovascular evaluation parallels the practices well established in cardiac diagnosis.

Current instrumentation has brought not only new kinds of information and new modes of therapy but also confusion and turmoil with regard to objectives and the delivery of services. The role models of the specialties which worked a decade ago will no longer suffice. A new clinical algorithm is required to integrate diagnostic information with clinical application to yield maximum patient benefit in an environment that is increasingly cost-conscious and critical. The system approach to brain ischemia and blood flow attempts to integrate the multiple factors involved which are of clinical significance into a practical working theory. Moreover, this approach functions at different levels of expertise from the basic level, where the principles are established, to the advanced level, where technical detail is used and sophisticated judgment made.

Critical Arterial Stenosis

The existence of pressure gradient within an artery is usually considered evidence of significant arterial obstruction (Tindall *et al.,* 1962; Wilkinson *et al.,* 1964; Jawad *et al.,* 1977). From this postulate evolved the concept of critical arterial stenosis. It is false that only atherosclerotic disease can produce significant obstructions, and that only the carotid bifurcation should be studied, that the determination of significance can exclude the intracranial vascular bed, or that the clinical decision can be based solely upon the angiogram.

Cardiac output, blood viscosity, the status of the arterial "runoff," the collateral capacity, the size of the vascular bed (Jawad *et al.,* 1977), and the volume of blood flow may markedly modify the pressure gradient (Rodbard and Kikuchi, 1976). If the flow is low, severe obstruction may not produce a pressure gradient at all, but high flow will create a marked gradient with the same perfusion pressure (Young *et al.,* 1977). Even a 50 percent arterial stenosis may become "critical" during low-pressure perfusion as encountered during cardiopulmonary bypass. Clinically, cardiac and vascular stress studies utilize high-blood-flow states to determine the significance of arterial obstruction. The hemodynamic consequences of obstruction, the functional disability, and the threat to life and to tissue are significant, and they should influence the interpretation of the angiogram.

The concept of critical arterial stenosis as it is applied to the highly collateralized cerebral vascular system falls short of the mark because it does not address critical issues: the impact on brain perfusion of total arterial occlusion (Nornes, 1973; Carney and Anderson, 1978b; Eikelboom, 1981; Prosenz *et al.,* 1974) or of dynamic obstructions. Similarly, it cannot be applied to the obstruction of short length (Eikelboom *et al.,* 1983), to the vertebral artery, or to vulnerable vascular beds. The angiogram of cervical arteries cannot predict the level of brain perfusion. Therefore, the significance of an obstruction of the carotid or vertebral artery should be determined by its impact on arterial flow (resting and reserve), brain perfusion, brain function, and brain structure.

When flow in both internal carotid arteries is studied simultaneously during the graded closure of one artery, the importance of the competitive increase of flow in the contralateral internal carotid artery and vertebral system immediately becomes apparent (Nornes, 1973; Nornes and Wikeby, 1977), the same way as the clamping of one aortocoronary graft will markedly affect the flow characteristics in the other (Reneman and Spencer, 1975).

Criteria of Significant Arterial Obstruction

An arterial obstruction is regarded as being significant when it compromises either brain perfusion, function, or structure. The obstruction may be static or dynamic. The dynamic obstruction induced by rotation or hyperextension of the head is characterized by its short length, duration, fluctuating severity, and fleeting pressure gradients. Acute catastrophic symptoms can be relieved by having the patient lie supine with the head in neutral position. Collateral channels do not develop in such situations.

Sites of predilection for trauma to the carotid artery are at the base of the skull and the atlas (Batzdorf *et al.,* 1979; Crissey and Bernstein, 1974; Sullivan *et al.,* 1973). Although entrapment usually occurs around peritonsillar inflammatory scars and lymph nodes (Wernick *et al.,* 1974), it may also be caused by anomalous muscle fibers (McMurtry and Yahr, 1966) or by the hypoglossal nerve (Mauersberger, 1974; Scotti *et al.,* 1978) [See also Chapter 14]. Compression of the vertebral artery may occur at the base of the skull (Bell, 1969), but is seen more often at the level of the second cervical vertebra. Compression by osteophytes may also occur within the cervical spine. Sympathetic fibers may also mechanically interfere with vertebral flow, usually at the level of the sixth cervical vertebra.

Head motion may also cause arterial occlusion by compression or stretching and can affect both the carotid and the vertebral arteries in adults and children. Under normal conditions, the circle of Willis compensates for such vascular occlusion which may occur at the skull base. This has been demonstrated by postmortem angiography which revealed occlusion after rotation (Brown and Tatlow, 1963) and after head hyperextension. This phenomenon is also well documented in vivo (Bauer, 1984b; Bell, 1969; Hope *et al.,* 1983). It has also been shown that sensitivity to head position is exaggerated in the presence of carotid occlusion (Bougousslavsky and Regli, 1983).

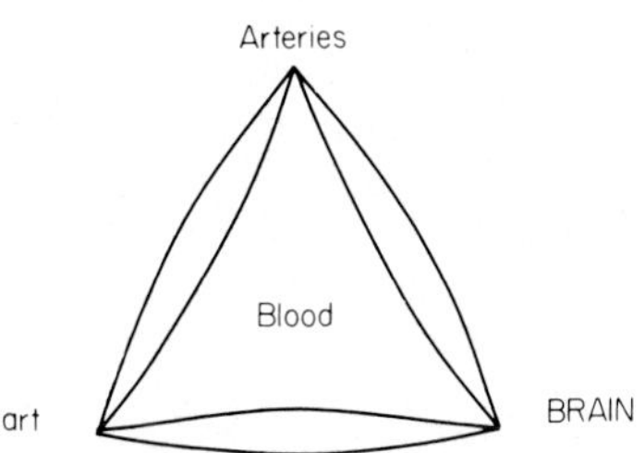

Figure 5-1. The SYSTEM approach to brain blood flow (registered trademark of Blood Flow Dynamics, Ltd.) consists not only of the brain and the arteries to the brain but also those factors that may critically affect regional perfusion. Depleted plasma volume, represented by the inner lines, is associated with reduced cardiac output and decreased brain perfusion. Overexpanded plasma volume, represented by the outer lines, increases cardiac output and the perfusion of the ischemic brain.

THE SYSTEM APPROACH TO BRAIN PERFUSION

Our fundamental concern in studying the circulation to the brain involves not only the blood flow through arteries and the brain tissues but also all those factors affecting the flow. The concepts of McDonald and Brain are extended to include the brain and the cardiovascular system. The objective of this approach is to provide a guide to the diagnosis and treatment of patients that will be most useful to the astute clinician.

Life is dynamic and full of stress. Walking erect, turning the head, and trauma are stresses commonly encountered. But there is a tendency to forget the stress owing to surgery and to disease. Cardiopulmonary bypass, anesthesia, blood loss, induced hypotension, and clamping of the carotid artery constitute formidable stress. The loss of cerebral "autoregulation" may make even the upright position extremely hazardous. Brain-stem ischemia does cause respiratory arrest and myocardial infarction does decompensate brain flow (see Figure 5-1).

Forebrain-Hindbrain Division

Just as in the case of the heart, brain anatomy is constant but the demand and supply of blood is variable. Although according to traditional anatomy the brain is divided into the supratentorial cerebral hemispheres and the infratentorial brain stem and cerebellum, according to vascular territory it is divided into the anterior and posterior circulation. The commonly used clinical designations "cerebral insufficiency" and "vertebral-basilar insufficiency" are not only confusing and inconsistent, but also impractical because symptoms are primarily related to the vascular tree. According to the latter, forebrain includes the territories of the anterior and middle cerebral arteries, and the hindbrain includes the territories of the posterior cerebral arteries and the branches of the vertebral and basilar arteries. Specifically, the frontal and parietal lobes constitute the forebrain, whereas the occipital and temporal lobes, the cerebellum, the pons, and the brain stem constitute the hindbrain.

Identifying regional ischemia establishes the organic nature of the problem. The localization suggests the pathological mechanism and the arteries involved, but it cannot by itself indicate either the side of arterial obstruction, the mechanism of flow reduction, or the most suitable method of revascularization. In addition, decision-making requires precise knowledge of the specific vascular tree of the head and neck defined by angiography, the hemodynamics involved (Carney *et al.,* 1981), and the functional disability of the patient.

Kramer (1912) repeated Willis's classic experiments by injecting methylene blue into the carotid and vertebral arteries in 50 dogs and three monkeys, killing the animals and observing the distribution of dye within the brain. "The results," Kramer reported, "were surprisingly constant." Specifically, injection of the carotid artery, when all other vessels were unobstructed, resulted in staining of the brain in the distribution of anterior and middle cerebral arteries, the anterior choroidal, and the posterior communicating artery. In the dog, only the posterior aspect of the occipital lobe lying on the tentorium remained unstained, but in the monkey, the posterior two thirds of the occipital lobes were stained.

Beside anatomical appearance and blood supply, the brain can also be divided according to the senses, because sensations, perceptions, and sense-organ functions are not vested in a single anatomical site. Small lesions of the brain can produce disability from apnea, sleep disorders, disequilibrium, deafness, and blindness. Vision involves the eye as well as multiple areas of the brain, each with a different blood supply. Up to this time, distinguishing brain ischemia from dysfunction of the end-organ has depended either upon end-organ testing or on demonstrating structural lesions in the cerebral hemisphere. The loss of balance, for example, may reflect either dysfunction of the normally perfused end-organ (the vestibular apparatus), dysfunction of the ischemic end-organ, regional brain-stem ischemia, or generalized brain ischemia.

Many medical specialties touch some aspect of a sense organ, cranial nerve, or the brain stem. Each has its own customs, its own terminology, and its own perception. The technical languages of the neurosciences separate one specialty from another. Some specialists quantitate disability in traditional terms of end-organ dysfunction (American Medical Association, 1977) and not in terms of brain ischemia. The measurement of brain perfusion and vessel flow now introduces a common language of hemodynamics, which is necessary to integrate these disciplines.

Normal Systems

McDonald and Potter (1951), following in Kramer's footsteps, found a similar and distinct pattern of blood-flow distribution to the brain in unobstructed vessels. In this regard, McDonald postulated that the definition for the circle of Willis must be extended to include the vertebral and basilar arteries and the four intracranial anastomotic sites: the two posterior communicating arteries, the anterior communicating artery, and the basilar artery. When flow is balanced, i.e., when the pressures are balanced, the point of no flow is termed the *dead point*. The dead point is, in fact, a floating point that rapidly moves with changing conditions to the point of lowest pressure.

Furthermore, McDonald demonstrated the division of flow within the basilar artery: blood from one vertebral artery will perfuse the ipsilateral side of the brain stem through the segmental branches of the basilar artery. Obstruction of one vertebral artery increases the flow from the other side and moves the dead point toward the side of obstruction. Increasing the flow and pressure in one vertebral artery moves the dead point in the direction of low flow.

Abnormal Systems

Like carotid compression, pressure injections during angiography disturb normal flow relationships. Yet both maneuvers are of clinical importance. Routine angiographic injections that visualize vascular patterns beyond those usually encountered should raise the question of reduced blood pressure or arterial obstruction in that particular area. On the other hand, inadequate visualization may be due to the inability of the pressure injection to overwhelm the high intravascular pressure.

In high-flow, low-resistance systems, as in arteriovenous malformations, the principle is the same. The dead point moves in the direction of the lowest pressure, i.e., the venous outflow tract. Despite high flow in the arteries, ischemia may result because an adequate tissue perfusion pressure cannot be maintained. In such a situation, the most severe ischemia may be either local or at a remote site.

Both Kramer and McDonald observed that the customary dye distribution was altered in the presence of multiple vessel occlusion. Ordinarily, because the pressure within the vascular bed of an occluded internal carotid artery is low, blood will flow to it from the higher-pressure carotid on the contralateral side through the anterior communicating artery. The dead point moves to the side of the obstruction, the side of lower pressure. Should this fail to occur, then either the remaining carotid is obstructed or significant flow is coming from the vertebral artery. Whenever a routine carotid injection fills the basilar artery, the pressure within the basilar artery is considered pathologically low and this merits explanation (see Figure 5–2).

Divisions and Levels

Brain (1957) recommended in the study of the nature of cerebral blood flow that we ac-

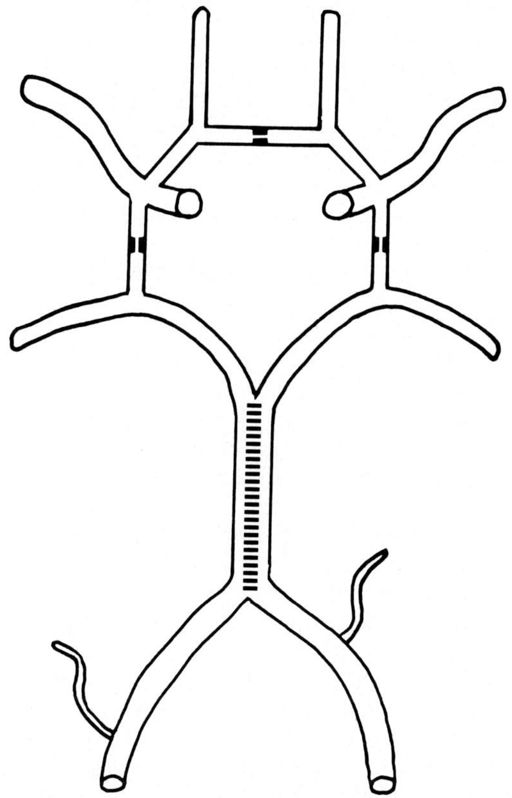

Figure 5–2. The circle of Willis and the vertebral arteries. The "dead" points" (marked by bars) are the sites at which pressure is balanced between supplying arteries and where there is no flow. When the flow is balanced between the vertebral arteries, the dead point divides the stream within the basilar artery longitudinally. Obstruction of one artery causes shifting of the dead point in the direction of low pressure until balance is achieved.

cept McDonald and Potter's hypothesis that the basilar artery and the vertebral artery constitute a critical part of the circle of Willis. He argued that, because the circle of Willis is present in all species of mammals, its purpose is surely to guarantee blood flow to the brain when one or the other artery is blocked by the posture of the blood.

Furthermore, he pointed out that the posterior cerebral arteries, which normally arise from the vertebral system and supply one or both of the occipital and temporal lobes, must be considered distinct from the cerebral hemisphere supplied by the carotid artery. Brain concluded that collateral systems exist on three levels: (1) the level of supply, proximal to the circle of Willis, (2) the circle of Willis per se, and (3) the level of the vascular bed, distal to the circle of Willis, where the territories of end-arteries meet.

Competitive Flow

Hardesty in 1960 demonstrated the reciprocal blood-flow relationship that exists between the two carotid arteries. When one is compromised, blood flow is increased in the contralateral vessel to maintain constant brain blood flow. Nornes (1973) showed that this relationship is not reciprocal but competitive and extends also to the vertebral artery. Toole and McGraw (1975) concluded that steal syndromes in reality constitute pressure-flow relationships between vascular trees, that "in some instances, the development of ischemic symptoms in the donor distribution led to false localization of the disease." Symptoms are the result of brain ischemia, the site of which may be remote from the site of arterial pathology. Furthermore, intrinsic brain pathology—tumors and arteriovenous malformations—may drastically alter the distribution of blood flow. Ischemic lesions in one hemisphere, e.g., cerebral infarction, may also cause ischemia in the contralateral hemisphere.

Isotope Techniques

The vascular bed perfused by the carotid artery in living human beings may be delineated by continually infusing Krypton 81m directly into the vessel and scanning the head with a gamma camera. Krypton 81m has a short half-life of 13 seconds and will never reach equilibrium within the brain because of its rapid decay. Its distribution reflects the new arrival of tracer, therefore regional perfusion from the vessel injected. By 1980, tomographic assessment with a rotating gamma camera permitted higher resolution of blood-flow distribution, delineation of localized areas of reduced or increased perfusion, and the definition of collateral pathways.

Taki and co-workers (1984) studied the vertebral artery by the Krypton 81m method. Four basic perfusion patterns emerged: ipsilateral, contralateral, bilateral, and mosaic. These observations are consistent with the varied anatomy of the region and with the clinical presentations of patients. This technique combined with balloon occlusion of vessels may greatly aid our further understanding of the dynamics of hindbrain perfusion.

Scanning by position emission tomography (PET) has also supported this hemodynamic approach to blood flow. PET data have shown that infarction in one site can alter the perfusion pattern in a nearby or remote site. Ischemia resulting from unilateral cerebral infarction has been shown to occur in both the contralateral hemisphere and the hindbrain.

From the foregoing, one may conclude that it is of practical importance to grasp the implications of the hemodynamic approach to the circulation of the brain and also to recognize the disadvantages and advantages of such an approach. For change, even from worse to better, is not made without inconvenience. It is not convenient to change from carotid stenosis and the angiogram to hemodynamics and perfusion. Observation and analysis are required. The carotid bifurcation becomes one tree in the forest. Brain perfusion, precise anatomy, and system hemodynamics must be understood, and new skills must be developed. Such endeavors alter our ways and our identity.

PERFUSION AND THRESHOLDS OF FUNCTION

In general, the function of the brain is directly related to perfusion. Progressive reduction of blood supply results in progressive deterioration, first of function and then of structure. Perfusion may decrease by two thirds of the normal before electrical dysfunction is noted. Metabolism is grossly disturbed when perfusion falls below 20 percent of the normal levels and cell death occurs shortly thereafter. What is notable is the wide range between optimal perfusion and cell death and the relatively narrow range between hypoperfusion and cell malfunction. The variables which may modify the course of these events include the metabolic activity of the cell, the particular function under consideration, the duration and type of stress, and the age of the individual. Both reduced perfusion and excessive perfusion are abnormal but they become pathological only if they compromise brain function, structure, growth or development (see Figure 5–3).

Transient Ischemic Attacks and Brain Infarction

The terms *stroke* and *transient ischemic attacks* (TIAs) in neurology are analogous to cardiological definitions of "heart attacks" and "acute chest pain." Precise information is replacing the latter terms with myocardial infarction and also supplies the location, such as "apex of the left ventricle" or "anteroseptal area." The objective of TIA and stroke management is the preservation of brain function and rehabilitation, just as the objective of cardiac management is the preservation of left ventricular function and rehabilitation. Caplan (1984) succinctly states the case: "We cannot continue . . . the grouping of patients only by temporal description of their symptoms, an idea which has an unsatisfactory past and no future."

In the past, the criteria for defining forebrain TIAs were generally agreed upon, though differences between observers were significant. Since the advent of the CT scan, the separation of focal ischemia from focal cerebral infarction with transient neurological findings has made conventional clinical diagnosis less certain. The distinction appears important, because TIA with brain infarction carries a worse prognosis. Moreover, patients may have a severe disturbance of the cerebral perfusion patterns for as long as six weeks without the occurrence of infarction. These recent developments raise the question of what exactly constitutes cerebral infarction?

Selective Brain Cell Infarction

In general, stroke implies a fixed and irreversible neurological deficit caused by infarction. There is, however, increasing recognition that neurological deficit may also be caused by hypoperfusion without infarction. A new type of brain lesion is now being recognized: ischemic insult to the brain under controlled hypotension. Ischemic hypoxia damages cells and structures in the order of decreasing metabolic activity. Gray matter is more vulnerable than white, and active cortical cells are damaged more easily and earlier than glial cells. The cortical cells of the occipital lobe are also more sensitive to insult than the Betz cells of the motor strip. This selective destruction of brain is more difficult to quantitate but is nonetheless increasingly important because function can be lost while gross structure is left intact (Lassen, 1982). CT, radioisotope, and NMR can now identify those ischemic lesions lacking the characteristics of infarction, thus making the analytical approach to treatment ever more relevant.

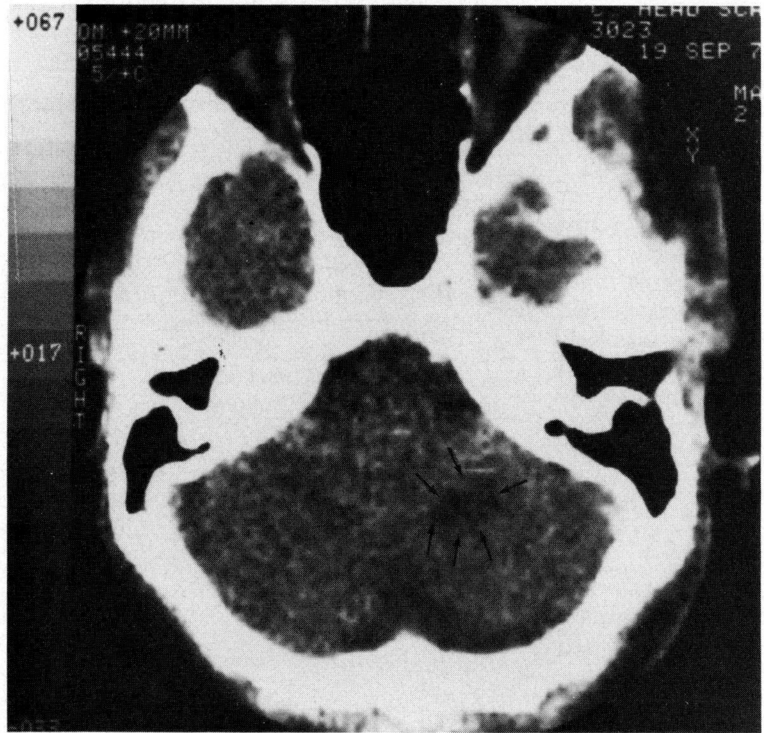

Figure 5–3. Avascular lesion and normal cerebellar perfusion. By means of 5 mm sections, the computed tomographic (CT) static study demonstrates a 5 mm focal lesion in the posterior fossa (arrows). CT dynamic scanning reveals the lesion to be avascular and the cerebellar perfusion to be normal. At surgery, a solitary cyst was removed. The ability to clearly image small foci in the posterior fossa is evident. From Mafee, M.F.; Anderson, E.M.; Carney, A.L.; *et al.*: Hindbrain evaluation. *Adv. Neurol.*, **30:**116–39, 1981, with permission.

Acute Hindbrain Ischemia

Because of the difficulty in separating sense-organ dysfunction from brain-stem ischemia, there are really no defined criteria for the clinical diagnosis of hindbrain TIAs. There is also lack of agreement whether to include vertigo, visual disturbances, alterations of cognition, memory, etc. For this reason, hindbrain TIAs were excluded in the cooperative aspirin study (Bauer, 1984a). Although the value of CT scanning is limited within the posterior fossa because of the dense cortical bone, it can indeed measure focal brain-stem perfusion. On the other hand, NMR is unencumbered by bone and can identify small (2 to 5 mm) ischemic lesions in the brain-stem.

AUTOREGULATION

Autoregulation has been defined as the ability of the brain to maintain tissue perfusion at a relatively constant level, irrespective of changes in the circulation that may occur during exercise or due to moderate changes in blood pressure. The loss of autoregulation due to brain infarction, tumor, ischemia, and aging permits hypotension to cause profound brain ischemia and hypertension which, in turn, may result in hemorrhagic infarction.

The major difficulty in understanding autoregulation is that it does not relate in a meaningful way to vascular anatomy, the distribution of the infarction, brain hemodynamics, or arterial obstruction; thus, it is difficult to consider it in clinical decision-making. Some of the specific situations where the pathology is both hard to understand and difficult to handle are (1) the brain with abnormalities of the circle of Willis that is vulnerable to infarction, (2) the loss of autoregulation in a specific vascular bed, and (3) the varying tolerance to carotid surgery. The explanation of these situations need not invoke a mystical mechanism but should be based on pressure-flow relationships, vascular configuration, and the local response of the vascular bed.

Vulnerable Vascular Beds

Intracranial vascular patterns are associated with brain dysfunction, ischemia, and infarctions in a consistent fashion. The development of techniques for measuring brain perfusion and precisely localizing infarctions requires a working theory that provides an explanation of observed phenomena. This requires the integration of vascular patterns and vessel blood flow with regional perfusion and brain function. Vulnerability also varies with metabolic activity. The active gray matter, for example, is more vulnerable than white, cells of the occipital cortex are more sensitive than those of the motor strip, and the vestibular system is less protected than the auditory system.

The Watershed

The watershed is the interface of adjacent vascular beds. Cerebral vascular beds compose circulation to the brain just as segments join to form an orange. One of the watersheds is located within the forebrain between the anterior and middle cerebral arteries; another lies between forebrain and hindbrain, between the parietal and the occipital and temporal lobes (Torvik, 1984). Electroencephalographic abnormalities are common in temporal lobe ischemia, and some are considered diagnostic of hindbrain ischemia (Maynard and Hughes, 1984). Decrease in blood flow to the watershed may be due to systemic hypotension (Adams *et al.,* 1966; Torvik, 1984), hypertension, increased intracranial pressure (Overgaard and Tweed, 1983), or to multiple arterial stenoses. Reduced perfusion in the watershed areas in the presence of systemic hypotension is especially associated with a poor prognosis (Overgaard and Tweed, 1983).

Vascular beds, particularly vulnerable, include the collateral bed, the overextended vascular bed, the artery of small diameter or high resistance, the hypoplastic system, and the artery of modified resistance. Areas perfused by arteries of small diameter and great length are especially exposed to ischemic damage (Carney and Anderson, 1981b).

Beside the vessels themselves, the blood and its volume and composition are integral components of the cardiovascular system which sustains the circulation to the brain. Adequate tissue perfusion requires cardiac output at a pressure that ensures appropriate blood flow to each vascular bed. The three items are of special concern (1) perfusion pressure, (2) blood flow, and (3) cardiac function.

Brain Perfusion Versus Brachial Pressure

When the patient is in the supine position, the pressure in the brachial artery does not reflect blood pressure in the intracranial arteries as well as does the pressure of the ophthalmic artery (Gee, 1982; Borras *et al.,* 1969). This discrepancy is the reason for using the ophthalmic artery pressure instead of the brachial blood pressure ratio to detect carotid obstruction. The upright or sitting position can also provoke intracranial arterial hypotension while the brachial blood pressure may remain normal (Carney *et al.,* 1981; Caplan and Sergay, 1976). One should concentrate upon brain perfusion and dysfunction; undue reliance on the brachial blood pressure may be misleading.

The Circle and the Postcircle

The configuration of the circle of Willis is variable (Wollschlaeger and Wollschlaeger, 1974; Krayenbuhl and Yasargil, 1968). Its functional capacity is best determined after one of the supplying vessels becomes occluded and the response of flow within the remaining arteries can be observed. Because a competitive relationship exists between the arteries supplying the circle, it might be expected that occlusion of one would result in increased flow in the rest (Nornes, 1973; Nornes and Wikeby, 1977). Compared with the arteries supplying the circle, the end-arteries to the brain have not received the attention that they deserve. Embolism and hypoperfusion are common in this segment, with vasospasm, aneurysm, dissection, and atherosclerosis assuming lesser roles (Spetzler *et al.,* 1983). The detection of disease at this level can be best done using conventional selective angiography rather than intravenous digital subtraction techniques.

The middle cerebral artery has been studied extensively (Corston *et al.,* 1984), primarily because of the interest in extracranial-intracranial bypass. The major cause of middle cerebral artery stenosis is embolism (Corston *et al.,* 1984) from the proximal carotid artery. Total occlusion of the middle cerebral artery has been found to resolve on second angiogram six weeks later in 44 percent of the patients. Demonstration of hypoperfusion, with a pressure gradient, has been found useful in predicting surgical outcome (Spetzler *et al.*, 1983). The anatomical complications that occur after superficial temporal to middle cerebral artery bypass are comparable to those after distal coronary bypass (Heros, 1984, Aldridge and Trimble, 1971).

Posterior cerebral artery occlusion is most often caused by emboli from the vertebral system. The emboli may lodge at the bifurcation and initiate the "top of the basilar" syndrome or enter the posterior cerebral artery and compromise the circulation to the occipital lobe.

Vascular Reserve Versus Collateral Flow

In the study of the coronary circulation, maximal capacity or the coronary vascular reserve may be measured by the increment of flow above resting level after transient coronary artery occlusion, exercise, or dilating agents. If the stimulus produces maximal dilatation, then the increase in flow will also be maximal (Hoffman, 1984). Mosher and associates (1964), who studied coronary autoregulation, concluded that the pressure-flow diagram was the best way to illustrate the coronary vascular reserve. This reserve capacity may also be measured by cardiac stress testing.

When referring to the circulation to the brain, collateral flow should be distinguished from vascular reserve. Whereas the former is defined as that which takes place in those secondary vascular channels indirectly supplying the circle of Willis and which slowly increases to meet demand, the definition of the latter is the flow in excess of resting flow in primary channels directly supplying the circle of Willis. This can rapidly increase to accommodate demand. When the vascular reserve is exhausted and the efficiency of the circle of Willis decreases by the loss of flow from primary vessels, secondary flow through collateral channels may increase, but the reserve capacity will not improve.

The vascular reserve of either carotid artery can be tested by temporarily occluding the contralateral carotid (Eikelboom, 1981, Tada *et al.*, 1975). If the vascular reserve is adequate, the blood flow through the patent carotid will increase and the perfusion pressure will be maintained in the vascular beds of both carotid and both ophthalmic arteries. If, however, the vascular reserve of the contralateral carotid is inadequate, ischemia of the brain will develop in one or both vascular beds. In either case, release of the temporary occlusion will result in increased flow above resting levels owing to reflex hyperemia.

Hyperperfusion

Sundt (1983) states that the primary cause for neurological complications after endarterectomy is ipsilateral hyperperfusion. In agreement with this, Schroeder and associates (1984) described a case of a 55-year-old man with an occluded right carotid who was operated upon for left carotid stenosis. Because clamping of the left carotid resulted in flattening and slowing of the electroencephalogram, a shunt was inserted. Marked bilateral hyperperfusion immediately followed endarterectomy, reaching 200 percent of the preoperative resting value. The patient became confused and developed a headache; his systolic blood pressure increased to 200 mm Hg from a preoperative value of 110 mm Hg. Decrease of blood pressure to normal levels was accomplished with medication, but it required one week for cortical perfusion to return to normal.

In this case, the vascular reserve of the right carotid was insufficient and only the vascular reserve of the vertebral system remained available to directly supply the brain. Temporary occlusion of one of the carotid arteries resulted in ischemia in both hemispheres and possibly in the brain stem as well. After carotid endarterectomy, the vascular reserve of the left carotid increased markedly, and the flow increased in both carotid beds. Because both lost ischemic autoregulation, reactive hyperemia provoked hyperfusion in both hemispheres.

THE CONCEPT OF CEREBRAL FLOW AND ITS REFLECTION TO DIAGNOSTIC APPROACHES

Since Egaz Moniz introduced cerebral angiography (Moniz, 1927), the method has been primarily structure-oriented, contributing much to our knowledge of vascular anatomy but less to brain perfusion.

Angiogram — Not the Gold Standard

The clinical value of the angiogram is coming increasingly under fire (Leeson *et al.*, 1983). Recent correlations of surgical findings with angiographic findings tarnished this gold standard. Thin-section, high resolution CT of the internal carotid artery now permits more accurate assessment of the extent of atherosclerotic plaque and the degree of luminal compromise (Comerota *et al.,* 1981) than angiography. Similarly, real-time B-mode carotid imaging has also improved our understanding of the dynamic anatomy and pathology not appreciated by static imaging. The ability to determine precisely peak Doppler velocities now permits functional calculation of obstruction (Payen *et al.,* 1982). As more brain perfusion studies become available, the limitations of angiography will be better appreciated.

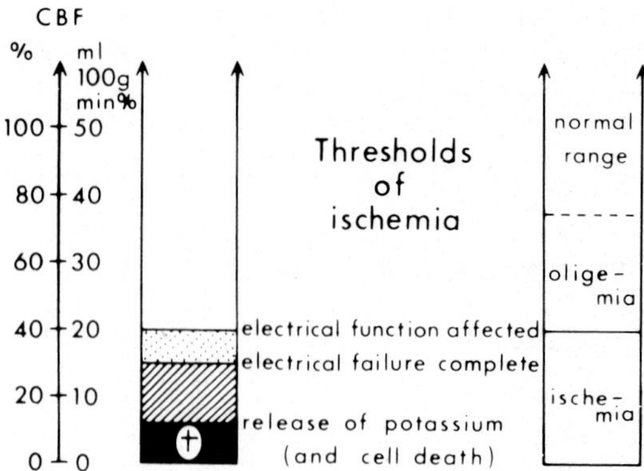

Figure 5–4. Thresholds of ischemia for electrical failure and for the release of cellular potassium. The regional cerebral perfusion was lowered by middle cerebral artery occlusion, and blood pressure was manipulated. The decrease in systemic blood pressure changed local cerebral blood flow proportionally in ischemic zones. The threshold of electrical response was measured by evoked potential in the cortex, but the actual values may vary for different functions and cover a large range depending upon metabolic rate. The direct relationship between systemic blood pressure and perfusion indicates a loss of autoregulation. From Astrup, J.; Symer, L.; Branston, N.M.; and Lassen, N.A.: Cortical evoked potential and extracellular K+ and H+ at critical levels of brain ischemia. *Stroke,* **8**:51–7, 1977, with permission.

Noninvasive Testing

In noninvasive testing, many reports have focused on the carotid bifurcation. As better methods of imaging of brain structure and determining brain perfusion are being utilized, noninvasive testing must also involve the brain itself. The blood velocity in the carotid arteries in the neck now can be related to cerebral perfusion (Risberg and Smith, 1980; Carney and Anderson, 1981a), and the combination of the range-gated Doppler and radioactive xenon perfusion studies of the brain has been used with success. The reduction of carotid velocity or significant asymmetry facilitates the selection of patients for further studies. Asymmetry of vertebral blood flow, however, is the rule, and its interpretation is more difficult.

Furthermore, as revascularization procedures extend in the carotid and vertebral artery at skull base and extracranial-intracranial microvascular procedures are used, the focus of noninvasive testing must shift to accommodate this area. Some of the probes are not suitable for these areas, but modifications of these probes will allow their use in the operating room and permit the imaging of the intact vessels, thus reducing the need for angiography (See also Chapter 7 on noninvasive diagnosis).

Total Cerebral Blood Flow Versus Regional Perfusion

Severe disability owing to abnormal regional brain ischemia could coexist with normal total cerebral blood flow. Radioisotope techniques, first reported in 1961 (Lassen and Ingvar, 1961), lacked practical application until the advent of microvascular reconstruction. By 1977, the use of Xenon 133 permitted better appreciation of perfusion in the accessible cortex, but diagnostic penetration into the brain substance and the posterior fossa was and remains poor.

Such terms as *physiologic activation, functional landscape,* and *luxury perfusion* were introduced to describe observations. But the concept of the threshold of ischemia (see Figure 5–4) and the relationship of the level of the brain perfusion to brain structure and function integrates these observations with a sense of order that was then extended clinically as the physiology of cerebral blood flow (Astrup *et al.,* 1977; Lassen and Christiansen, 1976). The men who participated in this work were research-oriented, labored under great handicaps, and often were concerned more with the theoretical impetus than with the clinical application.

Computed Tomography

In 1972, EMI, Ltd. announced the advent of computerized tomography (CT) (Hounsfield, 1973). The principal contribution of CT was the delineation of brain anatomy, i.e., structure, with a high degree of resolution. Contrast enhancement by infusion aided in visualization of blood vessels, mass lesions of the brain and areas of "luxury perfusion."

In 1977, pressure was brought to bear for more practical information regarding brain perfusion. This impetus came from two groups of surgeons: those performing superficial temporal-middle cerebral anastomoses and others performing vertebral artery surgery. The neurosurgeon sought to enhance flow to the middle cerebral artery by anastomosing it with the superficial temporal artery. Many questioned the value of this procedure. Surgeons responded by measuring brain perfusion in the territory of the middle cerebral artery with radioactive xenon and the critics by forming a study group to determine the efficacy of the procedure (ED/IC Bypass Study Group 1985). On the other hand, vertebral artery surgery was designed to enhance blood flow to the circle of Willis. Such an approach required a method to study brain perfusion in both the forebrain and the hindbrain (Carney and Anderson, 1978a). Reconstruction of the post-circle middle cerebral artery has been judged of limited value, reconstruction of the pre-circle vertebral artery still awaits evaluation.

Dynamic CT Scanning — Contrast Enhancement

By 1978, dynamic CT scans of the brain were being performed clinically, using iodinated contrast, a nondiffusible marker administered by bolus injection that is confined to the vessel lumen except in cases of disruption of the blood brain barrier, i.e., when luxury perfusion is not present. Contrast increases tissue density with the passage of the contrast bolus. Serial sections taken of the one level studied per injection permit the generation of a curve for each selected window. Interpretation is based on the mean transit time, which is qualitative, not quantitative.

One advantage of this technique is the larger number of scanners that could potentially perform the examination. The technique was applied clinically but drew little interest from radiologists who operated the scanners most often or from those studying brain perfusion who did not possess the scanners. Another advantage is the unique ability to penetrate the posterior fossa with high resolution for static imaging and dynamic scans.

Many radiologists, vascular surgeons, and clinicians came to accept angiography as the golden standard and carotid stenosis as the center of attention. Unexplained symptoms were attributed to embolism and treated as such, or labeled nonhemispheric and discounted. Discussion of critical arterial stenosis and the carotid bifurcation dominated medical and surgical meetings alike. Studies of brain perfusion would have changed this status quo but there was little interest in physiological evaluation and little was to be gained by change.

The 1970s saw an increasing number of clinicians entering diagnostic work because their need for physiological information exceeded that provided by existing services. Neurosurgeons have been by far the earliest and most active in the pursuit of applications of brain blood flow studies in clinical settings. It was a neurosurgeon who promoted the use of Xenon 133 for diagnosis and for use in the operating room. Its prime field of application was the accessible cerebral cortex, which correlated well with the electroencephalogram. Deep structures and the posterior fossa are not evaluated well by either technique.

Dynamic CT Scanning — Xenon Enhancement

In 1984, General Electric introduced the GE 9800 scanner, which had the ability to perform quantitative cerebral perfusion studies rapidly with low concentrations of stable xenon. Although there is significant experience with this technique, clinical experience with posterior fossa studies has yet to be reported. This was the first instrument to have commercially available software for this purpose. Stable xenon, which is administered by inhalation, is freely diffusible, and its solubility coefficient is utilized in calculating perfusion. It does not detect disruptions of the blood brain barrier but it does yield quantitative brain perfusion data.

Positron Emission Scanning

Positron emission tomography (PET) is a physiological instrument which has been used primarily in studies for metabolic problems and epilepsy. Time frames of study typically range in minutes. Stressing brain perfusion by dilating the vascular bed may require 30 to 40 minutes to achieve a steady state (Maziotta *et al.*, 1984). The scanners can utilize both diffusible and nondiffusible markers and can distinguish disruption of blood brain barrier (luxury perfusion) from focal hyperemia. Oxygen extraction is sometimes used as an index of tissue needs in low-flow areas. The assumption is that if oxygen extraction is high there is need for revascularization, and benefit would be derived.

Nuclear Magnetic Resonance

Nuclear magnetic resonance (NMR) scanners offer high-resolution image scans, unencumbered by cortical bone, which can be displayed in the transverse, sagittal, and coronal planes. The visualization of small infarctions in the posterior fossa and of spinal cord abnormalities exceeds the potentials of any other technique. The measurement of linear blood flow with this technique has been demonstrated by Mills and co-workers (1984). Though the ability to quantitate tissue perfusion is less likely, the estimation of regional patterns of flow appears possible. Interpretation of arterial obstruction may be difficult if the vessel is not imaged within a given section. Plaques are well visualized. Slowly flowing blood near the arterial wall is better visualized than high-velocity central flow. Turbulence increases the signal. The technical performance of NMR scanners is highly variable, even in scanners from the same manufacturer. Site preparation, maintenance, and personnel are key factors. Because the soft-tissue visualization is so good, potential application is wide. The use of NMR will offer increasing opportunities to clinicians.

As seen in the foregoing, as high-resolution measurement of brain perfusion and detailed structural information become more readily available, the precise knowledge of anatomy and pathology and an understanding of the system and brain hemodynamics are becoming practical necessities. Carotid surgery based upon angiography will give way to more advanced techniques of diagnosis and surgery.

HEMODILUTION

Increasing the intravascular blood volume with cell-free colloidal solutions, e.g., low-molecular-weight dextran, improves the perfusion of ischemic brain (Wood *et al.,* 1984). Hypervolemic hemodilution proved to be protective against cerebral infarction in experimental ligation of the middle cerebral artery (Wood *et al.,* 1984). It is believed that the hematocrit must decrease significantly to enhance brain preservation.

The therapeutic application of this process has been widespread among neurosurgeons in the treatment of brain ischemia and for the purpose of brain protection during surgery. It has been applied in the course of graded occlusion of the internal carotid artery and for initial treatment for acute neurological deficits (VanderArk and Pomerantz, 1973) as shown by the significant number of reports on the use of this technique. The physiological basis for hypervolemic hemodilution is based upon the increase in cardiac output and improvement of cerebral perfusion owing to the production of anemia and to the decrease in blood viscosity (Eisenberg, 1982).

Subarachnoid bleeding is a stimulus for intense vasospasm, which can cause severe brain ischemia. In 1967, the first reports (McMurtry *et al.,* 1967) described the use of blood volume expanders and induced hypertension in the treatment of brain ischemia due to vasospasm. Since then neurosurgeons, including Sundt (Sundt and Waltz, 1967), and Davis (Davis and Sundt, 1980), have been studying the cardiovascular effects of and relating cardiac and system hemodynamic changes to brain perfusion and function. Working with Xenon 133, neurosurgeons documented the response of cortical perfusion to manipulations of the system. The same investigators have also shown its adaptability by utilizing the hemodynamic instrumentation developed in cardiac surgery. Cardiovascular surgeons, however, have not applied the available instrumentation, either for the study of brain perfusion during surgery or for operative case selections. We believe that the measurement of brain perfusion (Aaslid *et al.,* 1984) definitely has a place in intraoperative monitoring.

Intracranial Pressure

The technique of hemodilution differs in cardiac and neurovascular surgery. Noncolloidal solutions used to prime the cardiopulmonary bypass result in an increase of tissue interstitial pressure and fluid retention, but the effects on intracranial pressure and cerebral edema are not known. While hypoosmolar solutions increase, hyperosmolar solutions, such as albumin, decrease edema, including cerebral edema (Little *et al.,* 1981). Wood recommends the use of the hyperosmolar, low-molecular-weight dextran; nevertheless, volume expansion increases intracranial pressure, possibly by increased cerebral blood volume (Wood *et al.,* 1982b).

Brain ischemia by itself causes cerebral edema (Hossman *et al.,* 1976), which in turn increases intracranial pressure and may further decrease brain perfusion. If the edema is marked and the perfusion pressure is low, deterioration of the cerebral circulation occurs, being first manifested in the watershed areas. Perfusion measured in these regions has been useful in detecting the development of ischemia and in predicting poor neurological prognosis (Overgaard and Tweed, 1983).

Isovolemic Hemodilution

Isovolemic hemodilution (Gejha, 1976) using albumin solution enhances brain perfusion and reduces cerebral edema during neurovascular surgery and in acute neurological deficits. In patients with high hematocrits the blood volume is first restored to normal. If the hematocrit remains high, phlebotomy is performed before surgery is undertaken. This approach has resulted in electroencephalographic stability during surgery and reduced the need for intraluminal shunting.

Heart Disease

Coronary artery disease almost triples the risk for stroke, and cardiac failure increases the risk five-fold (Kannel *et al.,* 1983). Atrial fibrillation with or without valvular involvement (Sage and VanUitert, 1983) carries by itself an inherent risk of embolism and stroke. Congenital cardiac anomalies and their correction also compromise brain perfusion (Adams *et al.,* 1984). This raises several questions: Is neurological dysfunction a symptom? If the cause of brain ischemia is cardiac, should the heart be treated in the absence of specific cardiac complaints (Adams *et al.,* 1984; Hertzer and Lees, 1981; Rokey *et al.,* 1984)? The decrease in cardiac output and brain ischemia may be the result of either disease or even be the consequence of medication. Although the overzealous use of cardiac medications should be tempered, the use of physiologic pacemakers, volume expansion, and anticoagulant therapy should be utilized whenever necessary.

In conclusion, technical advances in diagnostic and therapeutic instrumentation have made possible a novel hemodynamic approach to understanding and measuring brain perfusion, including flow through the arteries of the neck. This, combined with increased resolution imaging, permits objective evaluation of the circulation of both the forebrain and of the posterior fossa. Furthermore, objective demonstration of neurological dysfunction and regional ischemia provides the tools to determine adequacy of vessel flow in general.

The dynamic physiological approach to brain blood flow permits a rational clinical evaluation of brain ischemia. System hemodynamics also assume increased importance in both surgical and medical management of the acute neurological deficit. Now, in a symbolic sense, the brain can be held in the hand and examined.

REFERENCES

Aaslid, R.; Huber, P.; and Nornes, H.: Evaluation of cerebrovascular spasm with transcranial Doppler ultrasound. *J. Neurosurg.,* **60**:37–41, 1984.

Adams, H.P.; Kassell, N.E.; and Mazuz, H.: The patient with transient ischemic attacks—is this the time for a new therapeutic approach? *Stroke,* **15**:371–75, 1984.

Adams, J.H.; Brierly, J.B.; Connor, R.C.R.; and Treip, C.S.: The effect of systemic hypotension upon the human brain: clinical and neuropathological observations in 11 cases. *Brain,* **89**:235–68, 1966.

Aldridge, H.E., and Trimble, A.S.: Progression of proximal coronary saphenous vein grafting. *J. Thorac. Cardiovascular. Surg.,* **62**:7–11, 1971.

American Medical Association: *Guides to the Evaluation of Permanent Impairment,* 2nd ed. American Medical Association, Chicago, 1977.

Astrup, J.; Symer, L.; Branston, N.M.; and Lassen, N.A.: Cortical evoked potential and extracellular K^+ and H^+ at critical levels of brain ischemia. *Stroke,* **8**:51–7, 1977.

Batzdorf, U.; Bentson, J.R.; and Machledger, H.I.: Blunt trauma to the high cervical carotid artery. *Neurosurgery,* **5**:195–201, 1979.

Bauer, R.B.: Discussion regarding the cooperative aspirin study. In Berguer, R., and Bauer, R.B. (eds.): *Vertebrobasilar Arterial Occlusive Disease.* Raven Press, New York, 1984a.

Bauer, R.B.: Mechanical compression of the vertebral arteries. In Berguer, R., and Bauer, R.B. (eds.): *Vertebrobasilar Arterial Occlusive Disease.* Raven Press, New York, 1984b.

Bell, H.: Basilar artery insufficiency due to atlanto-occipital instability. *Am. Surg.,* **35**:695–700, 1969.

Borras, A.; Mendenez, M.S.; and Martinez, A.: Ophthalmic/brachial artery pressure ratio in man. *Am. J. Ophthalmol.,* **67**:684–88, 1969.

Bougousslavsky, J., and Regli, F.: Delayed TIAs distal to bilateral occlusion of carotid arteries—evidence for embolic and hemodynamic mechanisms. *Stroke,* **14**:58–61, 1983.

Brain, R.: Order and disorder in the cerebral circulation. *Lancet*, **2**:857–62, 1957.

Brown, B.St.J., and Tatlow, W.F.T.: Radiographic studies of the vertebral arteries in cadavers. *Radiology*, **81**:80–88, 1963.

Caplan, L.: Treatment of cerebral ischemia—where are we headed? *Stroke*, **15**:571–74, 1984.

Caplan L., and Sergay, S.: Positional cerebral ischemia. *J. Neurol. Neurosurg. Psychiatry*, **39**:385–91, 1976.

Carney, A.L.: Ocular plethysmography and suction ophthalmodynamography in the diagnosis of carotid disease. In Fein, J.M., and Reichman, O.H. (eds.): *Ischemia*. Springer Verlag, New York, 1978.

Carney, A.L: Vertebral artery surgery: historical development, basic concepts of brain hemodynamics, and clinical experience of 102 cases. *Adv. Neurol.*, **30**:249–82, 1981.

Carney, A.L., and Anderson, E.M.: Carotid distal vertebral artery bypass. *Clin. Electroencephalogr.*, **9**:105–109, 1978a.

Carney, A.L., and Anderson, E.M.: Collateral ophthalmic artery pressure (COAP) and the collateral ocular pulse (C)P). In Diethrich, E.B. (ed.): *Noninvasive Cardiovascular Diagnosis—Current Concepts*. University Park Press, Baltimore, Maryland, 1978b.

Carney, A.L., and Anderson, E.M.: Hypoglossal carotid entrapment. *Adv. Neurol.*, **30**:223–47, 1981a.

Carney, A.L., and Anderson, E.M.: The system approach to brain blood flow. *Adv. Neurol.*, **30**:1–30, 1981b.

Carney, A.L.; Anderson, E.M.; and Burns, E.: Cerebral hemodynamic evaluation. *Adv. Neurol.*, **30**:335–59, 1981.

Comerota, A.J.; Cranley, J.J.; and Cook, S.E.: Realtime B-mode carotid imaging in diagnosis of cerebrovascular disease. *Surgery*, **89**:718–29, 1981.

Corston, R.N.; Kendall, B.E.; and Marshall, J.: Prognosis in middle cerebral artery stenosis. *Stroke*, **15**:237–41, 1984.

Crissey, M.M., and Bernstein, E.F.: Delayed presentation of carotid intimal tear following blunt craniocervical trauma. *Surgery*, **75**:543–49, 1974.

Davis, D.H., and Sundt, T.M., Jr.: Relationship of cerebral blood low to cardiac output, mean arterial pressure, blood volume, and alpha and beta blockage in cats. *J. Neurosurg.*, **52**:745–54, 1980.

EC/IC Bypass Study Group: Failure of extracranial-intracranial arterial bypass to reduce the risk of ischemic stroke. *N. Engl. J. Med.* **313**:1191–1200, 1985.

Eikelboom, B.C.: *Evaluation of Carotid Artery Disease and Potential Collateral Circulation by Ocular Pneumoplethysmography*. Uitgeversmaatschappij Huisartsenpers BV, Utrecht, 1981.

Eikelboom, B.C.; Riles, T.R.; Mintzer, R.; Baumann, E.G.; DeFillip, G.; Lin, J.; and Imparato, A.M.: Inaccuracy of angiography in the diagnosis of carotid ulceration. *Stroke*, **14**:882–85, 1983.

Eisenberg, S.: Cerebral circulatory effects of acutely induced hypervolemia in human subjects. *Circ. Res.*, **10**:767–71, 1962.

Gee, W.: Carotid physiology with ocular pneumoplethysmography. *Stroke*, **13**:666–73, 1982.

Gejha, A.: Coronary and cardiovascular dynamics and oxygen availability during acute normovolemic anemia. *Surgery*, **80**:47–53, 1976.

Hardesty, W.H.; Roberts, B.; Toole, J.F.; and Royster, H.P.: Studies of carotid artery blood flow in man. *N. Engl. J. Med.*, **263**:944–46, 1960.

Heros, R.C.: Thromboembolic complications after combined internal carotid ligation and extra- to intracranial bypass. *Surg. Neurol.*, **21**:75–79, 1984.

Hertzer, N.R., and Lees, C.D.: Fatal myocardial infarction following carotid endarterectomy. *Ann. Surg.*, **194**:212–18, 1981.

Hoffman, J.: Maximal coronary flow and the concept of coronary vascular reserve. *Circulation*, **70**:153–59, 1984.

Hope, E.E.; Bodensteiner, J.B.; and Barnes, P.: Cerebral infarction related to neck position in an adolescent. *Pediatrics*, **72**:335–37, 1983.

Hossman, K.A., and Takagi, S.: Osmolarity in cerebral ischemia. *Exp. Neurol.*, **5**:124–31, 1976.

Hounsfield, G.N.: Computed transverse axial scanning (tomography). Description of system. *Br. J. Radiol.*, **46**:1016–22, 1973.

Jawad, K.; Miller, J.D.; Wyper, D.J.; and Rowa, J.O.: Measurement of CBF and carotid artery pressure compared with angiography. *J. Neurosurg.*, **46**:185–96, 1977.

Kannel, W.B.B.; Wolf, P.A.; and Verter, J.: Manifestations of coronary artery disease predisposing to stroke—the Framingham study. *J.A.M.A.*, **250**:2942–46, 1983.

Kety, S.S., and Schmidt, C.F.: The determination of the cerebral blood flow in man by the use of nitrous oxide in low concentrations. *Am. J. Physiol.*, **143**:653–56, 1945.

Kramer, S.P.: Function of the circle of Willis. *J. Exp. Med.*, **15**:348–63, 1912.

Krayenbuhl, H.A., and Yasargil, M.G.: *Cerebral Angiography*. Butterworths, London, 1968.

Lassen, N.A.: Incomplete cerebral infarction—focal incomplete tissue necrosis not leading to emollision. *Stroke*, **13**:522–23, 1982.

Lassen, N.A., and Christiansen, M.D.: Physiology of cerebral blood flow. *Br. J. Anaesth.*, **48**:719–34, 1976.

Lassen, N.A., and Ingvar, D.H.: The blood flow of the cerebral cortex determined by radioactive krypton. *Experientia*, **17**:42–43, 1961.

Leeson, M.D.; Cacayorin, E.D.; Hodge, C.J.; Culebras, A., and Iliya, A.R.: Atheromatous extracranial carotid arteries: CT evaluation correlated with arteriography and pathologic examination. *Radiology*, **156**:397–402, 1985.

Little, J.R.; Slugg, R.M.; Lachaw, J.P.; Lesser, R.P.: Treatment of acute focal cerebral ischemia with concentrated albumin. *Neurosurgery*, **9**:552–58, 1981.

Mafee, M.F.; Anderson, E.M.; Carney, A.L.; *et al.*: Hindbrain evaluation. *Adv. Neurol.*, **30**:116–39, 1981.

Mauersberger, W.: Cerebral Durchblutungsstörungen und Parese des Nervus hypoplossus bein extremer Schlingebildung der Arteria carotis interna. *Neurochirurgia (Stuttg)*, **17**:91–5, 1974.

Maynard, S.D., and Hughes, J.R.: A distinctive electrographic entity: bursts of rhythmical temporal theta. *Clin. Electroencephalogr.*, **15**:145–50, 1984.

Mazziota, J.C., and Engel, J., Jr.: The use and impact of positron computed tomography scanning in epilepsy. *Epilepsia*, **25** [Suppl 2]:S86–S104, 1984.

McDonald, D.A., and Potter, J.M.: The distribution of blood to the brain. *J. Physiol.*, **114**:356–71, 1951.

McMurtry, J.G., and Yahr, M.D.: Extracranial carotid occlusion by anomalous digastric muscle. *J. Neurosurg.*, **24**:108–10, 1966.

McMurtry, J.G.; Pool, J.L.; and Nova, H.R.: The use of Rheomacrodex in the surgery of intracranial aneurysms. *J. Neurosurg.*, **26**:218–22, 1967.

Mills, C.M.; Brant-Zawadzki, M.; Crooks, L.E.; Kaufman, L.; Sheldon, P.; Norman, D.; Bank, W.; and Newton, T.H.: Nuclear magnetic resonance: principles of blood flow imaging. *Am. J. Radiol.,* **142**(1):165–70, 1984.

Moniz, E.: L'encephalographie arterielle, son importance dans la localisation des tumors cerebrales. *Rev. Neurol.,* **2**:72, 1927.

Mosher, P.; Ross, J., Jr.; McFate, P.A.; and Shaw, R.F.: Control of coronary blood flow by an autoregulatory mechanism. *Circ. Res.,* **14**:250–59, 1964.

Nornes, H.: The role of the circle of Willis in graded occlusion of the internal carotid artery in man. *Acta Neurochir.* (Wien), **28**:165–77, 1973.

Nornes, H., and Wikeby, P.: Cerebral arterial blood flow and aneurysm surgery. 1. Local arterial flow dynamics. *J. Neurosurg.,* **47**:810–18, 1977.

Overgaard, J., and Tweed, W.A.: Cerebral circulation after head injury. 4. Functional anatomy and boundary-zone flow deprivation. *J. Neurosurg.,* **59**:439–46, 1983.

Payen, D.M.; Levy, B.I.; Menegalli, D.J.; Lajat, Y.I.; Levenson, J.A.; and Nicholas, F.M.: Evaluation of human hemispheric blood flow based on noninvasive carotid blood flow measurements using the range gated Doppler technique. *Stroke,* **13**:392–98, 1982.

Payen, D.M.; Giannotta, S.L.; Kindt, G.W.; McGillicuddy, J.E.; and Prager, R.L.: Treatment of patients with neurological deficits associated with vasospasm by intravascular volume expansion. *Neurosurgery,* **3**:364–68, 1978.

Prosenz, P.; Heiss, W.D.; Tschabitscher, H.; and Ehrmann, L.: The value of regional cerebral blood flow measurements compared to angiography in the assessment of obstructive neck vessel disease. *Stroke,* **5**:19–31, 1974.

Reneman, R.S., and Spencer, M.P.: The functional state of the coronary vascular system after aorto-coronary bypass surgery. In Norman, J.C. (ed.): *Coronary Artery Medicine and Surgery.* Appleton-Century-Crofts, New York, 1975.

Risberg, J., and Smith, P.: Prediction of hemispheric blood flow from carotid velocity measurements. A Study with the Doppler and ^{133}Xe Inhalation techniques. *Stroke,* **11**:399–402, 1980.

Rodbard, S., and Kikuchi, Y.: Arterial stenosis, pressure and flow. *J. Thorac. Cardiovasc. Surg.,* **7**:891–98, 1976.

Rokey, R.; Rolak, L.A.; Harati, Y.; Kutka, N.; and Verani, M.S.: Coronary artery disease in patients with cerebrovascular disease; a prospective study. *Ann. Neurol.,* **16**:50–3, 1984.

Sage, J.L., and VanUitert, R.L.: Risk of recurrent stroke with atrial fibrillation: differences between rheumatic and atherosclerotic heart disease. *Stroke,* **14**:537–40, 1983.

Schroeder, T.; Holstein, P.E.; and Engell, H.C.: Hyperperfusion following endarterectomy. *Stroke,* **15**:758, 1984.

Scotti, G.; Melancon, D.; and Olivier, A.: Hypoglossal paralysis due to compression by a tortuous internal carotid artery in the neck. *Neuroradiology,* **14**:263–65, 1978.

Spetzler, R.F.; Rosli, R.A.; and Zabramski, J.: Middle cerebral artery perfusion pressure in cerebrovascular occlusive disease. *Stroke,* **14**:552–62, 1983.

Sullivan, H.G.; Vines, F.S.; and Becker, D.P.: Sequelae of indirect internal carotid injury. *Radiology,* **109**:91–8, 1973.

Sundt, T.M., Jr.: The ischemic tolerance of neural tissue and the need for monitoring and selective shunting during carotid endarterectomy. *Stroke,* **14**:93–8, 1983.

Sundt, T.M., and Waltz, A.G.: Hemodilution and anticoagulation: effect on the microvasculature and microcirculation of the cerebral cortex after arterial occlusion. *Neurology* (Minneapolis), **17**:230–38, 1967.

Sundt, T.M.; Sharbrough, F.W.; Anderson, R.E.; and Michenfelder, J.D.: Cerebral blood flow measurements and electroencephalograms during carotid endarterectomy. *J. Neurosurg.,* **41**:310–20, 1974.

Tada, K.; Nukada, T.; Yoneda, S.; Kuriyama, Y.; and Abe, H.: Assessment of the capacity of the cerebral collateral circulation using ultrasonic Doppler technique. *J. Neurol. Neurosurg. Psychiatry.,* **38**:1068–75, 1975.

Taki, W.; Handa, H.; Higa, T.; Tanada, K.; Fukuyama, H.; Fujita, T.; Yonekawa, Y.; Kameyama, M.; and Torizuka, K.: Distribution of the blood flow supplied by the vertebral artery in humans as assessed by emission CT. *Stroke,* **15**:469–74, 1984.

Tindall, G.T.; Odom, G.L.; Cupp, H.B., Jr., and Dillon, M.L.: Studies on carotid artery flow and pressure. *J. Neurosurg.,* **19**:917–23, 1962.

Toole, J.F., and McGraw, C.P.: The steal syndromes. *Annu. Rev. Med.,* **26**:321–29, 1975.

Torvik, A.: The pathogenesis of watershed infarcts in the brain. *Stroke,* **15**:221–3, 1984.

VanderArk, G.D., and Pomerantz, M.: Reversal of neurologic signs by increasing the cardiac output. *Surg. Neurol.,* **1**:257–58, 1973.

Wernick, S.; Jerva, M.J.; and Guandique, M.A.: Extrinsic compression of the internal carotid artery by enlarged cervical lymph nodes. *Proc. Inst. Med. Chic.,* **30**:115–16, 1974.

Wilkinson, H.A.; Wright, R.L.; and Sweet, W.H.: Correlation of reduction in pressure and angiographic cross filling with tolerance of carotid occlusion. *J. Neurosurg.,* **22**:241–5, 1965.

Wollschlaeger, G., and Wollschlaeger, P.B.: The circle of Willis. In Newton, T.H., and Potts, D.G. (eds.): *Radiology of the Skull and Brain.* Vol. 2. C.V. Mosby, St. Louis, Missouri, 1974.

Wood, J.H.; Simeone, F.A.; and Snyder, L.L.: Cortical oxygen transport during hypervolemic hemodilutional therapy for focal cerebral ischemia (abstr.). *Neurosurgery,* **10**:781, 1982a.

Wood. J.H.; Simeone, F.A.; Fink, E.A.; and Golden, M.A.: Correlative aspects of hypervolemic hemodilution. Low molecular weight dextran infusions after experimental cerebral artery occlusion. *Neurology (Cleveland),* **34**:24–34, 1984.

Wood, J.H.; Simeone, F.A.; Kron, R.F.; and Litt, M.: Rheological aspects of experimental hypervolemic hemodilution with low molecular weight dextran: relationships of cortical blood flow, cardiac output and intracranial pressure to fresh blood viscosity and plasma volume. *Neurosurgery,* **11**:739–53, 1982b.

Young, D.F.; Cholvin, N.R.; Kirkeeide, R.L.; and Roth, A.C.: Hemodynamics of arterial stenosis at elevated flow rates. *Circ. Res.,* **41**:99–107, 1977.

6

Clinical Manifestations of Cerebral Ischemia

C. STEPHEN FORD and JAMES F. TOOLE

Ischemic cerebrovascular disease is manifested in a great variety of symptoms and signs. In many asymptomatic persons, a bruit heard over the carotid bifurcation or an embolus seen in the retinal vasculature is the only indication of such a potentially life-threatening condition. Others suffer devastating infarctions without previously having had symptoms or signs apparent to even the most astute observer.

The hallmark of symptomatic ischemic cerebrovascular disease is the focal neurologic deficit with an acute onset. Given the usual temporal profile and focal nature of the symptoms, the diagnosis of ischemic cerebrovascular disease is seldom open to question. Ischemic symptoms are maximal within minutes, hours or, very rarely, days of onset. A focal neurologic deficit which progresses steadily over the course of a week or longer is rarely related to ischemic cerebrovascular disease. The temporal profile of ischemia is usually also marked by improvement or resolution of the symptoms after having become maximal. By definition, if the symptoms and signs have resolved completely within 24 hours of onset, the episode is designated a *transient ischemic attack* (TIA). If a focal ischemic deficit persists for longer than 24 hours but resolves within two or three weeks, it is referred to as a *reversible ischemic neurologic deficit* (RIND). Focal ischemic deficits that last longer than three weeks are designated *cerebral infarctions.* Actually, these distinctions are arbitrary and often not helpful in the clinical management of patients. Although the primary significance of TIAs and RINDs lies in their capacity to predict a potentially devastating infarction, small cerebral infarctions often forebode larger, more devastating infarctions. In many ways TIAs, RINDs, and small cerebral infarctions are best considered a continuum of episodes of ischemia, all of which foretell possibly larger, more serious perfusion deficits. Beside a distinctive temporal profile, ischemic cerebrovascular disease also has a characteristic focal manifestation. In general, the underperfused region of brain corresponds to the area supplied by the diseased vessel, but many factors modify the extent of deficit caused by a given vascular lesion. Blood viscosity and oxygen concentration, for example, often play a role in the extent of cerebral infarction. Dehydration or other states of diminished cardiac output may also worsen infarctions. In internal carotid occlusion, collateral arterial supply to the region of ischemia is better if the occlusion develops slowly rather than abruptly and if the external carotid artery and the arteries of the circle of Willis are large and patent.

CLINICAL ARTERIAL SYNDROMES

Internal Carotid Artery

The syndromes of internal carotid artery disease have been described by Toole (1984), Meadows (1983), Marshall (1976), Adams and Victor (1981), and Fisher (1971). Disease of the internal carotid artery may be heralded by fleeting blindness of one eye owing to involvement of the ophthalmic artery, or may be signaled by hemispheric symptoms. Not infrequently, internal carotid occlusion at the level of the sinus is asymptomatic owing to extensive collateral flow through the circle of Willis.

The atheromatous but patent internal carotid origin often presents a greater risk than a completely occluded artery because of the chance of associated emboli. When cerebral infarction does occur in carotid sinus occlusion, the infarction is usually in the middle cerebral and, less frequently, in the anterior cerebral distribution. Occasionally, carotid occlusion induces a watershed infarction affecting the border zone between middle cerebral and anterior or posterior cerebral circulations. Such cases can sometimes be recognized by the presence of transcortical aphasia, in which repetition of spoken sentences is strikingly preserved.

Internal carotid occlusion with extension to the circle of Willis would be expected to cause more severe symptoms. Because of extensive orbital collaterals, persistent visual symptoms are rare in internal carotid occlusion, even when the origin of the ophthalmic artery is involved.

The effects of cessation of middle cerebral arterial blood flow vary with the site of occlusion. Obstruction at the origin is expected to cause infarction not only in the cortex (actually, the cortex is occasionally spared owing to leptomeningeal collaterals), but also in the regions supplied by the lateral striate arteries. The latter areas include part of the globus pallidus, caudate, the internal capsule, and optic radiations. Hemiparesis resulting from occlusion of the middle cerebral artery at its origin commonly affects the leg as well as the arm and face because the pyramidal tract fibers are equally affected in their internal capsular course. Middle cerebral cortical infarction that spares the deep structures, however, causes weakness in the face and arm, but may leave the motor function of the leg relatively unaffected. Middle cerebral stem occlusion may also cause a greater degree of spasticity in the affected extremities than cortical branch disease.

Distinction of the different clinical syndromes resulting from occlusion of the individual cortical branches of the middle cerebral artery is difficult and may not be helpful in serving practical clinical purposes. Neither the precise territories supplied nor the modes of origin of these branches are consistent among individual patients. Usually, however, a middle cerebral artery syndrome can be labeled as either anterior division or posterior division type. Occlusion of the anterior division results in apraxia and/or faciobrachial weakness and sensory loss. If the lesion involves the dominant hemisphere, there is often a Broca's aphasia (nonfluent, agrammatical, effortful, dysarthric speech), or, rarely, mutism or aphemia. Occasionally, after left-sided infarctions in the posterior part of the anterior division territory, patients present with conduction aphasia (fluent, paraphasic speech with good comprehension but markedly impaired repetition).

Infarctions in the distribution of the posterior division of the middle cerebral artery do not usually cause hemiparesis, though involvement of the more anterior and superior branches of the posterior division may occasionally lead to faciobrachial weakness and sensory loss. In the dominant hemisphere, posterior division infarctions affecting the angular gyrus may result in alexia with agraphia or features of the Gerstmann's syndrome (left-right disorientation, finger agnosia, dyscalculia, and agraphia). Infarctions affecting predominantly the posterior part of the superior temporal gyrus of the dominant hemisphere cause Wernicke's aphasia (fluent, paraphasic speech with poor comprehension and repetition).

Posterior division infarctions in the nondominant hemisphere do not generally induce aphasia but instead cause imperception or neglect of the contralateral body and extracorporeal space. This is manifested in a variety of ways. Patients with left hemiplegia may refuse to admit to being ill (anosognosia) or may deny ownership of their left-sided extremities. The abnormality of special perception may also cause difficulties in reproducing geometric figures (constructional apraxia), putting on clothes (dressing apraxia), or in learning directions in unfamiliar surroundings.

Posterior division infarctions often affect the optic radiations. Involvement of the optic radiations in the parietal lobe leads to a hemianopia which may affect predominantly the lower quadrant. Occlusion of the more posterior and inferior branches of the posterior division causes temporal lobe rather than parietal lobe infarction. Accordingly, the associated hemianopia may preferentially affect the superior rather than the inferior quadrant.

The syndrome of the anterior cerebral artery varies depending on the site of occlusion and the preexisting anatomic arterial pattern. The perfusion deficit caused by occlusion of the anterior cerebral artery proximal to the anterior communicating artery usually causes minimal deficit because of collateral flow through the anterior communicating artery. Occasionally, however, both anterior cerebral arteries are supplied by a common stem off the circle of Willis. Occlusion of this common anterior cerebral artery at its origin causes bilateral, extensive infarction. Usually, anterior cerebral artery syndrome occurs after occlusion distal to the anterior communicating artery. The resultant findings include a contralateral hemiparesis and a hemisensory deficit affecting the leg more than the arm. Urinary incontinence and abulia (slowness or lack of spontaneity of reactions) are sometimes seen. Left-sided infarction may cause speech abnormalities, including aphemia, mutism, or transcortical motor aphasia.

Vertebral-Basilar System

The clinical syndromes caused by vertebral-basilar ischemia have been described by Toole (1984), Adams and Victor (1981), Fisher (1971), Caplan (1980; 1981), Currier *et al.* (1961), Adams (1943), Gilman *et al.* (1981), Sypert and Alvord (1975), and Kubik and Adams (1946). Perfusion deficit within the vertebral-basilar circulation can be difficult to distinguish from ischemia occurring within the carotid distribution. Hemiplegia with an associated hemisensory deficit is, of course, the hallmark of ischemia caused by carotid disease; however, these are also often the presenting symptoms of vertebral-basilar disease. In such cases, progression of the deficit to involve both sides may indicate that posterior rather than anterior circulation ischemia is present. Other, more subtle signs and symptoms that may help distinguish vertebral-basilar from carotid ischemia are diplopia, vertigo, cerebellar ataxia, and deafness. Hemiplegia on one side of the body and cranial nerve signs on the opposite side (the so-called crossed or alternating hemiplegia) almost always indicate brain-stem disease. Likewise, a sensory deficit for pain and temperature which involves one side of the body and the opposite side of the face (the so-called crossed sensory deficit) is also characteristic of brain-stem pathology.

Atherosclerotic occlusion of the vertebral artery most commonly occurs at its origin where it is relatively benign because of collateral flow from the contralateral vertebral artery. Anastomotic channels from the thyrocervical, occipital, and deep cervical arteries also supply important collateral flow to the distal segment of the proximally occluded vertebral artery. It is notable that in 10 percent of the population, one of the vertebral arteries is so hypoplastic that it can be regarded as nonfunctional. Naturally, vertebral artery occlusion has more serious consequences when it occurs opposite such a hypoplastic vertebral. Vertebral artery occlusion is also more symptomatic when it occurs distally, especially if it involves paramedian and long circumferential branches or extends into the basilar artery.

Vertebral artery occlusion may lead to a variety of syndromes. If collateral flow from the opposite vertebral and both posterior communicating arteries is poor, the clinical presentation may be that of basilar artery occlusion. Vertebral artery occlusion also often causes cerebellar infarction, lateral medullary infarction, and, less frequently, medial medullary infarction.

The medial medullary syndrome results from cessation of flow in either of the two vertebral arteries or from occlusion of a paramedial penetrating branch of the vertebral or basilar artery. The resulting clinical syndrome consists of contralateral hemiplegia with impaired light touch and proprioceptive sensation with ipsilateral hypoglossal palsy.

The lateral medullary syndrome is also known as the syndrome of the posterior inferior cerebellar artery, even though it is caused by posterior inferior cerebellar artery occlusion in only 20 percent of cases and is associated with vertebral artery occlusion in 80 percent of the patients. The syndrome, produced by infarction of the dorsolateral medulla, is characterized by decreased sensation to pain and temperature over the opposite body half and the ipsilateral face. Dysphagia and dysarthria owing to damage to the ninth and tenth cranial nerves of the same side and vertigo due to involvement of the vestibular nucleus are some of the prominent symptoms. There is usually also ipsilateral appendicular ataxia caused by ischemia of the inferior cerebellar peduncle and ipsilateral Horner's syndrome owing to involvement of the descending sympathetic tract. Less frequent findings include hiccups and ipsilateral loss of taste.

In the lateral medullary syndrome, there is often some softening of the inferior aspect of the ipsilateral cerebellar hemisphere which is usually of little clinical significance. The subtle signs it may cause are masked by the more striking cerebellar signs owing to involvement of the ipsilateral inferior cerebellar peduncle. Vertebral artery occlusion on occasion, however, causes infarction primarily of the cerebellar hemisphere, sparing the dorsolateral medulla. Vertebral artery occlusion is, in fact, the most common cause of cerebellar infarction. The resultant clinical syndrome is distinctive but is often mistaken for a labyrinthine disorder. Patients with cerebellar infarction present with complaints of headache, difficulty with walking, dizziness, vertigo, nausea, and vomiting. Initial signs include truncal ataxia, ipsilateral gaze-evoked nystagmus and gaze-paresis, and ipsilateral appendicular ataxia. As time passes, the infarcted cerebellar hemisphere may become edematous, and brain-stem compression can occur. Hemiplegia, quadriplegia, and palsies of cranial nerves V through X may be seen as the result. The patient may even die, from extensive brain-stem infarction, obstructive hydrocephalus, tonsillar herniation, or ascending transtentorial herniation.

Basilar artery stenosis and occlusion present with variable findings, depending on the position and extent of the occlusion. Basilar artery thrombosis characteristically presents with pinpoint pupils, quadriplegia, and coma progressing to death. Less severe cases of basilar occlusion may develop with any combination of hemiplegia or quadriplegia, pseudobulbar palsy, vertigo, dizziness, ataxia, diminished consciousness, paresthesias, visual field deficits, and palsies of cranial nerves III through VIII. Occasionally, syndromes of isolated basilar branch occlusions may be recognized. Paramedian basilar branch occlusion can be diagnosed in patients with an ipsilateral abducens palsy, contralateral hemiplegia, and contralateral diminished light touch and proprioceptive sensation.

Clinical syndromes caused by occlusion of the anterior inferior and superior cerebellar arteries depend largely upon their size and the extent of collateral flow. The size of the area supplied by the anterior inferior cerebellar artery varies inversely with that perfused by the posterior inferior cerebellar artery. Anterior inferior cerebellar artery occlusion usually produces a syndrome identical to the lateral medullary syndrome except for the additional features of ipsilateral facial weakness and deafness. Occlusion of the superior cerebellar artery causes an ipsilateral Horner's syndrome, ipsilateral limb dystaxia with chorea, and contralateral decrease of pain and thermal sensation over the body and the face. Contralateral central facial weakness and partial deafness may also occur.

Recognition of a "top of the basilar" syndrome is useful because terminal basilar occlusion is usually caused by embolism, whereas lower basilar occlusion is commonly induced by atherothrombosis. The "top of the basilar" syndrome is characterized by visual, oculomotor, and behavioral abnormalities. Although hemiplegia or quadriplegia owing to involvement of the cerebral peduncles may occur, motor deficits are usually not prominent. Patients with such a syndrome are often agitated, even delirious, sometimes with formed visual hallucinations. Other behavioral abnormalities include somnolence, apathy, and amnesia. Homonymous hemianopia owing to occipital lobe infarction is common in "top of the basilar" syndrome. Bilateral occipital lobe infarction may cause complete or partial blindness, of which the patient is occasionally unaware. Oculomotor deficits seen include ptosis, skew deviation, third-nerve palsy, pupillary abnormalities, hyperconvergence, and disorders of vertical gaze.

LACUNAR INFARCTION

Lacunar infarctions are small subcortical strokes which, because of their unique pathogenesis, are distinct from other types of cerebral infarction. They account for up to 19 percent of all strokes. Though the maximum size of the lacunae has not been definitely established, most investigators consider their range to be from 2 to 15 mm in diameter. Some investigators, however, have included infarctions up to 35 mm in diameter (Fisher and Curry, 1965) within this category. Lacunar infarctions usually result from lipohyalinosis of small cerebral arteries from 20 to 400 μm in diameter usually associated with hypertension and diabetes. Arteries commonly involved include paramedian brain-stem branches of the basilar artery, lenticulostriate, and thalamoperforating arteries. Lacunar infarction is thus distinct from other cerebral infarctions, which are most commonly related to either cardiac emboli or atherosclerosis of larger arteries (Fisher, 1965; Miller, 1983). Victims of lacunar infarction have a past history of hypertension in 60 to 97 percent and diabetes in 11 percent of cases (Kase *et al.*, 1981). The most common sites of lacunar infarction in order of frequency are the lenticular nucleus, basis pontis, thalamus, caudate nucleus, and internal capsule (Miller, 1983). Lacunae are notably scarce in the cerebral and cerebellar hemispheres.

Just as the pathogenesis of lacunar infarction is distinct, so is its clinical presentation. A large proportion of lacunar infarctions are asymptomatic. When symptomatic, however, the stroke syndrome is remarkable for its lack of aphasia, visual field defects, and mental changes (Kase *et al.*, 1981). The prognosis for recovery in lacunar infarction is much better than that in cortical infarction, but the risk of recurrence is high.

Fisher (1965) described four stroke syndromes that are sufficiently unique to lacunar infarctions that the diagnosis at least can be suspected on clinical grounds alone. These four syndromes to be discussed are pure motor hemiparesis, pure sensory stroke, ataxic hemiparesis, and dysarthria–clumsy-hand syndrome. Since Fisher's initial description, he and other investigators have proposed additional lacunar syndromes, such as hemichorea (Kase *et al.*, 1981), pure dysarthria (Caplan, 1976), unilateral asterixis (Massey *et al.*, 1979), pure motor hemiparesis with contralateral gaze paresis (Fisher, 1971), and sensory motor stroke (Mohr *et al.*, 1977). None of these syndromes, however, has acquired as broad acceptance as have Fisher's original four categories (Miller, 1983). Although these four syndromes are highly suggestive of lacunar infarction, they are not absolutely diagnostic. The most common of the four syndromes, i.e., pure motor hemiparesis, has also been reported in association with cortical infarctions, intracerebral hematomas, metastatic tumors, subdural hematomas, and multiple sclerosis (Weisberg, 1979). Still, differentiating clinically between lacunar and cortical infarction is important, because the best treatment for the two conditions often differs.

Pure motor hemiparesis (Fisher and Curry, 1965) occurs in lacunar infarction of the contralateral basis pontis, internal capsule, or pyramid. The clinical findings consist of weakness affecting the face, arm, and leg, frequently in association with dysarthria. Although lacunae may present with weakness of one extremity, monoparesis as a pathognomonic symptom does not qualify because it is not as localizing or specific as is pure motor hemiplegia (Miller, 1983). Occasionally, patients with pure motor hemiplegia report sensory symptoms, but physical examination fails to reveal objective sensory abnormalities. A mild gaze paresis and nystagmus are rare accompaniments.

Pure sensory stroke (Fisher, 1978) results from infarction of the contralateral ventroposterior thalamic nuclei. The syndrome consists of paresthesias without weakness affecting the arm, leg, and usually also the face.

Ataxic hemiparesis (Fisher and Cole, 1965; Fisher, 1978), also known as the syndrome of "homolateral ataxia and crural paresis," is caused by infarction of the contralateral internal capsule or basis pontis. Clinical findings consist of hemiparesis affecting the leg more than the arm and ataxia of the same side. Although patients may occasionally report paresthesias, objective sensory findings are absent.

The dysarthria-clumsy-hand syndrome (Fisher, 1967) also occurs in infarctions of the contralateral internal capsule or basis pontis. The features are dysarthria and ataxia of one side, affecting the arm more than the leg. Facial weakness and extensor plantar responses may be seen on the affected side, but the sensory examination is normal.

TRANSIENT ISCHEMIC ATTACKS

Transient ischemic attacks (TIAs) are defined as episodes of focal neurologic dysfunction caused by ischemia that resolve completely within 24 hours. About 70 percent of TIAs last less than ten minutes (Fisher, 1976), and almost all TIAs resolve within six to eight hours (Pessin *et al.*, 1977).

By the definition of TIA, a patient presenting with a persistent focal neurologic deficit with a presumed vascular etiology could not be diagnosed as having a cerebral infarction until 24 hours had elapsed after the onset of the deficit. In practice, however, because TIAs usually present with mild deficits that last only minutes, distinguishing between a cerebral infarction and a TIA does not require such prolonged observation. Patients with severe hemiplegia which has not improved within an hour or two can usually be safely presumed to have a cerebral infarction rather than a TIA.

The focal neurologic abnormality of TIA is almost necessarily a "negative" dysfunction of that region of the brain. "Positive" phenomena, such as scintillating scotomata or tonic-clonic activity of an extremity, suggest a different pathogenetic mechanism and are only very rarely considered symptoms of TIA.

The definition of TIA also includes a provision that the focal neurologic deficit is due to ischemia. It is well documented that cerebral tumors, arteriovenous malformations, and even systemic abnormalities such as hypoglycemia can present with symptoms of transient focal neurologic deficit virtually identical to TIA. Such transient focal neurologic events are not appropriately classified as TIAs. Nonischemic causes of transient focal deficits must be excluded in every patient in whom the diagnosis of TIA is considered.

The neurologic dysfunction of TIA is said to be "focal," implying that only a circumscribed region of the brain is affected. The region of ischemia of TIA, however, need not be in the brain proper, for episodic monocular blindness (amaurosis fugax) owing to ischemia of the retina or optic nerve has, by common agreement, been classified as a TIA. Ideally, the focal nature of the symptoms of TIA should enable the clinician to name the small branch artery affected. While this is possible sometimes, more often it is not and the clinician can divide the symptoms only into a vertebral-basilar versus a left carotid or right carotid distribution. Even this distinction can be difficult in some cases (see Table 6–1).

Because the symptoms of TIA are said to be "focal," episodes of isolated syncope and/or dizziness are usually excluded. Syncope and dizziness owing to ischemia are much more frequently caused by global cerebral ischemia, such as seen in cardiac arrhythmias and postural hypotension. Still, many neurologists have seen rare patients with vertebral-basilar TIAs who, through involvement of the reticular activating system, had diminished consciousness as a manifestation of their TIAs. Almost all of these patients, however, also have other, more clearly focal neurologic symptoms associated with their episodes.

Table 6–1. Symptoms of Transient Ischemic Attacks (TIAs) Among 158 Patients by Arterial Distribution

	CAROTID	VERTEBRAL-BASILAR
Vertigo	12	48
Tinnitus	—	1
Visual field disturbance	14	22
Diplopia	—	7
Dysarthria	—	11
Facial paresthesiae	4	2
Drop attacks	—	16
Hemiparesis	31	8
Monoparesis	7	4
Hemianesthesia	33	9
Confusion	5	1
Dysphasia	20	—

From Marshall, J.: The natural history of transient ischemic cerebrovascular attacks. *Q. J. Med.*, **33**:309–24, 1964, with permission.

The possible connection between episodes of altered mentation and TIAs poses a difficult question. It is well established that a state of chronic dementia can result from multiple, recurrent focal infarctions (Hackinski *et al.*, 1975; Mayer-Gross *et al.*, 1969; Loeb and Gandolfo, 1983). There have also been several reports of improvement in postoperative neuropsychological testing in patients who have undergone carotid endarterectomy (Kelly *et al.*, 1980; Goldstein *et al.*, 1970; Perry *et al.*, 1975) or superficial temporal to middle cerebral artery bypass surgery (Gur *et al.*, 1983) [see also Chapter 23]. In general, however, acute episodes of confusion very rarely have a focal vascular etiology. Acute confusional states are much more frequently caused by metabolic encephalopathies, intoxication, withdrawal states, infection, head trauma, or postictal states (Adams and Victor, 1981). The astute clinician, however, must keep in mind a number of vascular syndromes which indeed may present with confusion. Amnesia without any other disorder of cortical function is sometimes seen in patients with lesions of both or, rarely, one medial temporal lobe or dorsal medial thalamic nucleus. Acute confusional states and delirium have also been reported as the dominant clinical features in infarctions in many different vascular distributions, including the anterior cerebral (Amyes and Nielson, 1955; Hyland, 1933), posterior cerebral (Horenstein *et al.*, 1967; Medina *et al.*, 1974), and right middle cerebral (Mesulam *et al.*, 1976) arteries. In such cases, associated physical findings and neuropsychological tests almost always establish the diagnosis of such vascular syndromes. Evaluating a history of a transient acute state of confusion after the episode has resolved, however, is infinitely more difficult. It is possible that many TIAs with the predominant symptom of confusion are misdiagnosed, but as a rule episodic confusion without other focal symptoms or signs is most appropriately considered a symptom of global cerebral dysfunction, not a symptom of TIA.

Table 6-2. Isolated Symptoms Not to be Considered TIA*

1. Altered consciousness or syncope
2. Dizziness, wooziness, or giddiness
3. Impaired vision associated with alteration of consciousness ("gray out")
4. Amnesia alone
5. Confusion alone
6. Tonic and/or clonic motor activity
7. March of motor and/or sensory deficits
8. Vertigo alone, with or without nausea or vomiting
9. Diplopia alone
10. Focal symptoms associated with migraine headache
11. Scintillating scotomata
12. Dysphagia alone
13. Dysarthria alone
14. Bowel or bladder incontinence

* Symptoms most often noted in patients without cerebrovascular disease, according to the Study Group on TIA Criteria and Detection of the Joint Committee for Stroke Facilities. Adapted, with permission, from the American Heart Association, Inc.

From Heyman, A.; Leviton, A.; Millikan, C.H.; *et al.:* Transient focal cerebral ischemia: epidemiological and clinical aspects. *Stroke,* **5**:277-287. 1974, with permission.

Many focal neurologic symptoms are rarely seen in isolation in TIAs, but are common in other nonischemic diseases. Therefore, they are traditionally not accepted as diagnostic for TIAs (see Table 6-2). The Study Group on TIA Criteria and Detection (Heyman *et al.,* 1974) thus urged that the transient occurrence of diplopia, dysphagia, or dysarthria, when presenting as an isolated symptom, should not be considered a manifestation of a TIA. For the same reason, isolated vertigo with or without nausea or vomiting and isolated bowel or bladder incontinence should also not be considered manifestations of TIA. The same study group also pointed out that certain features of some transient focal neurologic episodes suggest a different etiology than that of TIA. Thus, scintillating scotomata or any focal symptoms associated with migraine headaches should not be classified as manifestations of TIA. Episodes in which there is a gradual spread of motor and/or sensory symptoms consecutively over contiguous parts of one side of the body (a "march" of symptoms) are more likely to be migrainous accompaniments or partial seizures, not TIAs. Bilateral impairment of vision, when associated with an alteration of consciousness, should suggest global cerebral ischemia, not TIA. These recommendations regarding TIA symptoms are intended as general guidelines. Symptoms in individual patients, however, do not necessarily conform to such rules. Interpretation of individual histories, therefore, requires practiced judgment.

Prognosis of Transient Ischemic Attacks

The occurrence of TIAs is a predictor of subsequent cerebral infarction. Reports on the frequency with which patients with TIAs develop cerebral infarction vary greatly. The consensus, however, is that about one third of patients with TIAs will have infarctions within five years. This risk is unrelated to the age, sex, or race of the patient. TIAs in the distribution of a carotid artery are generally thought especially ominous predictors of subsequent infarction whereas vertebral-basilar TIAs usually run a more benign course (Toole, 1984).

In patients with TIAs who later have infarctions, the time between the onset of the TIAs and the subsequent infarction is usually brief (see Figure 6-1) with about 36 percent of the infarctions occurring within the first month after the onset of TIAs, and about 50 percent of the infarctions occurring within the first year (Toole, 1984). Furthermore, cerebral infarction usually happens after only a few TIAs. In most cases of cerebral infarction following TIAs, fewer than four TIAs precede the infarction (Wolf *et al.,* 1983). These data reinforce the significance of TIAs and suggest that TIAs are medical emergencies requiring immediate evaluation and prompt treatment. Patients with histories of one or two TIAs cannot be

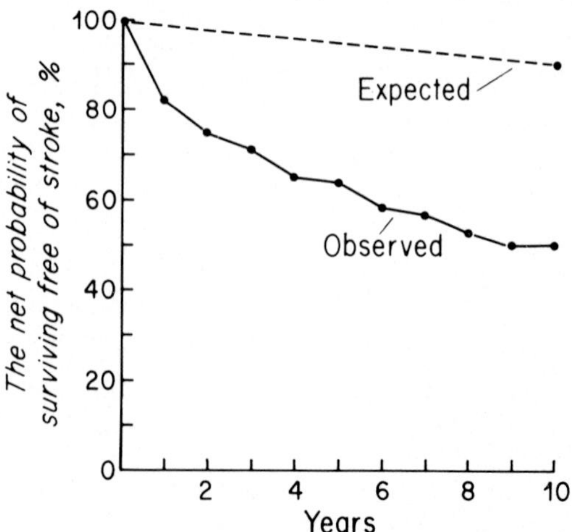

Figure 6-1. The conditional probability of surviving free of stroke after a first transient ischemic attack. Solid line: patients with TIA; dashed line: patients without TIA. Note the high incidence of stroke within the first year of TIA. (From Whisnant, J.P., Matsumoto, N.; and Elveback, L.R.: Transient cerebral ischemic attacks in a community: Rochester, Minnesota, 1955 through 1969. *Mayo Clin. Proc.,* **48**:194-198, 1973, with permission.)

observed safely to see whether they will have another TIA.

Beside being a predictor of subsequent cerebral infarction, TIAs are also indicators of more generalized atherosclerotic disease. Patients with TIAs are at strong risk of developing myocardial infarction. In fact, patients with TIAs die from heart attack twice as often as they die from cerebral infarction (Cartilidge *et al.*, 1977; Toole *et al.*, 1978). Aggressive evaluation for possible coronary artery disease is, therefore, indicated in all patients with TIAs.

THE ETIOLOGY OF TIA AND CEREBRAL INFARCTION

TIAs and infarctions occur whenever there is a temporary discrepancy between the metabolic requirements of neurons and the available supply of nutrients furnished by the circulation. Although almost all ischemic events are related to a vascular abnormality, the immediate cause can usually be determined as either hemodynamic or embolic. Hemodynamic TIAs are induced by hypoperfusion owing to an insufficient pressure gradient. More often, TIAs are caused by emboli from an atherosclerotic plaque in the carotid bifurcation or from an abnormal heart valve or chamber. TIAs with a hemodynamic etiology tend to be less abrupt in onset than embolic TIAs (Denny-Brown, 1960; Ross Russell, 1983). Some hemodynamic TIAs may occur in association with neck turning or neck extension because one or both vertebral arteries may be compressed by osteophytes, intervertebral disks, or fibrous bands in such maneuvers, compromising an already marginal blood supply. Hemodynamic TIAs, in contrast to embolic TIAs, are also prone to occur during periods of diminished cardiac output, such as postural hypotension, Valsalva maneuvers, and cardiac arrhythmias (Ross Russell, 1983).

Atherosclerosis

Atherosclerosis is the major cause of both TIAs and cerebral infarctions. Atherosclerotic plaques cause hemodynamic TIAs by obstructing arterial lumina and impeding the normal flow of blood. They may also cause embolic TIAs by providing a nidus for the aggregation of platelets and for the activation of the coagulation cascade (see also Chapter 16). The most common site for atherosclerotic plaques in the cerebral circulation is at the carotid bifurcation. Atherosclerosis also frequently occurs at the origins of the common carotids and in the osseous, cavernous, and intradural portions of the internal carotids. Vertebral-basilar atherosclerosis is most frequent in the origins and intraspinous portions of the vertebrals, but vertebral-basilar atherosclerosis tends to be more diffuse than carotid system atherosclerosis. Arteriolosclerosis or lipohyalinosis of small arteries (with diameters less than 400 μm) also is a common cause of both TIAs and infarction, particularly lacunar infarction.

Cardiac Causes

Over the past several decades, there has been a growing realization of the importance of cardiac causes of ischemic cerebrovascular disease. Previously, cardiac causes were felt to account for only 3 percent of cerebral infarctions (Whisnant *et al.*, 1973). Recent estimates range as high as 20 to 34 percent (Barnett, 1983) with most of these cases related to cardiogenic emboli. Whether the heart or atherothrombotic plaques of the carotid arteries are the more common source of cerebral emboli is still debated (Ross Russell, 1983; McGhee and Toole, 1982).

Emboli from the heart are pathophysiologically and clinically different from those originating from a carotid plaque. Although hyperaggregability of platelets and platelet activation play a prominent role in atherosclerotic cerebrovascular disease, in cardiogenic cerebrovascular disease platelet function may be normal and local hemodynamic alterations are felt to be more important factors (Uchiyama *et al.*, 1983). Emboli originating from heart valves and chambers are generally larger than those formed on atherosclerotic plaques. Cardiac emboli tend to lodge in and occlude larger arteries, such as the middle cerebral artery bifurcation and carotid artery junction within the circle of Willis. Artery-to-artery emboli, in contradistinction, usually block the more distal leptomeningeal branches of the cerebral circulation (Blackwood *et al.*, 1969; Soloway and Aronson, 1964) which have diameters less than 100 μm (Soloway and Aronson, 1964). These pathophysiologic differences between cardiac and atheromatous emboli are paralleled by dissimilarities in their clinical presentations. Cerebral emboli from the heart are more likely to cause infarction than TIA (Pessin *et al.,* 1977). When cardiogenic emboli do cause TIAs, the TIAs tend to last longer; hence, TIAs of several minutes' duration are likely to result from artery-to-artery embolism, whereas those lasting longer than one hour are very likely to result from cardiac embolism (Pessin *et al.,* 1977). Of course, associated carotid bruits or Hollenhorst plaques in the appropriate ocular fundi strongly suggest an atherosclerotic origin.

Although these differences in the general clinical presentation of atherosclerotic versus cardiogenic emboli are significant, they offer an uncertain differential diagnostic clue in any one particular patient. Cardiogenic emboli, though usually large, can also be small and present with a fleeting ischemic episode. Likewise, atheromatous emboli can on occasion be quite large. Coexisting clinical features of cardiac disease are fortunately more helpful. No clinical criteria unequivocally separate cardiac embolic events from atherosclerotic ones; however, the following clinical features, ranked in order of importance according to Barnett (1983), are strongly suggestive of cardiac embolic disease:

1. Symptoms, signs, or computed tomographic (CT) findings of emboli in multiple arterial distributions in the brain are present. The reverse of this rule is not necessarily true; that is, recurrent episodes of ischemia in an isolated arterial distribution are not necessarily of noncardiac etiology. Balloon catheters inserted into the carotid artery have been shown to be guided repeatedly by laminar flow to the same arterial branches (Gacs *et al.,* 1982).
2. The patient is under the age at which atherosclerosis commonly occurs.
3. The patient has a previous history of a cardiac disease that might resonably be considered a cause of cardiac emboli.
4. A cardiac disease that might cause emboli is identified by history or physical or by appropriate imaging and monitoring.
5. Angiography shows occlusion of the middle cerebral or posterior cerebral arteries or their major branches without evidence of concomitant atherosclerosis.
6. CT scan demonstrates hemorrhagic infarction (less common in thrombotic infarction).
7. There is clinical evidence of extracerebral, systemic embolization.
8. A cardiac cause of cerebral infarction is more likely if the deficit occurs abruptly without previous TIAs.

The cardiac diseases that have been associated with cerebral embolism are many. Rheumatic heart disease and coronary atherosclerosis have been said to account for the overwhelming majority of adult cases of cardiac emboli (Easton and Sherman, 1980), but with the declining incidence of rheumatic heart disease, this conception may change in the future.

Myocardial Infarction. Embolization of mural thrombus is the most common cause of cerebral infarction in association with myocardial infarction. Factors predisposing to embolization in acute myocardial infarction include the size of the infarction, involvement of the septum, associated congestive heart failure, and atrial fibrillation (Barnett, 1983; Easton and Sherman, 1980). The incidence of such emboli peaks during the second week, and 84 percent of all such emboli occur within the first month (Bean, 1938). In patients in whom there is a concomitant appearance of both cerebral and myocardial infarction, aortic dissection with occlusion of both the coronary ostia and great cerebral vessels must be considered. Cardiac dysrhythmias with associated cerebral hypoperfusion may also account for some of the cerebral infarctions seen early after myocardial infarction. In cerebral infarctions that occur more than one month after the occurrence of a myocardial infarction, the formation of a left ventricular aneurysm as the nest for thrombus formation must be suspected.

Rheumatic Heart Disease. Rheumatic heart disease commonly causes mitral stenosis and insufficiency, either of which may cause embolic disease (Barnett, 1983). Rheumatic lesions of the aortic valve are also common but probably do not cause emboli (McGhee and Toole, 1982). The subgroup of patients with mitral stenosis, left atrial enlargement, and atrial fibrillation is especially prone to cerebral embolization, having an incidence 17 times greater than that of the general population (Easton and Sherman, 1980; Wolf *et al.,* 1978). Whether rheumatic mitral stenosis without atrial fibrillation predisposes for embolization is debated (Easton and Sherman, 1980).

Atrial Fibrillation. Whether of rheumatic, arteriosclerotic, or unknown origin, atrial fibrillation predisposes to cerebral emboli, particularly when the atrial rhythm is changing, as in intermittent atrial fibrillation or in patients undergoing cardioversion (Toole, 1984).

Prosthetic Heart Valves. Prosthetic mitral and aortic valves can cause emboli, probably owing to turbulent flow, stasis, injury to blood components, and thrombosis at the junction of the valve with endocardium (Toole, 1984).

Cardiomyopathy. Cardiomyopathies, especially idiopathic and alcoholic cardiomyopathies, are associated with an increased incidence of cerebral embolism. Concomitant congestive heart failure or arrhythmia makes embolism particularly likely (Easton and Sherman, 1980).

Bacterial Endocarditis. Emboli associated with subacute bacterial endocarditis (SBE) most commonly manifest in infarction, but meningitis, subarachnoid hemorrhage, and toxic encephalopathy may also occur in SBE. Acute bacterial endocarditis can cause, in addition, multiple brain abscesses (Toole, 1984). Because valvulopathies are prone to develop endocarditis, their embolic potential is further enhanced.

Nonbacterial Thrombotic Endocarditis. Nonbacterial thrombotic endocarditis (NBTE) as a cause of cerebral embolism is being recognized with increasing frequency. The diagnosis of this condition is, however, exceedingly difficult to establish because associated carcinomas are present in less than half the patients, and cardiac murmurs are heard in only one third (Biller *et al.*, 1982). Antecedent valvular disease may predispose to the development of NBTE, which may then serve as a nidus for the development of SBE (McGhee and Toole, 1982; Biller *et al.*, 1982). The vegetations are so small that B-mode echocardiography usually fails to detect them. Associated thrombophlebitis or disseminated intravascular coagulation is often a clinical clue to NBTE as a cause of cerebral embolism (Biller *et al.*, 1982).

Prolapsing Mitral Valve. Prolapsing mitral valve occurs in 6 to 8 percent of the general population but is present 4.5 times as often in patients under the age of 45 who have cerebral infarctions (Barnett, 1983). Cardiac symptoms are not usually prominent in patients with mitral valve prolapse. Most patients who have strokes have been previously unaware of any heart disease. Embolism in mitral valve prolapse is not usually associated with arrhythmia. Occasionally, however, cerebral ischemic symptoms occur in conjunction with atrial fibrillation. Prolapsing mitral valve should be suspected in young patients with cerebral ischemia who have decreased anteroposterior diameter of the chest, scoliosis, or pectus excavatum (Barnett, 1983).

Left Atrial Myxoma. Up to one third of patients with left atrial myxoma present with symptoms of cerebral embolism. Beside cerebral embolism, atrial myxomas also present with symptoms of outflow obstruction and heart failure or with systemic symptoms, such as malaise, weight loss, lethargy, and fever. Helpful clues to the diagnosis of myxoma include the presence of anemia, leukocytosis, elevated erythrocyte sedimentation rate, and elevated serum and cerebrospinal fluid levels of gamma globulin (McGhee and Toole, 1982).

Other Cardiac Causes. Mitral annulus calcification probably accounts for many of the cerebral emboli in the elderly, but its significance is always difficult to assess because in the elderly persons in whom it occurs there are usually other possible causes of cerebral ischemia, most notably atherosclerosis. Mitral annulus calcification is the most frequent cause of systolic murmurs in the elderly. Calcific or platelet emboli to the retina are sometimes seen. Calcific aortic stenosis frequently causes syncope and other symptoms of global cerebral hypoperfusion but only very rarely causes cerebral embolism (Barnett, 1983). Cardiac decompensation of any cause can of itself lead to pulmonary venostasis with resultant thrombosis and embolism. Paradoxical embolus must be considered in any patient who presents with cerebral embolism associated with deep venous thrombosis. A patent foramen ovale or atrial or ventricular septal defect is the usual passageway through which venous emboli enter the cerebral circulation. Embolization of air, thrombi, and calcific material also occurs in the course of cardiac surgery. Cerebral emboli have also been reported as an uncommon complication in Libman-Sacks endocarditis.

Nonatherosclerotic Arterial Diseases

Nonatherosclerotic diseases of the cerebral arteries are relatively uncommon but must be considered as causes of ischemic symptoms, especially in young patients.

Fibromuscular Dysplasia. Fibromuscular dysplasia is a disease usually occurring in women in which there are alternate segments of stenosis and ectasia of arteries, giving the angiographic picture of a "string of beads" appearance. Various arteries throughout the body can be affected, including the internal carotid and vertebral arteries. The mean age of diagnosis for the cephalic disease is 58 years. One third of patients with fibromuscular dysplasia of the cerebral vasculature are asymptomatic; two thirds have neurologic symptoms. Neurologic symptoms are usually related to ischemia from hemodynamic compromise, spontaneous dissection, or thromboembolism, but may also result from subarachnoid hemorrhage from associated intracranial berry aneurysms (So *et al.*, 1981; Corrin *et al.*, 1981) [see also Chapter 17].

Aortic Arch Syndrome. Aortic arch syndrome (also known as "pulseless disease") is associated with many different arterial pathologies in which there is gradual occlusion of the vessels originating from the aortic arch. The syndrome usually evolves over several years before there are cerebral symptoms. The symptoms of pulseless disease are often related to focal or generalized cerebral ischemia, but may also be related to ischemia of the face, jaw musculature, or eyes (See also Chapters 28 and 29).

Moya-Moya. *Moya-Moya* (meaning "puff of smoke") *disease* refers to the characteristic angiographic appearance of a pseudoangioma composed of multiple small collateral channels bypassing an obstruction of the terminal carotid. The disease usually occurs in infants and young adults, especially among the Japanese. Consequences of Moya-Moya disease include cerebral infarction, seizures, mental retardation, and subarachnoid or intracerebral hemorrhage.

Other Nonatherosclerotic Vascular Diseases. Other causes of nonatherosclerotic cerebrovascular disease are numerous. Occasionally, thrombosis or occlusion of large cerebral vessels can be related to prior radiation exposure. Chronic or acute infections within the subarachnoid space are often associated with thrombosis of the basal portions of the cerebral circulation. Giant-cell arteritis has also been mentioned as a rare cause of cerebral infarction. Vasculitis associated with polyarteritis nodosa, systemic lupus erythematosus, rheumatoid arthritis, and scleroderma usually affect small arteries, but on occasion may involve large cerebral arteries, resulting in infarction. Intravenous drug abuse and trauma to the extracranial cerebral vessels can sometimes lead to cerebral infarction. Transient emboligenic aortoarteritis, thromboangiitis obliterans, and Behcet's disease account for other TIAs and infarctions.

Hematologic Abnormalities

Polycythemia. Polycythemia is clearly associated with cerebral infarction, whether the polycythemia is primary or secondary. Even spurious polycythemia (also known as stress polycythemia, relative polycythemia, apparent polycythemia, or pseudopolycythemia) clearly increases the risk of cerebral infarction. Furthermore, data from the Framingham study show that cerebral infarction is more common in those with high-normal hematocrits than in those with normal or low-normal hematocrits (Wolf *et al.*, 1983). Polycythemia predisposes to stroke by several mechanisms. Cerebral blood flow is decreased in almost all forms of polycythemia. Though it can be argued that the decreased blood flow is compensated (counterbalanced) by an increased oxygen-carrying capacity of polycythemic blood, sluggish blood flow is by itself probably conducive to coagulation and thrombogenesis. Polycythemia is probably also associated with enhanced platelet function, either because the platelets are forced to the periphery of the polycythemic column of blood, allowing for more platelet-vessel wall interaction, or because the platelets are activated by increased red blood cell adenosine diphosphate (ADP). Of course, many cases of polycythemia rubra vera are associated with thrombocytosis, with its resultant thrombotic tendency.

Paraproteinemia. Paraproteinemias are associated with both ischemic and hemorrhagic cerebrovascular complications. Curiously, the ischemic type tends to affect the vertebral-basilar circulation in preference to the carotid circulation. Cerebral ischemia in paraproteinemias is related to plasma hyperviscosity and can sometimes be aggravated by blood transfusions given to correct the associated anemia.

Thrombocytosis. Thrombocytosis is also associated with both ischemic and hemorrhagic cerebrovascular complications. Paradoxically, bleeding is more likely when platelet counts exceed abnormally elevated. Thrombosis is more common in cases which develop after splenectomy and in cases associated with polycythemia.

Other Hematologic Causes. Leukemia is more often associated with bleeding than thrombosis thus is rarely a cause of infarction.

Sickle-cell disease, hyperfibrinogenemia, oral contraceptive use, and paroxysmal nocturnal hemoglobinuria are also associated with cerebral infarction.

ASYMPTOMATIC CAROTID BRUITS

Frequently, patients without a previous history of cerebral infarction or TIA are found to have a bruit over the cervical carotid artery. Usually these asymptomatic carotid bruits indicate stenosis of the origin of the internal carotid artery. Patients with asymptomatic carotid bruits are two to three times more likely to have a stroke than age-matched patients without carotid bruits (Wolf *et al.*, 1981). In view of the fact that cerebral infarction is preceded by TIA in only 10 to 30 percent of cases (Kubik and Adams, 1946; Heyman *et al.*, 1974; Wolf *et al.*, 1983), it seems logical that listening for carotid bruits would be a good way of screening asymptomatic patients for possible prophylactic treatment against stroke.

Epidemiological studies of patients with asymptomatic bruits, however, have revealed the following limitations to this reasoning:

1. Although the occurrence of an asymptomatic carotid bruit does correlate with an increased risk of stroke, there is no correlation between the side of the bruit and the vascular distribution of the subsequent stroke (Wolf *et al.*, 1981; Heyman *et al.*, 1980). If carotid endarterectomy were the treatment recommended for asymptomatic carotid stenosis, presumably many strokes would not be prevented by treatment anyway.
2. Many investigators contend that most patients with asymptomatic carotid bruits who later have symptoms of cerebral ischemia have a TIA rather than infarction as the initial symptom (Durwood *et al.*, 1982). Therefore, in most patients with asymptomatic carotid bruits who are destined to have cerebral infarction, the danger of impending cerebral infarction is signaled by a TIA.
3. A bruit over the carotid bifurcation does not always imply severe stenosis of the internal carotid artery. Accordingly, not all patients with asymptomatic carotid artery bruits are at equal risk of having a cerebral infarction. Technological improvements in ultrasonic testing have made it possible to diagnose internal carotid stenosis safely and reliably. Unfortunately, most prospective studies of patients with asymptomatic cerebrovascular disease have reported the course of asymptomatic carotid bruits, not asymptomatic carotid stenoses. The significance and proper management of asymptomatic carotid stenosis is still open to question.

It is possible on routine physical examination to distinguish some patients with asymptomatic bruits who have particularly severe cerebral vascular disease. Such patients are probably more susceptible to stroke and are most likely to be helped by prophylactic therapy. Learning the subtleties of the neurovascular examination is, therefore, essential to physicians treating cerebral vascular disease.

Evaluation of Neck Murmurs by Physical Examination

Murmurs Heard at the Base of the Neck. Approximately one third of normal children and young adults have short, systolic bruits audible over the carotid arteries at the base of the neck (Allen and Mustian, 1962; Hurst *et al.*, 1980; Sandok *et al.*, 1982). These bruits are always soft and rarely transmitted distally up the carotid. They are of no significance. In middle-aged and elderly persons, carotid bruits that are maximal at the base of the neck are occasionally caused by atherosclerotic or other lesions of the common carotid artery near its origin. Also, atherosclerotic lesions of the subclavian or vertebral arteries at their origins will often present with bruits audible over the carotid arteries at the neck base; however, these bruits are almost always of greatest intensity in the supraclavicular fossa. Much more often, bruits loudest over the proximal carotid arteries are associated with radiated valvular heart murmurs or hyperdynamic circulatory states, such as anemia, fever, thyrotoxicosis, hemodialysis, or pregnancy. Valvular aortic stenosis is the most common cause of a heart murmur transmitted to the neck. Such a murmur usually decreases in intensity more distally in the carotids but can occasionally be of greater intensity at the neck base than at the right second intercostal space. Mitral insufficiency, coarctation of the aorta, and patent ductus arteriosus are other causes of radiated heart murmurs.

Jugular venous hums are extremely common in childhood and occasionally also occur in normal adults. A jugular venous hum is usually loudest along the medial ends of the clavicles at the anterior borders of the sternocleidomastoid muscles, more often on the right side than on the left. The murmur is low-pitched and continuous but increases in intensity during diastole. It can often be abolished by having the patient recline or perform a Valsalva maneuver or by applying gentle pressure over the jugular vein.

Carotid Bifurcation Murmurs. The common carotid artery bifurcates at the level of the hyoid bone or at the superior margin of the thyroid cartilage in 85 percent of humans (McAfee *et al.,* 1953). Bruits originating from a lesion of the proximal internal carotid are maximal at or slightly distal to this level. A higher frequency bruit implies a tighter stenosis (Allen and Mustian, 1962; Sandok *et al.,* 1982). Louder bruits suggest a greater degree of stenosis (Sandok *et al.,* 1982; David *et al.,* 1973), but the volume of a bruit also depends on the amount of subcutaneous tissue separating the stethoscope and the affected artery; obese persons tend to have softer bruits. Bruits tend to soften and often disappear altogether as the degree of stenosis in the affected artery approaches 85 to 90 percent (Toole, 1984). Bruits that are holosystolic or extend into diastole suggest that the pressure gradient across the stenosis persists into diastole, suggesting a high degree of stenosis. In internal carotid artery stenosis, there are usually large collaterals to the poststenotic segment of artery via the circle of Willis. An internal carotid artery bruit that extends into diastole suggests not only a high degree of internal carotid artery stenosis but also a lesion interrupting these normal collateral channels, such as an anomalous circle of Willis or a contralateral carotid occlusion (Allen and Mustian, 1962).

A bruit loudest over the carotid bifurcation correlates with a hemodynamically significant stenosis of the proximal internal carotid 75 to 90 percent of the time (Sandok *et al.,* 1982; Ziegler *et al.,* 1971). Stenosis of the proximal external carotid artery accounts for 5 to 10 percent of bruits over the carotid bifurcation (Toole, 1984). This is a relatively innocuous lesion that can be excluded as a cause of carotid bifurcation bruit by occluding the homolateral facial and superficial temporal arteries while listening to the bruit. A bruit caused by external carotid artery stenosis decreases in intensity or even disappears when this maneuver is performed (Reed and Toole, 1981). Occasionally, a carotid bifurcation bruit is heard even when both the external and internal carotid arteries are widely patent. Such bruits occur when there is augmentation of the normal flow carried in the carotid because it is serving as a collateral channel for an occluded artery elsewhere in the cerebral vasculature. Such "augmentation" bruits of the carotid artery most commonly signify contralateral carotid occlusion.

In 30 to 40 percent of internal carotid arteries with hemodynamically significant stenosis, no bruit is audible over the carotid bifurcation (David *et al.,* 1973; Ziegler *et al.,* 1971; Ueda *et al.,* 1979). In most of these cases, the absence of a bruit can be explained on the basis that bruits often become softer and eventually disappear as the degree of stenosis approaches 85 to 90 percent. In such cases of near or total occlusion, many physical signs other than bruit are important. Patients with internal carotid occlusion have a diminished internal carotid pulse in the pharynx. They also often have augmentation bruits from increased flow in the contralateral carotid artery. These bruits are audible both over the neck and over the orbit, where turbulent flow in the cavernous carotid is heard. In carotid occlusion, collateral channels through the ipsilateral external carotid become more prominent, manifested by an increased pulse in the ipsilateral superficial temporal artery. Ipsilateral facial pulses not present in normal persons may appear at the angle of the nose, above the brow, just below the orbit, and along the nasolabial fold (Fisher, 1970). Dilated episcleral blood vessels on the side of the lesion (Countee *et al.,* 1978), unilateral arcus senilis on the side opposite the lesion (Bagla and Golden, 1975), and decreased severity of hypertensive retinal changes ipsilateral to the carotid lesion (Hollenhorst, 1962) are all signs suggestive of internal carotid occlusion or near occlusion. By searching for these signs of carotid occlusion and by listening for carotid bruits, physicians can sensitively detect cerebral atherosclerotic disease (for evaluation of asymptomatic carotid bruits by noninvasive studies, see Chapter 7).

REFERENCES

Adams, R.D.: Occlusion of the anterior inferior cerebellar artery. *Arch. Neurol. Psychiatry,* **49**:765–70, 1943.

Adams, R.D., and Victor, M.: *Principles of Neurology,* 2nd ed. McGraw-Hill, New York, 1981.

Allen, N., and Mustian, V.: Origin and significance of vascular murmurs of the head and neck. *Medicine,* **41**:227–47, 1962.

Amyes, E.W., and Nielson, J.M.: Clinicopathologic study of vascular lesions of the anterior cingulate region. *Bull. Los Angeles Neurol. Soc.,* **20**:112–30, 1955.

Bagla, S.K., and Golden, R.L.: Unilateral arcus corneae senilis and carotid occlusive disease. *J.A.M.A.,* **233**:450, 1975.

Barnett, H.J.M.: Heart in ischemic stroke—a changing emphasis. *Neurol. Clin.,* **1**:291–315, 1983.

Bean, W.B.: Infarction of the Heart. III. Clinical course and morphological findings. *Ann. Intern. Med.,* **12**:71–94, 1938.

Biller, J.; Challa, V.R.; Toole, J.F.; *et al.*: Nonbacterial thrombotic endocarditis: a neurologic perspective of clinicopathologic correlations of 99 patients. *Arch. Neurol.,* **39**:95–98, 1982.

Blackwood, W.; Hallpike, J.F.; Kocen, R.S.; *et al.*: Atheromatous disease of the carotid arterial system and embolism from the heart in cerebral infarction: a morbid anatomical study. *Brain,* **92**:897–910, 1969.

Caplan, L.R.: Lacunar infarction: a neglected concept. *Geriatrics,* **31**:71–5, 1976.

Caplan, L.R.: "Top of the basilar" syndrome. *Neurology,* **30**:72–9, 1980.

Caplan, L.R.: Vertebrobasilar disease: time for a new strategy. *Stroke,* **12**:111–14, 1981.

Cartilidge, N.E.F.; Whisnant, J.P.; and Elveback, L.R.: Carotid and vertebral-basilar transient cerebral ischemic attacks: a community study, Rochester, Minnesota. *Mayo Clin. Proc.,* **52**:117–20, 1977.

Corrin, L.S.; Sandok, B.A.; and Hauser, O.W.: Cerebral ischemic events in patients with carotid artery fibromuscular dysplasia. *Arch. Neurol.,* **38**:616–18, 1981.

Countee, R.W.; Gnanadev, A.; and Chavis, F.: Dilated episcleral arteries—a significant physical finding in assessment of patients with cerebrovascular insufficiency. *Stroke,* **9**:42–5, 1978.

Currier, R.D.; Giles, C.L.; and DeJong, R.N.: Some comments on Wallenberg's lateral medullary syndrome. *Neurology,* **11**:778–91, 1961.

David, T.E.; Humphries, A.W.; Young, J.R.; and Beven, E.G.: A correlation of neck bruits and arteriosclerotic carotid arteries. *Arch. Surg.,* **107**:729–31, 1973.

Denny-Brown, D.: Recurrent cerebrovascular episodes. *Arch. Neurol.,* **2**:194–210, 1960.

Durwood, Q.J.; Ferguson, G.G.; and Barr, H.W.K.: The natural history of asymptomatic carotid bifurcation plaques. *Stroke,* **13**:459–64, 1982.

Easton, J.D., and Sherman, D.G.: Management of cerebral embolism of cardiac origin. *Stroke,* **11**:433–42, 1980.

Fisher, C.M.: Ataxic hemiparesis: a pathological study. *Arch. Neurol.,* **35**:126–28, 1978.

Fisher, C.M.: Cerebral ischemia—less familiar types. *Clin. Neurosurg.,* **18**:267–336, 1971.

Fisher, C.M.: Discussion: transient ischemic attacks—an update. In Scheinberg, P. (ed.): *Cerebrovascular Diseases, Tenth Princeton Conference.* Raven Press, New York, 50, 1976.

Fisher, C.M.: Facial pulses in internal carotid artery occlusion. *Neurology,* **20**:476–78, 1970.

Fisher, C.M.: A lacunar stroke: the dysarthria–clumsy-hand syndrome. *Neurology,* **17**:614–17, 1967.

Fisher, C.M.: Lacunes: small, deep cerebral infarcts. *Neurology,* **15**:774–84, 1965.

Fisher, C.M.: Thalamic pure sensory stroke: a pathological study. *Neurology,* **28**:1141–44, 1978.

Fisher, C.M., and Cole, M.: Homolateral ataxia and crural paresis: a vascular syndrome. *J. Neurol. Neurosurg. Psychiatry,* **28**:48–55, 1965.

Fisher, C.M., and Curry, H.B.: Pure motor hemiplegia of vascular origin. *Arch. Neurol.,* **13**:30–44, 1965.

Gacs, G.; Merei, F.T., and Bodosi, M.: Balloon catheter as a model of cerebral emboli in humans. *Stroke,* **13**:39–42, 1982.

Gilman, S.; Bloedel, J.F.; and Lechtenberg, R.: *Disorders of the Cerebellum.* F.A. Davis, Philadelphia, 1981.

Goldstein, S.; Kleinknecht, R.; and Gallo, A.: Neuropsychological changes associated with carotid endarterectomy. *Cortex,* **6**:308–22, 1970.

Gur, R.C.; Gordon, J.; and Reivich, M.: Neuropsychological consequences of superficial temporal to middle cerebral artery bypass surgery (abstr.). *Neurology,* **33** [Suppl. 2]:164, 1983.

Hackinski, V.C.; Iliff, L.; Zilhka, E.; Boulay, G.H.; McAllister, V.L.; Marshall, J.; Russell, R.W.; and Symon, L.: Cerebral blood flow in dementia. *Arch. Neurol.,* **32**:632–37, 1975.

Heyman, A.; Leviton, A.; Millikan, C.H.; *et al.*: Transient focal cerebral ischemia: epidemiological and clinical aspects. *Stroke,* **5**:277–87, 1974.

Heyman, A.; Wilkinson, W.E.; Heyden, S.; *et al.*: Risk of stroke in asymptomatic persons with cervical arterial bruits: a population study in Evans County, Georgia. *N. Engl. J. Med.,* **302**:838–41, 1980.

Hollenhorst, R.W.: Carotid and vertebral-basilar arterial stenosis and occlusion: neuro-ophthalmologic considerations. *Trans. Am. Acad. Ophthalmol. Otolaryngol.,* **66**:166–80, 1962.

Horenstein, S.; Chamberlain, W.; and Conomy, J.: Infarction of the fusiform and calcarine regions: agitated delirium and hemianopia. *Trans. Am. Neurol. Assoc.,* **92**:85–89, 1967.

Hurst, J.W.; Hopkins, L.C.; and Smith, R.B.: Noises in the neck (editorial). *N. Engl. J. Med.,* **302**:862–63, 1980.

Hyland, H.H.: Thrombosis of the intracranial arteries. *Arch. Neurol. Psychiatry,* **30**:342–56, 1933.

Kase, C.S.; Maulsby, G.O.; deJuan, E.; *et al.*: Hemichorea-hemiballism and lacunar infarction in the basal ganglia. *Neurology,* **31**:452–55, 1981.

Kelly, M.P.; Garron, D.C.; and Javid, H.: Carotid artery disease, carotid endarterectomy, and behavior. *Arch. Neurol.,* **37**:743–48, 1980.

Kubik, C.S., and Adams, R.D.: Occlusion of the basilar artery: a clinical and pathological study. *Brain,* **69**:73–121, 1946.

Loeb, C., and Gandolfo, C.: Diagnostic evaluation of degenerative and vascular dementia. *Stroke,* **14**:399–401, 1983.

Marshall, J.: The natural history of transient ischemic cerebrovascular attacks. *Q. J. Med.,* **33**:309–24, 1964.

Marshall, J.: *The Management of Cerebrovascular Disease,* 3rd ed. Blackwell Scientific Publisher, London, 1976.

Massey, E.W.; Goodman, J.C.; Stewart, C.; *et al.*: Unilateral asterixis: motor integrative dysfunction in focal vascular disease. *Neurology,* **29**:1180–82, 1979.

Mayer-Gross, W.; Slater, E.; and Roth, M.: *Clinical Psychiatry,* 3rd. ed. Baillier, Tindall and Carssell, London, 1969.

McAfee, D.K.; Anson, B.J.; and McDonald, J.J.: Variation in the point of bifurcation of the common carotid artery. *Bull. Northwest. Univ. Med. Sch.,* **27**:226–29, 1953.

McGhee, T.B., and Toole, J.F.: Cerebrovascular disease and neurologic manifestations of heart disease. In

Hurst, J.W.; Logue, R.B.; Schlant, R.C.; and Wenger, N.K. (eds.): *The Heart, Arteries and Veins,* 5th ed. McGraw-Hill, New York, 1486–98, 1982.

Meadows, J.C.: Clinical features of focal cerebral hemisphere infarction. In Ross Russell, R.W. (ed.): *Vascular Diseases of the Central Nervous System,* 2nd ed. Churchill Livingstone, New York, 169–84, 1983.

Medina, J.L; Rubino, F.A.; and Ross, A.: Agitated delirium caused by infarction of the hippocampal formation and fusiform and lingual gyri: a case report. *Neurology,* **24:**1181–83, 1974.

Mesulam, M.M.; Waxman, S.G.; Geshwind, N.; *et al.:* Acute confusional states with right middle cerebral artery infarctions. *J. Neurol. Neurosurg. Psychiatry,* **39:**84–89, 1976.

Miller, V.T.: Lacunar stroke: a reassessment. *Arch. Neurol.,* **40:**129–34, 1983.

Mohr, J.P.; Caplan, L.R.; Melski, J.W.; *et al.:* The Harvard cooperative stroke registry: a prospective registry. *Neurology,* **28:**754–62, 1978.

Mohr, J.P.; Kase, C.S.; Meckler, R.J.; *et al.:* Sensorimotor stroke due to thalamocapsular ischemia. *Arch. Neurol.,* **34:**739–41, 1977.

Perry, P.M.; Drinkwater, J.E.; and Taylor, G.W.: Cerebral function before and after carotid endarterectomy. *Br. Med. J.,* **4:**215–16, 1975.

Pessin, M.S.; Duncan, G.W.; Mohr, J.P.; *et al.:* Clinical and angiographic features of carotid transient ischemic attacks. *N. Engl. J. Med.,* **296:**358–62, 1977.

Reed, C.A., and Toole, J.F.: Clinical technique for identification of external carotid bruits. *Neurology,* **31:**744–46, 1981.

Ross Russell, R.W.: Pathogenesis of transient ischemic attacks. *Neurol. Clin.,* **1:**279–90, 1983.

Sandok, B.A.; Whisnant, J.P.; Furlan, A.J.; *et al.:* Carotid artery bruits: prevalence survey and differential diagnosis. *Mayo Clin. Proc.,* **57:**227–30, 1982.

So, E.L.; Toole, J.F.; Dalal, P.; *et al.:* Cephalic fibromuscular dysplasia in 32 patients: clinical findings and radiologic features. *Arch. Neurol.,* **38:**619–22, 1981.

Soloway, H.R., and Aronson, S.M.: Atheromatous emboli to the central nervous system. *Arch. Neurol.,* **11:**657–67, 1964.

Sypert, G.W., and Alvord, E.C., Jr.: Cerebellar infarction: a clinicopathological study. *Arch. Neurol.,* **32:**357–63, 1975.

Toole, J.F.: *Cerebrovascular Disorders,* 3rd ed. Raven Press, New York, 1984.

Toole, J.F.; Yuson, C.P.; and Janeway, R.: Transient ischemic attacks: a prospective study of 225 patients. *Neurology,* **28:**746–53, 1978.

Uchiyama, S.; Takeuchi, M.; Osawa, M.; Kobayashi, I.; Maruyama, S.; Aosaki, M.; and Hirosawa, K.: Platelet function tests in thrombotic cerebrovascular disorders. *Stroke,* **14:**511–7, 1983.

Ueda, K.; Toole, J.F.; and McHenry, L.C., Jr.: Carotid and vertebrobasilar transient ischemic attacks: clinical and angiographic correlation. *Neurology,* **29:**1094–1101, 1979.

Weisberg, L.A.: Computed tomography and pure motor hemiparesis. *Neurology,* **29:**490–95, 1979.

Whisnant, J.P.; Matsumoto, N.; and Elveback, L.R.: Transient cerebral ischemic attacks in a community: Rochester, Minnesota, 1955 through 1969. *Mayo Clin. Proc.,* **48:**194–98, 1973.

Wolf, P.A.; Dowber, T.R.; Tholmas, H.E.; *et al.:* Epidemiologic assessment of chronic atrial fibrillation and risk of stroke: the Framingham Study. *Neurology,* **28:**973–77, 1978.

Wolf, P.A.; Kannel, W.B.; Sorlie, P.; and McNamara, P.: The asymptomatic carotid bruit and risk of stroke: the Framingham Study. *J.A.M.A.,* **245:**1442–45, 1981.

Wolf, P.A.; Kannel, W.B.; and Verter, J.: Current status of risk factors for stroke. *Neurol. Clin.,* **1:**317–43, 1983.

Ziegler, D.K.; Zileli, T.; Dick, A.; and Sebaugh, J.L.: Correlation of bruits over the carotid artery with angiographically demonstrated lesions. *Neurology,* **21:**860–65, 1971.

7

Noninvasive Diagnosis of Carotid Artery Disease

JEFFREY K. RAINES and FREDERICK WALBURN

During the past decade, noninvasive technology for the diagnosis of extracranial cerebrovascular disease advanced at a rapid pace. This progress is due to a number of factors, including improvement in surgical technique, increased understanding of arterial hemodynamics, and steady advancement in electronic and computer technology. At least two other facts also deserve mention: First, patients are presenting with extracranial arterial disease at an increasing rate. This can be traced to declining cardiac morbidity and mortality secondary to better risk-factor control, newly developed pharmacological substances, and coronary reconstructive surgery. Since we have uncovered no basic mechanism to alter the generalized atherosclerotic process, with decreasing cardiac morbidity and mortality atherosclerotic patients are expected to survive in increasing numbers; in many, extracranial arterial disease will develop. Also, government agencies and other third-party insurers are now pressing the medical community to provide early and accurate diagnoses with maximum efficiency and at minimal cost and to do so in outpatient facilities whenever possible.

For these reasons, since 1972 more than 3,000 clinically oriented vascular laboratories have been opened in the United States. They are found not only in major university medical centers and larger private groups, but also in small vascular practices where physicians wish to enhance the quality of vascular diagnosis. As a rule, these laboratories begin on a limited scale concentrating primarily on lower extremity arterial occlusive disease and using only functional testing. Later, however, they gradually expand to cover most if not all areas of vascular practice.

The development of imaging technology supplemented functional and hemodynamic information, and has proved particularly helpful in the extracranial cerebrovascular territory.

IMPORTANCE OF IDENTIFYING EXTRACRANIAL CEREBROVASCULAR DISEASE

Although this topic is covered in more detail in other chapters of this volume, a brief comment is appropriate here to focus on the reasons why physicians should routinely perform noninvasive testing on their patients when extracranial cerebrovascular disease is suspected.

There are nearly 1.8 million persons living in the United States who have a history of acute stroke (American Heart Association, 1982). The economic impact of this fact is enormous—an annual cost to society of approximately $7.4 billion. Up to one half of all strokes are caused by surgically accessible lesions in the cervical carotid arteries. It has also been reported that there is a 20 percent initial mortality rate for the first stroke caused by carotid artery disease. In addition, one half of all persons who have an acute stroke from the carotid system eventually die from the same cause (Callow, 1982). Finally, carotid endarterectomy has become a widely accepted and most effective treatment for selected patient groups with extracranial arterial disease.

With such background information, it would appear that for a vascular laboratory to be considered helpful in the area of cerebrovascular disease it must have the effect of reducing the occurrence of stroke. It can indeed accomplish this goal by identifying the presence of extracranial arterial disease accurately, safely, and at minimal expense. Furthermore, to augment its use, the vascular laboratory should also provide information that aids in patient management; this should include the matter of surgical versus medical therapy and, if surgery is decided upon, its optimal timing.

HEMODYNAMIC CONSIDERATIONS

Before proceeding with the discussion on the technique of noninvasive evaluation, a brief outline of important hemodynamic considerations is proper. More extensive treatment of these topics can be found in engineering (fluid mechanics) and medical reports (Grady, 1984; Strandness and Sumner, 1975).

Symptoms

Symptoms secondary to extracranial arterial disease may be caused by carotid artery lesions that either reduce perfusion on a chronic or transient basis or have the capability of producing emboli. Well-known symptoms characterize each of these settings. There is much debate over whether flow-limiting or emboli-producing lesions are more important. We believe that (1) most symptoms are caused by embolic phenomena, (2) as a lesion progresses anatomically, so does its embolic potential, and (3) even small lesions (25 percent by diameter) can produce emboli, but the incidence of this is low.

Pressure Reduction

Owing to high resistance to flow in the small vessels, stenosis in the large arterial territories must be "high grade" to reduce blood flow and pressure in a particular vessel. The definition of "high grade" is a function of the flow rate itself. In the internal carotid artery, decrease in pressure generally does not occur unless 75 percent of the lumen becomes obstructed. The length of the lesion has relatively little effect on the pressure gradient. Pressure reduction across a stricture is also a function of velocity, as is systolic pressure, because the local velocity is near maximum at peak systole.

Velocity

As mentioned previously, a stenosis can progress up to a point without causing any change in flow rate. Velocity, however, does increase with decreasing luminal area. Increased velocity can produce local turbulence in the bloodstream, which in turn induces small pressure fluctuations at the compliant arterial wall, causing it to vibrate and to produce a bruit.

Shear Stress

When any fluid flows along a boundary, it exerts a force along the interface, known as *shear stress*. This stress increases with velocity. Therefore, in arterial stenosis significant force may be exerted on the vessel wall. If this force is strong enough, it can dislodge loosely attached material (e.g., platelets, thrombus) and cause emboli.

METHODS

It should be recognized that in noninvasive testing, as in many other areas of clinical investigation, there are alternative ways to arrive at similar results. What follows is based on the senior author's 17-year experience with noninvasive vascular testing, which includes more than 50,000 patient evaluations carried on concurrently with the development and direction of vascular laboratories at Massachusetts General Hospital and at the Miami Heart Institute. We believe the following recommendations regarding instrumentation and interpretation represent the state of the art. Modifications for individual strong and weak points within laboratories can be anticipated. However, a word of warning is given: No matter what the initial results of a particular modality may seem to promise, unless it is based on sound physical and hemodynamic principles, it will ultimately fail the test of time.

We have also learned that no single noninvasive test can "stand by itself" in the extracranial vascular territory. We therefore combine four modalities (three functional, one anatomical) with history taking and physical examination. The accuracy and effectiveness of this approach has been proven in many centers and with thousands of patients.

History

It is desirable to have complete vascular testing performed by a well-trained vascular technologist. We prefer to have nurses in this role, inasmuch as their training includes knowledge of medical terminology, ability to handle emergencies, and in-depth training in concomitant diseases which are often present in vascular patients. The technologist is the eyes, ears, and hands of the laboratory director, who must interpret test results in light of the clinical situation.

The vascular technologist should inquire whether the patient has a history of smoking, hypertension, diabetes, elevated blood lipid levels, obesity, myocardial infarction, angina, claudication, or previous extracranial arterial surgery. Details should be provided as indicated.

If the patient has already had a cerebrovascular accident, complete history of this event should be obtained. The patient should be carefully questioned regarding headaches, dysphasia, vertigo, syncope, visual disturbances, and other relevant symptoms.

Physical Examination

The brachial blood pressure should be measured in both arms. We recommend that the carotid, temporal, and facial pulses also be graded by palpation. The presence of murmurs over the chest and the subclavian and the carotid arteries is noted. If a carotid bruit is believed to be partly or totally transmitted from the subclavian artery, it should also be evaluated while the proximal subclavian artery is compressed.

Ophthalmic Artery Pressure

Due to anatomical proximity and hemodynamic function, the ophthalmic artery pressure usually provides a reliable index of pressure in the distal internal carotid artery and its major branches. In the past, ophthalmodynamometry has been used to estimate retinal artery pressure. This technique involves the application of a measured lateral pressure to the sclera while directly observing retinal pulsations. Many physicians now believe that this technique is inaccurate and subjective owing to poor resolution inherent in the procedure, variability in examiner skill, or presence of retinal lesions.

Owing to the primary efforts of Gee and colleagues (1974), an accurate method of measuring ophthalmic artery pressure is now available. The method is a variant of suction ophthalmodynamometry and is referred to as oculoplethysmography (OPG), or oculopneumoplethysmography.

The physical basis of the technique is rather simple and is illustrated in Figure 7–1. A rigid cup (14 mm in diameter) is placed on the lateral aspect of the sclera. As vacuum is applied to the cup, the sclera is pulled into it, thus increasing intravascular pressure. At the same time, a sensitive transducer records the volume fluctuations encountered within the cup. During the normal cycle, the size of the eyeball is variable, reaching its peak at systole and its ebb at diastole. As increased vacuum is applied, intraocular pressure rises. In this sequence, a level is reached at which intraocular pressure equals the ophthalmic artery systolic pressure, and blood flow to the eyeball ceases. At this point, volume fluctuations in the eye are no longer present. Careful experiments have been performed to correlate vacuum level at the point of the first volume fluctuation with systolic artery and intraocular pressure. This correlation has been verified by several investigators who found a direct relationship between ophthalmic artery systolic pressure and the point at which volume fluctuations appear on the eyeball.

This technique must not be confused with another form of OPG, in which ophthalmic artery pressure is not measured (Kartchner *et al.,* 1976). In the latter technique, a heated sa-

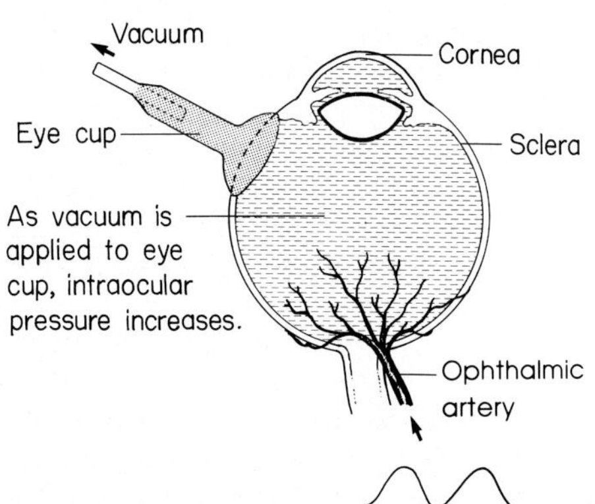

Figure 7–1. The measurement of ophthalmic artery pressure by oculopneumoplethysmography.

line solution-filled system is used with eyecups placed on the cornea of both eyes. This is done in an effort to predict hemodynamic significance of internal carotid artery lesions on the basis of wave-speed delay and volume-time contour alterations measured over the cornea (one side compared with the other). The technique has been criticized for the following reasons:

1. Delay in pulse-wave arrival even in presence of high-grade lesions is extremely short and difficult to measure.
2. The parameters that affect pulse-wave speed in the range of interest (vascular length, diameter, and compliance) are variable from one side to the other. These variants may produce hemodynamic alterations that are inherently more significant than those produced by stenotic lesions themselves.
3. Pulse-wave phenomenon is a path function and provides no information regarding compensation, collateralization, or perfusion.
4. The presence of bilateral disease may delay the ocular pulse equally.

For these reasons and for other considerations, we believe that OPG should be used to measure opthalmic artery pressure instead of pulse-wave phenomena.

The application of OPG provides an accurate evaluation (generally within 2 mm Hg) of the systolic pressure within the ophthalmic artery. Because the ophthalmic artery originates proximal to most major intracranial vessels, it provides a measure of system perfusion pressure to the respective hemisphere.

Ophthalmic artery pressure in the presence of internal carotid artery disease may be modified by collateralization via the ipsilateral external carotid circulation, from the contralateral hemisphere through the circle of Willis, and through the vertebral-basilar system. As a rule, compensation by these channels is not stimulated until a lesion produces a pressure gradient. Significant gradient develops in the internal carotid artery only if stenotic lesions produce about a 50 percent reduction in lumen diameter (75 percent by area). Therefore, OPG alone cannot be expected to identify lesions in the internal carotid artery obstructing less than 50 percent of its diameter. It does, however, give an accurate measure of maximum hemispheric perfusion pressure of the hemodynamic deficit, and of the degree of compensation. Present instrumentation does not allow the measurement of ophthalmic artery pressure above 145 mm Hg. However, because the measured value is usually considerably lower than systemic systolic pressure, it is not a severe limitation of the technique.

Uncompensated internal carotid artery lesion is suspected when the following criteria are met:

1. A difference of 5 mm Hg or more is detected in ophthalmic artery pressure between the two eyes. Although the vast majority of patients meet this criterion, it may fail in the presence of symmetrical bilateral disease. For this class of patients, a second criterion is given:
2. If ophthalmic artery pressures are within 5 mm Hg and the pulse amplitudes are within 2 mm at their measured pressure levels, the test shown in Figure 7–2 is used to define individual compensation. The present accuracy of this test in pa-

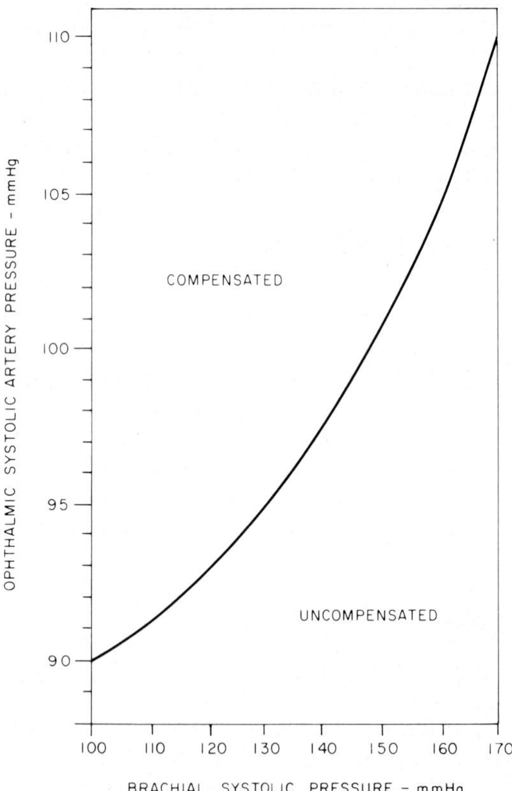

Figure 7–2. Criteria used to differentiate between compensated and uncompensated internal carotid artery disease in patients with symmetrical bilateral disease using the blood pressure measured in the brachial and ophthalmic arteries as guidelines. From Cullen, S. et al.: Clinical sequelae in patients with symptomatic carotid bruit. *Circulation,* **68**(Suppl. II): 83–87, 1983, with permission.

tients meeting the second criterion is approximately 92 percent.

Carotid Audiofrequency Analysis

Carotid audiofrequency analysis (CAA) is similar in technique to phonocardiography, but is taken over cervical carotid arteries rather than over the heart. Signals are recorded at three positions along the length of the neck: at the common carotid artery level, over the carotid bifurcation, and above the carotid vessels distal to the bifurcation. The equipment for CAA includes the following:

1. A specifically designed microphone with a frequency range of 50 to 750 Hz
2. A headset for audio interpretation
3. A cathode-ray tube for visual display
4. A computerized, permanent chart recording system.

As the arterial wall becomes rough and narrow owing to the presence of an atherosclerotic plaque, separation and increased velocity produce turbulence in the bloodstream. This in turn causes the wall of the vessel to vibrate and emit bruits, which can be heard at the skin level if the attenuation between the source and the receiver is not too great. Although the dynamics of sound generation in turbulent arterial flow constitute a complex subject, clinically useful guidelines have been established for many years and have been verified by recent investigations.

It should be emphasized that although audio frequency analysis by CAA is helpful in identifying early lesions (25 percent reduction in diameter) and in estimating anatomical severity (from 25 to 80 percent by diameter), it fails to provide information regarding compensation, collateralization, and perfusion. This fact underlines the importance of other complementary tests, especially OPG and cerebral Doppler evaluation.

The major diagnostic CAA parameters include the presence or absence of the first and second heart sounds, the level of frequency content in systole or systole and diastole, and the differential character of the three traces taken on each side. Critics of CAA assert that experienced vascular specialists can obtain similar information with a simple stethoscope. This may be true; however, several points should be emphasized:

1. The sensitivity, amplification, quantitation, and frequency range of CAA are well above the capacity of the human ear. It also allows appreciation of bruits that cannot be heard through a stethoscope alone.
2. In the setting of a vascular laboratory, the examiner is usually not a vascular specialist but rather a nurse who will later present the test results to the specialist for interpretation. The advantages of quantitation and hard copy are obvious.
3. CAA is helpful even for the experienced examiner in identifying transmitted murmurs.

As mentioned, although CAA will not provide information regarding compensation, collateralization, or perfusion, it can detect lesions at an early stage of development and estimate anatomical severity. Figure 7–3 can be used as a guide for interpretation. It should be applied to tracings obtained at each of the three levels. Stenosis of the internal carotid artery may cause abnormal recordings at all three levels; however, most often, lesions in the internal carotid artery produce increased sound abnormalities as the microphone is moved more distally. For example, a normal record obtained at the base of the neck but with indications of stenosis at the midneck and under the mandible suggests a lesion at the carotid bifurcation.

For the most part, CAA cannot distinguish between external and internal carotid artery stenosis. Because the internal carotid artery is of primary interest and most bifurcation lesions involve the internal carotid artery, it is suggested that all CAA abnormalities be interpreted as internal carotid artery stenosis. This assumption will produce very few false-positive results. Also, external carotid artery flow changes direction in diastole; internal carotid artery flow does not. Therefore, bruits heard only in diastole can be assumed to be generated in the internal carotid artery.

In most centers the mean age of patients undergoing cerebral vascular evaluation is about 70. This group often has concomitant cardiovascular disorders which may produce murmurs transmitted to the carotid system. These must be differentiated from turbulence generated by carotid artery stenosis. In a series published by the Vascular Laboratory of the Miami Heart Institute, 35 percent of the patients referred to the laboratory with the diagnosis of asymptomatic carotid bruits actually had transmitted murmurs (Cullen *et al.*,

% STENOSIS By Dia.	By Area	DESCRIPTION	CPA TRACING
0-25	0-44	1) Normal 1st and 2nd heart sounds with no significant audiofrequency content (amplitude, intensity) during either systole or diastole. Note: absence of only the 1st heart sound does not suggest abnormal carotid artery pathology.	
25-40	44-64	2) The first heart sound is obliterated; high frequency content is noted at the initiation of systole. As the lesion becomes more severe the audiofrequency content extends over a longer portion of systole.	
40-80	64-96	3) The 1st and 2nd heart sounds are obliterated; high frequency content is observed throughout systole and extends partially into diastole. As the lesion becomes more obstructive the audiofrequency content extends over a longer portion of diastole.	
80-100	96-100	4) When the lesion becomes severe enough to significantly reduce blood velocity, turbulence is also reduced, and the abnormal audiofrequency content is lost. In this case the CPA tracings may be normal. In some patients the heart sound amplitude is reduced.	

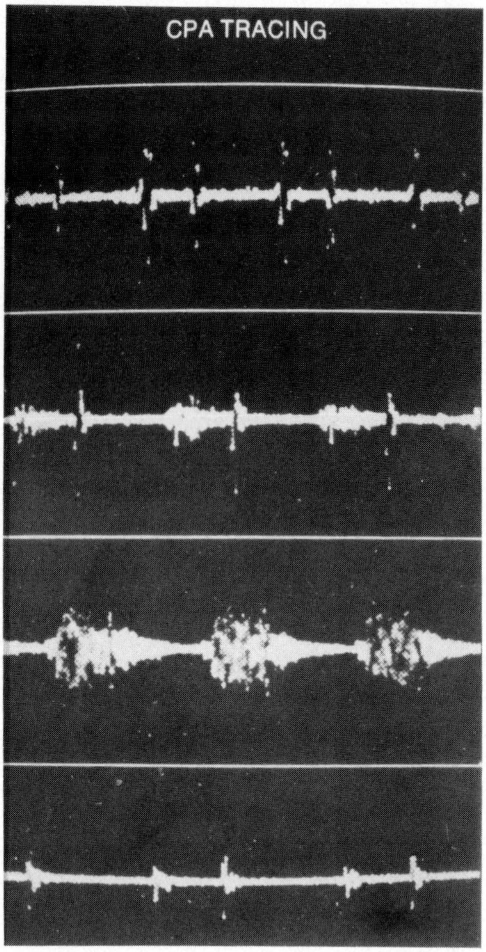

Figure 7-3. Guide for carotid audiofrequency analysis.

1983). CAA can be very helpful in differentiating these lesions, but to do so, the examiner should always listen over the chest and subclavian arteries. If murmurs are heard, their character should be compared with that of murmurs present over the carotid systems. Valvular murmurs transmitted to the carotid system have increased audiofrequency content at the base of neck and diminish in both frequency and intensity as the microphone moves more distal. This is in contrast to lesions in the carotid system. It is possible, of course, that these lesions may coexist. This same pattern may also be observed with subclavian artery stenosis, except that the intensity at the base of the neck is generally not as marked as in valvular disease. Subclavian artery compression with CAA (midneck level) may provide the diagnostic clue when such a lesion is suspected.

Doppler Evaluation

Continuous-wave ultrasound has been used for noninvasive evaluation of peripheral and cerebral vascular diseases for many years. In this test, an electronic oscillator is used to resonate a piezoelectric crystal at a particular frequency. Frequencies in the range of 9 MHz have been shown to be most effective in the study of the supraorbital, carotid, and vertebral arteries. During the study, the ultrasonic wave is directed toward a blood vessel. When the wave front strikes a moving object such as an erythrocyte, it is reflected back to the crystal at a different frequency (Doppler effect). By appropriate filtering, a third signal equalling the difference between the entry and returning frequencies may be produced and converted to an audible signal or chart recording. Furthermore, with additional electronic circuitry, it is possible for ultrasound to determine the direction of blood velocity.

Doppler systems can be used in the extracranial arterial system to obtain patency estimates in specific arterial vessels and qualitative estimates of changes in blood velocity with various maneuvers. In determination of the direction of flow, the probe is placed over the supraorbital artery near the orbital notch of the side being examined. The probe's orientation is adjusted to produce a crisp audio signal with minimal background interference. The quality of the signal and its direction are noted. While maintaining the position of the probe, the operator palpates the superficial temporal artery, occluding it by digital pressure, and notes the changes in the audio signal and flow direction. With the same probe position, the compression procedure may also be repeated over the facial artery near the mandibular notch.

Using the probe, the operator next identifies the quality of the audible signals over the common, external, and internal carotid arteries. The operator starts by palpating the common carotid artery, positioning the probe (45 degrees toward the direction of flow), and maximizing the signal. The common carotid artery has a biphasic signal with a "thumplike" sound heard at the initiation of systole. Moving distally along the common carotid, the signal will change character as the bifurcation is reached. The signal over the external carotid artery is also biphasic but does not have the thumplike character in its cycle. It is generally situated anteriorly when compared with the common carotid artery. After the external carotid artery is identified, the probe is slowly moved posteriorly. In this plane, if the angle of the bifurcation is wide, all sound will disappear until the course of the internal carotid artery is intersected. The signal over the internal carotid artery is generally lower-pitched and is always monophasic.

The vertebral artery is evaluated next. Again, the common carotid artery is located by palpation and by using the probe. From this point, which is at the base of the neck, the probe is slowly moved posteriorly and laterally until it intersects the course of the vertebral artery. The signal over the vertebral artery is often lower-pitched and may be either mono- or biphasic. If possible, the direction of flow should be noted.

The foregoing cerebral Doppler evaluation is not suitable for evaluating the severity of internal carotid artery disease. Used in combination with OPG and CAA, it is, however, helpful in three areas:

1. Differentiating total internal carotid artery occlusion from high-grade stenosis (75 percent by area), both of which may produce identical results using OPG (reduced ophthalmic artery pressure) and CAA (normal). Establishing the true anatomy in this situation is very important for surgical considerations. Inability to identify the internal carotid artery by Doppler signals implies total occlusion of that vessel.
2. Determining the source of collateralization. The direction of velocity in the supraorbital artery is normally anterograde. When the diameter of the internal carotid artery is reduced by more than 50 percent, a pressure gradient develops across the lesion which in turn activates various collateral channels. Primary collateralization, via the ipsilateral external carotid circulation, will produce retrograde velocity in the supraorbital artery and/or reduced supraorbital artery velocity with superficial artery and/or facial artery compression. Primary collateralization can also be provided by the contralateral internal carotid circulation. Under such conditions, supraorbital artery velocity remains anterograde and is not affected by ipsilateral compression. One further note on collateralization: Although it has not been reported, it is theoretically possible to have a normal OPG evaluation with abnormal carotid Doppler evaluation. Such a finding suggests a well-compensated lesion with collateralization via the ipsilateral external carotid circulation.
3. Qualitative evaluation of flow through the vertebral arteries is often difficult due to its orientation and surrounding bony structures, but qualitative patency assessment is indeed possible. If a strong velocity signal is easily identified, patency is highly probable. A weak signal (particularly when compared with that of the contralateral vertebral artery) indicates diffuse disease. If the vertebral artery cannot be identified, occlusion is probable. If the direction of the blood velocity is retrograde, subclavian steal syndrome may be present. Flow reversal is

rarely found unless significant differences (35 mm Hg) in brachial blood pressure between the two arms are present.

Imaging Techniques

Although evaluations based upon functional hemodynamic procedures have been very successful in contributing to the management of patients with cerebral vascular disease, these evaluations are even more useful in conjunction with anatomical data. Various ultrasonic imaging techniques have been developed: continuous-wave Doppler (Kristensen *et al.,* 1971), pulsed Doppler (Griffith *et al.,* 1977), and ultrasonic B-mode imaging (Blue *et al.,* 1972; Comerota *et al.,* 1981). However, Doppler imaging systems have a number of limitations. To image along the length of an artery, the Doppler probe must be positioned sequentially. This results in images that are subject to artifacts owing to minor patient motion. In addition, the procedure is time-consuming. Ultrasonic B-mode imaging (see Figure 7–4) has been used in our vascular laboratory since April 1978. Many other centers are now using this technique as well.

During carotid imaging, the patient sits in a swivel chair with the examiner either behind or beside him. The studies are first made in the anterior oblique view. The probe is placed on the patient's clavicle to visualize the common carotid artery, then moved distally, keeping the carotid artery in focus. The carotid bulb and bifurcation are now identified. The internal carotid artery is usually easily visualized because it lies in the same plane with the common carotid artery (see Figure 7–4). The external carotid artery is located anteriorly and is usually smaller than the internal carotid. If the operator is not sure which branch is being visualized, the built-in audible pulsed Doppler unit may be used. The Doppler may be directed to the anatomical location in question and the velocity signal recorded. As stated previously, the signal over the internal carotid artery is biphasic. Each branch is followed distally until further movement of the transducer is stopped by the mandible.

The common, internal, and external carotid arteries can also be visualized in the posterior

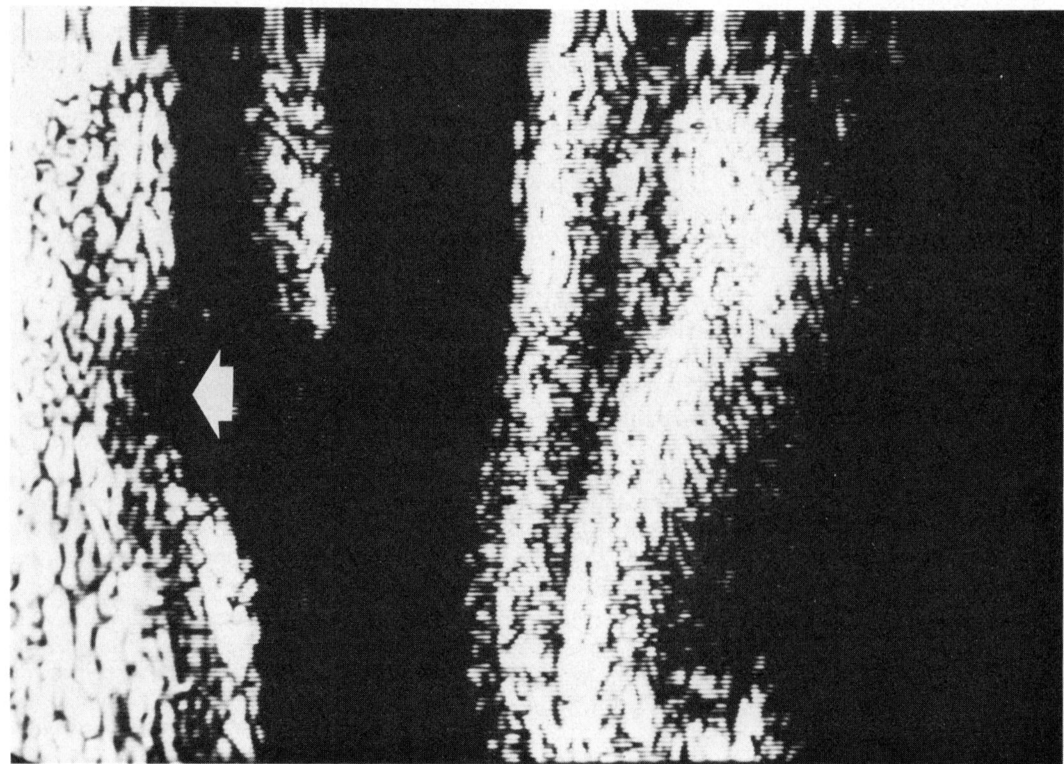

Figure 7–4. Ulcerated plaque at the orifice of the external carotid artery (arrow) as shown by B-mode imaging.

oblique view. To do this, the transducer is placed behind the external head of the sternocleidomastoid muscle. The common carotid artery is identified proximally, and the arterial tree is traced as described previously. The vessel can usually be followed distally in the posterior oblique view. The entire procedure is then repeated for the left extracranial arterial territory. We routinely use the anterior and posterior views and have found that "fanning" the probe in either position is helpful in some cases to elucidate the anatomy of a particular arterial segment. We have not found the transverse view to yield valuable data. The resolution of the latter is poor compared with that of the longitudinal view; therefore, we do not recommend routine transverse imaging.

Two important points can be made regarding B-mode imaging: (1) B-mode imaging alone may be misleading, and (2) information gained from B-mode imaging and noninvasive functional testing is complementary. Our experience also indicates that it is preferable to perform functional studies before B-mode imaging is attempted because they provide important guidelines. In addition, the results of functional studies are required to interpret B-mode images appropriately. This has been a consistent finding of ours and others. For this reason, if B-mode imaging is performed as the only diagnostic test, it may be misleading. B-mode imaging provides important information in the setting of the noninvasive evaluation owing to its ability to document disease that has not been detected by functional evaluations.

In a study performed at the Vascular Laboratory of the Miami Heart Institute in patients with specific lateralized cerebral symptoms, we found 233 arterial territories that were functionally normal according to hemodynamic criteria. These arteries were also evaluated with B-mode imaging (Calderon-Ortiz *et al.,* 1984). The diseases identified by B-mode imaging in these arteries ranged from ulceration (9 percent of patients) to measurable atherosclerotic stenosis (45 percent). These data demonstrate the usefulness of B-mode imaging as an adjunct to hemodynamic functional testing. Our experience now includes real-time B-mode imaging of more than 5,500 patients for extracranial arterial disease. In April 1981, our laboratory was chosen to be one of the clinical centers for the B-Scan Assessment Program of the National Institutes of Health (NIH). The purpose of this program was to establish the sensitivity, specificity, repeatability, and variability of the scans and to determine quantification parameters of clinically relevant lesions documented by real-time B-mode imaging using angiographic, surgical, and pathological findings as standards of comparison. The main B-Scan Assessment Program terminated enrollment in April 1984 with results to be published. The laboratory is presently involved in the NIH B-Scan Assessment Follow-Up Program, which will extend to December 1, 1986 and which should provide important information regarding the natural history of carotid artery disease.

AUTOMATED PROCEDURES LABORATORY

The use of microcomputers in the medical diagnostic field is expanding rapidly. Vascular laboratories are ideally suited for microcomputer technology because the procedures are limited in number and standardized.

Recently, microcomputer technology has been added to the armamentarium of the noninvasive peripheral vascular laboratory in the form of the automated procedure laboratory (APL)* (Raines, 1983). The APL is geared for noninvasive evaluation of the leg arterial and venous systems and the extracranial cerebral circulation. We are using it routinely in our vascular laboratory to identify the presence of arterial disease, measure its severity, and follow its course.

The APL system consists of a measurement unit (MU) and an analysis unit (AU). The MU is mounted on a mobile cart and contains automated versions of the pulse volume recorder, continuous-wave Doppler, dual-channel OPG, and CAA. The mobility of the MU also allows for studies to be performed at bedside or in the recovery room. During the evaluation, the operator is prompted for data input, measurements, and procedures. After the evaluation has been completed, the data are stored on a floppy diskette which can either be placed in the analysis unit, or transmitted via a modem.

The AU consists of an IBM-AT microcomputer with a 20 MB hard disk and an Okidata 193 dot-matrix graphic printer. A menu-driven protocol guides the operator through

* Life Sciences Inc., Greenwich, CT.

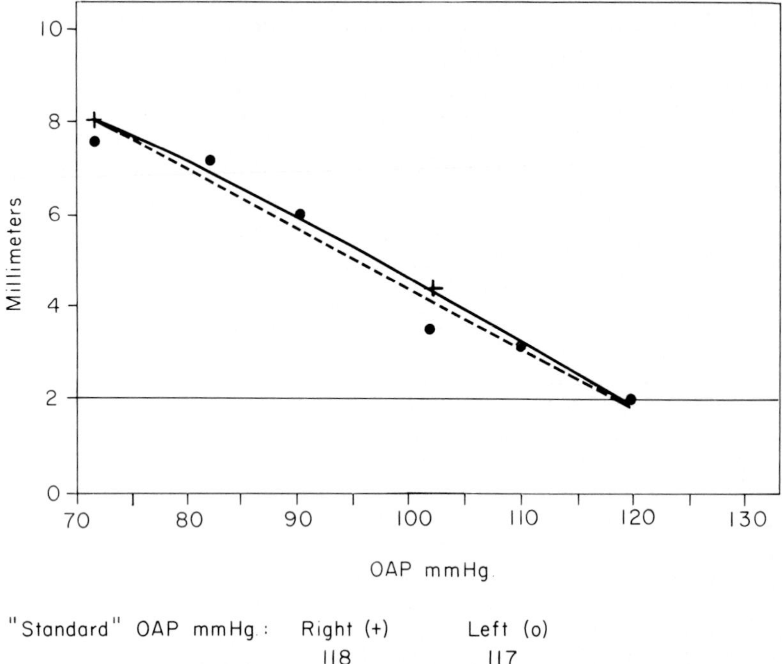

Figure 7–5. Least squares regression lines used to determine ocular pneumoplethysmographic pressure (OAP = ophthalmic artery pressure).

the procedure, which includes reviewing the data entered into the MU, entering B-mode imaging data, positioning cursors to measure OPG amplitudes and the duration of increased frequency in the CAA traces, and responding to other system signals. A regression procedure is used to determine automatically the OPG pressure (see Figure 7–5). When the data analysis is completed, an automated interpretation package provides a final diagnosis on the screen. The operator has the options of changing or adding to this interpretation.

OTHER SELECTED MODALITIES

Many other modalities for noninvasive evaluation of the extracranial arterial circulation have also been proposed over the years. These range from very simple devices, such as continuous-wave Doppler, to more complex and expensive methods, such as B-mode imaging and even forms of thermography. It is beyond the scope of this chapter to list them all. Because of their widespread use, however, two deserve brief elaboration.

Doppler Imaging

As previously mentioned, we believe that carotid imaging is best performed combining B-mode imaging with pulsed Doppler. Early imaging technology used continuous-wave and pulse-wave Dopplers. These systems were slow, had extremely poor resolution, and often produced artifactual images. For these reasons, examiners relied on sound and velocity tracing analysis rather than the images after the introduction of B-mode imaging. Doppler can now differentiate internal and external carotid arteries and distinguish stenosis from total occlusions.

Spectral Analysis

A number of laboratories use spectral analysis of auscultatory and especially Doppler signals to derive parameters useful for diagnostic purposes. We have not found this method to offer significant advantages over CAA. However, with additional use and with more efforts of clinical correlation meaningful algorithms may emerge.

Effect of DVI Arteriography

A discussion of noninvasive extracranial arterial evaluation would not be complete without a few comments regarding its relation to digital venous injection (DVI) arteriography. Over the last five years, we have monitored the effect of DVI arteriography on our vascular laboratory and have arrived at a number of conclusions. First, the number of functional studies has increased. This is due to several factors: (1) physicians accustomed to functional diagnoses continue to obtain this information before proceeding with anatomical definition, and (2) physicians not accustomed to obtaining functional data now use the vascular laboratory to supplement the "less than standard" anatomical data provided by DVI. We have also found the vascular laboratory to be particularly helpful when deciding whether a patient should have standard arteriography or DVI arteriography. For example, if the patient presents with a transient ischemic attack and the functional studies indicate significant carotid bifurcation disease, DVI arteriography may be all that is needed to proceed to the next step. However, if low-grade disease is suggested, a more definitive arteriographic procedure may be indicated.

INTERPRETATION AND ACCURACY

Noninvasive evaluation of extracranial arterial disease is intended to obtain certain basic information. First, based on functional measurements and imaging procedures, the degree of obstruction (percent of stenosis) should be estimated. In some circumstances, B-mode imaging can also reveal whether characteristics suggesting ulceration are present. In cases of common or internal carotid artery disease, it is also helpful to know whether the lesion is compensated or uncompensated. An uncompensated internal carotid artery lesion is one that triggers significant functional hemodynamic alterations, such as reduced distal pressure, which in turn induces the development of significant collateral circulation. Such lesions have high potential for significant emboli, rapid progression, and acute occlusion, the consequences of which in the presence of already compromised hemodynamics may be disastrous. Total internal carotid artery occlusion is especially likely to produce uncompensated hemodynamic situations. In such cases, it is most important to preserve existing collateral channels, especially if the contralateral internal carotid artery is diseased. The testing should also indicate collateralization patterns and provide quantitative information regarding vertebral artery disease and the presence or absence of subclavian steal syndrome.

Using the combined modality we have achieved the following accuracy levels in estimating common carotid or internal carotid artery disease: total accuracy, 90 percent; false-positive results, 5 percent; and false-negative results, 5 percent. These percentages were obtained by using arteriography as control.

PERIPHERAL VASCULAR REGISTRY

With increasing surgical and medical therapeutic modalities, need for credentials, and improving noninvasive techniques, the necessity of careful follow-up of study of vascular patients is evident. The advances in microcomputer technology mentioned previously make data storage and retrieval practical. Our laboratory has developed a comprehensive and easy-to-use microcomputer-based Peripheral Vascular Registry (Raines, 1983) consisting of a state-of-the-art data-base management system (DATAEASE) and specifically designed data input screens. The Registry consists of ten files: lower-extremity venous laboratory data, lower-extremity venography, lower-extremity arterial laboratory data, lower-extremity arteriography, cerebral laboratory data, cerebral arteriography, compact surgical record, complete follow-up record, vascular laboratory/angiography codes, and surgical follow-up codes.

After the analysis and printout of the clinical report on the AU, cerebral laboratory data are stored on a hard disc and then fed into the Vascular Registry at appropriate intervals (daily in our laboratory) using the DATAEASE import facility and our procedure files. In addition to saving time, this procedure avoids entry errors that can occur when data are entered by hand. The hard disk in the IBM-AT can store approximately 20,000 patient records for review of vascular history and prior noninvasive evaluations of patients scheduled for future evaluations. The registry can also be used in a research mode to identify and follow patients presenting with identical symptoms to determine their long-term clinical outcomes.

Many investigators believe that major advances in clinical patient management are more likely to occur due to careful monitoring and recording of noninvasive data rather than by the further developments of new techniques of sophisticated measurements. Registry technology assists in this undertaking.

REFERENCES

American Heart Association: *Heart Facts,* 1982.

Blue, S.K.; McKinney, W.M.; Barnes, R.; and Toole, J.F.: Ultrasonic B-mode scanning for study of extracranial vascular disease. *Neurology,* **22**:1079–85, 1972.

Calderon-Ortiz, M.; Holtzhauser, C.; Correa, M.C.; Forster, J.; and Walburn, F.: Role of real-time ultrasonic B-mode imaging in the management of patients with lateralized cerebral symptomatology. *Proceedings of the 7th Annual Meeting of the Society of Noninvasive Vascular Technology,* Atlanta, Georgia, June 1984.

Callow, A.D.: Risk factors in current status of carotid endarterectomy. *Int. Angiol.,* **1**:95–108, 1982.

Comerota, A.J.; Cranley, J.J.; and Cook, S.E.: Real-time B-mode carotid imaging in diagnosis of cerebrovascular disease. *Surgery,* **89**:718–29, 1981.

Cullen, S.J.; Correa, M.C.; Calderon-Ortiz, M.; Walburn, F.J.; and Raines, J.: Clinical sequelae in patients with asymptomatic carotid bruits. *Circulation,* **68** (Suppl. 2):83–7, 1983.

Gee, W.; Smith, C.A.; Hinsen, C.E.; and Wylie, E.J.: Ocular pneumoplethysmography in carotid artery disease. *Med. Instrum.,* **8**:244–48, 1974.

Grady, P.A.: Pathophysiology of extracranial cerebral arterial stenosis—a critical review. *Stroke,* **15**:224–36, 1984.

Griffith, J.M.; McLead, F.D.; and Leroy, A.F.: The pulsed Doppler ultrasound flowmeter: experimental evaluation of velocity accuracy and range resolution. *Med. Instrum.,* **11**:139–43, 1977.

Kartchner, M.M.; McRae, L.P.; Crain, V.; and Whitaker, B.: Oculoplethysmography: an adjunct to arteriography in the diagnosis of extracranial carotid occlusive disease. *Am. J. Surg.,* **132**:728–32, 1976.

Kristensen, J.K.; Eiken, M.; and Von Wowern, F.: Ultrasonic diagnosis of carotid artery disease. *J. Neurosurg.,* **35**:40–44, 1971.

Raines, J.: Second-generation vascular laboratory with registry. *Vascular Lab. Rev.,* **1**:10–37, 1983.

Strandness, D.E., and Sumner, D.S.: *Hemodynamics for Surgeons.* Grune & Stratton, New York, 1975.

8

The Eye in the Diagnosis and Treatment of Extracranial Cerebrovascular Disease

MARTIN J. KRESHON

A thorough study of the visual system can lead to discovery of pathological occurrences in the extracranial vascular tree. Microembolization to or impaired perfusion of the retina and its connections produces characteristic episodic symptoms. This chapter presents a review of anatomical, physiological, and clinico-diagnostic features of the eye and relates them to findings in patients with extracranial vascular problems. Such ocular symptoms are present in about 65 percent of patients with carotid insufficiency.

THE OCULAR CIRCULATION

The caliber of the internal carotid artery, which provides blood supply to both the eye and to the visual pathways (see Figures 8-1 and 8-2), decreases immediately after giving off the ophthalmic artery, therefore directing a high proportion of carotid flow into the ophthalmic artery. This arrangement, combined with the fact that the ophthalmic artery is also comparatively short, creates a slightly higher pressure in the retinal and uveal arteries compared with that of most peripheral vessels of similar order. It also allows a higher blood pressure to be transmitted directly to the interior of the eye. The retinal blood pressure may be estimated by ophthalmodynamometry. The accuracy of this technique is discussed later. Its major clinical use is in comparing the pressures between the two eyes of the same patient.

The intraocular venous pressure is believed to be slightly higher than the intraocular pressure; otherwise, the veins, which do not have rigid walls, would collapse. The venous pressure, which approximates a level 2 mm above the normal intraocular pressure, varies with the intraocular pressure (Adler, 1959).

The volume of blood present in the eye at one time has been estimated to be 211 cu mm, and the blood flow through the eyes of rabbits has been judged to be in the neighborhood of 0.32 ml/min/g, which is 46 percent of the volume estimated for cerebral blood flow.

In the central retinal artery, the intima is comprised of a layer of epithelium, the nuclei of which, lying in the long axis of the vessel, project somewhat into the lumen. It is surrounded by a subendothelial layer, which increases in thickness with age. It is composed of connective tissue fibers and the circular elastic fibers, the coat being enclosed in a fenestrated internal elastic membrane. The media is represented by circularly arranged smooth-muscle cells with the nuclei at right angles to the axis of the vessels, interwoven with small amounts of connective tissue and elastic fibers, and surrounded by a nondescript external elastic membrane.

The adventitia is made up of connective tissue and elastic fibers running in bundles both longitudinally and circularly. Externally, it is bounded by a network of astrocytes. This sheeting is essentially a continuation of the pial and glial coverings which the vessels carry with them into the optic nerve when they enter behind the globe and form the septa.

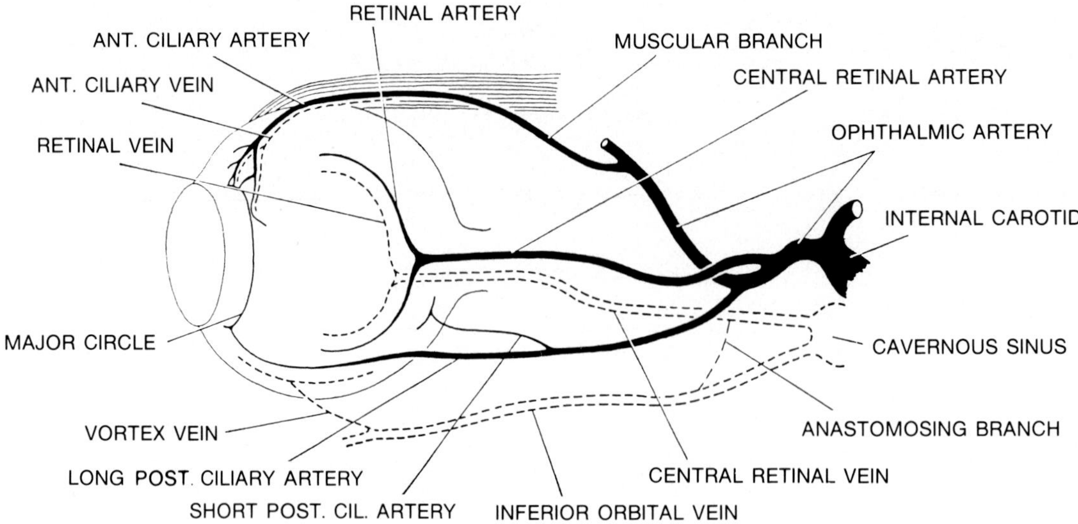

Figure 8-1. The retinal and the uveal circulation. (Modified after Duke-Elder, 1976.)

The veins have thin walls which also conform in structure to that of other medium-sized veins in other parts of the body. They have an endothelial lining, a tenuous subepithelial layer, a media composed largely of elastic fibers with sparse muscle cells, and a thin adventitia mainly composed of fibrous connective tissue, but no elastica either in the external or internal layers.

The arterial venous crossings in the retina are unique, for they are intimate. The artery may cross superficially to the vein, or the reverse arrangement may be seen; but in either case, a confluence of the vascular sheath is present, which gives them a common fibrous coat surrounded by the usual insulating glial tissue. Involvement of the arterial wall in various conditions produces the ophthalmoscopic sign of "banking of blood" at the arterial venous crossing.

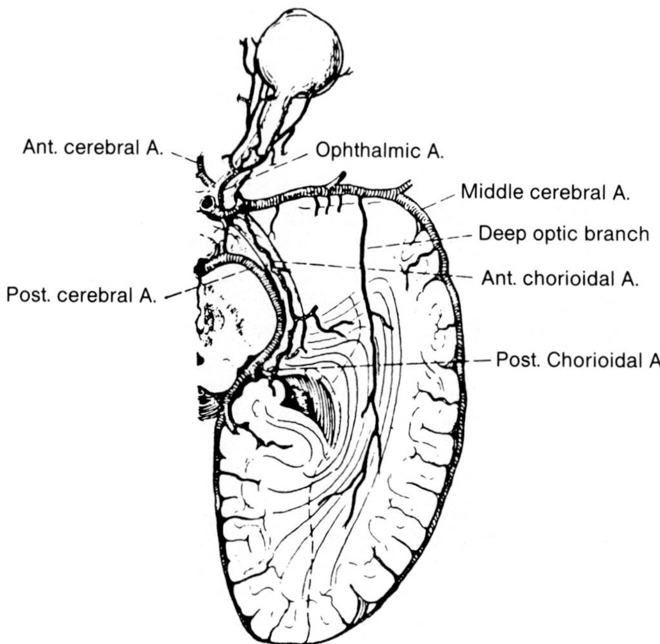

Figure 8-2. Blood supply to the visual pathways. The deep optic branch of the middle cerebral artery has been enlarged for emphasis. Reproduced with permission from Kreshon, M.J.: *Physiology of the Eye,* 4 ed. C.V. Mosby, St. Louis, 1965, page 307.

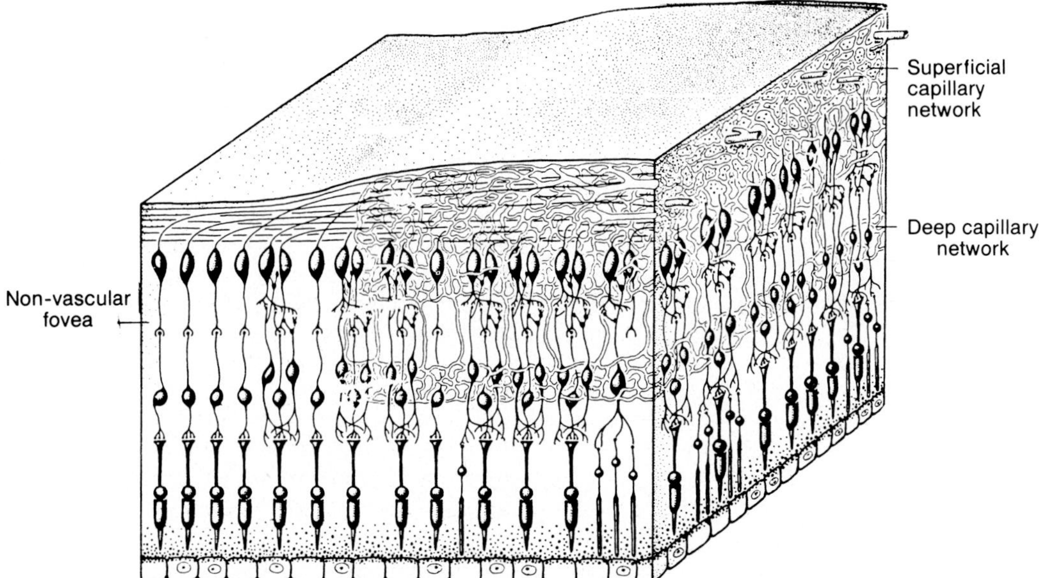

Figure 8–3. Stereogram of retina in the macular region showing the synapses between the various cellular components. The superficial and deep capillary plexi are shown in the right half of the picture only, because the vessels do not enter the uveal area. Reproduced with permission from Kreshon, M.J.: *Physiology of the Eye,* 4 ed. C.V. Mosby, St. Louis, 1965, page 307.

The deep capillary network of the retina is more complex than the superficial one and lies in the boundary plane between the inner nuclear layer and the outer plexiform layer. The superficial capillary network is found in the nerve fiber layer at the level of the retinal artery and vein. Anastomotic capillaries run from one layer to the other.

Surrounding each artery is a zone normally free of capillaries which extends on either side of the artery for an average of 15 μm. There is no capillary-free space around the veins.

In the macular region, the two layers are replaced by a three-layered pattern. This area appears more vascularized than the region outside the macula owing to a closer capillary mesh and the appearance of the third capillary layer (see Figure 8–3). The fovea shows a completely avascular area varying from 0.4 to 0.5 mm in diameter. Blood to the fovea is supplied entirely from the choriocapillaries.

CLINICAL EXAMINATION OF THE CIRCULATION OF THE EYE

Major arteries and veins are easily distinguishable by ophthalmoscopic examination. Arteries are smaller and brighter red than veins and run a more linear course. They usually lie superficially in the retina and anterior to the veins at the arteriovenous crossings. With advancing age, the angulation of the crossing becomes more of a right angle. The finer vascular pattern is obscured ophthalmoscopically by the orange background of the choroidal vessels. Because walls of the vessels are transparent, the blood columns within the vessels are easily visible under normal circumstances. When the vessels become sclerotic, the wall appears as a thin streak that enlarges as arteriosclerosis progresses until the blood column is obscured, producing "copper" or "silver wiring" of the arterial tree.

Because retinal diastolic pressure is well above the intraocular pressure, the retinal artery shows no expansile pulsation under normal conditions. The retinal vein, however, usually pulsates at its exit from the disk which is the site of the lowest venous pressure. This pulsation reflects changes in the intraocular pressure with each cardiac beat rather than a change in the venous pressure itself. The vein collapses as the intraocular pressure exceeds that within the vein. Venous pulsation is of limited clinical significance; however, if it is present, it rules out increased intracranial pressure in questionable cases of papilledema. Spontaneous pulsation of the artery, on the other hand, is always of pathological significance, indicating either an abnormally low retinal diastolic pressure or an excessive intraocular pressure.

Methods of Examination

Ophthalmoscopy. The ophthalmoscope is the most commonly used instrument for direct examination of the fundus of the eye. It contains a series of lenses in varying dioptic power to permit sequential focusing from the front to the back of the eye. It is best to start with +8 to +10 diopter lenses several inches from the eye to determine the clarity of the media and to allow time for the patient to steady his gaze. Moving closer to the eye, the lens power is decreased as the disk comes into view. The magnification of the direct ophthalmoscope is 15 times the normal size of 1.5 mm (Cogan, 1974).

Indirect ophthalmoscopy may be also used to obtain a stereoscopic view of the fundus. The instrument used for this purpose consists of a collimated light source strapped to the examiner's forehead with a focusing lens of 20 to 25 D which the examiner places between his own eyes and those of the patient. The advantages of the indirect ophthalmoscope include, in addition to the three-dimensional visualization feature, a larger field available for examination, a greater accessibility of the peripheral fundus, and a greater penetrability of cloudy media with a bright light. These advantages become especially valuable when ophthalmoscopy is performed in uncooperative patients or in those who have nystagmus, incipient cataracts, cloudy vitreous, detached retinas, tumors, etc. The disadvantages of indirect ophthalmoscopy include the inverted image of the fundus, which necessitates dilating the pupils and requires extensive experience in the use of the method.

Slit-Lamp Biomicroscopy. This method is used chiefly to examine the anterior parts of the eye but may be adapted with special lenses for supplemental examination of the fundus in three dimensions.

Fluoroangiography of the Fundus. This method was introduced in the early 1960s as a means of visualizing the vessels in the back of the eye. The customary technique consists of injecting fluorescein into the antecubital vein and then taking photographs of the fundus in rapid sequence to show the entrance and transmission of the fluorescein through the vessels. Two or more pictures are taken per second with special filters to eliminate extraneous light. The pictures illustrate the vascular patterns, including capillary plexus, and are comparable to the histologic preparation of flat mounts. They also provide information on hemodynamics that would be impossible to obtain otherwise (see Figure 8–4).

The fluorescein dye is essentially nontoxic, but I have observed transient nausea and mild allergic reactions. Because of reports of more

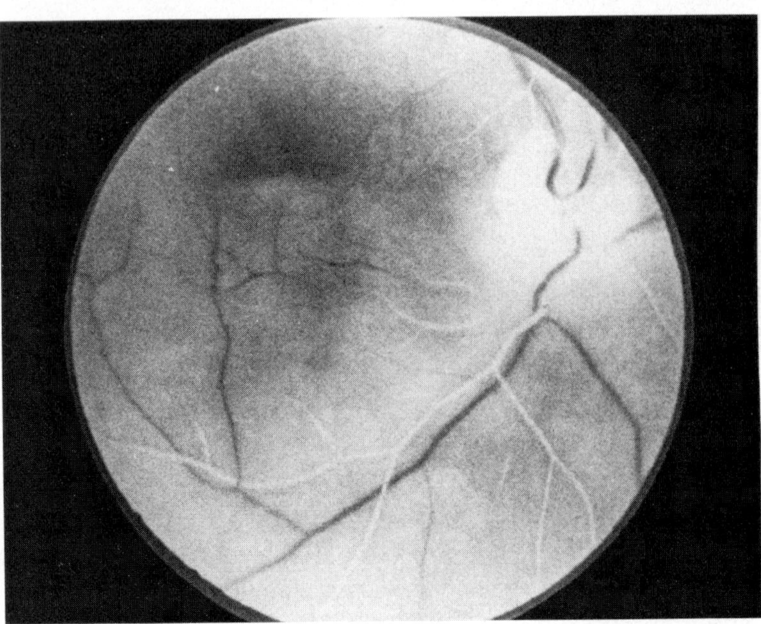

Figure 8–4. Fluorescein angiogram showing superior branch occlusion.

serious complications, such as bronchospasm, emergency resuscitation measures should be available.

The fluorescein enters the eye 8 to 12 seconds after the injection is begun. The entire fundus lights up as the fluorescein enters the choroid, but the central fundus is darker owing to the greater amount of pigment in this area. As the choroid lights up, fluorescein enters the retinal arteries, and within one to two seconds is passed into the veins.

The fluorescence clears from the retinal vessels in five to ten minutes, leaving a faint glow of protein-bound fluorescein in the bloodstream. It does not normally leak out of the retinal vessels but does leak out of choroidal vessels. This leakage produces a luminous background in the choroid and the nerve head that persists for an hour or more. Recent modifications have been made with different colors in the dye and with other filters, but the basic fluorescein solution is still commonly used.

The principal value of a retinal angiogram is the detection of obstruction to flow, defects in the pigment epithelium, pathological vessel formation, and, especially, abnormal leaks from the choroidal and retinal blood vessels. Retinal vascular anomalies are demonstrated most vividly.

Ophthalmodynamometry. By applying an external force to the sclera and observing the arterial pulsation on the nerve head, the blood pressure of the retinal arteries can be measured. The first induced pulsation corresponds with the diastolic pressure, whereas the eventual elimination of pulsation and sustained collapse of the artery corresponds to the systolic pressure. The Bailliart ophthalmodynamometer is the most popular instrument used for this purpose. It has a spring-loaded plunger within a sliding barrel. The scale is calibrated in millimeters of mercury and corresponds approximately to the intraocular pressure which in turn is exerted on the wall of the artery. Comparative measurements of the two eyes are the main goal of this type of testing (Heyman *et al.*, 1957; Kempczinski, 1979).

To initiate the procedure, local anesthetic is instilled in the eye, and the footplate of the dynamometer is placed on the sclera several millimeters behind the limbus. Indirect ophthalmoscopy with a dilated pupil is usually used, and the end points are read off the scale as the pressure on the sclera is gradually increased. The diastolic end points are easy to obtain. The systolic end point is more difficult to determine and causes some discomfort to the patient because of the amount of pressure necessary to close the artery. In addition, there is danger of trauma from slippage of the footplate on the sclera or even of permanent occlusion of the central retinal artery. Unless it is especially indicated, therefore, systolic pressures are not obtained routinely. In the absence of an ophthalmodynamometric measurement, arterial pressure may be roughly estimated by manual pressure against the lid during ophthalmoscopy.

The pressures are usually measured with the patient in the sitting position; however, comparative measurements in the supine and standing position are occasionally indicated, especially in cases of suspected postural hypotension. While pressure levels may vary from person to person, they are normally equal to within 15 percent in the two eyes of any one individual. They usually amount to 50 to 75 percent of the brachial pressures. What is actually determined is the pressure in the ophthalmic artery rather than that in the normal retinal artery, because the act of arresting the circulation automatically increases the pressure to that of the feeding vessel. The observed pressure in the retinal arteries is probably 14 to 17 mm higher than the normal pressure in the retinal artery.

Retinal blood pressures are important in revealing retinal artery occlusion, but their chief value lies in the study of carotid occlusive disease. A difference of arterial pressure greater than 20 percent between the two eyes or significant difference in pulse pressures suggests carotid disease. Collateral circulation from either the ipsilateral carotid artery or the contralateral internal carotid, however, may maintain normal ophthalmic artery pressures despite the carotid occlusion.

Ophthalmodynamometry is based on the assumption that central retinal artery pressure reflects internal carotid pressure because the ophthalmic artery is a branch of the internal carotid artery and the central retinal artery is an end-artery. It measures pressure and not blood flow through the central retinal artery system. Reasons for false-positive results in ophthalmodynamometry include the following:

1. The end points are subject to measurement error.
2. Cardiac arrhythmia may cause inaccurate readings.

3. Generalized atherosclerosis in the aortic arch and its branches may alter pressure-flow relationships in the internal carotid artery.
4. A stenosed or occluded ophthalmic artery lowers the pressure on that side, whereas a carotid obstruction distal to the origin of the ophthalmic artery may increase the reading.

Arterial pulsation occurs when the retinal diastolic pressure is lower than the intraocular pressure, that is, when it is less than 20 mm Hg. It is thus encountered with aortic regurgitation, carotid stenosis, aortic arch disease, and vasometer collapse. Spontaneous arterial pulsation may also occur in the presence of a normal arterial pressure when the intraocular pressure is sufficiently elevated, as in glaucomatous eyes.

Obstruction of the ophthalmic artery can usually be distinguished from that of the carotid by the quality of pulsation induced by ophthalmodynamometry. With ophthalmic artery obstruction, the pulsation is weak or absent. As diastole is approached, the artery collapses and then refills slowly as the external pressure is released. The pulsation does not have the snapping quality which is normally present and which may be present even with carotid stenosis.

Electroretinography, Electrooculography, and Cortically Evoked Potentials. Although usually available only in centers for specialized services, these electrical tests can provide important information on retinal function. The electroretinogram (ERG) is a measure of a transient millivoltage change in the electrical potential between the cornea and the retina in response to a flash of light. Its presence indicates that the photoreceptive layer of the retina is intact but it gives no indication of the status of the inner retinal layers. Thus, the graph may be normal despite loss of the entire inner portion of the retina from central retinal artery occlusion but will be weak or absent with choroidal vasculopathies or degenerations that destroy the outer portion of the retina (see Table 8-1). It is not a sensitive test; extensive portions of the outer layers must be lost before reliable changes in the electroretinogram can be detected.

The electrooculogram (EOG) depends on stationary differences in potential between the retina and the cornea rather than on changes induced by light. It is usually measured by use of bitemporal or nasotemporal electrodes which record changes in potential with horizontal movements of the eye. The EOG has much the same application as the ERG and is particularly useful in defining degenerative diseases rather than vasculopathies. For obvious reasons it is especially adaptable for tracking eye movements.

Cortically evoked potentials are recorded by tapping off changes in the occipital potentials that result from exposing the eye to flashes of light. This method has been made possible by integrative techniques that select and summate the significant signals from a noisy background. It supplements the ERG and EOG methods in detecting disease of the neural conduction system. Cortically evoked potentials

Table 8-1. Findings of Electroretinography in Retinal Circulatory Abnormality

ABNORMALITY	FINDINGS
Extraocular	
Carotid artery occlusion	Diminished b-wave, especially to flicker
Temporal arteritis	Most commonly diminished b-wave, but may have enhanced a-wave
Ophthalmic artery occlusion	Absent ERG
Intraocular	
Hypertension	Normal in grade 1 or 2, normal or subnormal ERG in grades 3 or 4 K-W*
Arteriosclerosis	No typical picture, most commonly a diminished b-wave
Retinal artery occlusion	
Central	Generally reduced or negative ERG; may find initial elevation of b-wave
Branch	Generally normal
Retinal vein occlusion	
Central	Varies from sub- to supernormal; prognosis better in cases with normal or supernormal ERG
Branch	Normal
Diabetic retinopathy	Usually normal; occasionally supernormal, possibly owing to venous stasis; abnormal oscillatory potentials even before visible retinopathy

* Keith-Wagener classification of hypertensive retinopathy. From Keith, N.M.; *et al.*; Some different types of essential hypertension, their course and prognosis. *Am. J. Med. Sci.*, **197**: 332, 1939, with permission.

are unelicitable with loss of the inner retinal layers even though the ERG and EOG are normal. It further supplements the ERG, which is responsive to large areas of photoreceptor loss only, by being especially sensitive to loss of macular vision. The macular response is due to the disproportionate contribution that macular vision makes to the electrical activity of the occiput.

Measurement of cortically evoked potentials is important for evaluating visual functions, especially if the presence of opaque media would prevent ordinary means of testing, but it has no specific relevance to vascular disease.

Ocular Pneumoplethysmography. This technique requires the application of suction to the sclera as a method of increasing the intraocular pressure (Duke *et al.,* 1979; Gee *et al.,* 1976). Through a small cup, suction is applied to the sclera lateral to the cornea. There is a precise relationship between the degree of vacuum applied and the resulting increase in intraocular pressure. If the intraocular pressure exceeds the systolic pressure and the ophthalmic artery pressure, blood flow to the eye will cease and the eye itself will pulsate no longer. Of the three transducers contained in the instrument, two are designed to sense the return of ocular pulsation as the intraocular pressure induced by the applied vacuum falls to a level below the systolic pressure in the respective ophthalmic arteries. The third transducer measures the degree of vacuum applied simultaneously to both eyecups. The instrument is portable. With the development of newer diagnostic techniques, ocular pneumoplethysmography is used less frequently.

Doppler Imaging of the Carotid and Doppler Ophthalmic Tests. The Doppler ophthalmic test was introduced by Brockenbrough in 1970. It is based on the fact that supraorbital artery flow is anterograde in normal subjects and in persons with internal carotid stenosis less than 75 percent by diameter, but reverts if the internal carotid is more severely stenosed or occluded completely (Hedges *et al.,* 1983; LoGerfo and Mason, 1974). The test uses a directional Doppler flowmeter to determine the direction of supraorbital artery flow. It is of clinical value in screening stroke patients and in the evaluation of patients undergoing carotid endarterectomy (Check, 1984; Kempczinski, 1979). However, retrograde flow is not always an index of the clinical significance of carotid stenosis. Ultrasonography reveals carotid stenosis in nearly 50 percent of cervical bruit cases (Lemak and Fields, 1976). Doppler imaging of the carotid, including real-time ultrasonography, is described elsewhere in this volume (Moore *et al.,* 1977; Otis *et al.,* 1979) (See also Chapter 7 on noninvasive diagnosis).

OCULAR SYMPTOMS AND SIGNS OF EXTRACRANIAL ARTERIAL INSUFFICIENCY

In 1856, Virchow (1962) provided the first description of carotid artery thrombosis in a patient who had lost all vision in his ipsilateral eye. Gowers (1875) described a patient with the clinical syndrome of monocular blindness and contralateral hemiplegia in whom postmortem examination revealed mitral stenosis, clots in the auricular appendices, an embolus in the left middle cerebral artery, and several small emboli in the central artery of the retina. He stressed the importance of examining the retinal vessels in any patient in whom carotid thrombosis is suspected.

In 1905, Chiari published a report that stands as a landmark in the medical literature on cerebrovascular thrombosis. He found that soft thrombi in major intracranial branches of the carotid artery often rise from mural thrombi on an atheromatous plaque situated at the carotid bifurcation. He also stipulated that disease in the main carotid trunk was a prime source of the emboli causing strokes in elderly patients.

Fisher (1951) reawakened interest in the whole problem of carotid thrombosis when he stressed that patients with this disease may have isolated fleeting episodes of monocular blindness and then, months later, develop catastrophic hemiplegia on the opposite side of the body.

Since that time, a voluminous amount of material has been written concerning ocular symptoms and signs of carotid and vertebrobasilar artery disease (see Table 8-2). One of the most common visual symptoms is amaurosis fugax. It is usually the result of embolism from an atheromatous plaque in the carotid artery. Three common types of emboli have been identified: (1) fibrin and platelet, (2) cholesterol lipid (Hollenhorst plaques), and (3) calcific or fibrinoid (see Tables 8–3 and 8–4). Cholesterol plaques are the most common, followed by the fibrin-platelet and then the calcific plaques (Pfaffenbach and Hollenhorst, 1972).

Table 8-2. Ocular Signs in Carotid Vascular Disease

SITE	SIGN
Retina	
	Emboli
	Vessel-wall changes after emboli
	Central retinal artery occlusion
	Branch retinal artery occlusion
	Unilateral retinopathy
	Unequal retinal hypertensive change
Optic disk	
	Ischemic optic neuropathy
	Optic atrophy
Iris	
	Ipsilateral Horner's syndrome
	Transient dilatation and loss of reactivity
Cornea	
	Unequal arcus senilis
Sclera	
	Ipsilateral dilation of episcleral vessels
	Visual loss

From Till. J.S.: Ophthalmologic aspects of cerebrovascular disease. In Toole, J.F. (ed.): *Cerebrovascular Disorders*. Raven Press, New York, 1984, 231-50, with permission..

In 1961 and 1962, Hollenhorst described 31 patients of a series of 328 subjects with either carotid or vertebrobasilar artery disease each of whom had one to several dozen brightly refractile plaques in the retinal arteries (Hollenhorst, 1961, 1962).

Amaurosis Fugax

Amaurosis fugax (fleeting blindness) occurs without warning and usually without any obvious precipitating factor. The patient has a sudden, painless loss of vision in a single eye. This is usually described as either a sudden "dimming" or "graying out" of the field of vision, or a "gray or black curtain," descending from the top of the field and rapidly lowering to cover the inferior field. Gray or black

Table 8-3. Features of Common Retinal Microemboli

	TYPE OF EMBOLI		
FEATURE	PLATELET-FIBRIN	CHOLESTEROL-LIPID	CALCIFIC OR FIBRINOID
Color	White, nonrefractile	Orange-yellow, orange, or bright metallic gold refractile, usually at bifurcation, often without infarction	Gray-white, dull, nonrefractile
Shape	Long, smooth segments with flat discrete ends	(1) Globular, containing bright crystals, and with indistinct interface with blood; (2) small rectangular flakes alone	Ovoid, discrete, and filling arterial lumen
Apparent caliber	Same as blood column	Larger than blood column	Same or slightly larger than proximal blood column
Mobility	Highly mobile; jerks from one bifurcation to the next	Amoeboid-gelatinous movement with massage of eye; moves or breaks up over a period of days	Fixed
Location in retinal artery	Usually in motion	At bifurcations of medium and small vessels, unless large and mixed with stable fibrin	In unbranched segments of main or medium-sized retinal arterioles
Ischemic changes	Transient slowing of blood flow	Dilated vein indicating mild hypoxia; retinal infarction from multiple plaques variable in density and without clear borders	Usually a dense, sharply delimited retinal infarct; small ischemic hemorrhages
Vessel changes	No damage seen	Gray-white segmental mural opacity at bifurcation; slow appearance	Segmental mural change with narrowing, collateral capillary shunts or both
Source and significance	Mural or "tail" thrombus in carotid occlusion (acute or imminent)	Eroding atheroma in carotid bifurcation; carotid patent and often without stenosis	Calcific valvular disease (apparent in x-ray of heart); rheumatic heart disease; myocardial disease; mitral valve prolapse

From Till. J.S.: Ophthalmologic aspects of cerebrovascular disease. In Toole, J.F. (ed.): *Cerebrovascular Disorders*. Raven Press, New York, 1984, 231-50, with permission.

Table 8–4. Other Retinal Microemboli

EMBOLI	APPEARANCE	SOURCE
Endogenous		
Bacteria	White-centered hemorrhages (Roth's spots)	Subacute bacterial endocarditis and drug addiction
Tumor	Central retinal artery occlusion, (usually left eye)	Atrial myxoma or bronchogenic carcinoma
Amniotic fluid	Retinal edema and pallor with later degeneration of pigment epithelium	Complicated delivery or pregnancy
Parasites and fungi	Appearance varies greatly according to organism	Cysticercus, *Angiostrongylus cantonensis, Schistosoma mansoni,* Mucor, and others
Exogenous		
Silicone	Multiple small emboli	Heart valve prosthesis, plastic surgery of the nose and face
Air and mercury	Multiple small emboli	Accidental emboli at surgery
Oil	Glistening dots	Hysterosalpingography contrast media
Talc and cornstarch	Red-yellow glistening particles near macula, cotton-wool patches	Methylphenidate injection by drug abusers
Glass beads	Central retinal artery occlusion	Injected into carotid to close cerebral aneurysms

From Henkind, P., and Chambers, J.: Arterial occlusive disease of the retina. In Duane, T.D. and Jaeger, E.A. (eds.): *Clinical Ophthalmology.* Harper and Row, New York, 1984, 3–14, with permission.

areas rise from the inferior field and ascend to cover the superior portions of the visual field. This loss of vision occurs in a matter of seconds and most frequently involves the entire field, which becomes totally gray or black. This usually resolves rapidly with complete return of vision in five to ten minutes.

Most current evidence indicates that amaurosis fugax and other carotid territory transient ischemic attacks are caused by emboli (see Figure 8–5). Angiographic studies in patients in the age group appropriate for atherosclerotic vascular disease have shown that amaurosis fugax predicts angiographically sig-

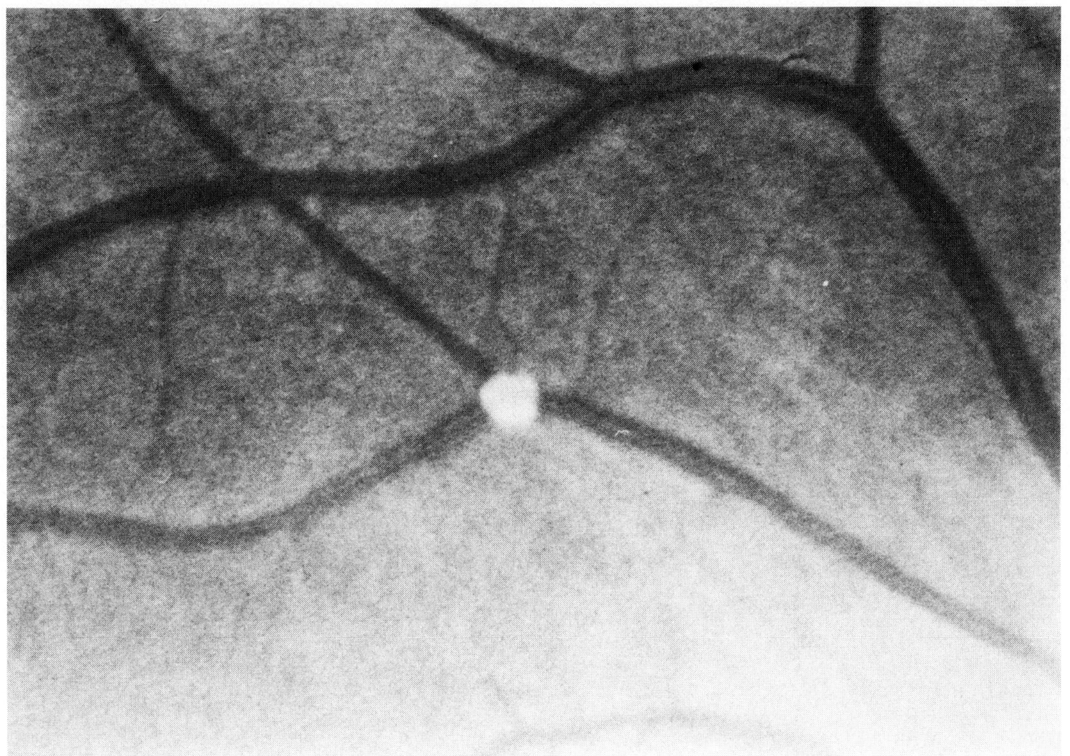

Figure 8–5. Cholesterol embolus in retinal artery branch.

nificant ipsilateral carotid disease (occlusion, significant stenosis, or ulcerated plaque) with a 70 to 97 percent accuracy; thus, it is useful in predicting the future risk of stroke. Pfaffenbach and Hollenhorst (1972) followed 24 patients with amaurosis fugax and cholesterol emboli for six to ten years and found a 37.5 percent incidence of permanent visual loss or stroke.

Adams and associates (1983), in studying the result of arteriography in 59 patients, found that only 34 percent with amaurosis fugax had no carotid abnormality and that fewer than 39 percent had carotid stenosis. Their conclusion was that all patients with transient monocular blindness should be assumed to have carotid artery disease until other causes such as emboli from other sites can be proven. They summarized ten other series in the literature in the past 20 years which showed normal angiograms in 3 to 41 percent of patients with amaurosis fugax.

In considering possible causes of amaurosis fugax, one must be aware of all conditions which can produce it (see Table 8-5). In addition, there are many causes of transient monocular visual loss, including direct insults to the central nervous system and the cardiovascular system (see Table 8-6).

Table 8-5. Possible Etiology of Amaurosis Fugax

Emboli
Heart, vegetation, myxoma, postsurgical occlusion, postcoronary occlusion
Carotid—atheromatous plaques
Bone fracture (fat emboli)
Exogenous emboli—intravenous drug abuse

Other causes
Carotid stenosis
Vasculitis
Polyarteritis
Giant-cell arteritis
High ratio of intraocular pressure to retinal blood pressure
Sickle-cell disease
Ischemic optic neuritis
Aortic arch and steal syndrome (blood for vertebral system)
Retrolental fibroplasia
Hyperviscosity syndromes (cryoglobulinemia, macroglobulinemia, polycythemia)
Homocystinuria
Papilledema
Drusen of the optic disk with bleeding
High myopia (nearsightedness)
Dysplasias of the optic disk (pseudopapilledema)
Retinal migraine
Arteritis or Raynaud's phenomenon
Anemia
Coagulopathies
Dural arteriovenous malformation
Optic-nerve tumors
Sphenoidal sinus dysplasia
Hypertensive crisis
Intermittent elevations of intraocular pressure
Postcataract extraction intermittent bleeding
  From wound vascularization
  From pseudophakic irritation of iris

Table 8-6. Causes of Transient Monocular Visual Loss

CENTRAL NERVOUS SYSTEM	CARDIOVASCULAR SYSTEM
Traumatic	Inflammatory
Closed head injuries	Endocarditis
Subarachnoid hemorrhages	Polyarteritis
Nutritional	Temporal arteritis
Beriberi	Raynaud's disease
Degenerative	Reflex
Schilder's disease	Angiospasm
Multiple sclerosis	Traumatic
Devic's disease	Hemorrhage into optic nerve
Tumor	Degenerative
Sarcoma of choroid	Atherosclerosis
Visuopsychic	Carotid ulcerated plaque
Hysteria	Pathophysiological
Migraine	Hypotension
Pregnancy	Digital pressure
Other	Hemorrhage
Myopia	Glaucoma
Polycythemia	Metabolic
Thrombocythemia	Diabetes mellitus
Papilledema	Anatomic
	Vasodilation of orbital veins
	Takayasu's disease
	Biochemical
	Migraine

Approximately 6 to 20 percent of patients with amaurosis fugax will eventually have occlusion of the central retinal artery or its branches (see Figure 8-6). The involved retinal area is initially hazy but soon becomes milky white. The arteriolar area narrows, but the veins maintain their caliber. Blood within the veins stagnates and oscillates to-and-fro ("boxcar-type segments") (see Figure 8-7). Within weeks these signs disappear, and the inner retinal layers are replaced by a thin, transparent glial scar. The artery remains irregularly narrowed. More than 90 percent of retinal artery branch occlusions are secondary to emboli. A central retinal artery occlusion may be either thrombotic or embolic with a clear differentiation possible only if some emboli are visible in the peripheral retinal arteriole tree.

The signs and symptoms of central retinal artery occlusion include sudden, painless loss of vision in the affected eye. The pupil on the same side is fixed or sluggish to direct light stimulation but usually responds consensually. Ophthalmoscopic findings usually in-

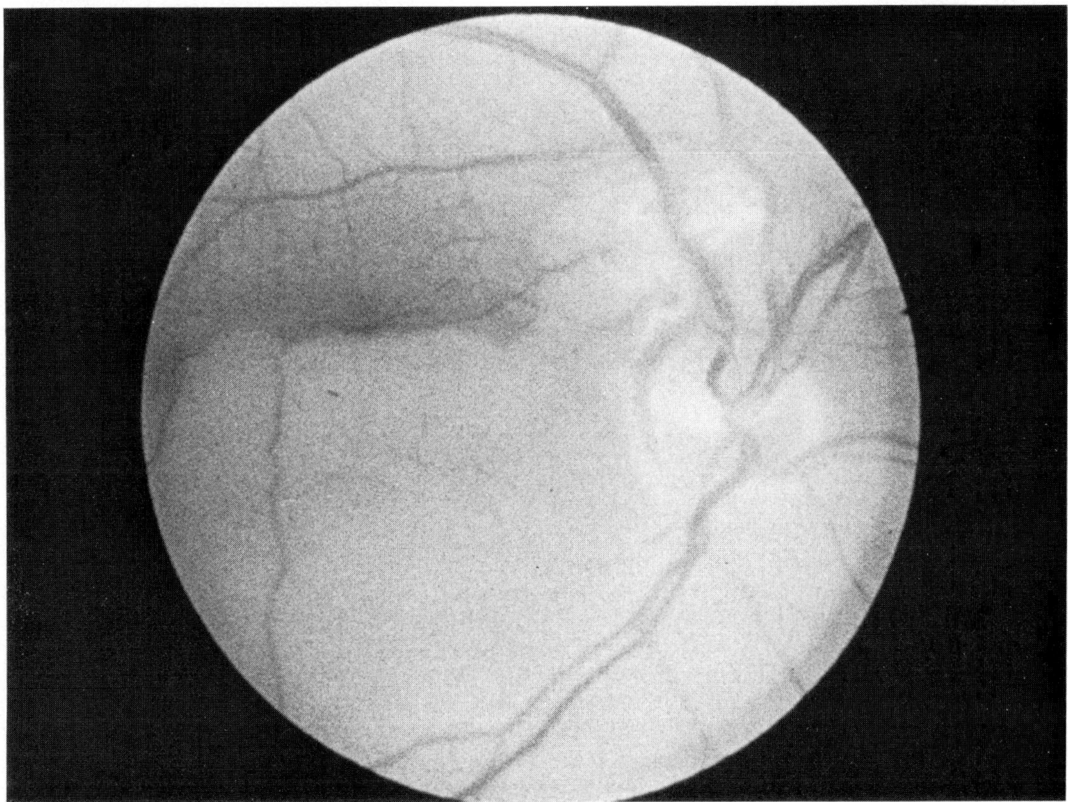

Figure 8–6. "Pale fundus" in a case of retinal branch occlusion.

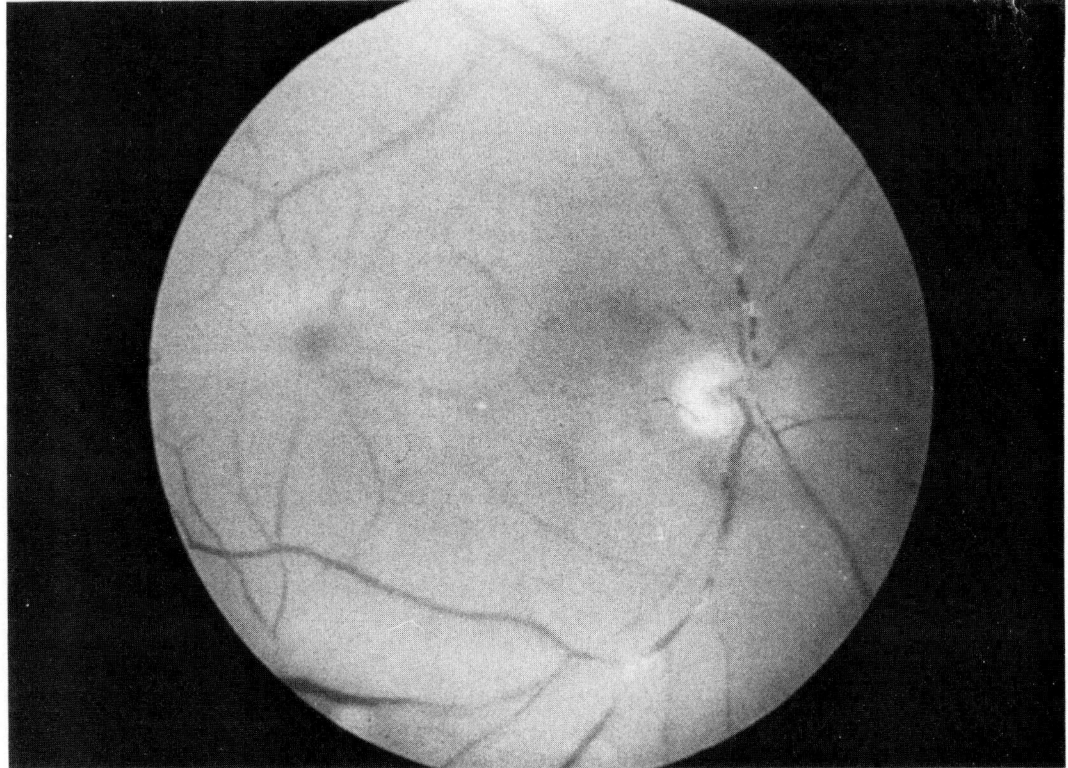

Figure 8–7. Retinal artery occlusion with "boxcar" phenomenon.

clude a pale disk with attenuated arterioles and veins; a cloudy, gray retina; and cherry-red maculae. If circulation is not restored quickly, permanent blindness will result, and with time there will be atrophy of the inner retinal layers. The disk will remain pale and the retinal arterioles will become attenuated and pale, and the veins less distinct. A mild ache in the eye may be present; severe pain suggests involvement of the ophthalmic artery as well. Of the many causes of retinal artery occlusion, atheromatous involvement of the central artery and the optic nerve and embolus are most common. However, central retinal artery spasm has been seen in patients with transient monocular blindness due to retinal migraines; it could also result in retinal damage during the vasospastic phase of the migrainous attack (Ellis, 1964). Temporal arteritis and thromboangitis obliterans may also cause central retinal artery occlusion. Dental anesthesia with injection about the alveolar region of the maxilla may cause embolisation of air, fat, or other foreign substance into the central retinal artery. The embolus may pass through the anastomoses between the facial and internal maxillary arteries with the ophthalmic artery. Such emboli have also been seen after injections of steroids containing long-acting medroxyprogesterone acetate products into the sinuses. Intravenous drug addicts may embolize talc or other debris.

The diagnosis of central retinal artery occlusion includes strong consideration of atherosclerotic disease in the ipsilateral carotid bifurcation and internal carotid artery and requires an evaluation at least by noninvasive carotid studies. The erythrocyte sedimentation rate should be taken to rule out the possibility of giant cell arteritis or temporal arteritis (Henkind and Chambers, 1984), and a complete blood count including platelets should be taken to evaluate the patient for polycythemia, thrombocythemia, and hyperviscosity syndromes. After these initial steps, four-vessel arteriography should be considered. Other occlusive arterial diseases of the retina include "steal" syndromes, in which blood is robbed from the retina; orbital masses; homocystinuria, in which the retinal artery participates with other arterial disease; and collagenoses.

Treatment of acute retinal artery occlusion, though frequently unrewarding, must be directed toward an immediate attempt to dislodge the embolus toward the periphery by either dilating the central retinal artery or by softening the eye (Wolff, 1948). When the circulation is completely obstructed, treatment must be undertaken before irreversible necrosis of the ganglion cells of the retina occurs. In humans, this happens in approximately 1½ hours. Fortunately, complete obstruction is rare, and if there is even minimal retinal circulation, it is still possible to obtain considerable recovery for as long as to 24 hours (see Figure 8–8). Decreasing the pressure by digital massage with the patient in the supine position is the simplest way of mechanically moving the clot along. The massage should be continued for at least four to five minutes with intermittent stops to observe the fundus. Digital massage may be accompanied by retrobulbar injection of 2 percent lidocaine with hyaluronidase to lower the ocular pressure. This also relieves the sympathetic constricting effect in the intraneural central retinal artery.

Massage may be combined with inhalation of 95 percent oxygen and 5 percent carbon dioxide. There is some controversy about whether or not 5 percent carbon dioxide can produce vasodilatation. Carbon dioxide, however, does widen the plasma zone surrounding the red-cell column and the retinal vessels but does not increase the width of the red-cell column itself (Bulpitt *et al.,* 1970; Deutsch *et al.,* 1983). Hyperventilation has been demonstrated to prolong the mean retinal circulation time. Oxygen saturation can increase 3 to 4 percent during hyperventilation.

Paracentesis of the anterior chamber was recommended in 1877 by Secondi. In 1881, Samuelson suggested the use of amyl nitrate by inhalation with the patient supine. Although retrobulbar injections of acetylcholine, atropine, and tolazoline have been described in the past, these, like most retrobulbar drug injections, have been abandoned. Intravenous injection of 20 mg of tolazoline is useful as well as intravenous acetazolamide or mannitol to lower the intraocular pressure.

Attempts to dissolve the clot by intravenous steptokinase have usually been ineffective because it is not delivered in high enough concentrations to the site of the obstruction.

Treatment by injections of antispasmodic or thrombolytic agents into the supraorbital artery, which arises from the ophthalmic artery close to the origin of the central retinal artery, has been advocated, especially by Watson (1959) and by Younge (1978). Approximately one third of patients so treated recovered vision.

After initiation of emergency treatment, in-

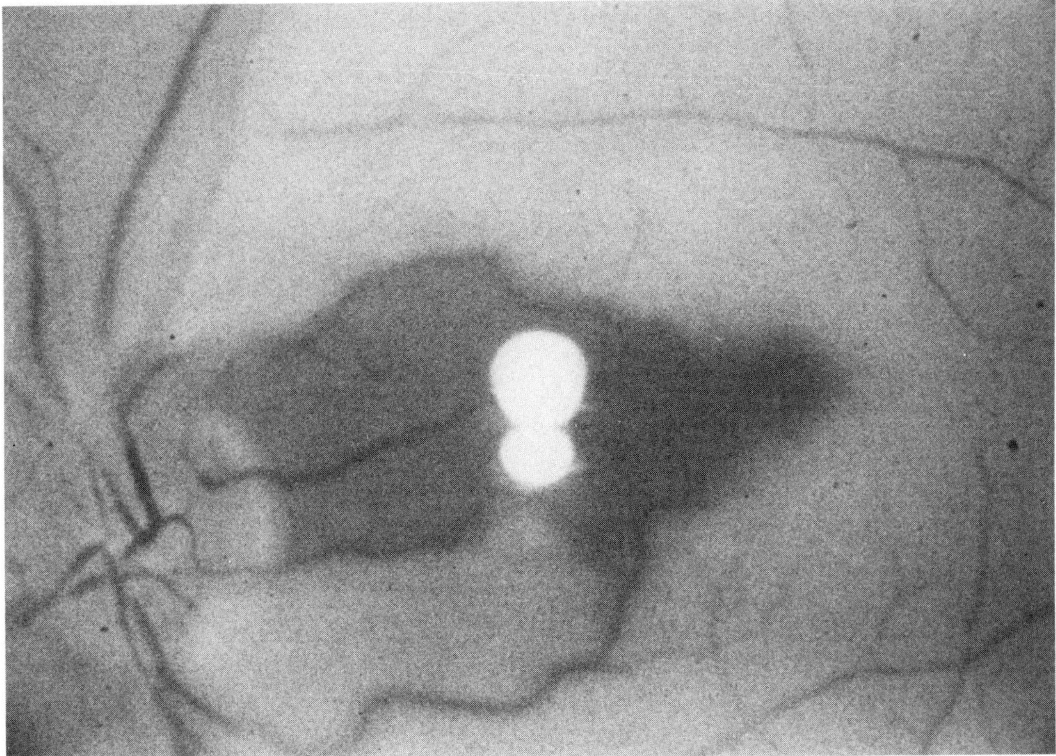

Figure 8-8. Sparing of the cilioretinal circulation in retinal artery occlusion.

cluding softening of the eye by digital massage, retrobulbar injection, and/or intravenous acetazolamide and mannitol, the patient should be given heparin and later sodium warfarin if there is no medical contraindication. During this period, a thorough search should be made for the source of the embolus. Long-term anticoagulation is usually not necessary unless there is some other medical indication.

Miscellaneous Syndromes

Takayasu's Disease (Aortic Arch Syndrome, or Pulseless Disease). Takayasu's disease is an uncommon condition in which the major vessels of the aortic arch become progressively obliterated, causing reduction of blood flow to the head and arms (see also Chapter 29).

The ocular findings of Takayasu's disease relate directly to the decreased blood flow to the eyes, and the findings are similar to those of carotid insufficiency. The findings, however, are almost always bilateral and are more severe than those found in isolated carotid artery disease, and have been labeled as hypotensive or ischemic optic neuropathy (see Figure 8-9). The prolonged and slowly progressive retinal ischemia produces retinal changes beginning in the periphery. Microaneurysms and arterial obliteration are seen early, along with arteriovenous shunts. After the retinal periphery is lost, there is involvement of the posterior pole where neovascularization, peripheral arteriovenous anastomoses, cotton-wool spots, microaneurysms, and secondarily dilated retinal veins may ensue. Late in the course of the condition, rubeosis of the iris and cataracts may develop.

The ophthalmologist must also be aware of the nonocular manifestations of Takayasu's disease. The patient has cold hands, paresthesias, and claudication of the arms in exercise. Radial pulses are weak or absent. The patient may have transient attacks of syncope, hemiplegia, headaches, seizures, deafness, and coma. These are sometimes precipitated by elevating or turning the head. Associated signs are cranial arterial insufficiency, including orbital and facial muscle atrophy, nasal septal defects, and loss of hair.

Treatment of the ocular findings secondary

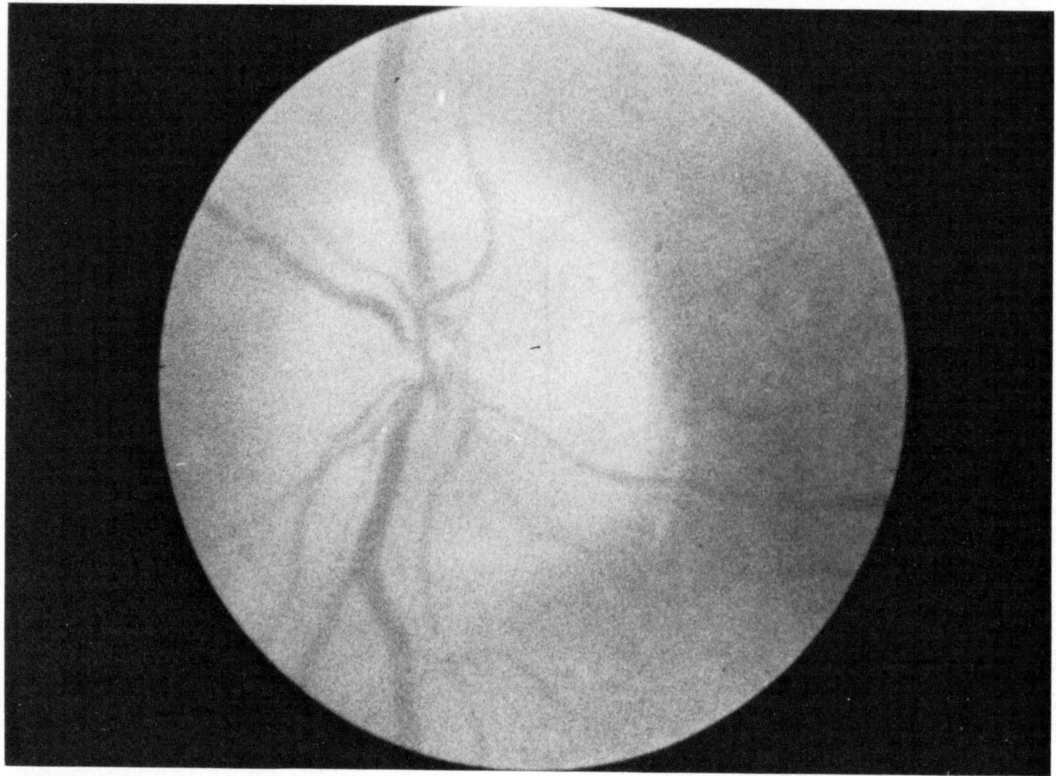

Figure 8-9. Ischemic optic neuropathy.

to Takayasu's disease depends solely on eliminating the cause of the decreased blood flow to the head. Steroids and anticoagulant therapy may also be beneficial in selected cases.

Signs and symptoms that differentiate carotid from vertebral disease are given in Tables 8-7 and 8-8.

Giant-Cell Arteritis. Giant-cell arteritis (also called temporal arteritis or cranial arteritis) is a chronic inflammatory disease of the elderly which has an extremely high incidence of ocular involvement (Henkind *et al.,* 1984). The disease is often listed with autoimmune connective tissue disorders. Histological findings of the involved arteries include thickening, reduced lumen, inflammatory cell infiltration of the median adventitia degeneration of the smooth-muscle cells, and fragmentation and loss of the internal elastic lamina. Inflammatory cells are mainly lymphocytes, but plasma cells, leukocytes, macrophages, and giant cells are also found. Rarely, an ischemic anterior segment syndrome or central retinal artery occlusion occurs. More often, ischemic optic neuropathy is seen.

The patient may have headaches, intermit-

Table 8-7. Signs and Symptoms of Cerebral Ischemia caused by Carotid Artery Disease*

Absence of scintillations
Monocular amaurosis fugax, usually altitudinal, "like a veil coming down over the eye"
Horner's syndrome (infrequent)
Absence of diplopia
Perioral paresthesias (rare)
Extremity signs crossed to eye
Diabetes (occasional)
Lowered ophthalmodynamometric values
Some giddiness (occasional; true vertigo rare)
Bright plaques of Hollenhorst
Bruit on ipsilateral carotid, 70+ percent of patients; on contralateral eye, 10 to 15 percent of patients
Fundus picture of central artery occlusion (10 percent of patients)
Corneomandibular reflex, pseudobulbar palsy (bilateral carotid disease, when well developed)
Asymmetric carotid pulses
No positional nystagmus
No vertical nystagmus
"Carotid sinus syndrome" (occasional)
Normal caloric responses
Supranuclear conjugate gaze lesions
Symptoms mimicking those of a tumor (papilledema, pineal shift, localized swelling)
Dysphasia
No cranial nerve palsies except central facial

* Positive carotid compression test helpful in unequivocal cases.

Table 8-8. Signs and Symptoms of Cerebral Ischemia caused by Vertebral Artery Disease.

Scintillations (common)
Binocular amaurosis fugax (may be horizontal as a hemianopia spreads across eyes)
Horner's syndrome (common)
Diplopia (frequent)
Perioral paresthesias (frequent)
Bilateral involvement (common)
Diabetes (70+ percent of patients)
Ophthalmodynamometric values equal in both eyes
True vertigo (very common)
Presence of bright plaques evidence of concomitant carotid disease
Carotid and ocular bruits (uncommon)
Normal findings with carotid compression test
Corneomandibular reflex, basilar sign
Equal carotid pulses
Positional nystagmus (frequent)
Vertical nystagmus (common)
"Carotid sinus syndrome" (rare)
"Dead labyrinth" response
Infranuclear conjugate gaze lesions
Symptoms mimicking those of a tumor (uncommon)
Dysarthria
Cranial nerve palsies (common)

tent claudication of the jaw while eating, and scalp tenderness. Palpation may reveal tortuous thickened temporal arteries with decreased or absent pulses. The diagnosis of giant-cell arteritis is made from the patient's history and physical findings. In an elderly patient, mental deterioration coupled with the visual findings already described is highly suggestive of this entity. Characteristically, patients with this disease have a significantly elevated erythrocyte sedimentation rate.

Temporal artery biopsy can confirm the presence of giant-cell arteritis and should be performed promptly in any patient in whom the diagnosis is suspected. A positive biopsy establishes the diagnosis beyond dispute, but a negative biopsy finding does not rule out the presence of the disease.

Cranial arteritis is treated with corticosteroids. The therapy is directed not at reversing the damage already done, for lost vision is rarely regained, but at preventing further loss of vision. Administration of corticosteroids should be in doses of 60 to 120 mg of prednisone or its equivalent per day; however, the crucial indicator of the adequacy of the dosage is the erythrocyte sedimentation rate. If the erythrocyte sedimentation rate remains high after a day or so of therapy, the dose must be increased. Only when the erythrocyte sedimentation rate has fallen to normal can the dose be slowly decreased. Corticosteroids should be maintained at the lowest level for at least four to six months, but even then the patient must be watched closely for signs of reactivation of the disease. Owing to the hazards of steroid therapy, particularly in the elderly, it is wise to have patients who are prescribed corticosteroids followed by a physician who is well versed in their use.

Syndromes With Pupillary Manifestations. Ocular sympathetic fibers travel along the internal carotid artery to the dilating muscle of the iris. With carotid artery disease, these fibers are occasionally damaged, producing an ipsilateral Horner's syndrome, ptosis, miosis, and enophthalmos. During an attack of amaurosis, orbital ischemia can give rise to iridoplegia with a dilated nonreactive pupil.

Other rare signs of carotid disease include ipsilateral dilatation of the episcleral vascular network ("red eye") and a unilateral corneal arcus senilis contralateral to a stenotic carotid artery (Pavlou and Wolff, 1959).

In carotid disease, the visual field is defective and enhanced with dark borders, usually picked up by confrontation technique. Unilateral field cuts vary from sharply demarcated sector field defects seen in branch artery occlusion, altitudinal field cuts (loss of the upper or lower half of the visual field) in ischemic optic neuropathy, to total or nearly total visual loss from central retinal artery occlusion (Parker, 1979).

Ischemic Optic Neuropathy. Approximately 50 percent of patients with ischemic optic neuropathy have hypertension, diabetes, or acute circulatory failure (Repka and Schatz, 1974). The disease is thought to result from impaired blood supply to the posterior ciliary arteries at the circle of Zinn together with some involvement of the ophthalmic artery. The patient appears with a swollen disk with small hemorrhages and soon develops quadrantal or altitudinal field defects (see Figure 8-9). Erythrocyte sedimentation rate is normal and treatment is disappointing. Aspirin given daily combined with dipyridamole is the only known treatment. A complete physical examination is mandatory.

Monocular Hypoxic Syndrome. This syndrome, described first by Knox (1961), is occasionally seen in patients with severe internal carotid stenosis or occlusion without adequate collateral flow to the eye. It may also be seen in patients with more proximal common carotid occlusions. The patient has pain, and there is chronic ocular injection. The cornea becomes edematous, the anterior chamber is hazy from the cellular reaction of a low-grade iritis, and lens opacities are usually present. The iris becomes deeply pigmented and atrophic, and the pupil is poorly reactive. On ophthalmoscopy, segmental venous dilatation, scattered cotton-wool patches and hemorrhages, and comma-shaped microaneurysms in the equatorial periphery of the retina can be seen. Neovascularization may be observed in the iris in the form of rubeosis, in the angle of the anterior chamber at the optic disk, and occasionally in the retina. These newly formed vessels are quite fragile and can bleed into the anterior chamber or into the vitreous body. The intraocular pressure may be either elevated or depressed. Chronic hypoxic syndrome often leads to progressive ocular infarction with eventual blindness.

NEUROOPHTHALMOLOGIC CHANGES SECONDARY TO INVOLVEMENT OF END BRANCHES OTHER THAN THE OPHTHALMIC ARTERY OF THE CAROTID IN THE BRAIN

Anterior Cerebral Arteries

The blood supply to the deep sagittal cortical matter and narrow parasagittal strips of cortex on the superior aspect of the cerebrum is derived from the anterior cerebral arteries. Horizontal saccadic eye movements are coordinated in Brodmann's area 8, and disruption of vascular flow here can result in chronic eye deviations to the ipsilateral side. This eye sign may be fleeting and resolve after a few days, when the intact contralateral frontal gaze center apparently takes control. Contralateral hemiparesis, with the leg more often involved than the arm, and some contralateral sensory change may also occur with this type of vascular occlusion.

The anterior cerebral arteries may become hardened and compress the optic nerves and the chiasma, producing a slowly progressive bitemporal hemianopia.

Anterior Choroidal Arteries

The lateral aspect of the lateral geniculate body and the optic tract receive most of their vascular supply from the anterior choroidal arteries. An ischemic infarction of the optic tract results in incongruous homonymous hemianopia with sloping margins. If the blood supply to the lateral geniculate body over its lateral aspect is interrupted, the visual field defect one would expect would be homonymous upper quadranopia on the contralateral side. This could be associated with hemiparesis and hemihypesthesia, also contralateral to the side of the arterial occlusion because of the proximity of the internal capsule and thalamus.

Middle Cerebral Artery

The optic radiations are supplied by several arteries. The deep optic artery which passes through the putamen and internal capsule supplies blood to the initial portion of the optic radiation. The inferior temporal-occipital artery, which is another branch of the middle cerebral artery, supplies the temporal radiation. The superior temporo-occipital artery, an artery with dual supply (from both the middle and the posterior cerebral arteries), is the major blood supply of the posterior radiation. This dual supply explains the relatively common occurrence of sparing of macular fibers which are supplied by this artery. Occlusion of any of these vessels can result in homonymous hemianopia, but visual acuity is usually spared. Cortical damage in this distribution of the middle cerebral artery includes cortical ptosis.

Balint's syndrome is a form of ocular motor ataxia (Cogan, 1956). There is usually an associated ataxia of the head and sometimes of the legs. Paradoxical preservation of random movements with loss of purposeful movements often gives rise to the erroneous impression of hysteria or blindness in such a patient. The patient may be unable to perform visually guided operations (optic ataxia) and may have hemispheric paralysis of visual fixation. For example, the patient's head turns in the correct direction when a loud auditory signal is given, but he is unable to look in that direction or at a particular object. There may be a disturbance of visual attention wherein the patient is unable to respond to threatening visual stimuli. The parieto-occipital cortical areas are involved bilaterally, and in some instances the frontal lobes are also involved. Embolic infarction in the distribution of the middle cerebral artery can produce contralateral ptosis.

Posterior Communicating Arteries

Interruption of the posterior communicating arterial supply is usually caused by aneurysms. A change of blood supply in these arteries usually produces a contralateral homonymous hemianopia with macula sparing and intermittent diplopia. Palsy of the ocular motor nerve can be associated with aneurysm of the posterior communicating arteries.

As can be seen in Table 8-1, obstruction will affect ocular performance depending upon the site of interference of circulation to the optic radiations beginning in the retina and ending in the occipital cortex.

In summary we state our hope that this short review of clinical symptoms and signs of ocular and neuro-ocular involvement secondary to carotid vascular disease is of help in recognizing their basis in the extracranial circulation. Rapid, thorough evaluation of the patient's ocular status is helpful in choosing the appropriate diagnostic test, which will then allow initiation of precise treatment before irreversible ocular or intracranial sequelae occur.

REFERENCES

Adams, H.; Putnam, S.; Corbett, J.J.; Sires, B.P.; and Thomspon, H.S.: Amaurosis fugax: results of angiography in fifty-nine patients. *Stroke,* **14**:742-44, 1983.

Adler, F.: *Physiology of the Eye: Clinical Application,* 3rd ed. C.V. Mosby, St. Louis, Missouri, 1959.

Bulpitt, C.J.; Dollery, C.T.; and Kohner, E.M.: The marginal plasma zone in the retinal microcirculation. *Cardiovasc. Res.,* **4**:207-12, 1970.

Check, W.: Ultrasound shows carotid stenosis in just half of carotid bruit cases. *J.A.M.A.,* **252**:593-94, 1984.

Chiari, H.: Über das Verhalten des Teilungswinkels der Carotis communis bei der Endarteritis chronica deformans. *Verh. Dtsch. Ges. Pathol.,* **9**:326-330, 1905.

Cogan, D.: *Neurology of Ocular Muscles.* Charles C Thomas, Springfield, Illinois, 1956.

Cogan, D.: *Ophthalmic Manifestations of Systemic Vascular Disease.* W.B. Saunders, Philadelphia, 1974.

Deutsch, T.; Read, J.; Ernest, J.; and Goldstick, T.: Effects of oxygen and carbon dioxide on the retinal vasculature in humans. *Arch. Ophthalmol.,* **101**:1278-80, 1983.

Duke, L.; Slaymaker, E.; and Wright, C.: Results of ophthalmosonometry and supraorbital photoplethysmography in evaluating carotid arterial stenosis. *Circulation,* **60**:127-31, 1979.

Ellis, P.P.; Lende, M.D.: Induced spasm in the retinal arterioles of cats. II Influences of physical factors and drugs. *Arch. Ophth.* **71**:706, 1964.

Fisher, C.M.: Transient monocular blindness associated with hemiplegia. *Trans. Am. Neurol. Assoc.,* **154**:147, 1951.

Gee, W.; Oller, D.; and Wylie, E.: Noninvasive diagnosis of carotid occlusion by ocular pneumoplethysmography. *Stroke,* **7**:18-21, 1976.

Gowers, W.R.: A case of simultaneous embolism of central retinal and middle cerebral arteries. *Lancet,* **2**:794-96, 1875.

Hedges, T.; Giegre, G.; and Albert, D.: *Arch. Ophthalmol.,* **101**:1251-54, 1983.

Henkind, P., and Chambers, J.: Arterial occlusive disease of the retina. In Duane, T.D., and Jaeger, E.A. (eds.): *Clinical Ophthalmology.* Harper and Row, New York, 1984, pages 3-14.

Heyman, A.; Karp, H.R.; and Bloor, B.M.: Determination of retinal artery pressure in diagnosis of carotid artery occlusion. *Neurology,* **7**:97-104, 1957.

Hollenhorst, R.: Significance of bright plaques in the retinal arterioles. *J.A.M.A.,* **178**:23-29, 1961.

Hollenhorst, R.W.: Carotid and vertebral-basilar arterial stenosis and occlusion: neuro-ophthalmologic considerations. *Trans. Am. Acad. Ophthalmol. Otolaryngol.,* **66**:166-80, 1962.

Keith, N.M.; Wagener, H.P.; Barker, N.W.: Some different types of essential hypertension, their course and prognosis. *Am. J. Med. Sci.,* **197**:332, 1939.

Kempczinski, R.: A combined approach to the noninvasive diagnosis of carotid artery occlusion disease. *Surgery,* **85**:689-94, 1979.

Knox, D.L.: Ocular signs of cervical vascular disease. *Surv. Ophthal.* **13**:245-62, 1961.

Kreshon, M.J.: *Physiology of the Eye,* 4 ed. C.V. Mosby, St. Louis, 1965, page 307.

Lemak, N., and Fields, W.: The reliability of clinical predictors of extracranial artery disease. *Stroke,* **7**:377-78, 1976.

LoGerfo, E., and Mason, R.: Directional Doppler studies of supraorbital artery flow in internal carotid stenosis and occlusion. *Surgery,* **76**:723-28, 1974.

Moore, W.; Bean, B.; Burton, R.; and Goldstone, J.: The use of ophthalmosonometry in the diagnosis of carotid artery stenosis. *Surgery,* **82**:107-15, 1977.

Otis, S.; Smith, R.; Dalessio, D.; Kroll, A.; Rush, M.; and Dilley, R.: Ineffectiveness of the Doppler ophthalmic test in post-endarterectomy evaluation. *Stroke,* **10**:396-99, 1979.

Parker, L.: Neurophthalmological aspects of cerebrovascular disease. *Stroke,* **10**:69-89, 1979.

Pavlou, A., and Wolff, H.: The bulbar conjunctival vessels in occlusion of the internal carotid artery. *Arch. Intern. Med.,* **104**:69-76, 1959.

Pfaffenbach, D., and Hollenhorst, R.: The significance of bright plaques in the retinal tree. *Trans. Ophthalmol. Soc.,* **70**:337-49, 1972.

Repka, M.J., and Schatz, N.J.: Clinical profile of long term implications of anterior ischemic optic neuropathy. *Am. J. Ophthalmol.,* **78**:137-42, 1974.

Samuelson, R.: *Zbl. Prakt. Augenheilkd.* **5**:200, 1881.

Secondi, R.: *Ann. Ottal.* 5-6, 1877.

Till, J.S.: Ophthalmologic aspects of cerebrovascular disease. In Toole, J.F. (ed.): *Cerebrovascular Disorders.* Raven Press, New York, 1984, pages 231-250.

Virchow, R.: Quoted in Hager, J.: Der Diagnose der Karotisthrombose durch den Augen. *Klin. Monatsbl. Augenheilkd.,* 141, 1962.

Watson, P.G.: Treatment of acute retinal artery occlusion. In MacKenzie, W. (ed.): *Centenary Symposium of Ocular Circulation in Health and Disease.* C.V. Mosby, St. Louis, Missouri, 1959, page 234.

Wolff, E.: *The Anatomy of the Eye and Orbit.* W.B. Saunders, Philadelphia, 1948.

Younge, B.: Treatment of acute central retinal artery occlusion. *Mayo Clin. Proc.,* **53**:408-10, 1978.

9

The Arteriographic Diagnosis of Extracranial Cerebrovascular Disease

CHRISTOPHER G. ULLRICH,
ARL V. MOORE, JR. and
R. GREGORY PARSONS

Effective treatment of cerebrovascular disease requires a precise knowledge of the patient's vascular anatomy. Arteriography is the radiographic method that best delineates normal vascular structures, identifies the morphologic characteristics of abnormalities, and demonstrates collateral blood flow patterns. Catheter arteriography has become the "gold standard" against which other methods of cerebrovascular evaluation are compared. Unlike noninvasive techniques, arteriography does carry a small but definite risk of worsening the patient's condition. This chapter reviews the principal indications and technical considerations for arteriography as well as the risks and complications that may be encountered. Both normal and pathological arteriographic anatomy are discussed in detail.

HISTORICAL PERSPECTIVES

At the meeting of the Neurologic Society of Paris in 1927, Egas Moniz first presented the diagnostic method of human cerebral arteriography. After his initial attempts were technical failures, he abandoned percutaneous puncture in favor of direct surgical exposure of the common carotid artery. Moniz first used strontium bromide as the contrast agent, but after his sixth patient died following the examination, he changed to a 25 percent solution of sodium iodide. A "satisfactory" cerebral arteriogram was finally obtained in his ninth patient. Subsequent studies reported seizures, strokes, and deaths due to sodium iodide. In 1931, Moniz and Lima began using colloidal thorium dioxide, an agent which produced excellent angiograms and fewer neurological side effects. The disadvantage of thorium dioxide was that it caused a painful local granulomatous reaction if extravasated, and, being a colloid, it was retained by the reticuloendothelial cells. Because of its radioactive properties, thorium dioxide-induced cancers of the bone marrow and liver were reported years later. Cerebral angiography thus remained a potentially hazardous diagnostic procedure and was practiced in only a few centers before and during World War II.

After the development of less toxic water-soluble contrast agents in the 1950s, Scandinavian researchers were able to achieve good results with carotid-cerebral arteriography, still using direct carotid puncture. The technique for percutaneous introduction of a catheter into the vascular system was described by Seldinger in 1953. From then on, the evolution of carotid-vertebral-cerebral arteriography to the currently favored transfemoral selective catheter techniques closely parallels the development of such sophisticated equipment as the image intensifier, television, contrast injectors, catheters, guide wires, and programmable film changers. The development and radiographic adaptation of many of these items were spurred on by expanding neurovascular diagnostic needs (Lingren, 1974; Taveras and Wood, 1976). Today, digital subtraction angiographic systems have significantly reduced the volume and concentration of contrast agent necessary to produce an acceptable angiogram. Nonionic water-soluble contrast agents (iohexol, iopamidol) promise improved patient comfort and perhaps fewer adverse effects. Progress in polymer chemistry is now allowing the production of smaller caliber, high flow-rate catheters. All of these present and future advances are contributing to make arteriography a safe and widely available diagnostic tool.

The increasing complexity of the radiographic equipment and skill needed to perform and interpret cervicocerebral arteriography has led to the emergence of neuroradiology as a subspecialty. The neuroradiologist devotes a major portion of his time to maintaining the skills required to safely perform and interpret arteriographic studies accurately. He works with a supporting team of highly trained radiographic technologists. In consultation with the primary physician and other medical specialists, the neuroradiologist determines and performs the appropriate arteriographic examination for the particular clinical situation encountered.

INDICATIONS AND CONTRAINDICATIONS

The most common clinical indications for carotid and/or vertebral angiography are clinical symptoms and signs of cerebrovascular occlusive disease, such as a transient ischemic attack (TIA), a bruit, or an absent pulse. Completed stroke, blunt or penetrating trauma, head and neck tumor, and vasculitis are less common indications.

A TIA is a transitory neurologic deficit which lasts from a few minutes to no more than 24 hours. Amaurosis fugax, transient monocular blindness, is a form of TIA reflecting inadequate ophthalmic artery perfusion. Vertebral-basilar insufficiency is a TIA in the posterior cerebral circulation. Patients presenting with recurring TIAs or progressively more frequent (crescendo) TIAs occurring despite medical therapy, a progressively advancing neurologic deficit (stroke in evolution), or fluctuating neurological deficit (unstable state) may also be candidates for immediate arteriography. Patients with fixed neurological deficit (completed stroke) in whom precise vascular diagnosis is required or patients in whom surgical intervention is contemplated should be studied only after their general condition stabilizes.

Patients with asymptomatic carotid bruits are often studied angiographically. Those with unequivocally normal Doppler evaluations performed in a reliable laboratory seldom require arteriography even in the presence of carotid bruits. Conversely, patients with abnormal noninvasive test findings should be arteriographically studied to define precisely the vascular lesions present and to guide possible therapy. The indications for arteriography in trauma and tumor are self-evident. Inflammatory lesions in the cervical vessels usually resemble atherosclerosis. The distinctive angiographic pattern of inflammatory segmental stenoses and dilatations is often more readily recognizable in the intracranial cerebral circulation.

Although the foregoing indications seem straightforward, the decision to perform an arteriographic examination must also take into account the patient's wishes and general medical condition. Arteriography is rarely justifiable in a patient who is not a potential candidate for surgery.

There are no absolute medical contraindications for arteriography. Relative contraindications include compromised renal function, multiple myeloma, iodine allergy, hypo- and hypercoagulative states, and severe hypertension.

Because compromised renal function is common in candidates for cerebral angiography, particularly in the elderly, blood urea nitrogen (BUN) and serum creatinine values should be routinely obtained before elective, and if time allows, even before emergency arteriography. In patients with elevated values, hydration before angiography, judicious use of contrast media, and the administration of diuretic agents during and after the procedure will usually prevent subsequent renal complications. On the following day, BUN and creatinine values should be rechecked to assess any changes in renal function. Patients with multiple myeloma and sickle cell disease should be handled in a similar fashion to minimize the risk of renal impairment. Persons dependent on renal dialysis should be dialyzed soon after the arteriogram. Iodine contrast allergy is usually a manageable problem.

Intraarterial injection of contrast agent is less hazardous than intravenous administration. Premedication with steroids, cimetidine, and diphenhydramine for 48 hours before the examination may be helpful in preventing allergic reactions. Appropriate resuscitative facilities should be readily available in the angiographic suite at all times. Anesthesia standby is warranted in patients with a history of severe respiratory or cardiovascular reactions.

General conditions that predispose the patient to bleeding at the puncture site during and after arteriography should be corrected before the procedure. The prothrombin time and partial thromboplastin are used to evaluate these situations; patient values should be within three seconds of the control values. Heparin administration is discontinued at least four hours before the angiographic study or reversed with protamine immediately before the procedure. Patients treated with warfarin may require vitamin K or fresh frozen plasma to correct their clotting function. Patients with advanced hepatocellular dysfunction may also require the administration of fresh frozen plasma. After the arteriogram, prolonged compression of the puncture site may be necessary to obtain hemostasis. The patient's vital signs and access site should be checked regularly for up to 24 hours after the procedure to detect late bleeding complications, particularly if anticoagulation therapy is resumed.

Patients whose diastolic blood pressure exceeds 110 mm Hg also have increased incidence of hematoma formation at the puncture site during and after arteriography. Therefore, if possible, blood pressure should be pharmacologically controlled before the procedure. Hypotensive patients are poor candidates for arteriography unless their blood pressure has been stabilized at a normotensive level.

TECHNICAL CONSIDERATIONS

This section briefly considers the equipment, radiographic imaging, catheter, and direct puncture angiographic techniques as they are applied in neurovascular radiology. For in-depth discussions, we refer the reader to the reports by Newton and Potts (1974), Taveras and Wood (1976), and Osborn (1980). Regardless of the equipment and techniques used, the goal is to obtain the best possible anatomical information at the lowest possible risk to the patient.

The equipment used in the modern neuroangiographic suite is complex and can be arranged in a variety of configurations. Image-intensified fluoroscopy, preferably with a variable field of view, is an absolute necessity. Video monitors, spot-film camera, and digital subtraction angiography capability are very useful. Biplane programmable rapid-sequence film changers interfaced with automated contrast-media injectors which control the volume, rate, and pressure of injection are necessary. Small focal spot x-ray tubes (0.3 mm) driven by 1,200 mA, three-phase generators will facilitate high-quality geometric magnification filming. A "floating-top" examination table allows the patient to be moved smoothly between fluoroscopy and biplane filming.

Radiographic Evaluation

Radiographic projections employed for the evaluation of cerebrovascular disease include the single-plane right posterior oblique (RPO) view usually used for the aortic arch study. The patient is positioned so that the top of the aortic arch, the origins of the brachiocephalic vessels, and the neck are included in the field of view. Biplane films using anteroposterior (AP) and lateral views of the carotid bifurcation and of the cerebral vessels are also routinely obtained. In vertebral angiography, we prefer the AP Townes and magnification lateral views. Supplemental radiographic projections, including zero-degree AP, Waters, submentovertex, and oblique views, are also used as needed to unfold overlapping vessels and better demonstrate pathology. Stereoradiography, which produces a three-dimensional image when properly viewed, can be very helpful too, particularly in assessing complex abnormalities, such as arteriovenous malformations and highly vascular tumors.

The film sequence is guided by the clinical situation. To visualize the carotid bifurcation, a rate of two films per second for four seconds will suffice. In the course of a cerebral study, a rate of two films per second for three seconds and one film per second for four seconds permits the arterial and venous phases to be properly recorded. In lesions associated with high blood-flow, such as arteriovenous malformations, a rate of six films per second may be desirable. For slow blood – flow lesions, such as near occlusion of the internal carotid artery a rate of one film per second for 10 to 15 seconds might be necessary to demonstrate the pertinent anatomy.

Overlapping bone and soft-tissue densities can obscure small but important angiographic details. Subtraction films may overcome this difficulty by displaying the contrast-filled vas-

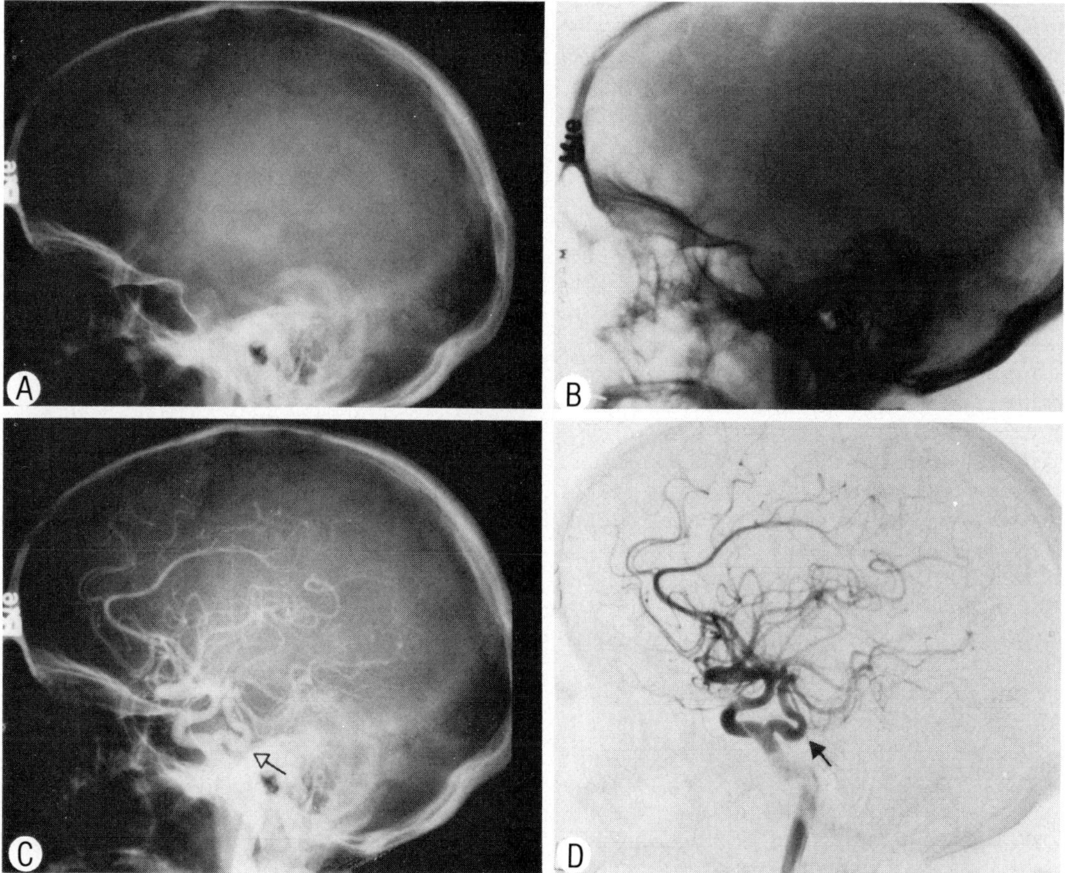

Figure 9–1. Subtraction angiography. *(A)* The first radiograph in any film sequence is timed in a way that no contrast media is present. *(B)* A reversal image or mask is prepared from the first radiograph. *(C)* The mask is precisely superimposed on a radiograph with intravascular contrast media present. *(D)* This paired set of radiographs is rephotographed to produce the subtraction film. All preexisting bone and soft-tissue density has been "subtracted," leaving an isolated vascular-system image. Digital subtraction angiographic equipment performs a similar process using computer-based techniques. The lateral-view subtraction (*D*) best demonstrates the primitive trigeminal artery (arrow).

cular system devoid of its surrounding structures. To facilitate the film-subtraction process, the first radiograph in any sequence is timed so that no contrast media are present. A reversal film (mask) is then prepared from this first radiograph. The subtraction film is then produced by rephotographing this mask film superimposed on the contrast angiogram (see Figure 9–1). Preexisting bone and soft-tissue densities are thus "subtracted," leaving only the vascular system opacified by the contrast media. Acceptable subtraction films require exact registration between the mask and the angiographic film. Patient motion degrades the quality of the subtraction. Small ulcerations and very high-grade stenotic lesions are often best demonstrated with the subtraction technique (Newton and Potts, 1974).

Subtraction images may also be prepared by computer techniques using recently available digital subtraction angiography (DSA) equipment. These systems, rather than recording the angiogram on a film, digitize and store the analog image from the image intensifier. Compared with a film, a large improvement in contrast resolution is obtained at the expense of lower spatial resolution. However, small lesions, such as endothelial ulcers, may go undetected.

Given the improved contrast resolution, reduced contrast media doses can be used with intraarterial digital subtraction angiography (IA-DSA). IA-DSAs can substitute for film-recorded angiograms in many instances. In our practice, IA-DSA is used primarily in situations where limitation of contrast-media dose is important or when selective vessel catheterization is deemed inadvisable (e.g., a stenotic vertebral artery orifice). DSAs high-contrast sensitivity also allows arterial studies to be produced using large-volume venous injections (IV-DSA) of contrast media. Typically, 40 ml of 76 percent contrast agent is injected directly into a brachial vein or through a catheter inserted into the vena cava or the right atrium.

IV-DSA avoids complications particular to catheter arteriography and can be easily performed on an outpatient basis. Because these images are analogous to arterial aortic arch injections, superimposition of vascular shadows is a major limitation with this technique, particularly at the base of the skull. The large amount of contrast material needed with IV-DSA also limits the number of views that can be obtained. For a successful study, the patient must also be very cooperative because patient motion severely degrades these subtraction images. Inadequate arterial vascular opacification is produced when low cardiac output causes excessive dilution of the contrast bolus. These constraints make IV-DSA suitable as a screening test for carotid and vertebral disease, but not as a definitive diagnostic procedure.

Doppler ultrasound carotid artery evaluation is often preferable to IV-DSA for screening purposes. It is totally noninvasive, is more cost-effective, and avoids the known hazards of radiation and intravascular contrast agents (see also Chapter 7 on noninvasive diagnosis of carotid disease).

Catheter Arteriography

Basic to catheter arteriography is the Seldinger method of percutaneous introduction of a catheter into the vascular system. The technique is initiated by percutaneous vessel puncture with a hollow needle. A guide wire is inserted through this needle and into the vascular lumen, then the needle is withdrawn, leaving the guide wire in place. The catheter is then advanced over the guide wire into the vascular lumen. After manipulation into an appropriate position, the guide wire is removed, leaving the intravascular catheter ready for contrast injection. Catheters, needles, and guide wires for cerebral angiography are available in a wide variety of shapes, sizes, and materials. The selection is made according to personal preference, prior training, the puncture site, and the particular vessel(s) to be catheterized.

Most neuroangiographic procedures used today are performed by femoral arterial puncture. This site is readily accessible for catheter insertion and can be easily compressed to maintain hemostasis after catheter removal. It is subjectively less traumatic than direct cervical vessel puncture and is associated with a very low incidence of major complications. Local complications, such as hematoma, spasm, thrombosis, and subintimal dissection, do not produce central neurological sequelae. A single puncture allows evaluation of the aortic arch and selective catheterization of all of the craniocervical vessels. Success rates of 95 to 98 percent have been reported for transfemoral bilateral selective common carotid catheter arteriograms (Vitek, 1973).

Femoral puncture should be generally avoided in most patients with aortofemoral bypass grafts or advanced aortoiliac arteriosclerotic disease. In such patients, using the right axillary artery puncture site and appropriate catheters, aortic arch and selective right and left common carotid artery and right vertebral artery (VA) catheterization can be achieved. With left axillary artery puncture, selective right carotid-vertebral catheterization may sometimes be technically impossible. Selective internal-external carotid artery studies are also very difficult, even with the right axillary artery approach. Local complications of this technique are similar to the femoral approach, but brachial plexus injury may also occur from hematoma or from the puncture itself.

A translumbar puncture can be used to perform aortic arch and selective carotid-vertebral arteriography in patients whose femoral and axillary artery sites are unsuitable. As an alternative method, direct cervical vessel puncture techniques could also be used in such cases. IV-DSA, though limited in its intracranial vascular evaluation, can also be useful in some of these patients.

Direct Puncture Carotid Arteriography

Percutaneous direct puncture of the carotid artery is now rarely performed in institutions where sophisticated catheter angiography facilities are available. Patients with advanced generalized occlusive disease or very tortuous great vessels, however, may occasionally benefit from this approach. This technique does not require highly specialized equipment and is the fastest and least expensive method if a single-vessel study will suffice. As in selective catheter angiography, only a small volume of contrast material is required to obtain a satisfactory arteriogram.

Disadvantages of percutaneous direct puncture of the carotid artery are numerous. The inevitable hematoma may complicate subsequent surgery. Damage to the vessel could cause neurologic deficit, the highest risk being associated with advanced atherosclerotic disease (Allen *et al.*, 1965). Carotid punctures also tend to be painful, and multiple penetrations are required for a complete cerebral study. The aortic arch cannot be studied. Also, supplemental projections, such as the submentovertex view, may be difficult to perform without dislodging the needle.

Percutaneous puncture of the VA not only has all the disadvantages of the carotid study but is also technically more difficult to perform because the artery is smaller and cannot be palpated. This technique has been virtually abandoned.

In retrograde brachial arteriography the brachial artery is percutaneously cannulated. Rapid large-volume retrograde injection of contrast media (30 to 50 ml) causes a transient reversal of blood flow, and allows opacification of carotid and vertebral vessels. The technique is easy to perform and is as safe as any other remote arterial puncture, but the injection is very painful. Other disadvantages of the approach are that with right brachial artery injection, both the carotid and VA usually fill simultaneously and produce overlap of the vessels, particularly in the AP cerebral view. Left brachial artery injection opacifies the left VA unless it anomalously arises directly from the aortic arch (5 percent of cases). An additional direct puncture of the left carotid artery is required for a complete cervicocerebral arteriographic study. The aortic arch cannot be adequately demonstrated with this technique. The intracranial vessels may also be suboptimally visualized owing to dilution of the contrast agent. For all of these reasons, this technique is now rarely applied.

NORMAL ARTERIOGRAPHIC FINDINGS

A thorough understanding of the normal radiographic vascular anatomy and possible congenital variants is fundamental to the interpretation of an angiographic study in carotid and VA disease. A brief overview of this vital topic is presented here; detailed discussions are found in Wylie and Ehrenfeld (1970), Newton and Potts (1974), Krayenbuhl and Yasargil (1968), Taveras and Wood (1976), and Osborn (1980).

The detailed anatomical features of the extracranial cerebral vessels are described in Chapter 3, as seen at postmortem examination or at the operating table. Below is described the way these vessels are visualized on the angiogram.

Aortic Arch and Brachiocephalic Vessel Origins

In the commonly used RPO projection, the normal aorta forms a smooth arch in the superior mediastinum as it arises from the heart to the right of the midline, courses upward anterior to the trachea and esophagus, passes over the left mainstem bronchus, and descends through the left hemithorax posterolateral to the esophagus and anterolateral to the spine. Aortic arch anomalies are often associated with congenital heart disease. Various forms of right aortic arch, double aortic arch, and cervical aortic arch are described (Haughton and Rosenbaum, 1974). These anomalies result either from failure of primitive vessel involution or from vascular involution occurring at unexpected sites.

In about 75 percent of the population, the innominate artery, left common carotid artery, and left subclavian artery arise successively from the aortic arch. The innominate and left common carotid artery share a common origin from the aortic arch in 16 percent of the population (see Figure 9–2). The left VA arises directly from the aortic arch between the left common carotid artery and the left subclavian artery in 5 percent of patients (see Figure 9–3; Haughton and Rosenbaum, 1974). The RPO projection is best for demonstrating these individual brachiocephalic vessel origins.

The innominate artery bifurcates to form the right subclavian and right common carotid arteries. If the right subclavian artery arises directly from the aortic arch distal to the left subclavian artery, it is termed "aberrant" (see Figure 9–4). In such cases, as the vessel courses rightward, it usually passes posterior to the trachea and esophagus, but on rare occa-

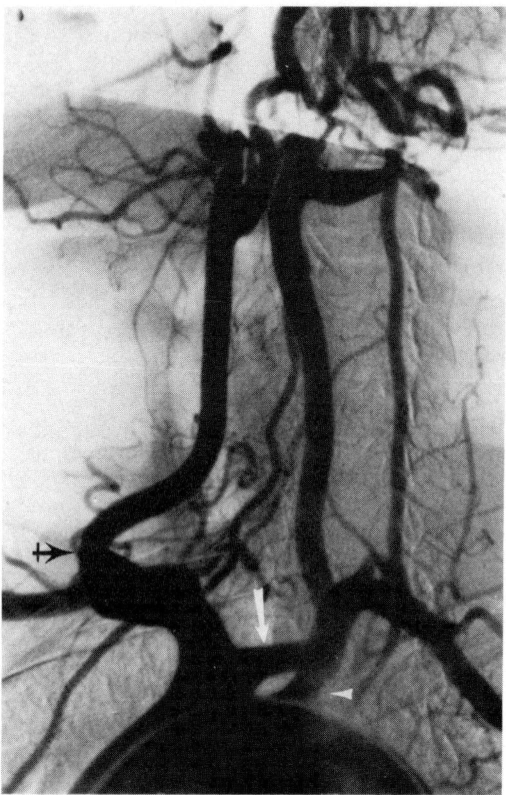

Figure 9–2. A left common carotid artery (white arrow) arising from the innominate artery. This 55-year-old woman had a "pulsatile mass" in the right supraclavicular area caused by tortuous right innominate and proximal common carotid arteries (crossed arrow). A small, smooth atherosclerotic plaque is noted at the origin of the left subclavian artery (white filled arrowhead).

sions its course runs between these structures. (Robicsek *et al;* 1968). A barium esophagogram or intravenous contrast-enhanced computed tomographic (CT) scan can define this relationship between the artery and the esophagus. A shared right and left common carotid artery origin (bicarotid trunk) occurs in 29 percent of patients with aberrant right subclavian (Haughton and Rosenbaum, 1974) arteries. Virtually any imaginable combination of aortic arch vessel origin can occur, but these variants are rare (bi-innominate trunk, congenitally absent left common carotid artery, etc.).

Common Carotid Artery and Its Bifurcation

The length of the common carotid arteries is variable. Although the carotid bifurcation is located most often at the C4 vertebral body level, it may be found at any level in the neck. An abnormally low carotid bifurcation (C6 or C7) may make safe selective catheterization technically difficult. The use of direct puncture technique is also hazardous in such a situation.

Internal Carotid Artery

In conjunction with selective common carotid artery catheterization or indirect puncture, AP and lateral views are routinely obtained to evaluate the internal carotid artery

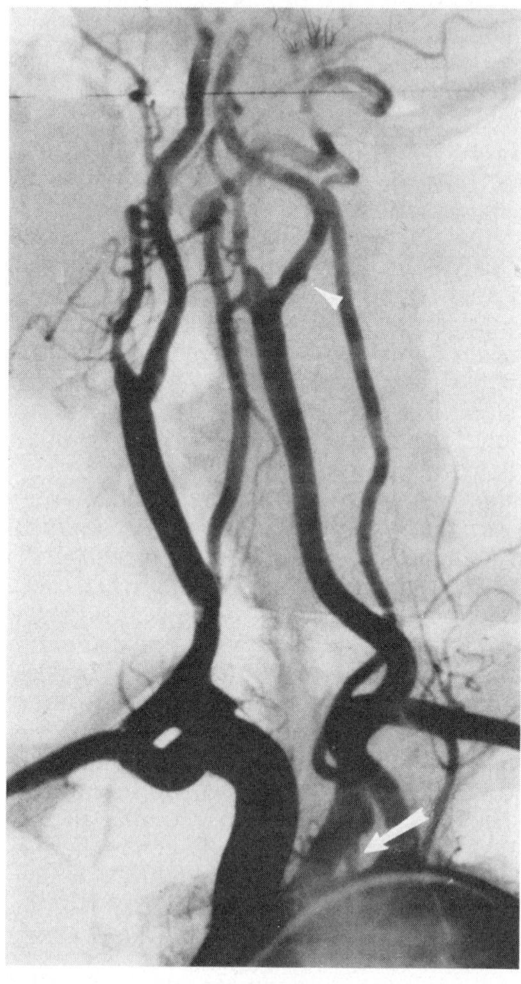

Figure 9–3. In 5 percent of patients, the left vertebral artery (white arrow) rises directly from the aortic arch between the origin of the left common carotid and subclavian arteries. A mild stenosis of the left vertebral artery orifice and a small ulceration (white filled arrowhead) of the proximal left internal carotid artery are clearly shown in the RPO projection aortic arch subtraction film.

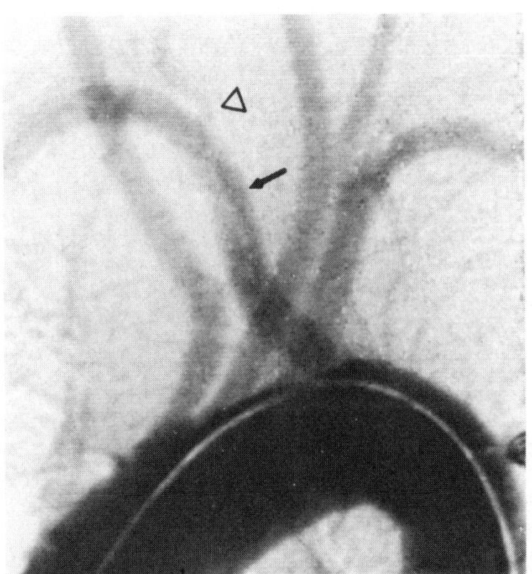

Figure 9–4. Aberrant right subclavian artery (arrow) arising from the aortic arch distal to the left subclavian artery in an IA-DSA image made in the RPO projection. In this patient, the right vertebral artery (open arrowhead) rises from the right subclavian artery. The right and left common carotid arteries originate separately from the aortic arch.

(ICA), while oblique views are commonly needed to "unfold" the carotid bifurcation.

The *cervical segment* extends from the bifurcation to the base of the skull. The origin of the ICA is usually posterolateral to the external carotid artery (ECA) origin. The carotid sinus is the mild dilatation of the lumen of the ICA origin. A gentle curving course is normally present, but "looping" and "coiling" occur in 5 to 15 percent of cases (see Figure 9–5). This redundancy may be developmental, but atherosclerosis and hypertension appear to play a role in some patients. The normal cervical ICA has no branches, but anomalous ECA branch vessel origins including the ascending pharyngeal and occipital arteries have been described (Teal *et al.,* 1973). These anomalous vessels are most easily recognized in the lateral view.

The *petrous segment* of the ICA initially traverses the petrous bone vertically anterior to the jugular fossa. At the level of the tympanic cavity and the cochlea, the vessel assumes a horizontal anteromedial course. A thin plate of bone or dura separates the ICA from the middle-ear cavity.

The *cavernous segment* is composed of presellar and juxtasellar subsegments. The short portion of the ICA which ascends vertically from the carotid canal to the posterior clinoid process constitutes the presellar subsegment. The meningohypophyseal artery arises near the apex of the presellar portion to supply the tentorial dura and the pituitary gland. In the lateral view, the juxtasellar ICA courses forward and slightly inferior along the sphenoid sinus and then turns sharply upward and posterior to pass beneath the anterior clinoid process (see Figure 9–6). This juxtasellar subsegment is also named the *carotid siphon* (see Figure 3–6). In the AP view, the carotid siphon is foreshortened and partly superimposed, its posterior aspect being more medial in position. The lateral main-stem artery originates from the inferolateral aspect of the proximal carotid siphon and provides a collateral flow pathway to the maxillary, ophthalmic, and meningeal vessels. Lateral-projection geometric magnification radiography is usually required to demonstrate the normally very small meningohypophyseal and lateral main-stem arteries.

The *intracranial (supraclinoid) segment* of the ICA extends from the anterior clinoid process to the bifurcation of the anterior and middle cerebral arteries. Anatomically, the segment begins where the ICA pierces the dura. The origin of the ophthalmic artery, the first major branch of the intracranial carotid, is intradural in 89 percent of patients (Punt, 1979). The lateral view best demonstrates the origin of the ophthalmic artery, while the supraclinoid carotid bifurcation is optimally seen in the AP view (see Figure 9–6A). The posterior communicating artery connects the supraclinoid carotid artery with posterior cerebral circulation. This portion of the circle of Willis is a major intracranial collateral vessel.

External Carotid Artery

The ECA, which is normally the smaller branch of the common carotid bifurcation, lies anterior and medial to the ICA. The numerous ECA branches which supply the face and neck are most easily distinguished in the lateral projection. The occipital artery is quite tortuous as it courses along the posterior aspect of the skull. The ECA terminates in the superficial temporal and internal maxillary arteries. The former follows a meandering path over the lateral surface of the skull. The middle meningeal artery, the largest branch of the internal maxillary artery, enters the skull through the foramen spinosum. Unlike the superficial temporal artery, it courses in relatively straight grooves along the inner table of the skull. The

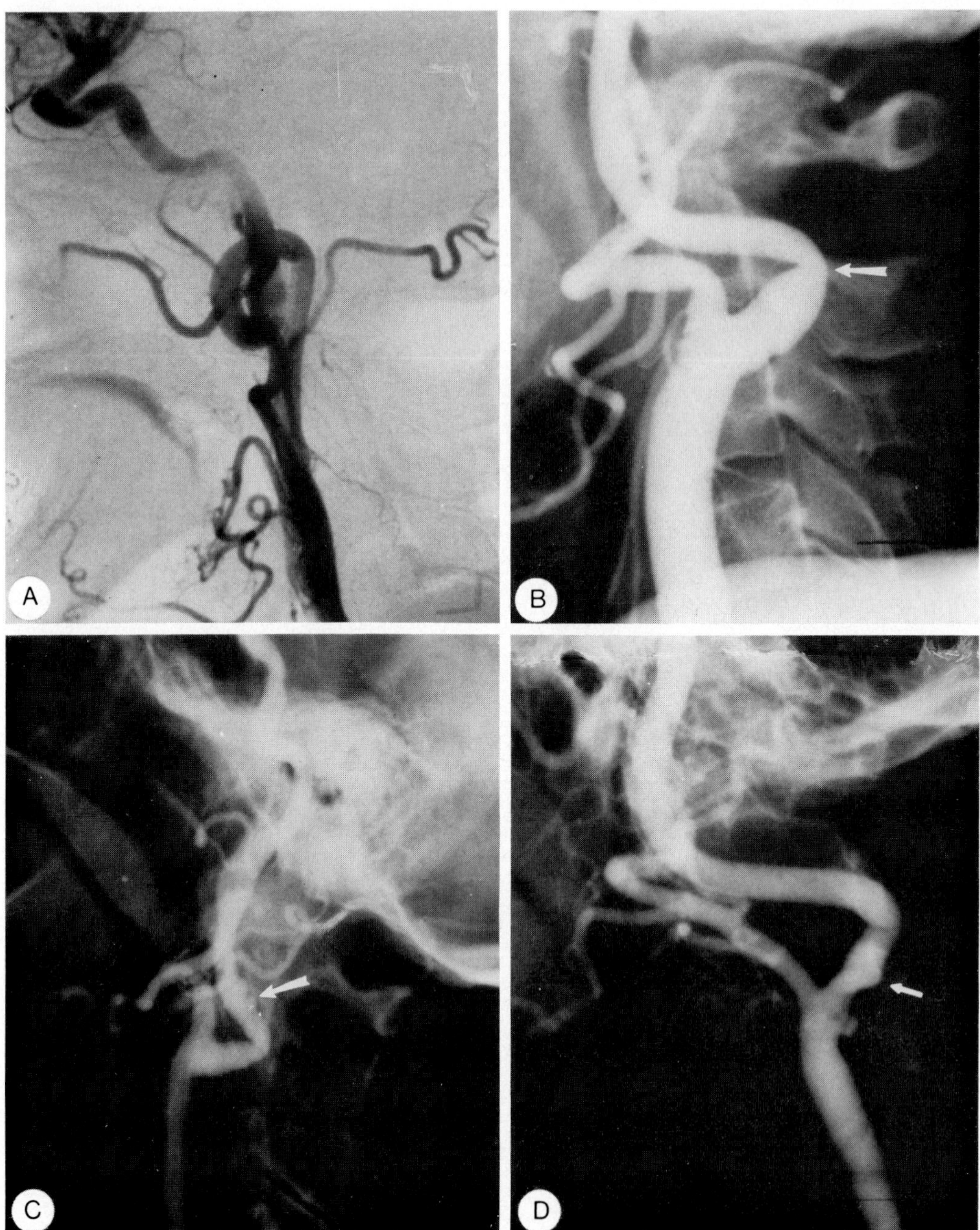

Figure 9–5. Internal carotid artery loops and kinks. *(A)* Asymptomatic redundant ICA loop without stenosis. *(B)* Left ICA kink with a moderate stenosis (arrow) in a 55-year-old hypertensive woman with transient ischemic attacks. *(C)* ICA fibromuscular hyperplasia (arrow) and a kink in a hypertensive 70-year-old woman with an ipsilateral temporal lobe infarction. *(D)* Ulcerated atherosclerotic plaque (arrow) at the carotid bifurcation associated with a nonstenotic ICA kink in a 61-year-old woman with amaurosis fugax.

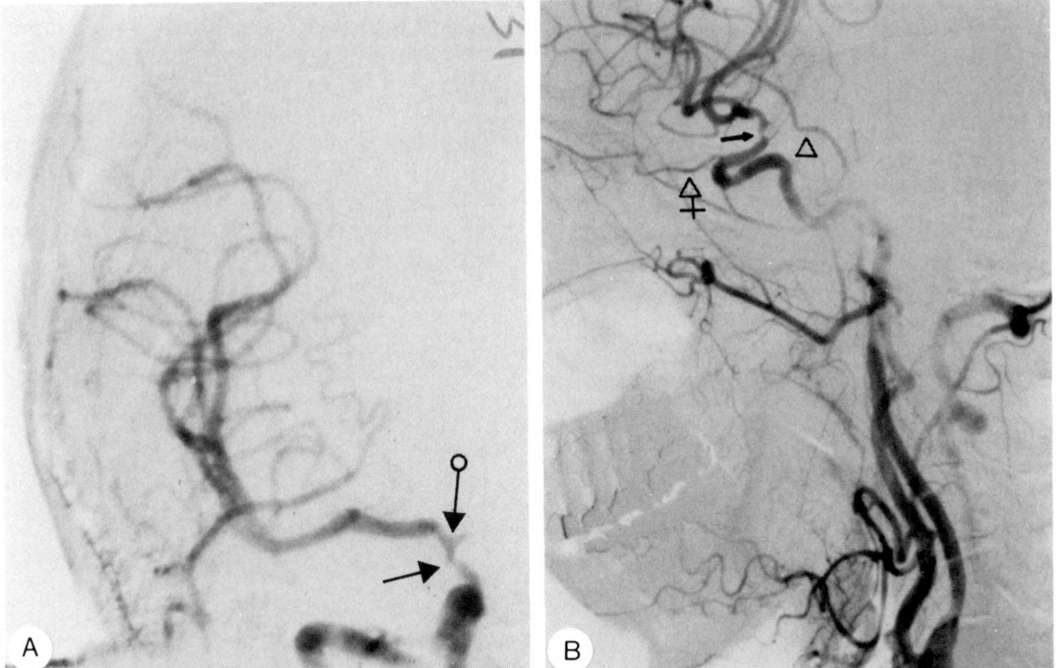

Figure 9-6. Clinically unsuspected right supraclinoid internal carotid artery stenosis (arrow) in (*A*) AP (*B*) lateral views in a 55-year-old woman with a left carotid bruit. The supraclinoid bifurcation (open circle with arrow) into anterior and middle cerebral arteries is best seen in the AP view, while the carotid siphon (open arrowhead and ophthalmic artery (open crossed arrow) are best demonstrated in the lateral projection. Both anterior cerebral arteries filled from the left carotid injection (not shown).

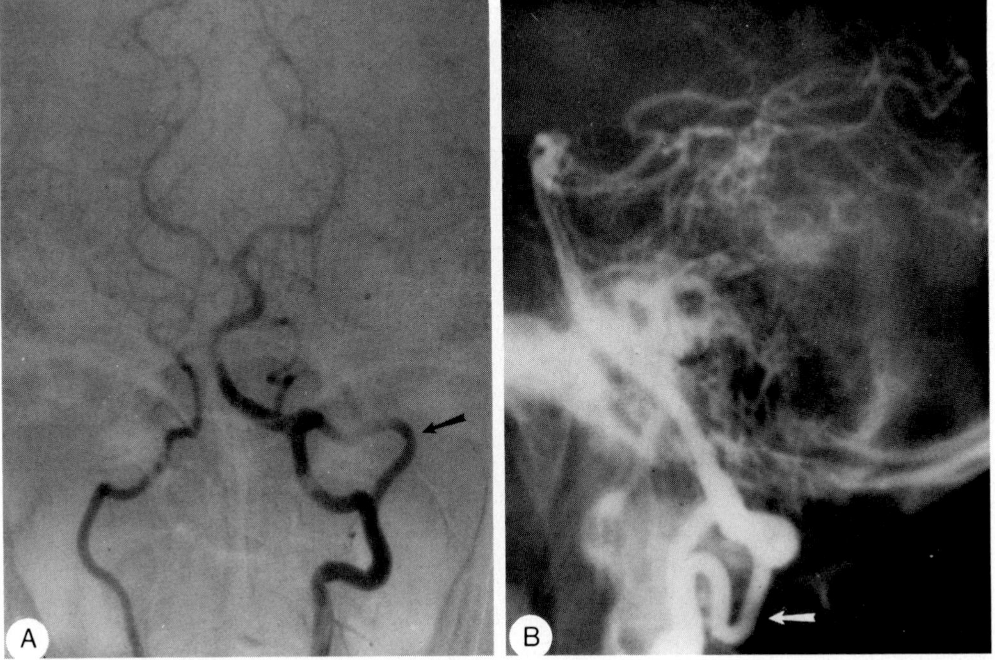

Figure 9-7. Duplication or "fenestration" of the third segment of the vertebral artery (arrow) in AP (*A*) and lateral (*B*) views of two different patients. This anatomic variant is seldom clinically significant.

infraorbital branch of the internal maxillary artery angiographically delineates the roof of the maxillary sinus and provides collateral pathways to the facial and ophthalmic artery territories.

Vertebral Artery

The VA is normally the first branch of the subclavian artery. In approximately 80 percent of patients the left VA is larger than or equal in size to the right VA (vertebral dominance). The left VA arises directly from the aortic arch in 5 percent of cases (see Figure 9–3). In extremely rare instances the right VA may rise from the aortic arch, the right common or ICA, or the right subclavian artery distal to the thyrocervical trunk. Duplicate origins or segments of either VA may also occur (see Figure 9–7).

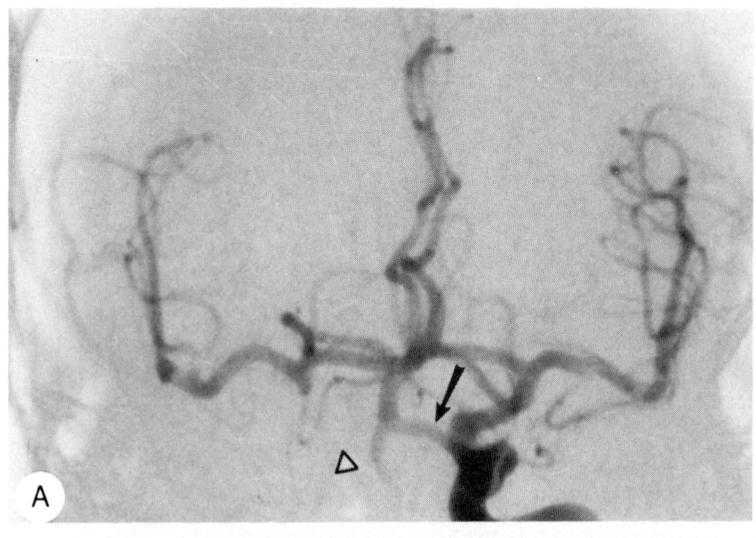

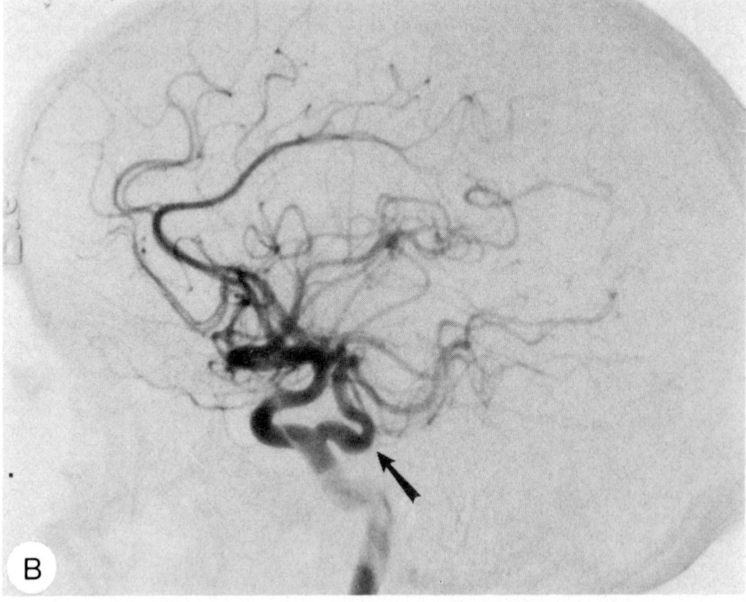

Figure 9–8. Left primitive trigeminal artery (arrow) in AP (*A*) and lateral (*B*) views found in a 40-year-old man with traumatic right ICA occlusion. This artery connects the presellar ICA to the midportion of the basilar artery. In the AP view (*A*), collateral blood flow to the right middle cerebral artery through the anterior communicating artery is seen due to the right ICA occlusion. The proximal basilar artery (open arrowhead) is hypoplastic. This trigeminal artery (arrow) is best seen in the lateral projection (*B*).

Anatomically and radiographically, the VA is divided into four parts. The *first segment* designates the VA from its origin to the level at which it enters the foramen transversarium, usually at C6. Tortuosity is common in the first segment. The *second segment* of the VA passes straight upward through the foramen transversaria from C6 to C2. Muscular branches from this segment provide potential pathways for collateral circulation in proximal vertebral occlusive disease. The *third segment* lies between C2 and the dural entrance point above the posterior arch of C1. The intradural portion of the VA constitutes the *fourth segment.* The posterior inferior cerebellar artery (PICA) originates from the fourth segment. The fourth segments of the two VAs normally unite near the midline to form the basilar artery. Very rarely a VA ends in the posterior inferior communicating artery (PICA).

The vertebral arteries are optimally studied arteriographically by selective vertebral artery or subclavian artery catheterization. We prefer the AP Townes and the lateral projection for studying the third and fourth VA segments and the basilar artery. Occasionally, AP transorbital or Waters views may be employed. Standard AP and lateral views may be used for the cervical portions of the VA. The RPO projection demonstrates well the right VA and left PICA vascular origins. The left posterior oblique (LPO) projection will best demonstrate the origins of the left VA and right PICA.

Persistent Embryonic Carotid-Basilar Anastomotic Vessels

These vessels are not "anatomic curiosities" but provide important pathways for collateral flow and may explain paradoxical posterior circulation symptoms in patients with carotid occlusive disease. The lateral projection is often the most helpful for identifying the presence of these vessels, whereas AP and oblique projections may be necessary to study them in detail.

The *primitive trigeminal artery,* the most common of these vessels (0.1 to 0.2 percent incidence on angiography), arises near the junction of the presellar and juxtasellar subsegments of the ICA and courses posteriorly either through the dorsum of the sella or adjacent to it to anastomose with the VA. Proximal to this anastomosis, the VA is usually hypoplastic (see Figure 9–8). The *persistent proatlantal intersegmental artery* arises from the cervical ICA (rarely from the ECA) and unites with the ipsilateral vertebral artery at the foramen magnum after passing over the posterior arch of C1. In a similar fashion, the *primitive hypoglossal artery* extends from the cervical ICA, courses through the ipsilateral hypoglossal canal, and unites with the proximal basilar artery. The *primitive stapedial artery* extends from the petrous ICA through the middle ear and continues upward to form the middle meningeal artery; the foramen spinosum is absent in these cases. The extremely rare *optic artery* rises from the petrous ICA then passes through the internal auditory canal.

PATHOLOGIC ARTERIOGRAPHIC FINDINGS

The pathophysiology of the carotid-vertebral arterial system and the clinical symptoms produced by these lesions are described in other chapters in this volume. This section emphasizes the arteriographic findings associated with these various lesions.

Atherosclerotic Disease

Atherosclerosis is a systemic disease with an uneven distribution. Clinically symptomatic lesions tend to occur at arterial bifurcations. Atherosclerotic *stenoses* are predisposed to the following vessel origins, listed in descending order of frequency: internal carotid, vertebral, left subclavian, external carotid, innominate, right subclavian, and left common carotid arteries.

Arteriographically, the atherosclerotic vessel lumen appears either narrowed or elongated (see Figures 9–9 to 9–12). Ulceration of the lesion is common (see Figure 9–13). Since these lesions are often eccentric, a stenosis should be visualized in at least two projections made at 90 degree angles to each other. Failure to do this may result in either over- or underestimation of the severity of a lesion (see Figure 9–9). A 50 percent reduction in lumen diameter corresponds to a 75 percent reduction in lumen cross-sectional area. In such cases blood flow becomes significantly reduced. The stenosis may be described as a percentage of the original lumen cross-sectional area but descriptive terms, such as "mild" (less than 30 percent), "moderate" (30 to 70 percent), and

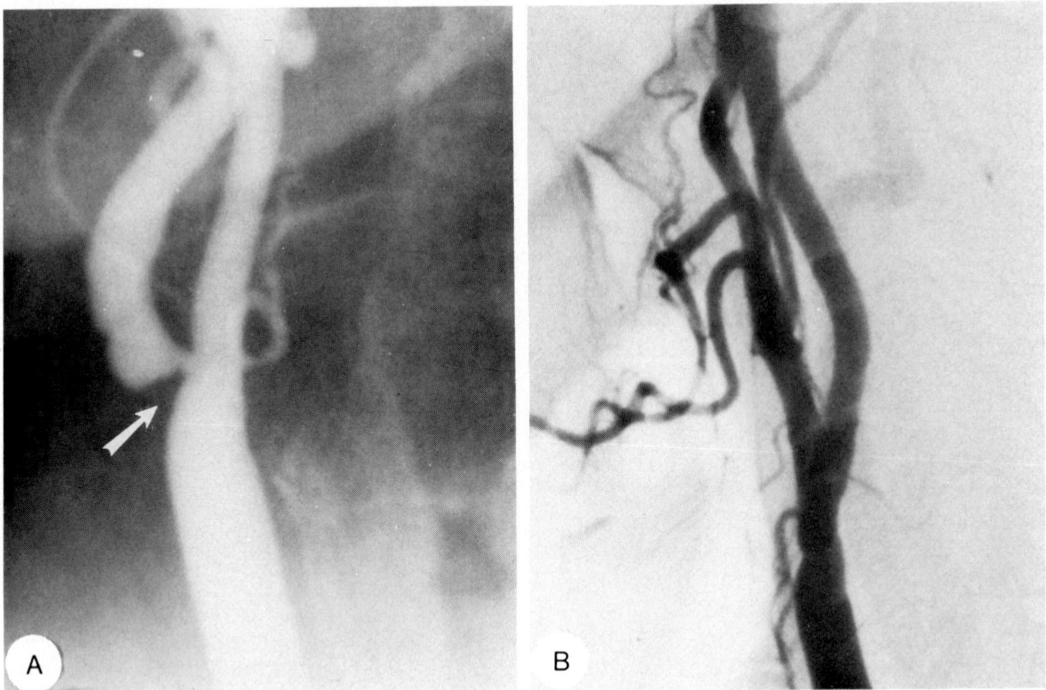

Figure 9–9. Severe internal carotid stenosis (arrow) seen in the AP projection (*A*) but not in the lateral view (*B*). The residual lumen measures less than 1 mm. This case emphasizes the critical importance of obtaining at least two views of each bifurcation to ensure accurate evaluation. By means of fluoroscopy, the optimal angle of view to "unfold" the carotid bifurcation can be easily determined for each patient.

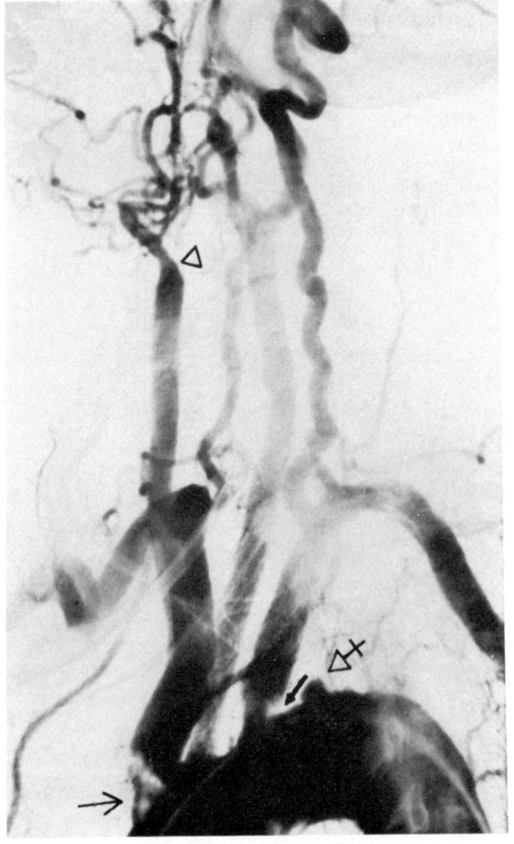

Figure 9–10. Large irregular atherosclerotic plaques (arrows) involving the origin of the right innominate and left subclavian arteries, producing moderate stenoses and making selective catheterization hazardous for this patient. The right ICA is totally occluded (open arrowhead). The left VA is dominant and tortuous. A large ulcerative lesion of the aorta is noted distal to the left subclavian artery origin (open crossed arrow).

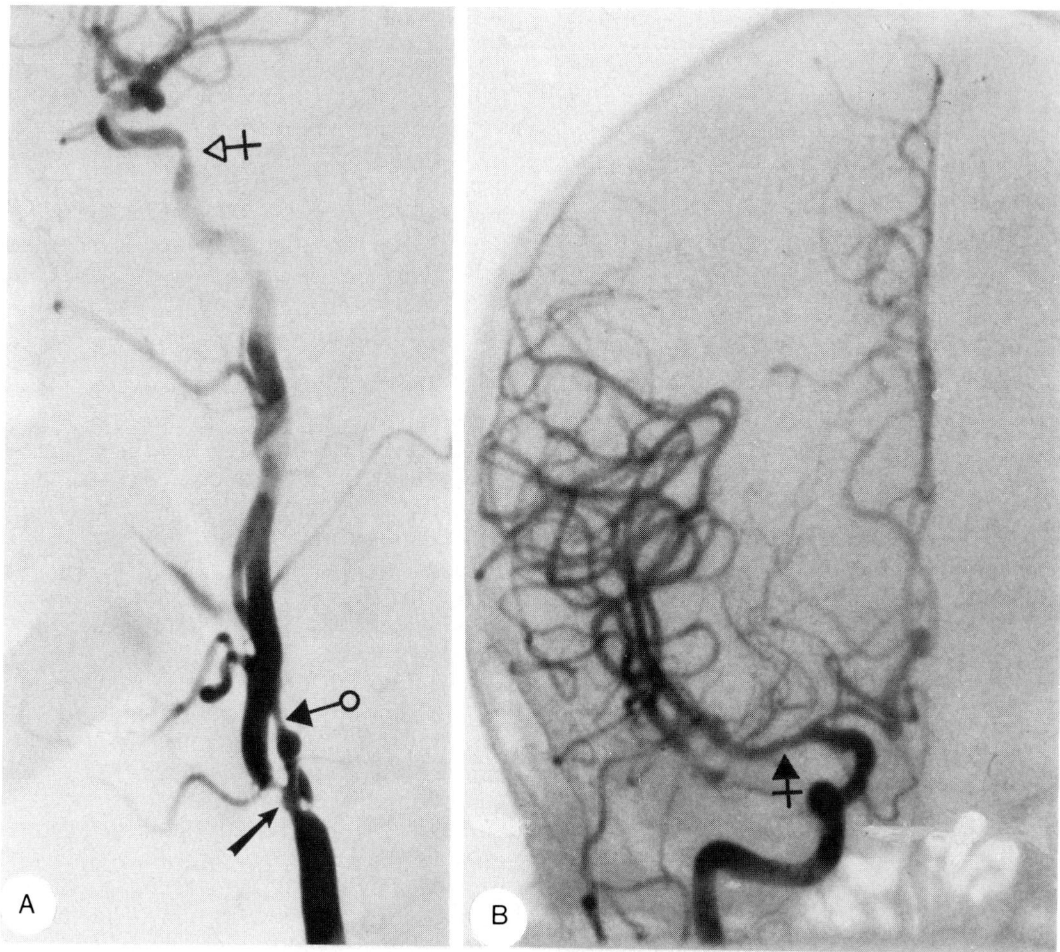

Figure 9–11. Successive atherosclerotic stenoses. *(A)* Left common carotid arteriogram lateral view demonstrates a severe ulcerated stenosis (arrow) of the carotid bifurcation and proximal internal and external carotid arteries in a 55-year-old patient with carotid bruits and an abnormal Doppler vascular evaluation. Subsequent severe stenoses of the proximal (open circle with arrow) and presellar portion (open crossed arrow) of the ICA are also identified. *(B)*: On the right common carotid arteriogram AP cerebral view, a moderate stenosis of the right middle cerebral artery (crossed arrow) is seen. A thorough examination of both intracranial and cervical vessels is necessary for complete evaluation of patients with cerebrovascular disease.

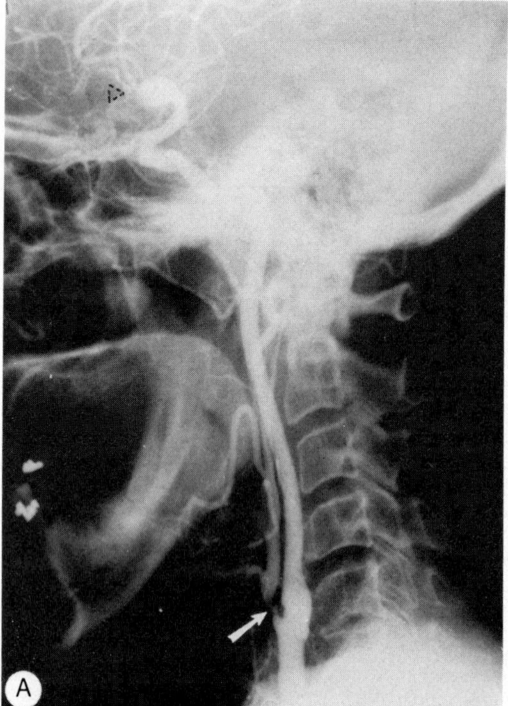

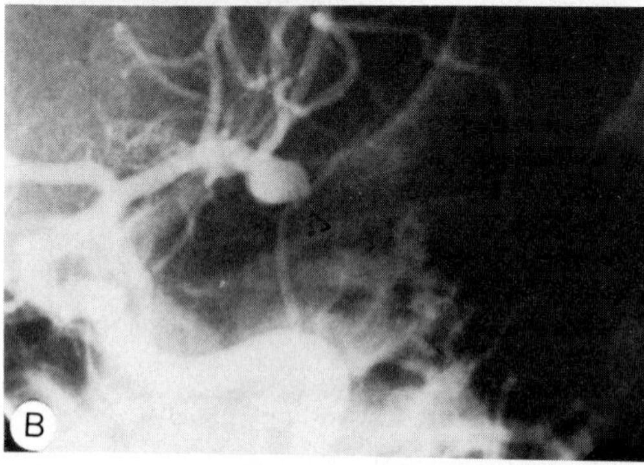

Figure 9–12. Severe right ECA stenosis (arrow) with a large right middle cerebral artery aneurysm (dashed open arrowhead) found in a 67-year-old man with TIAs (*A*). The aneurysm is better demonstrated in an LPO projection (*B*). When an intracranial aneurysm is discovered, a complete cerebral arteriographic examination is indicated to exclude additional lesions.

"severe" (greater than 70 percent) stenoses, are often used as well.

In *complete occlusion* there is no contrast flow within the vessel (see Figures 9–13 and 9–15). The lumen distal to the occlusive site is usually thrombosed to the site of the nearest collateral inflow. For example, if the left common carotid artery occludes at its origin, thrombus will initially fill the lumen to the area of the carotid bifurcation, where collateral flow from the ECA or ICA will maintain patency (see Figure 9–13). Similarly, if the proximal left subclavian artery becomes occluded, blood flow will reverse in the left vertebral artery to maintain flow in the left upper extremity. If enough blood flow is diverted ("stolen") from the right vertebral and basilar arteries into the left vertebral artery, symptoms of vertebral-basilar insufficiency occur. The term *subclavian steal* is applied to this condition (see Figure 9–14). An analogous situation occurs less frequently on the right side (see Figure 9–15). The RPO projection of the aortic arch arteriogram using an extended film sequence is usually best for demonstrating subclavian steal or common carotid artery occlusion. Selective carotid or vertebral artery catheterization may be necessary to show collateral flow patterns in some patients.

An occlusion of the ICA origin usually produces thrombosis up to the level of the petrous carotid segment, a site which for practical purposes is surgically inaccessible. Complete occlusion must be distinguished from cases of *subocclusion* or *near occlusion* in which very slow forward flow produces a thin stream of contrast ("string sign"). Patients with these conditions are potential operative candidates (see Figure 9–16). Selective common carotid angiography (catheter or direct puncture) with prolonged film sequences is often necessary to demonstrate this phenomenon. A lateral projection, which includes the head and neck, best demonstrates the pertinent angiographic findings. Doppler vascular examination and IV-DSA may be misleading. The overlapping vessel shadows which occur on arch aortography can obscure a near occlusion and the associated collateral flow patterns.

While a slowly progressing stenosis is often clinically well tolerated, a sudden increase in the degree of vascular stenosis may produce acute cerebrovascular insufficiency if the collateral circulation is inadequately developed. Hemorrhage within the arterial wall beneath an already existing atherosclerotic plaque is a common cause of such a sudden change. This phenomenon is consistently observed only at the carotid bifurcation and can be suspected in an appropriate clinical setting when an angiographically smooth but severe stenosis is noted on one side while the opposite carotid bifurcation is relatively normal in appearance.

Emboli, usually of cardiac origin, can also produce sudden occlusion of the carotid or

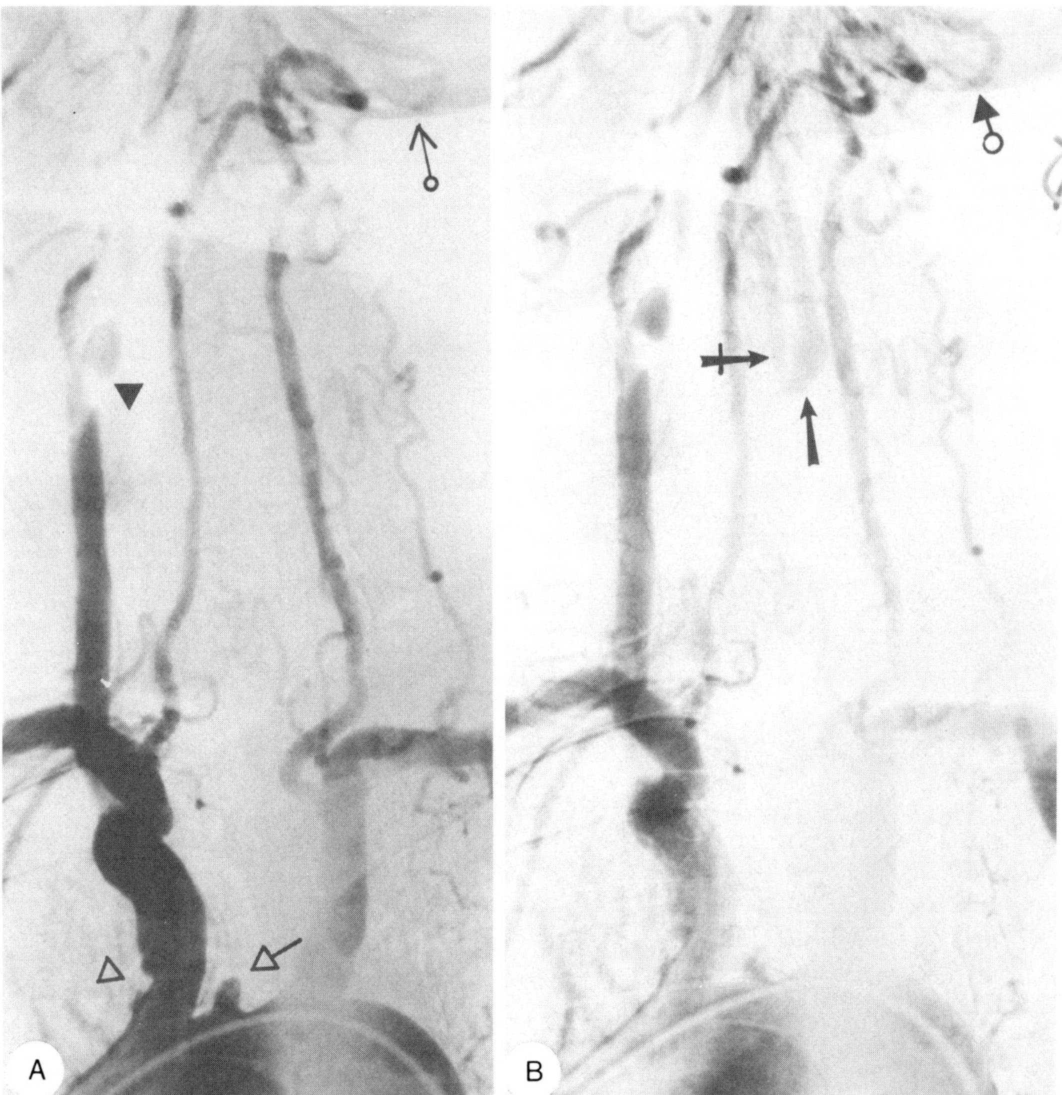

Figure 9–13. Extensive atherosclerotic vascular disease with left common carotid artery occlusion shown by aortogram in the RPO projection. An early arterial phase image (*A*) reveals proximal left common carotid artery occlusion (open arrow), a plaque at the innominate artery origin (open arrowhead), and a poorly shown severe stenosis of the right carotid bifurcation and proximal internal carotid artery (filled arrowhead) with ulceration. Late arterial phase image (*B*) demonstrates opacification of the left ICA (arrow) and ECA (crossed arrow). The film sequence (*B*) suggests retrograde blood flow down the ICA. The occipital artery also opacified early (filled arrow with circle) and may have been the dominant collateral flow pathway in this case.

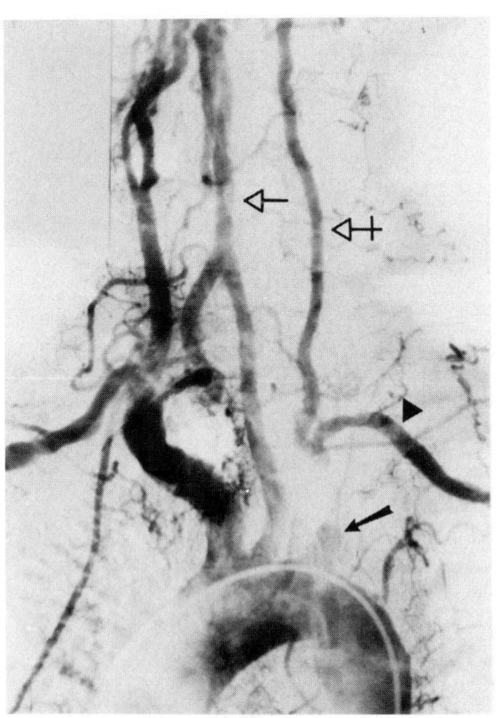

Figure 9–14. Left subclavian steal syndrome. Late arterial phase aortogram in the RPO projection shows proximal occlusion of the left subclavian artery (arrow) and retrograde flow through the left VA (open arrow) to fill the distal left subclavian artery (arrowhead). Symptoms of vertebrobasilar insufficiency will occur if this collateral flow diverts ("steals") too much blood from the posterior fossa. The superimposition of the right VA and left common carotid artery bifurcation (open arrow) prevents adequate evaluation of these structures in this RPO projection.

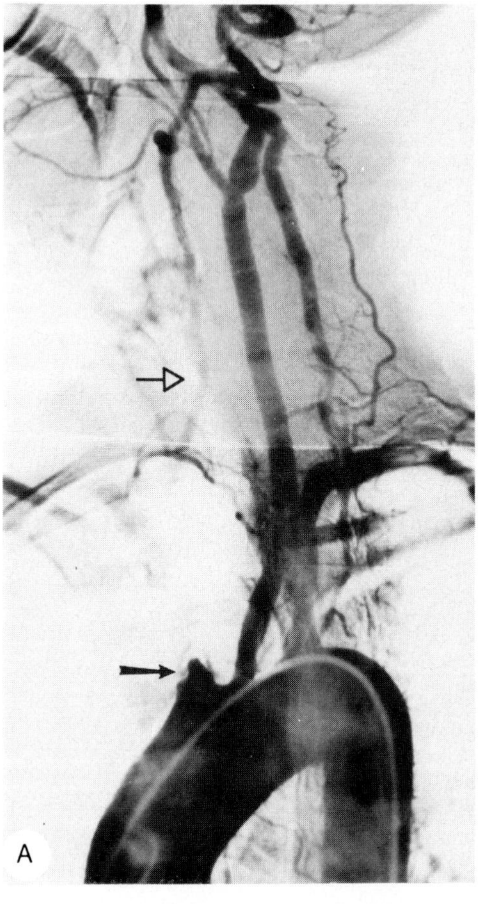

A

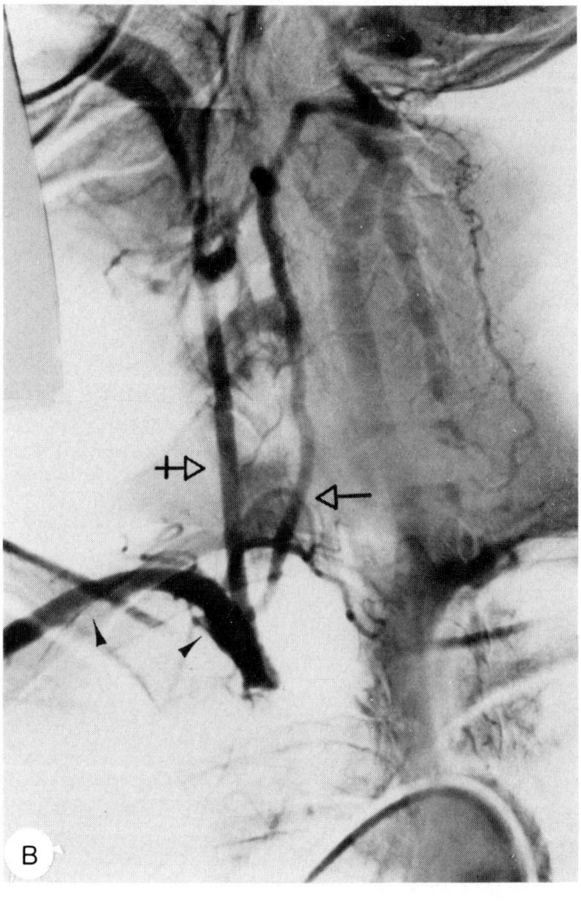

B

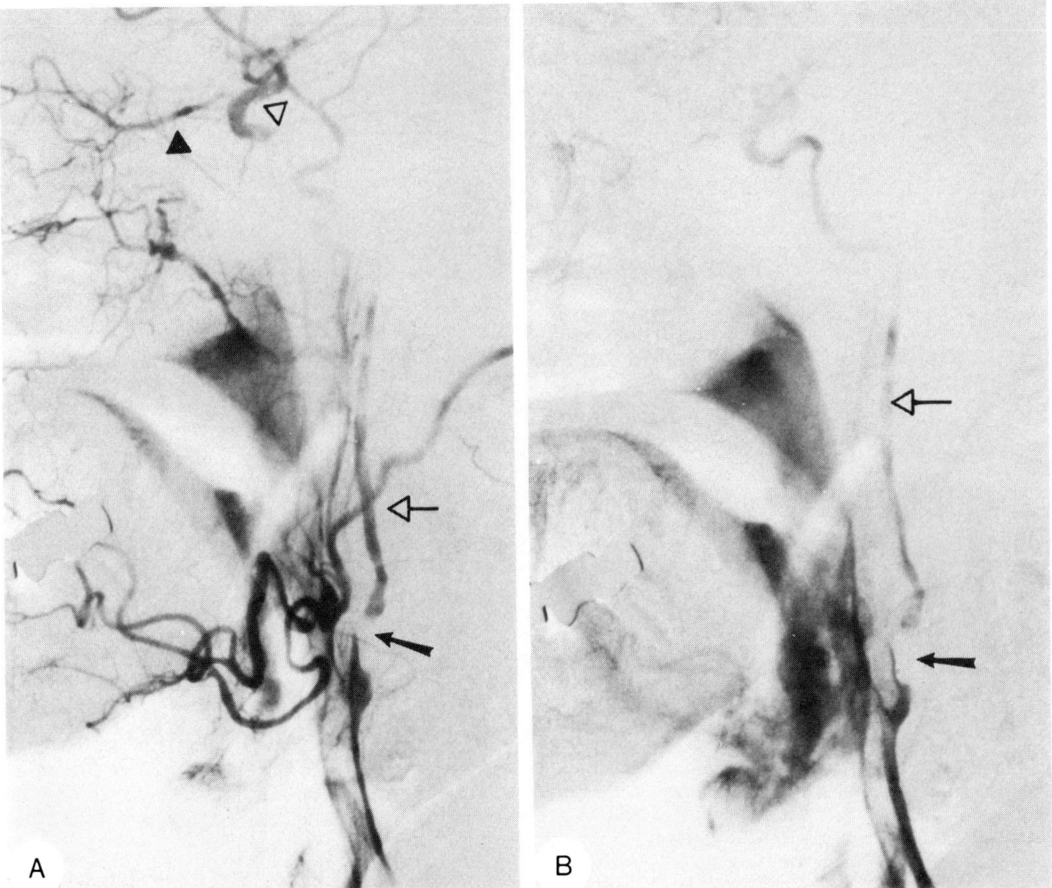

Figure 9-16. A late arterial phase lateral view (*A*) of a selective common carotid arteriogram shows extensive collateral blood flow from the internal maxillary to the ophthalmic artery (closed arrowhead). Retrograde flow through the ophthalmic artery opacifies the carotid siphon (open arrowhead) and the middle cerebral artery. Near occlusion of the proximal ICA (arrow) is also noted, with slow forward blood flow above this site (open arrow). The venous phase lateral view (*B*) again shows near occlusion of the proximal ICA (arrow) and slow forward blood flow ("string sign") opacifying the partially collapsed vessel (open arrow).

vertebral vessels. This can be arteriographically recognized by the sharp cutoff it creates in the contrast-filled lumen (see Figure 9-17). A portion of the embolus may protrude into the lumen causing a filling defect in the contrast column. Slowly progressive and longstanding atherosclerotic occlusion often displays a mildly tapered but abrupt blunt convex end to the vascular lumen (see Figures 9-14 and 9-15). In contrast, subintimal hemorrhage and intimal flaps tend to produce a much longer, smoothly tapered occlusion.

Ulceration of atherosclerotic plaques occurs when the endothelium breaks down, exposing the medial layer. Ulcerative plaque has the arteriographic appearance of a smooth outpouching or spiculated recess from the vascular lumen (see Figures 9-18 and 9-19). Small surface ulcerations and ulcers filled with debris may go undetected by angiography even when geometric magnification techniques are used (Edwards *et al.*, 1979; Eikelboom *et al.*, 1983). Ulcerations may or may not be associated with hemodynamically significant stenosis

Figure 9-15. Right innominate artery occlusion. Early arterial phase image from RPO projection aortogram (*A*) shows atherosclerotic occlusion of the right innominate artery (arrow), with widely patent left common carotid and subclavian arteries. There is retrograde flow through the right VA (open arrow). (*B*) reveals retrograde flow through the right VA, which in turn provides antegrade flow in the distal right subclavian (filled arrowheads) and the right common carotid arteries (crossed open arrow) (*B*).

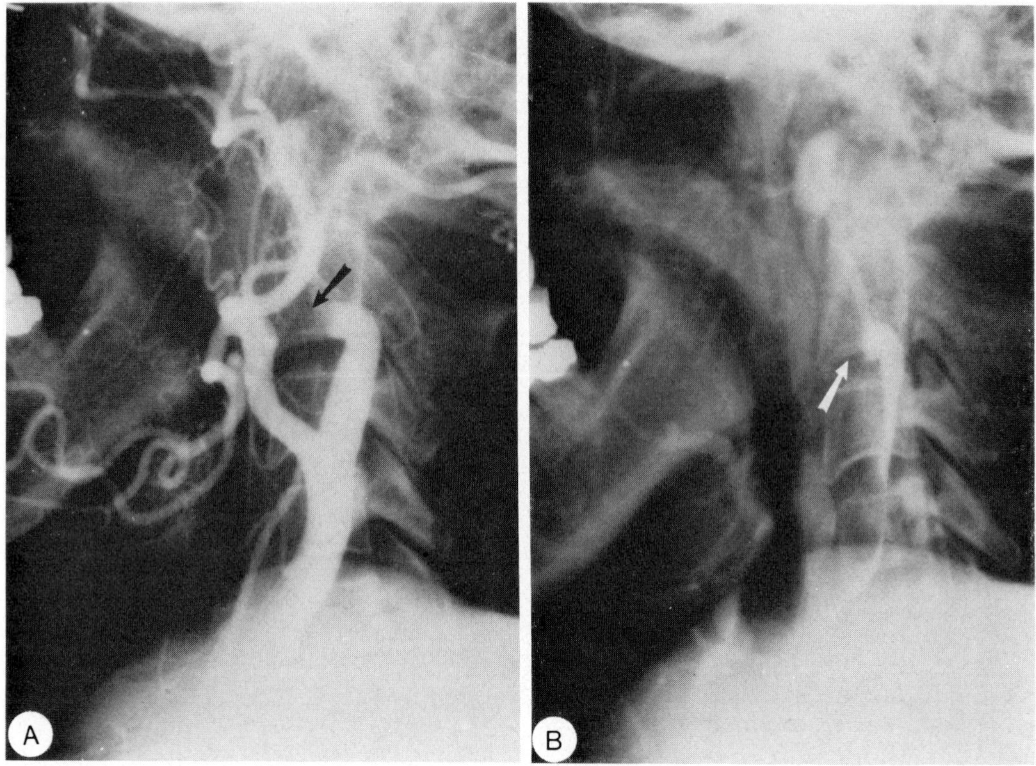

Figure 9–17. Embolic occlusion of the ICA. Lateral projection early arterial (*A*) and late venous phase (*B*) images of a selective left common carotid arteriogram reveal abrupt occlusion of the ICA by a thrombus (arrow) originating in the heart. The embolus indents the end of the contrast column, whereas atherosclerotic occlusions usually have a blunt, tapered appearance (see Figures 9–14 and 9–15).

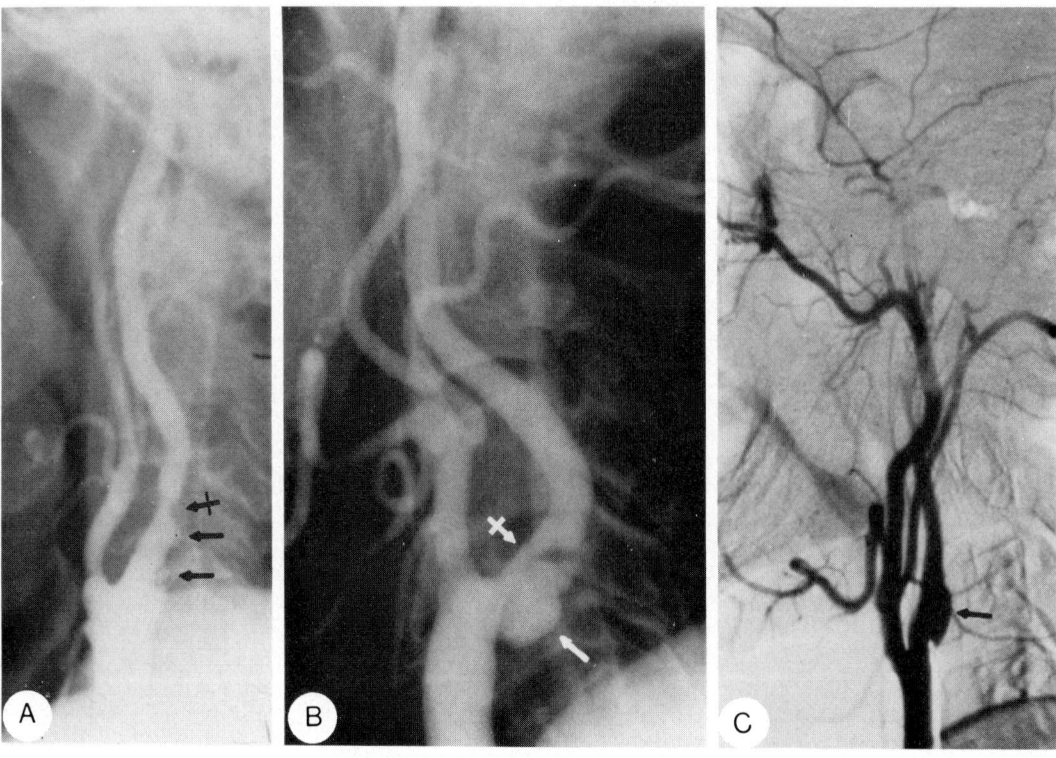

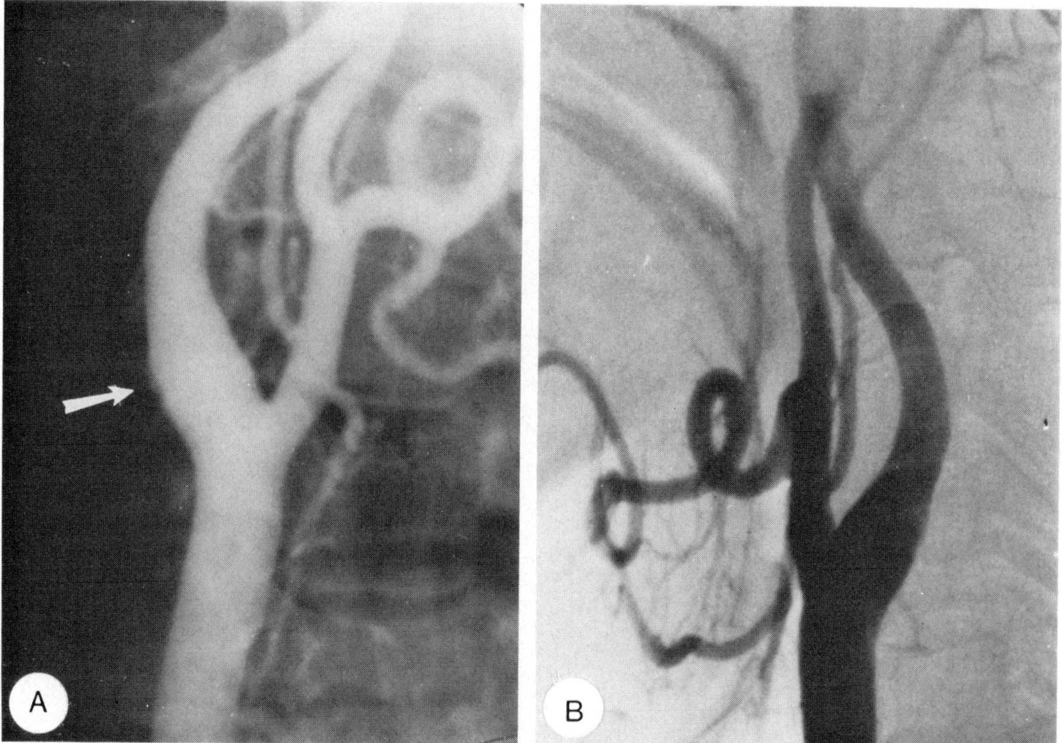

Figure 9–19. A small carotid ulcer (arrow) without vascular stenosis identified in the oblique-view spot-film (*A*), but not in the lateral projection (*B*). Complete angiographic evaluation requires that each vessel be examined in at least two different radiographic projections, usually made at 90 degree angles to each other.

Thrombi may form distal to a tight stenosis even in the absence of ulceration (see Figure 9–20). The ICA origin is the most frequent site of ulceration; symptomatic ulcers also occur in the proximal subclavian and innominate arteries and much less frequently in the greater curvature of the ascending aorta. Atherosclerotic plaques at the vertebral artery origins virtually never ulcerate.

The goal of carotid endarterectomy is to reestablish the vascular lumen and remove ulcerative plaques. Arteriography performed immediately after surgery usually demonstrates an enlarged, smooth undulating vascular lumen. An abrupt transition zone to "normal endothelium" at the upper and lower limits of the operative field may be observed. In time, endothelium will regrow at the operative site, producing a smoother and more normal arteriographic appearance. Atherosclerotic lesions may recur, producing new ulceration and/or stenosis. If an artery is occluded immediately after surgery, it is usually caused by an intimal flap (See Figures 9–21 and 9–22).

Nonatheromatous Vascular Lesions

Many of these lesions have an angiographic appearance that is indistinguishable from atherosclerosis; typical lesions, however, allow definite diagnosis. In other cases, the diagnosis must be based on clinical presentation, serologic findings, and biopsy results.

Fibromuscular hyperplasia (FMH) is an angiopathy of unknown etiology occurring predominantly in young women. Angiographically, FMH most commonly involves the midcervical ICA and spares the carotid bifurcation and the petrous-cavernous ICA in al-

Figure 9–18. ICA ulcerations seen on selective common carotid arteriograms in three different patients. Two ulcers (arrows) and a severe stenosis (crossed arrow) of the ICA (*A*). One large ulcer (arrow) with a moderae-to-severe ICA stenosis (crossed arrow) (*B*). Large ulcer (arrow) of the proximal ICA without hemodynamically significant stenosis (*C*).

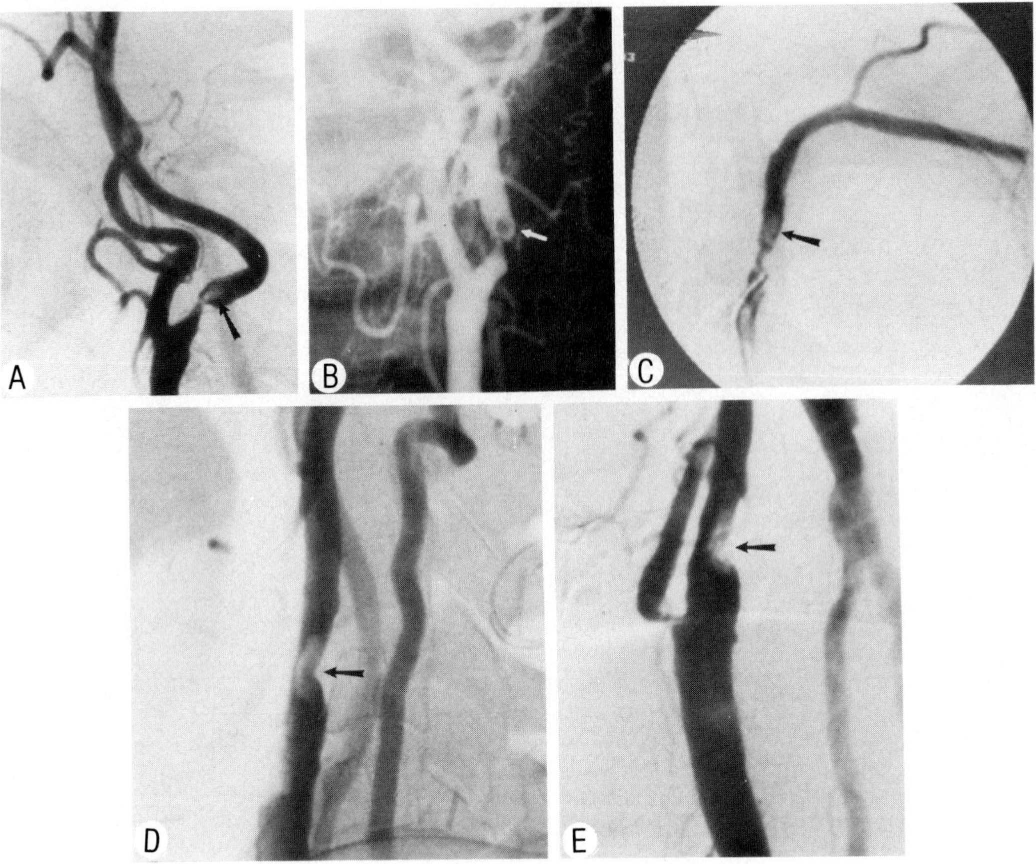

Figure 9-20. Intraluminal thrombus associated with vascular stenosis in four different patients. Severe ICA stenosis with thrombus (arrow) (*A*). A second patient with similar findings (*B*). Severe left subclavian artery stenosis with thrombus (arrow) seen with selective injection IA-DSA study. The left VA is occluded (*C*). Lateral and oblique views (*D* and *E*) show the probable thrombus (arrow) associated with a moderate vascular stenosis.

most all cases. Intracranial aneurysm is seen in approximately one third of the cases. Bilateral disease is frequent. Vertebral artery lesions are less common but, when present, usually occur at the C1-C2 area. In 80 percent of cases, irregularly spaced focal concentric stenoses with interposed areas of arterial dilatation produce the characteristic "string of beads" appearance on angiography (see Figures 9-23 and 9-24). *Vascular spasm* can resemble FMH on arteriograms, but the constrictions tend to be more evenly spaced, and the intervening vessel is not dilated (New, 1966). FMH presenting as a long tubular stenosis may be difficult to distinguish, by arteriographic criteria alone, from arterial hypoplasia, diffuse vascular spasm, arteritis, or extensive subintimal dissection. Pseudoaneurysm formation is a rare presentation for FMH (see also Chapter 17 on fibromuscular dysplasia).

The term *arteritis* includes a wide spectrum of diseases. Giant-cell arteritis and arteritis caused by amphetamine abuse may manifest as segmental vascular stenoses and dilatations seen primarily in the intracranial circulation. Radiation could cause either long tubular stenoses resembling FMH or a focal stricture. Takayasu's disease produces occlusions at the origins of the brachiocephalic vessels.

Positional obstructions may involve both the carotid and the vertebral (see Figure 9-25) system (see also Chapter 22 on positional obstructions).

Spontaneous *dissection* with or without aneurysm formation can also cause vascular compromise. Angiographically, a smooth tapering of the lumen is present even if the vessel is occluded. An intimal flap may be apparent as a linear filling defect. Rarely, a double lumen may be observed. The aortic arch and

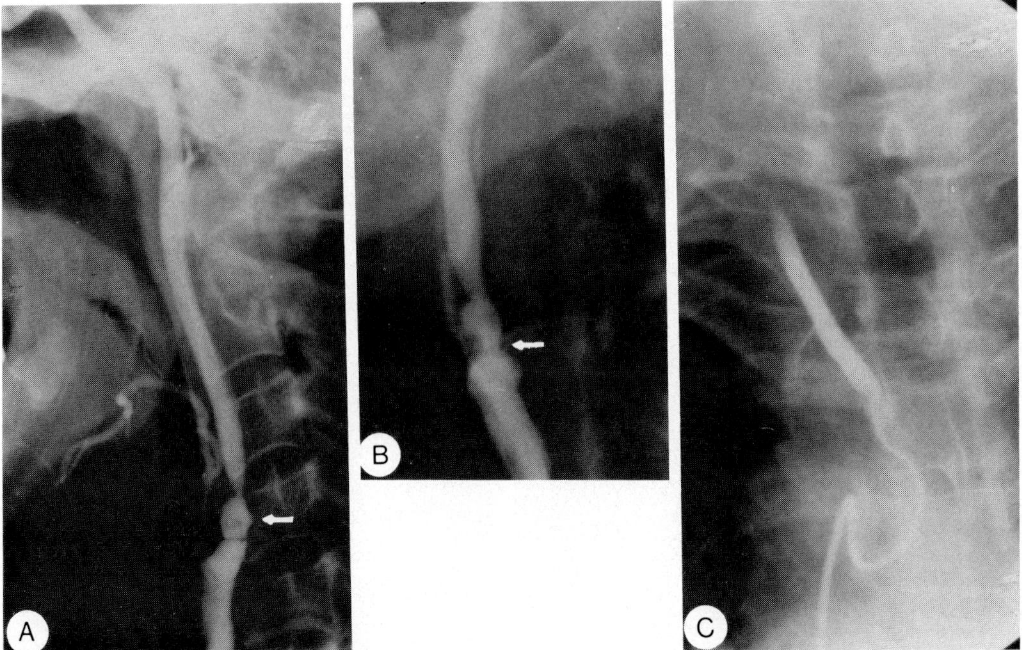

Figure 9–21. A postoperative stricture after carotid endarterectomy. Lateral and LPO projections (*A* and *B*) show severe ICA and ECA stenoses, with ulceration and possible thrombus in the ICA (arrow). A selective common carotid artery injection (*C*) immediately after surgery shows a smooth, tapered occlusion of the midportion of the vessel. The angiographic appearance is compatible with an intimal flap, which was surgically confirmed.

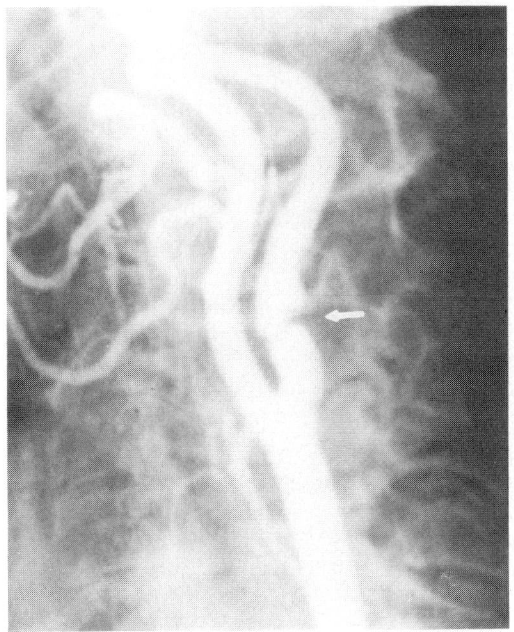

Figure 9–22. Intimal flap. This 75-year-old man presented with clinical symptoms of left amaurosis fugax. A left carotid endarterectomy had been performed ten years before this study. A selective RPO projection left common carotid arteriogram shows stenosis of the proximal ICA. At least two discrete lines (arrow) are faintly seen in the contrast column, which may represent intimal flaps. The patient's symptoms were relieved after a second carotid endarterectomy.

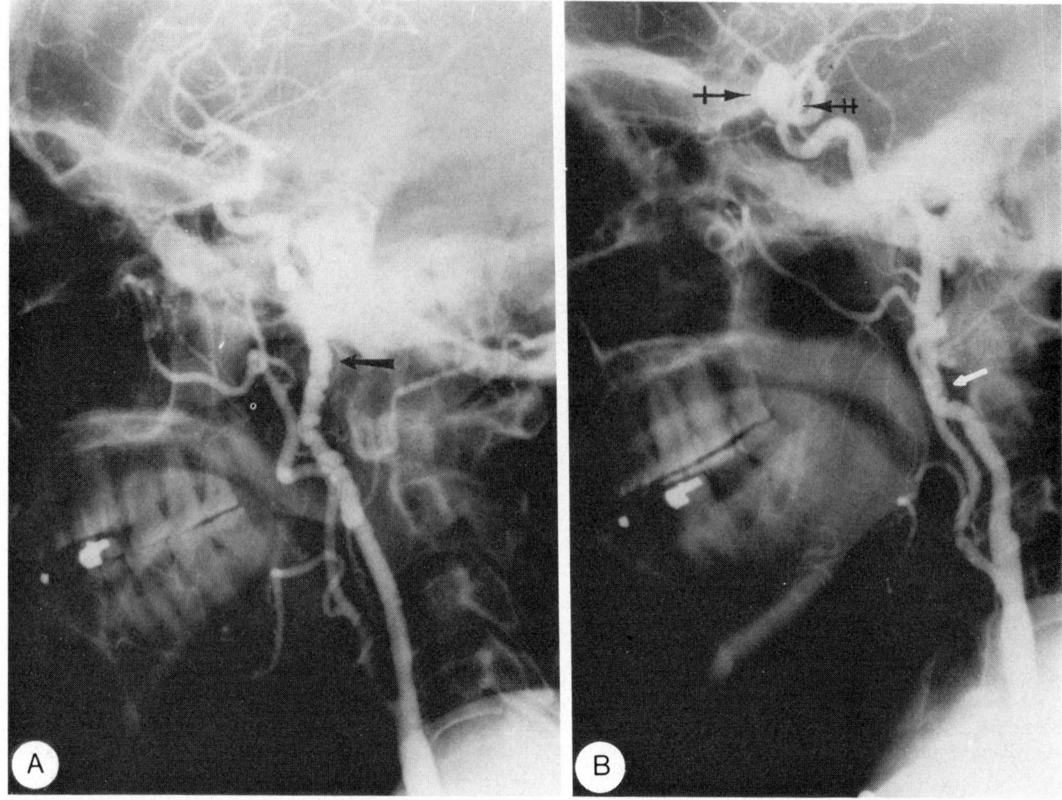

Figure 9-23. Fibromuscular hyperplasia. Selective right common carotid arteriography reveals typical concentric stenoses with interposed areas of dilatation ("string of beads") (arrow). The upper cervical ICA is most involved (*A*). Selective left common carotid arteriogram of the same patient (*B*) shows a less impressive string of beads (arrow), a large ophthalmic artery aneurysm (crossed arrow), and a smaller supraclinoid carotid aneurysm (double crossed arrow).

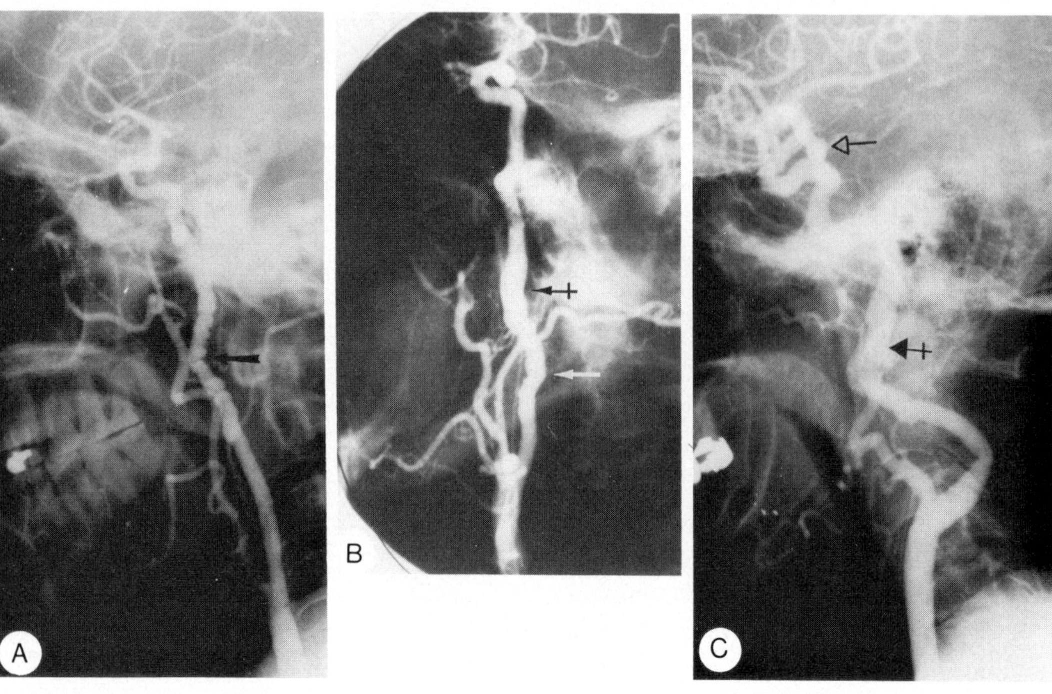

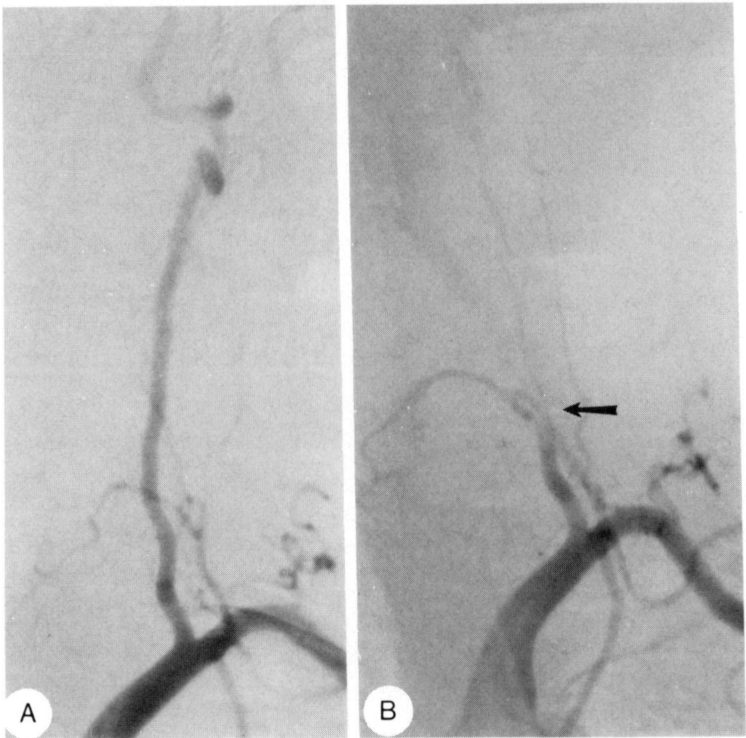

Figure 9–25. Positional occlusion of the left VA. This 44-year-old woman noted dizziness and blurred vision when she turned her head to the right. Selective left subclavian artery injection with the patient's head turned to the left (*A*) reveals a normal left VA. Repeat left subclavian artery injection with the patient's head turned to the right (*B*) shows left VA occlusion near C6 (arrow). The right VA (not shown) was hypoplastic.

cervical ICA are most commonly involved, while vertebral artery dissection is very rare (Bradac *et al.*, 1981) (see also Chapter 25 on carotid dissection).

Aneurysm of the cervical vessels is uncommon. Margolis *et al.* (1972) reported 20 patients with cervical ICA aneurysm, of which five were caused by atherosclerotic disease, seven were congenital, six were posttraumatic, and two were secondary to local infection. Radiotherapy, FMH, cystic medial necrosis, and angiographic trauma may also lead to aneurysm formation. Arteriographically, these lesions are either fusiform or saccular in configuration and they may contain mural thrombi (see Figure 9–26). AP, lateral, and oblique views are often necessary to fully assess these lesions. If an intracranial aneurysm is discovered (see Figures 9–12 and 9–24), a complete cerebral arteriographic examination is warranted to exclude additional lesions (see Chapter 25 on aneurysms).

Carotid body tumors may clinically mimic aneurysms but can be easily diagnosed by their characteristic angiographic appearance (see Figure 9–27).

Trauma may produce stenosis, occlusion, arteriovenous fistula, or aneurysm (see Figures 9–28 and 9–29) in the cervicocerebral vessels. Basal skull fracture may be associated with both carotid-cavernous fistula and ICA occlusion. Blunt injury to the neck may cause dissection, particularly in the cervical ICA. Penetrating trauma (e.g., bullet or knife) may grossly sever a vessel (see Figure 9–29). Traumatic occlusion of the ICA usually produces a

Figure 9–24. Fibromuscular hyperplasia manifested as a fusiform ICA aneurysm. Selective left common carotid arteriogram (*A*) shows a midcervical ICA string of beads (arrow). Selective right common carotid arteriogram (*B*) shows a fusiform aneurysm of the cervical ICA (crossed arrow) associated with "string of beads" (arrow). Arteriogram of another patient (*C*) with a fusiform cervical ICA aneurysm (crossed arrow) associated with fibromuscular hyperplasia. A posterior communicating artery saccular aneurysm (open arrow) and a milk kink of the cervical ICA are also seen.

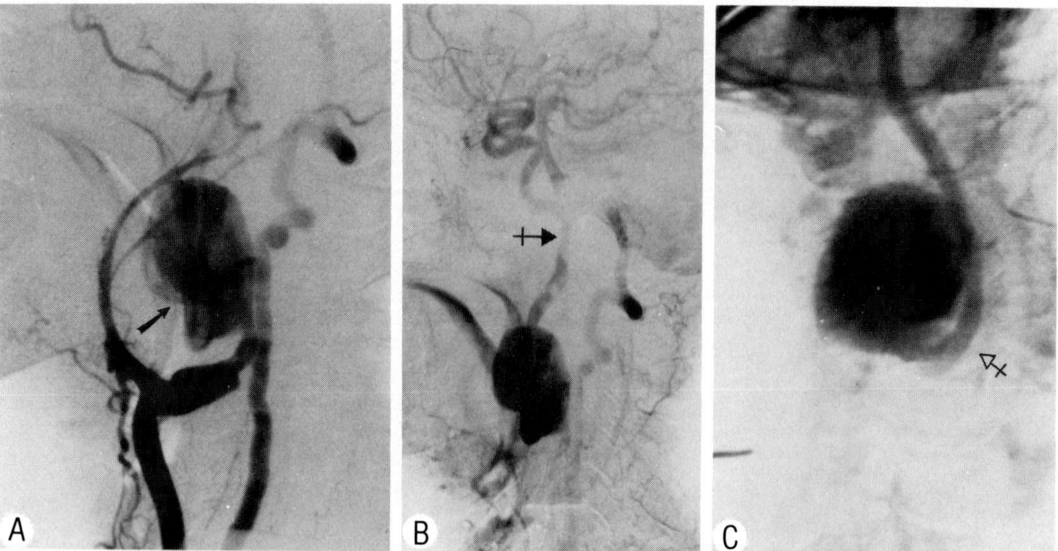

Figure 9–26. Aneurysm of the ICA. This 71-year-old woman noted a painless pulsatile mass which progressively enlarged over a three-month period. A selective right innominate artery injection demonstrates a large saccular right ICA aneurysm (arrow) which widens the carotid bifurcation (*A*); later film (*B*), shows the distal ICA (crossed arrow) emerging from the aneurysm. A selective right common carotid artery IA-DSA study (*C*) demonstrates the relationship of the aneurysm to the distal ICA.

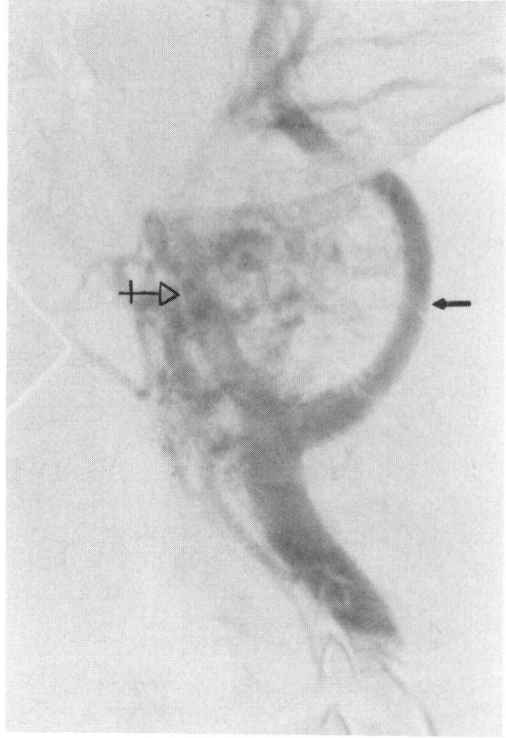

Figure 9–27. Carotid body tumor. This 37-year-old patient had had a slowly enlarging mass in his right neck for 15 years. The typical arteriographic findings of a highly vascular tumor as well as splaying apart the ICA (arrow) and ECA (crossed open arrow) are present.

rapid thrombosis of the vessel from the carotid bulb to the ophthalmic artery (see Figure 9–30). Traumatic injury to the vertebral arteries has also been described due to cervical spine fractures, after chiropractic manipulations (Miller and Burton, 1974) or yoga exercises (Hanus *et al.,* 1977). Angiographic findings are similar to those already described (see Chapter 24 on trauma).

Patterns of Collateral Blood Flow

The ECA is an extensive source of collateral blood flow in ICA and VA occlusive disease (see Figure 14–17). The most common pattern seen with ICA occlusive disease is blood flow from the distal pterygopalatine branches of the maxillary artery to the ethmoidal branches of the ophthalmic artery. Reversal of blood flow in the ophthalmic artery allows filling of the supraclinoid ICA (see Figure 9–31). The distal facial artery and anterior branches of the superficial temporal artery (STA) anastomose with orbital vessels and may provide additional blood flow as well. The superficial temporal artery can be surgically anastomosed to an opercular branch of the middle cerebral artery (STA-MCA bypass) to provide collateral flow to the brain (see Figure 9–32). By utilizing selective catheterization of the ipsilat-

Figure 9–28. Small pseudoaneurysm of the left common carotid artery (arrow) caused by a shotgun injury. One pellet entered the vessel at this point and embolized to the left middle cerebral artery (not shown).

eral common carotid artery and prolonged filming sequence, these collateral vessels can be identified most easily in the lateral projection. Crossover collateral flow to the brain on the occluded ICA side through the anterior communicating artery is best judged in the AP view during selective injection of the contralateral common carotid artery (see Figure 9–8). Similarly, collateral flow through the posterior communicating arteries is best assessed by selective vertebral-subclavian artery injection (see Figure 9–33).

In VA occlusive disease, the occipital artery along with the costocervical and thyrocervical branches of the subclavian artery form an anastomotic network in the posterior cervical musculature capable of reconstituting the VA with antegrade flow above the occlusion. These vessels can be well demonstrated by either aortic arch or selective arterial injections (see Figures 9–34 and 9–35). The contralateral VA and the posterior communicating arteries are also important sources of collateral flow to the vertebral-basilar system and are best evaluated by use of selective arterial injections.

In common carotid artery occlusion, reversal of flow in the ICA may provide antegrade ECA flow (see Figure 9–13). Occasionally, collateral circulation through the ECA will supply antegrade ICA flow in these patients.

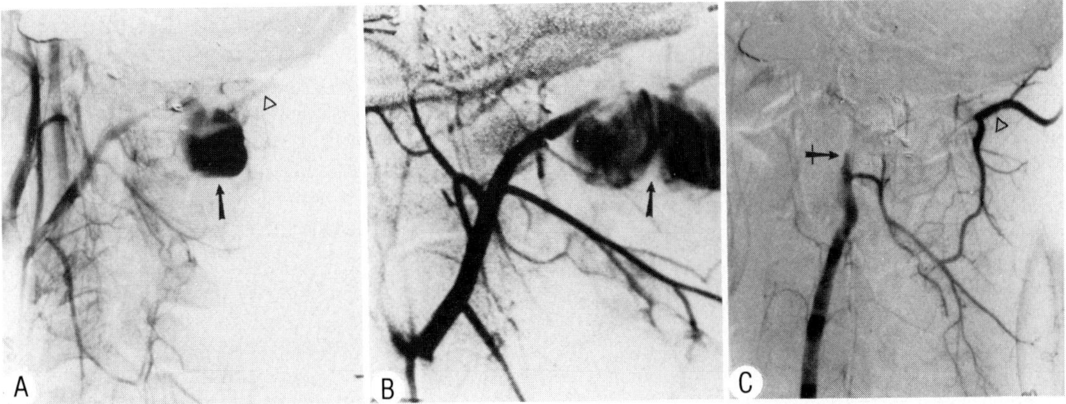

Figure 9–29. Pseudoaneurysm caused by a gunshot injury. In this 23-year-old man, a painless pulsatile mass developed behind the left ear two months after he was shot with a single large-caliber bullet. The patient remained intact neurologically. Selective left occipital arteriogram (*A*) demonstrates a large pseudoaneurysm (arrow) and filling of the distal occipital artery (open arrowhead). Selective left occipital arteriogram. (*B*) 1A-DSA image shows a two-lobed pseudoaneurysm (arrow). Selective left vertebral arteriogram (*C*) reveals traumatic occlusion of the VA at C2 (crossed arrow). A large muscular collateral vessel opacifies the distal occipital artery (open arrowhead) but not the pseudoaneurysm.

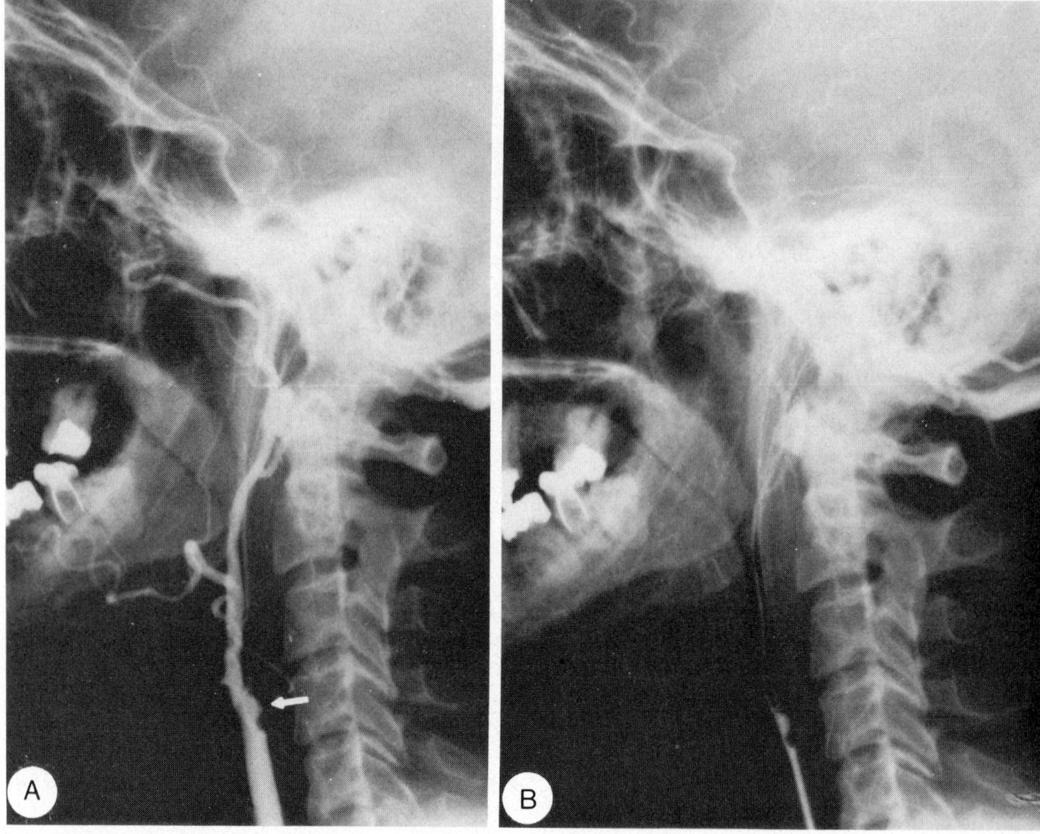

Figure 9–30. Acute ICA occlusion. This 40-year-old man sustained blunt neck trauma and acute right ICA occlusion developed. Selective right common carotid arteriogram (*A*) shows eccentric occlusion of the ICA at its origin (arrow). Late arterial phase image (*B*) shows no evidence of collateral flow reopacifying the distal ICA. Collateral pathways are often poorly developed when sudden occlusion of a previously normal vessel occurs. The neurological deficits associated with an acute vascular occlusion may improve as collateral blood flow develops.

With proximal subclavian artery occlusion, reversal of the flow in the ipsilateral VA provides collateral circulation to the arm which may clinically manifest itself as the subclavian steal syndrome (see Figures 9–14 and 9–15). All these situations can be well shown angiographically by use of aortic arch injections with prolonged filming sequences.

COMPLICATIONS OF CAROTID-VERTEBRAL ANGIOGRAPHY

Variations in patient populations studied and the use of different definitions for complications make direct comparison between published series difficult. Major arteriographic complications include death, permanent neurological deficit, and arterial occlusion requiring surgery. Minor complications consist of transient neurologic deficit, hematoma, and urticaria. One well-documented series of 5,000 catheter angiography procedures reported a 0.16 percent major complication rate (Mani *et al.*, 1978). Another series reported a 0.13 percent major complication rate in 6,000 studies performed from 1971 to 1978, and a 0.02 percent major complication rate in 1,500 studies performed from 1978 to 1982 (Bradac and Oberson, 1982). This improvement was attributed to increased experience and better patient selection. In another series of 301 patients, no major complications occurred with the use of transfemoral catheter techniques (Eisenberg *et al.*, 1980). Minor complications occurred in the range of 1 to 4 percent in these studies. Somewhat higher complication rates have been encountered with direct carotid puncture techniques (Hass *et al.*, 1968; Miller *et al.*,

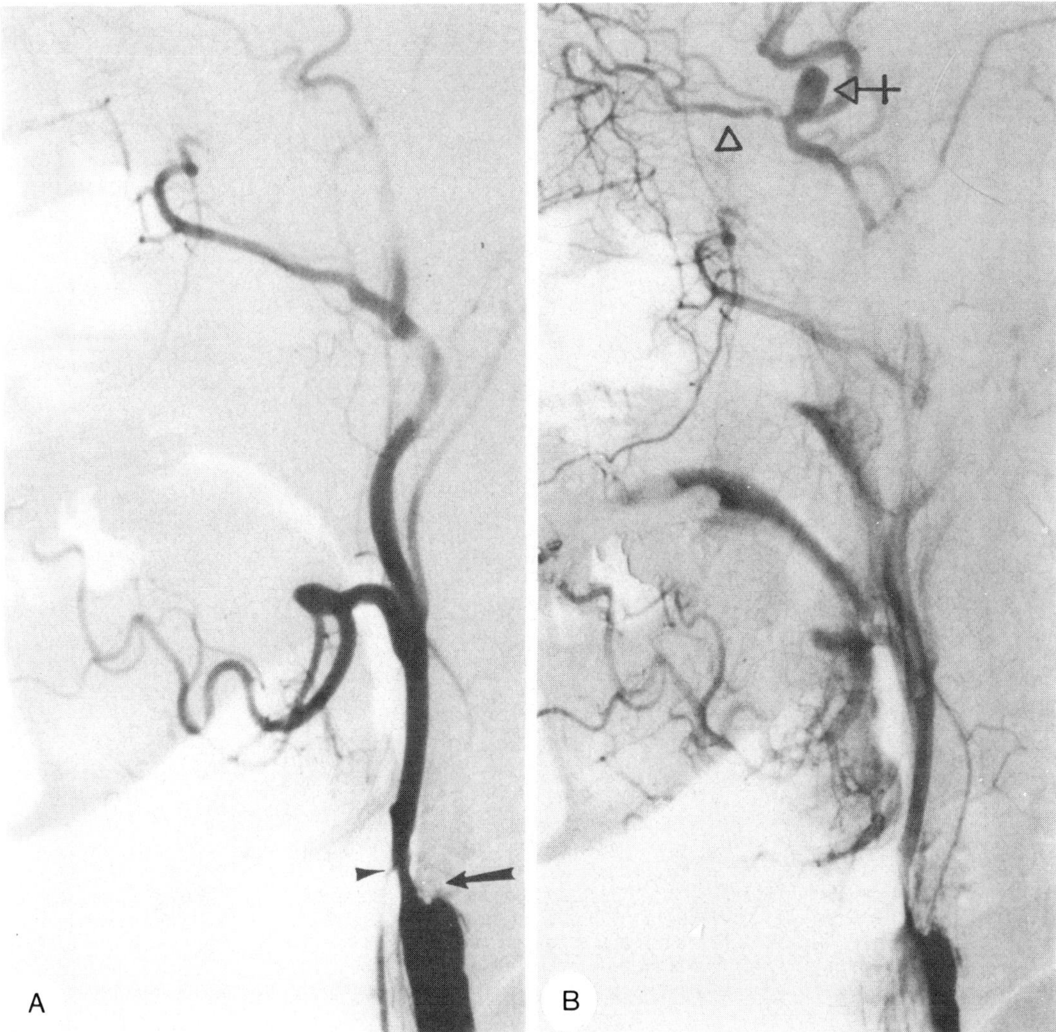

Figure 9–31. ICA occlusion and collateral blood flow. Selective right common carotid arteriogram (*A*) shows complete ICA occlusion (arrow) and a moderate stenosis of the proximal ECA (filled arrowhead) late arterial phase image (*B*) demonstrates a network of collateral vessels from ECA providing blood flow to the ophthalmic artery (open arrowhead) and the cavernous-supraclinoid ICA. A large opthalmic artery aneursym is also noted (crossed arrow).

1977). Risk factors predisposing to complications include long procedure times, large contrast doses, angiographer inexperience, large catheters, and multiple catheter exchanges. Patients with advanced cerebrovascular occlusive disease, recent stroke, subarachnoid hemorrhage, migraine, or posttraumatic or postoperative conditions tended to have more complications.

Local Complications

Hematoma is the most frequent local complication of arteriography. Good technique and effective puncture-site compression will make its development less likely. Patients with impaired blood-clotting function, severe hypertension, or advanced atherosclerotic disease are especially predisposed to hematoma formation. The use of large catheters, prolonged catheter manipulation, and multiple catheter exchanges also contribute to hematoma formation. With direct axillary or brachial artery puncture, a hematoma can damage the median nerve and the brachial plexus. Horner's syndrome may result from a hematoma associated with direct carotid artery puncture. If the artery of Adamkiewicz is dam-

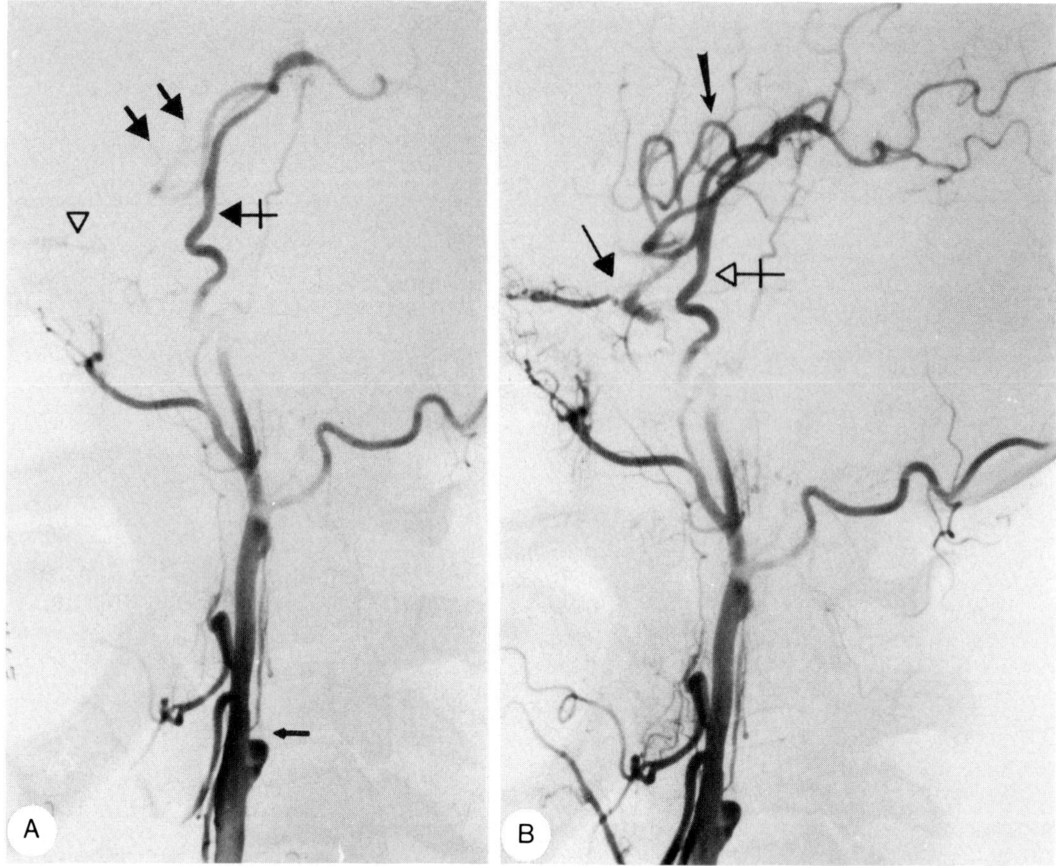

Figure 9-32. Superficial temporal-middle cerebral artery bypass. Selective left common carotid arteriogram (*A*) shows complete ICA occlusion (arrow), early filling of the ophthalmic artery (open arrowhead) from collateral vessels, and the superficial temporal artery (crossed arrow) supplying left middle cerebral artery opercular branches (filled arrows). Later arterial phase (*B*) reveals moderate stenosis of the proximal ophthalmic artery (arrow) with opacification of the cavernous-supraclinoid ICA. Progressive filling of the middle cerebral artery (small arrow) from the superficial temporal artery (crossed open arrow) is also present.

aged during the translumbar approach, distal spinal cord infarction may occur.

Arterial thrombosis is the most common local major arteriographic complication. Vascular spasm, multiple punctures, large catheters, prolonged catheter manipulation, and multiple catheter exchanges can contribute to its occurrence. An intimal flap raised during initial arterial puncture can also cause vascular occlusion. Occasionally, atherosclerotic debris is dislodged and occludes vessels distal to the puncture site. Thrombi can form on the catheter itself and embolize in a similar fashion. In the peripheral vascular system, intraarterial streptokinase-urokinase therapy may be helpful in some cases. Most of the time, however, surgical intervention is needed.

Other less frequent complications include clinically symptomatic *venous occlusion* or compression secondary to hematoma or inadvertent puncture. *Infection, arteriovenous fistula,* and *false aneurysm* formation are very rare late complications of arterial puncture.

Systemic Complications

Systemic reactions to iodine contrast agents include a transient *sensation of warmth,* "burning discomfort," *nausea* and *vomiting.* These require no specific therapy. Urticaria, itching, and nasal stuffiness may occasionally occur and can be suppressed with 25 to 50 mg of diphenhydramine (intramuscular) or 300 to 600 mg of cimetidine (intravenous). Severe *allergic reactions,* such as laryngospasm, angioedema, and anaphylaxis, must be recognized

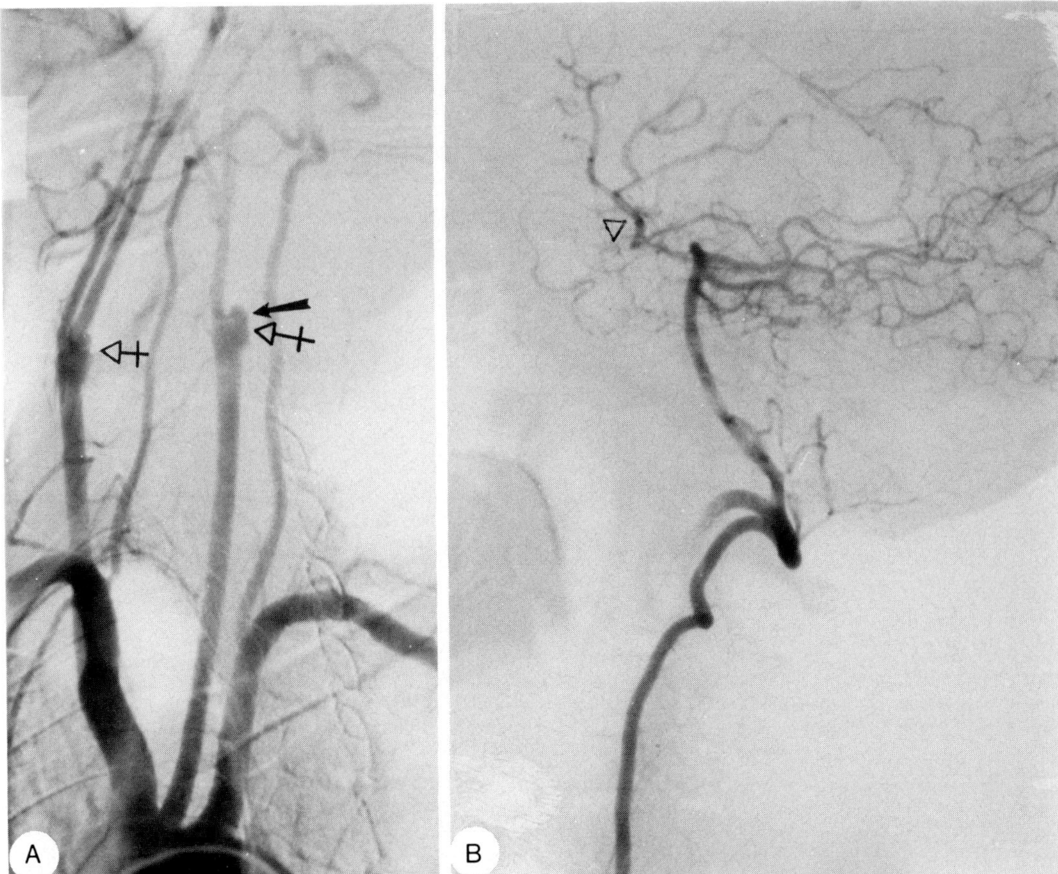

Figure 9–33. Occlusion of the ICA with collateral blood flow through the posterior communicating artery. Arch aortogram in RPO projection (*A*) shows left ICA atherosclerotic occlusion (arrow), bilateral carotid bifurcation ulcerated plaques (crossed open arrow), and a mild right VA origin stenosis. Selective right vertebral arteriogram (*B*) displays left middle cerebral artery opacification (open arrowhead) via the posterior communicating artery. Washout in the left middle cerebral artery indicates that additional collateral blood flow may be coming through the ophthalmic artery and/or the anterior communicating artery.

immediately and treated with appropriate resuscitation measures. Fatal reaction to intravenous iodine contrast is reported to occur in one in 10,000 to 20,000 cases (Shehadi, 1975). Some evidence suggests that intraarterial administration is less hazardous than the intravenous route.

Intravenous atropine sulfate given in 0.4 mg increments to a maximum dose of 2 mg is used if bradycardia develops during the procedure. If the stress of the procedure precipitates angina in susceptible patients, sublingual nitroglycerin should be given to abolish the pain.

Iodine contrast media may impair renal function or even cause complete *renal failure,* particularly in patients with preexisting renal disease. As has already been stated, BUN and serum creatinine values obtained before the examination will identify these patients. Adequate hydration before arteriography, judicious use of contrast media, and the administration of diuretic agents during or after the procedure usually prevent subsequent renal complications. BUN and serum creatinine values may be obtained on the following day to evaluate postarteriogram renal function. Patients with multiple myeloma should be handled in a similar fashion but they still remain at high risk for renal complications. Renal dialysis-dependent patients should be dialyzed after the arteriogram.

Neurologic Complications

Contrast media may not only penetrate the already abnormal blood brain barrier of pa-

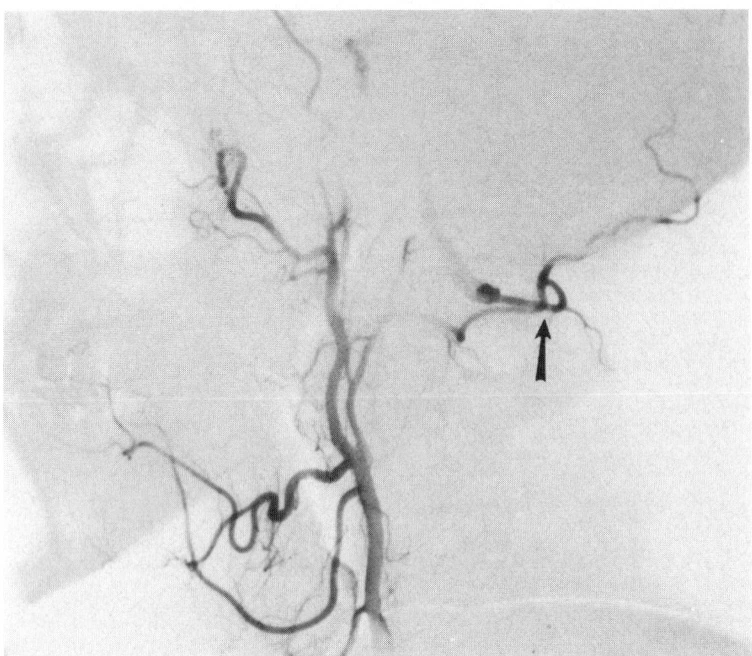

Figure 9–34. Anastomotic channel between the occipital and vertebral arteries. A selective left ECA injection in lateral view reveals a large collateral vessel (arrow) connecting the occipital artery and the third portion of the VA at C1. The VA may either provide or receive collateral blood flow through this vascular connection with the occipital artery.

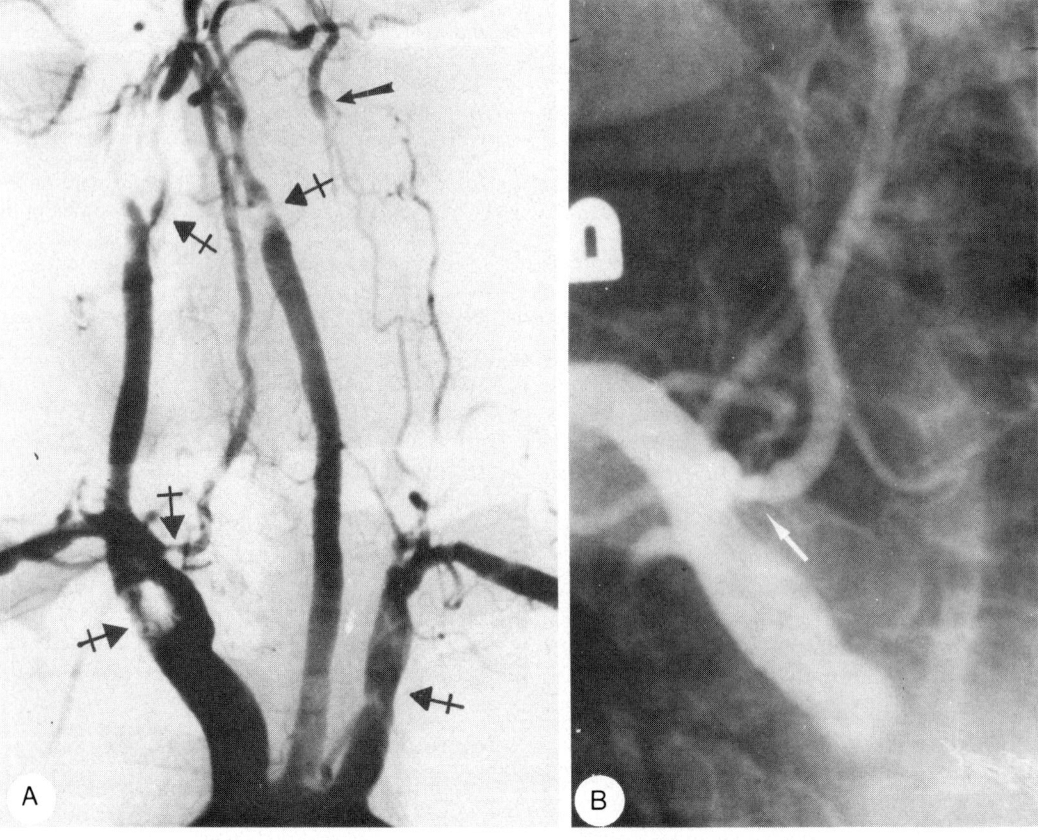

tients with recent infarction, trauma, or surgery but it can disrupt even the normal vascular endothelium. Chemical composition, osmolarity, contact time, and the dose of the contrast media are all factors contributing to this phenomenon. Brain edema associated with the direct toxic effects of the contrast media itself may produce a new or worsen a preexisting neurological deficit. Angiographically induced cortical blindness has been reported and was attributed to contrast media toxicity to the calcarine cortex (Morawetz *et al.,* 1984). Adequate hydration and the judicious use of contrast agents reduce the risk of contrast media-induced neurological deficits (Eisenberg *et al.,* 1980).

New neurological deficit after arteriography is most commonly caused by embolization of atherosclerotic debris, by thrombi formed on the catheter, or by intimal flaps. Anticoagulation therapy may be helpful when an intimal flap occurs, but it is of no proven benefit in the event of embolization. Some intimal flaps may be appropriately treated by surgery. These risks are minimized by meticulous attention to technique and prudent judgment by the angiographer regarding selective catheterization and direct arterial puncture.

The angiographic procedure should be immediately discontinued whenever a neurological complication is identified. Although most cerebral complications are transient, resembling TIAs, in approximately one in 1,000 patients an angiographically induced permanent neurological deficit will occur (Mani *et al.,* 1978). Skillfully performed transfemoral catheter cervicocerebral arteriography appears to offer the lowest risk of neurological complications.

REFERENCES

Allen, J.H.; Parera, C.; and Potts, D.G.: The relation of arterial trauma to complications of cerebral angiography. *A.J.R.,* **95**:845-51, 1965.

Bradac, G.B.; Kaenback, A.; Bolk-Weischedel, D.; and Finck, G.A.: Spontaneous dissecting aneurysm of cervical cerebral arteries. Report of six cases and review of the literature. *Neuroradiology,* **21**:149-54, 1981.

Bradac, GB, and Oberson, R.: *Angiography and Computed Tomography in Cerebro-Arterial Occlusive Diseases,* 2nd ed. Springer-Verlag, New York, 1982.

Edwards, J.H.; Kricheff II; Riles, T.; and Imparato, A.: Angiographically undetected ulceration of the carotid bifurcation as cause of embolic stroke. *Radiology,* **132**:369-373, 1979.

Eikelboom, B.D.; Riles, T.R.; Mintzer, R.; Baumann, F.G.; DeFillip, G.; Lin, J.; and Imparato, A.M.: Inaccuracy of angiography in the diagnosis of carotid ulceration. *Stroke,* **14**:882-85, 1983.

Eisenberg, R.L.; Bank, W.D.; and Hedgcock, M.W.: Neurologic complications of angiography in patients with critical stenosis of the carotid artery. *Neurology,* **30**:892-95, 1980.

Hanus, S.H.; Homer, T.D.; and Harter, D.H.: Vertebral artery occlusion complicating yoga exercises. *Arch. Neurol.,* **34**:574-75, 1977.

Hass, W.K.; Field, W.S.; North, R.R.; Kirchett, I.I.; Chase, N.E.; and Bauer, R.B.: Joint study of extracranial arterial occlusions. II. Arteriography, techniques, sites and complications. *J.A.M.A.,* **203**:961-68, 1968.

Haughton, V.M.; and Rosenbaum, A.E.: The normal and anomalous aortic arch and brachiocephalic arteries. In Newton, T.H.; Potts, D.G. (eds.): *Radiology of the Skull and Brain.* Vol. 2. C.V. Mosby, St. Louis, 1974, pages 1145-1163.

Krayenbuhl, H., and Yasargil, M.G.: *Cerebral Angiography,* 2. ed. W.B. Saunders, Philadelphia, 1968.

Lingren, E.: A history of neuroradiology. In Newton, T.H.; and Potts, D.G. (eds.): *Radiology of the Skull and Brain. The Skull.* C.V. Mosby, St. Louis, 1974, pages 1-25.

Mani, R.L.; Eisenberg, R.L.; McDonald, E.J., Jr.; Pollock, J.A.; and Mani, J.R.: Complications of catheter cerebral angiography: analysis of 5,000 procedures. I. Criteria and incidence. *A.J.R.,* **131**:861-65, 1978.

Margolis, M.T.; Stein, R.L.; and Newton, T.H.: Extracranial aneurysms of the internal carotid artery. *Neuroradiology,* **4**:78-89, 1972.

Miller, R.G., and Burton, R.: Stroke following chiropractic manipulation of the spine. *J.A.M.A.,* **229**:189-90, 1974.

Miller, J.D.R.; Grace, M.G.; Russell, D.R.; and Zacks, D.J.: Complications of cerebral angiography and pneumography. *Radiology,* **124**:741-44, 1977.

New, P.F.J.: Arterial stationary waves. *A.J.R.,* **97**:488-99, 1966.

Newton, T.H., and Potts, D.G. (eds.): *Radiology of the Skull and Brain.* Vol. 2. C.V. Mosby, St. Louis, 1974.

Osborn, A.G.: *Introduction to Cerebral Angiography.* Harper & Row, New York, 1980.

Punt, J.: Some observations on aneurysm of the proximal internal carotid artery. *J. Neurosurg.,* **51**:151-54, 1979.

Robicsek, F.; Sanger, P.W.; and Daugherty, H.K.: The angiographic picture of dysphagia lusoria. *Vasc. Surg.,* **2**(1):29-40, March 1968.

Shehadi, W.H.: Adverse reactions to intravascularly administered contrast media: a comprehensive study

Figure 9-35. VA occlusion with collateral blood flow. Right axillary artery puncture was used to perform this examination. Arch aortogram in the RPO projection (*A*) demonstrates left VA occlusion with cervical muscular arteries reconstituting the vessel at C3 (arrow). Extensive atherosclerotic disease is producing stenosis at the right VA origin, the proximal right common carotid and internal carotid artery, the left carotid bifurcation, and the midportion of the left subclavian artery (crossed arrows). Selective right subclavian artery injection in the RPO projection (*B*) shows the severe right VA origin stenosis (arrow) more clearly than the aortic arch study.

based on a prospective survey. *A.J.R.,* **124:**145–52, 1975.

Taveras, J.M., and Wood, E.H.: *Diagnostic Neuroradiology.* Vol. 2. William & Wilkins, Baltimore, 1976.

Teal, J.S.; Rumbaugh, C.L.; Segall, H.D.; and Bergeron, R.T.: Anomalous branches of the internal carotid artery. *Radiology,* **106:**567–73, 1973.

Vitek, J.J.: Femoro-cerebral angiography: analysis of 2,000 consecutive examinations, special emphasis on carotid arteries catheterization in older patients. *A.J.R.,* **118:**633–46, 1973.

Wylie, E.J., and Ehrenfeld, W.K.: *Extracranial Occlusive Cerebrovascular Disease: Diagnosis and Management.* W.B. Saunders, Philadelphia, 1970, pages 25–53.

10

The Assessment of Carotid Artery Disease by Computed Tomography

E. RALPH HEINZ

Film and screen angiography has long been accepted as the "gold standard" for the evaluation of carotid artery disease. Recently, however, several reports have been critical of traditional angiography, pointing out some of its flaws (Countee and Vijayanathan, 1979). Edwards and associates (1979) showed that of 50 consecutive patients who had carotid endarterectomy for embolic disease of that hemisphere, the carotid angiogram was negative in 40 percent. However, intimal disease was discovered in the postsurgical pathology endarterectomy examination in these patients. A number of investigators have pointed out that ultrasound is a more sensitive method for detection of atheroma in the neck. It has the advantage of Doppler measurement of flow and is complemented by B-mode imaging. Finally, increasing numbers of reports indicate that the carotid artery may occasionally appear to be occluded on the angiogram but at operation the artery distal to the point of occlusion is actually open and carotid endarterectomy can be accomplished (Clark *et al.*, 1971; Riles *et al.*, 1984; Yonas and Meyer, 1982).

COMPUTED TOMOGRAPHIC SCANNING IN THE NECK

During the past decade, investigation in electronic imaging in diagnostic radiology led to the development of the computed tomography (CT) scanner and then digital subtraction angiography. Both techniques utilize radiation detectors instead of film, and in both methods digitization of the data allows subsequent image processing. Cross-sectional reconstruction or digital subtraction gives comparable information to film-screen imaging at lower radiation doses. Furthermore, the contrast sensitivity, which is the capacity to detect small or low levels of iodine in the bloodstream, is enhanced. In this chapter we present early work indicating that transverse CT images of arteries utilizing this enhanced contrast sensitivity can show highly detailed pictures of vascular pathology without resorting to angiography.

A CT scan of the carotid arteries in the neck visualizes the carotid arteries with a low concentration of contrast material and then takes sequential cross-sectional images of them, much like visualizing multiple short segments of the carotid artery at the postmortem table.

Technique

The patient is placed supine on the scanner and is told to hold his breath for each scan and not to swallow. Methylglucamine diatrizoate is infused intravenously at 50 to 60 drops/minute and the scan sequence begins. Rapid scanning of the neck requires about five minutes with the General Electric (GE) 9800 and eight minutes with the GE 8800; the infusion is discontinued when the last scan is completed. The average study requires about 70 g of iodine. A continuous infusion throughout the study is required because of the rapid drop in

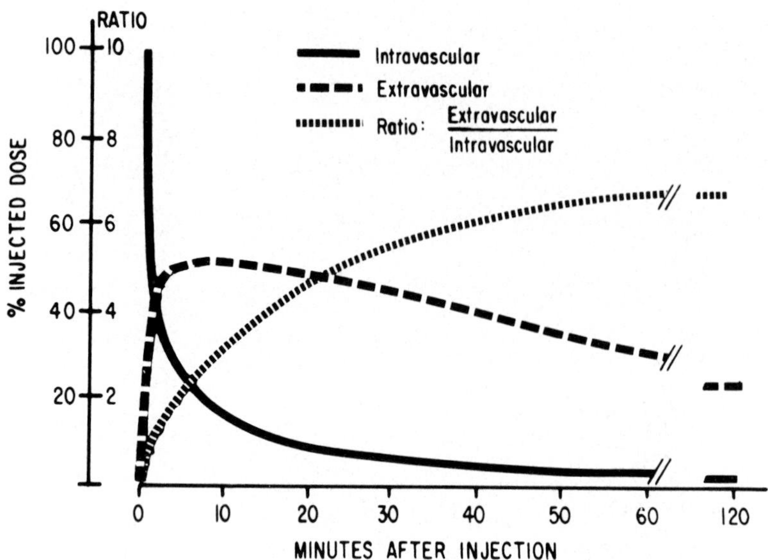

Figure 10–1. The blood level of intravascular contrast material after bolus injection. The solid curve indicates the rapid fall of intravascular contrast material given by rapid injection. When arteries are to be imaged by CT scanning, multiple scans must be made in the first five minutes after injection by dynamic CT scanning, even if the intravenous infusion continues after scanning is initiated (From Newhouse, J.: Fluid compartment distribution and intravenous cothalamate in the dog. *Invest. Radiol.*, **12**:364, 1977, with permission.)

intravascular contrast concentration (see Figure 10–1). Twenty-four to 36 contiguous slices are taken 1.5 mm apart along the course of the common carotid artery, the bifurcation, and the internal and external carotid arteries. This is done by scanning the neck from C6 to C3. Each scan requires 9.6 seconds at 160 mA, with prospective soft-tissue target software reconstruction (GE software program). More recently we have been using the GE 9800, which requires only about 50 g of iodine to be infused. Twelve 3 mm CT slices were obtained with the GE 9800 with a 3 mm table increment between scans. Each GE 9800 scan requires 2 seconds at 300 mA. The kilovoltage was 120 with each machine. CT scans illustrating the normal carotid artery are seen in Figure 10–2.

The scans are displayed sequentially on 14 × 17 in film. The spacing of the scan is shown by the numerical value for the consecutive table positioning for each scan. Sagittal or other paraxial reformations of the scans displayed on top of one another can be made with the ARRANGE* software program, but with experience the scans are simply reviewed in sequence on the 14 × 17 in film, and the artery is reformed in the mind's eye.

Phantom Studies

CT sections of human carotid arteries correspond closely to cross-sections of the same artery prepared as macrosections for pathology. Three studies of human postmortem carotid arteries were performed. In one of these specimens there was a recent, organizing thrombus closely adherent to the internal carotid intima (see Figure 10–3A,C). Erythrocytes trapped in the thrombus confirmed its recent formation. The thrombus could not be detected in the barium gelatine injection specimen resembling a carotid arteriogram. The thrombus, however, was easily demonstrated on the CT specimen study (see Figure 10–3B and C). We have not, however, attempted to differentiate atheroma from thrombus by this technique.

The Normal Cervical Carotid

Using either 1.5 or 3 mm consecutive slices, the common carotid, carotid bifurcation, and internal carotid arteries can be easily and clearly seen with this technique. In the more proximal scans the carotid artery, while immediately adjacent to the jugular vein in the ca-

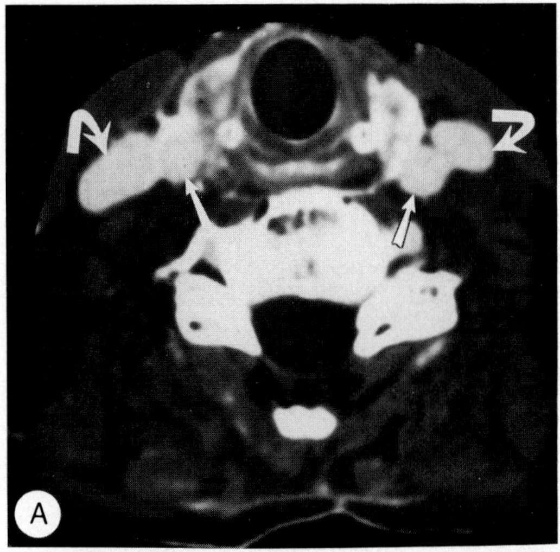

Figure 10–2. Normal carotid CT examination. Ten 3 mm CT slices with table increment of 3 mm were completed within five minutes on the GE 9800 CT unit. Normal common carotid artery CT section at C6 (*A*) shows round common carotid artery (arrows). The internal jugular vein (curved arrows) lies immediately adjacent to the carotid artery and anterolateral, lateral, or posterolateral to it. A normal carotid bifurcation at the lower half of C4 (*B*). Note the oval configuration to the left carotid bifurcation (arrow). The smaller external carotid is seen anteriorly (white arrowheads). Two veins are to join together to form the internal jugular vein, so it is septated on this scan (curved arrows). The larger left and smaller right vertebral arteries are demonstrated (open arrowheads). Normal internal and external carotid arteries at the uper half of C4 (*C*). Note that the internal carotid arteries (arrows) are slightly larger than the external carotid (white arrowheads) and lie posteromedial to it. At this level, which is cephalad to the bifurcation, the arteries usually lie at some distance from the internal jugular veins (curved arrows).

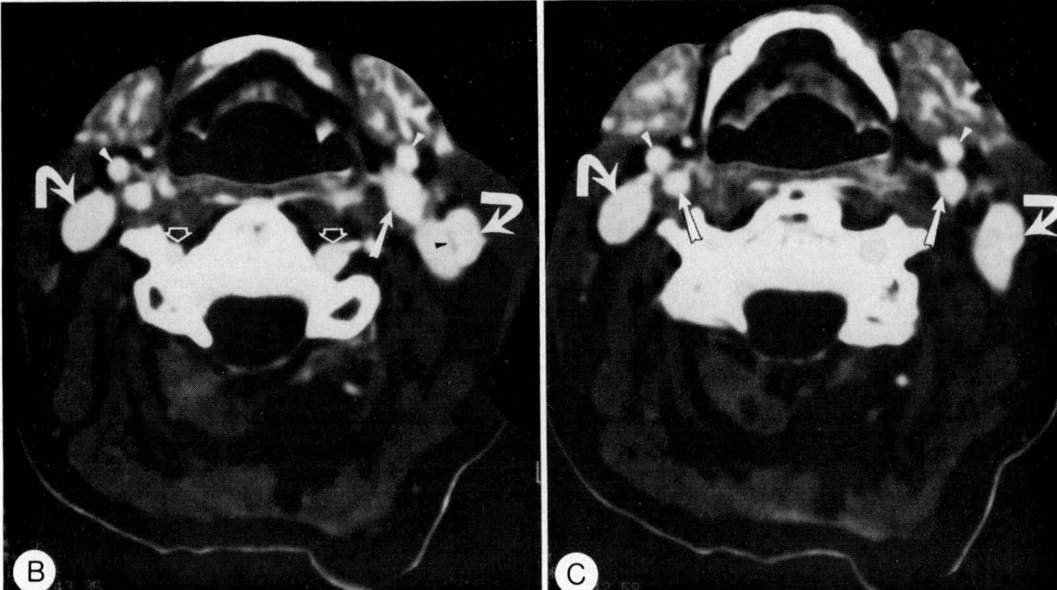

rotid sheath, can always be separated from the vein. The artery and the vein form two discrete circles contiguous with one another, and are filled with dense iodine contrast material. The carotid artery lies anteromedially with respect to the larger jugular vein. The arterial wall usually shows a thin, hypodense rim around the intraluminal contrast within the artery. The wall of the jugular vein is too thin to be visualized (see Figure 10–2). In the areas where the vein does not overlap the carotid artery, the arterial wall is readily distinguishable from the surrounding fat (low density). Although arterial pulsation might be anticipated to hinder the arterial imaging, in fact, the carotid images are quite sharp (see Figures 10–2 and 10–4).

At the bifurcation, the carotid artery is oval in configuration. The anteromedial portion of this oval represents the beginning of the external carotid artery. Distal to the bifurcation, the internal carotid continues to run adjacent to the jugular vein. The external carotid, which gives off several smaller branches, passes anteriorly and medially to the internal carotid.

These consecutive images can be displayed

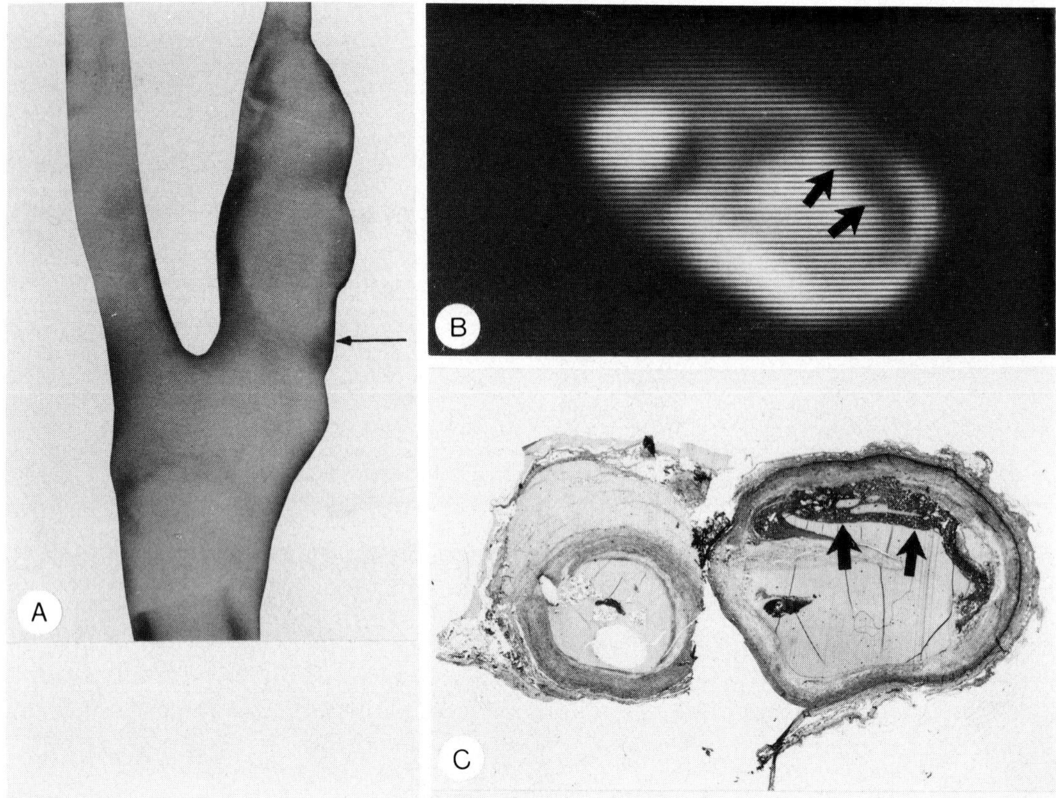

Figure 10–3. A radiological-CT-pathological correlation study of a human carotid artery. Postmortem radiogram of a carotid artery from a 60-year-old man; barium gel injection (*A*). Note the subtle transverse band of increased density (arrow) at the origin of the internal carotid artery. A CT scan of the same carotid artery in a 25 cm water phantom (*B*). Note the low density area which parallels the internal carotid wall (arrows). This is an extensive, organizing thrombus, which is of low density compared with the arterial wall. The pathologic specimen of the same carotid artery (*C*). Note the organizing thrombus (arrows) which parallels the internal carotid artery wall. This closely corresponds to the low density area visualized in the CT section above. Microscopic analysis revealed red blood cells trapped in fissures within the clot, confirming that this was a recent, organizing thrombus adherent to the carotid intima.

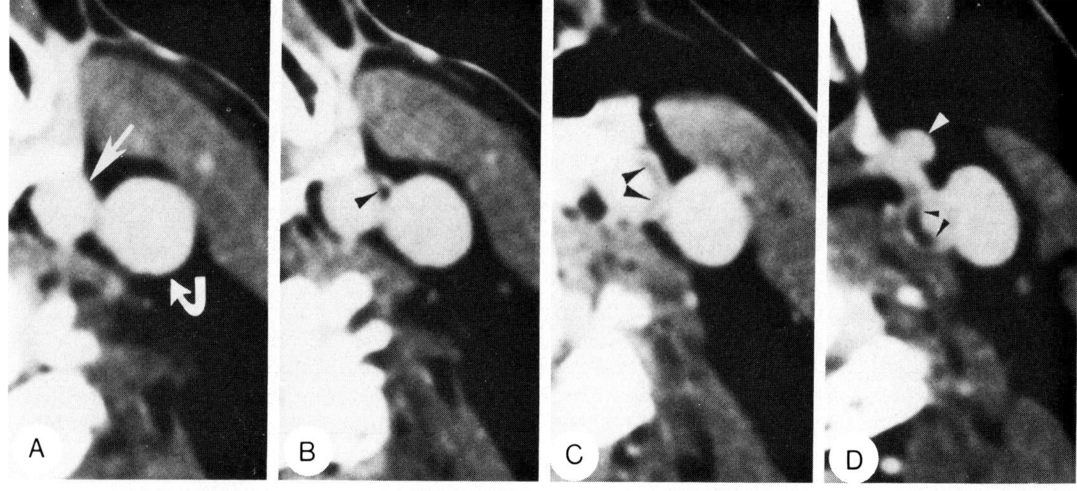

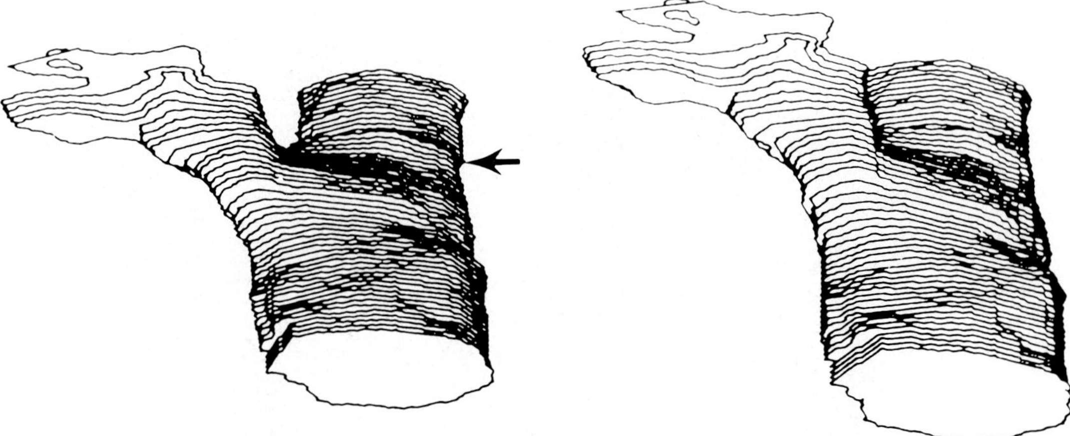

Figure 10–5. Two views of a computer reconstruction by the edge detection and boundary search program of the carotid bifurcation which are 15 degrees apart. This reconstruction of a fairly normal appearing carotid bifurcation shows the proximal internal and external carotid arteries at 15-degree increments. Note the slight motion artifact (arrow). (From Heinz, E.R.; Pizer, S.M.; Fuchs H.; Fram, E.K.; Burger, P.; Drayer, B.P.; and Osborne, D.R.: Examination of the extracranial carotid bifurcation by thin-section dynamic CT: direct visualization of intimal atheroma in man (part 1). *Am. J. Neuro. Radiol.* **5**:355–59, 1984b, with permission.)

in sequence on a GE multiformat camera using 14 × 17 in films. Although clinicians are accustomed to seeing the carotid artery displayed along its long axis, these pictures, which resemble the cross-sectional pictures of the carotid artery seen at the postmortem table, will quickly become familiar and make longitudinal display unnecessary. Figure 10–5 shows a simple longitudinal display method which could be performed using the CT computer (Heinz *et al.,* 1984b).

Pathological Characteristics of the Cervical Carotids as Seen by Computed Tomographic Examination

Angiography shows thrombus or atheromatous lesions by *indirect* means, because we see only the contrast material on the radiogram, rather than the plaque or thrombus itself. Thin-section CT examination of the carotid artery in the neck can *directly* image atherosclerosis or thrombus within the carotid lumen. These pathological areas of atheroma or thrombus are hypodense with respect to the arterial wall and the iodine-filled lumen (Heinz *et al.,* 1984a). Calcification is not usually seen in the atheroma or in the organizing clot within the lumen (Heinz *et al.,* 1984a). In angiography, because one relies on seeing such an indirect expression of the atheromatous lesion, one must rely on tangential views to see the multiple edges that are present. Obviously it is possible to miss the best tangential view of a given lesion. Although the abnormality might be seen in an *en face* projection, if the iodine contrast is dense enough it may obscure the lesion. In contrast, the CT examination shows the transverse section of the image and one can see the walls in a 360 degree panorama with less chance of missing a lesion.

We studied eight consecutive patients with transient ischemic attacks (TIAs) using CT scanning of the neck and compared the results with both the angiographic picture and the operative situs (see Figures 10–6 and 10–7). These findings are summarized in Table 10–1. Six of the eight patients had additional or more

Figure 10–4. Direct imaging of carotid artery atheroma by CT. These four images, which were selected from a series of 12, were made using a 3 mm slice thickness, a table increment of 3 mm, and an interscan time of 8 seconds and were completed in less than five minutes. Cross section of the left common carotid (straight arrow) (*A*). Cross section of a common carotid artery at the upper half of C6, just proximal to the carotid bifurcation (*B*). Note the low density filling defect on the lateral wall, which represents a discrete atheroma (arrowhead). Cross-section through the proximal carotid bifurcation at C5 (*C*). Note the atheroma (arrowheads) following the contour of the intima laterally. Cross section of internal and external carotid arteries at the distal bifurcation (white arrowhead) (*D*). Note the atheroma adjacent to the intima all 360 degrees of the artery (arrowheads).

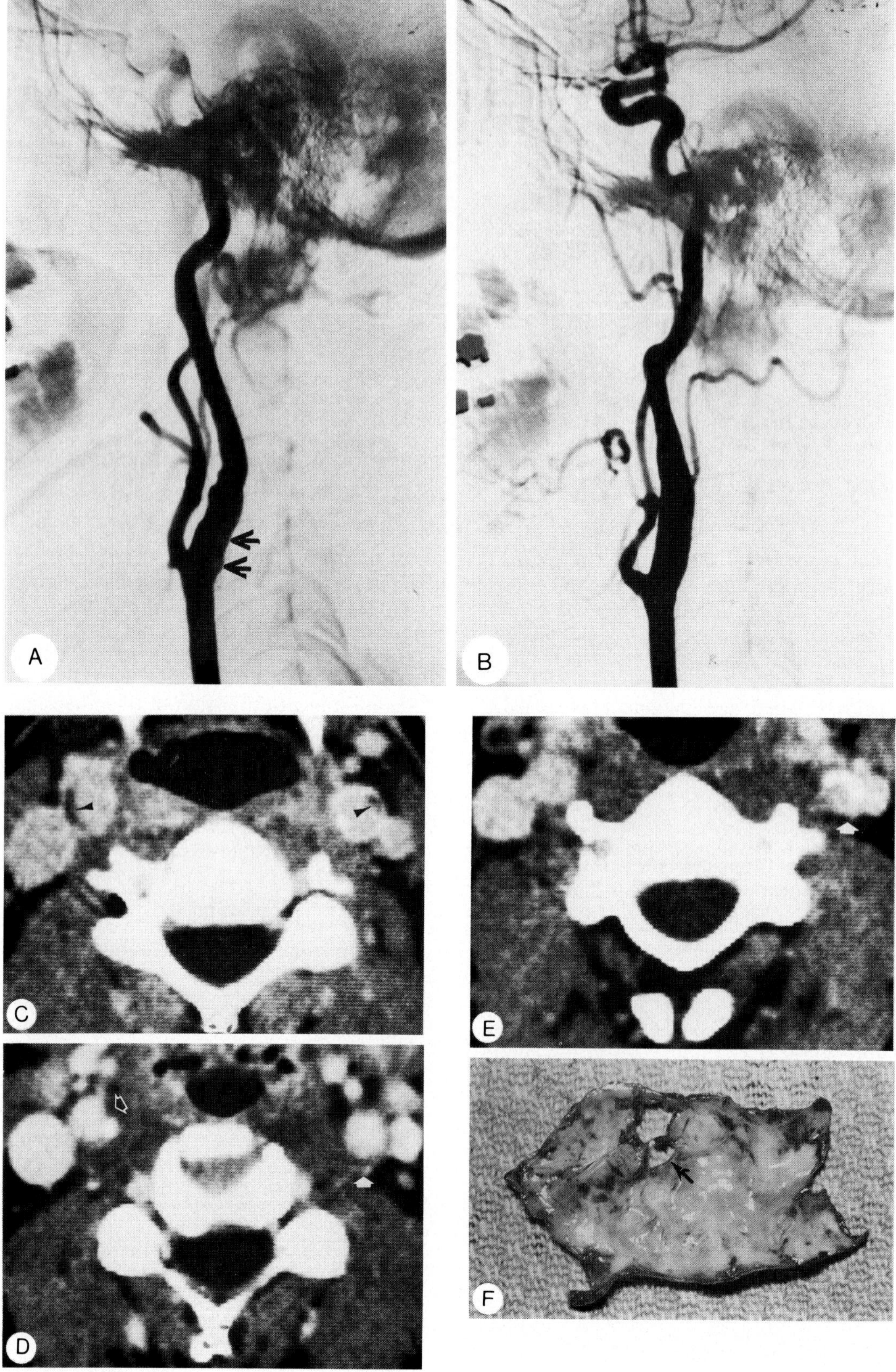
A
B
C
D
E
F

Table 10-1. Cervical CT versus Angiography in the Detection of Carotid Intimal Disease

Clinical condition case no. (side)	Right carotid		Left carotid		Comments
	CT	Angiography	CT	Angiography	
Amaurosis fugax: 1 (L)	Bifurc. lateral wall: 1+; RIC medial wall: 1+	Normal	CC lateral wall: 1+; bifurc.: post. wall dissection; LIC: 3+ atheroma	Bifurc. 1+; LIC 1+	Atheroma lat. wall CC: dissection at bifurc. L; and LIC atheroma not detected by angio; RCC and RIC atheroma not shown by angio.
4 (R)	RIC: 1+	Normal	CC: 2+; bifurc.; 2+; LIC: normal	Normal	CT detects 1+−2+ atheromas digital subtraction misses
5 (R)	CC: 1+ post. wall atheroma	Normal (not selective)	Normal	Normal	CT detects atheroma; angio. does not
Carotid TIAs: 2 (R)	CC: 3+ medial wall; bifurc.: 2+ medial wall; RIC: 2+ ant. wall	CC: 2+; bifurc.: 1+; irregularity ant. wall; normal RIC	CC: 1+; bifurc.: post. wall 2+; LIC: 1+	Post. wall: 1+	CT CC shows 40% (3+) narrowing RC; angio. 2+ bifurc. medial wall atheroma not shown on angio.; RIC: CT showed 2+ atheroma; angio. neg.
6 (L)	CC: 2+; bifurc.: 2+; RIC: 4+	40% narrowing large excavation; RIC narrowing not seen	CC: 4+ atheroma, almost complete occlusion; extends from below bifurc. to prox. LIC	98% occlusion	RIC: 4+; narrowing not appreciated on angio.
7 (L)	RIC: 2+	Normal	LIC: 1+ post. wall	LIC: post. wall 1+ plaque	CT detects CC post. wall atheroma and internal carotid atheroma missed by angio. (R)
3 (L)	Normal	Normal	2+ post. wall atheroma	Bifurc.: subtle post. wall plaque	CT atheroma is much larger than angio. lesion
8 (R)	Normal	Normal	Normal	Normal	

* R = right, L = left; TIAs = transient ischemic attacks; bifurc. = bifurcation; RIC = right internal carotid; CC = common carotid; post. = posterior; LIC = left internal carotid; angio. = angiography; ant. = anterior; prox. = proximal; lat. = lateral; neg. = negative; 1+ = 1–10% narrowing; 2+ = 11–25% narrowing; 3+ = 26–50% narrowing; 4+ = 51–90% narrowing.

Source: Heinz, E.R.; Fuchs, J.; Osborne, D.; Drayer, B.; Yeates, A.; Fuchs, H.; and Pizer, S.: Examination of the extracranial carotid bifurcation by thin section dynamic CT: direct visualization of intimal atheroma in man (part 2). *Am. J. Neurol. Radiol.*, **5**:361–6, July/August, 1984a, with permission.

Figure 10-6. A 60-year-old man with repeated episodes of left amaurosis fugax. Left (*A*) and right (*B*) carotid angiogram, CT studies (*C*, *D*, and *E*), and endarterectomy specimen of the left carotid bifurcation (*F*). Proximal left internal carotid artery angiogram shows posterior wall changes of 1+ (arrows) which are confirmed by extraluminal dissection on the CT (arrowheads). Specimen from left carotid shows area of dissection (arrow). The right (asymptomatic) carotid artery does not appear narrowed on the angiogram but has an unusual shape. There is 1+ change in lateral wall at bifurcation (arrowheads) and 1+ change in the medial wall of the internal carotid artery which is not seen on the angiogram but is visible on CT (arrow). (Partially reproduced from Heinz, E.R. *et al.*: Examination of the extracranial carotid bifurcation by thin-section dynamic CT: Direct visualization of internal atheroma in man (part 2). *Am. J. Neurol. Radiol.* **5**:361–66, July/August, 1984a, with permission.)

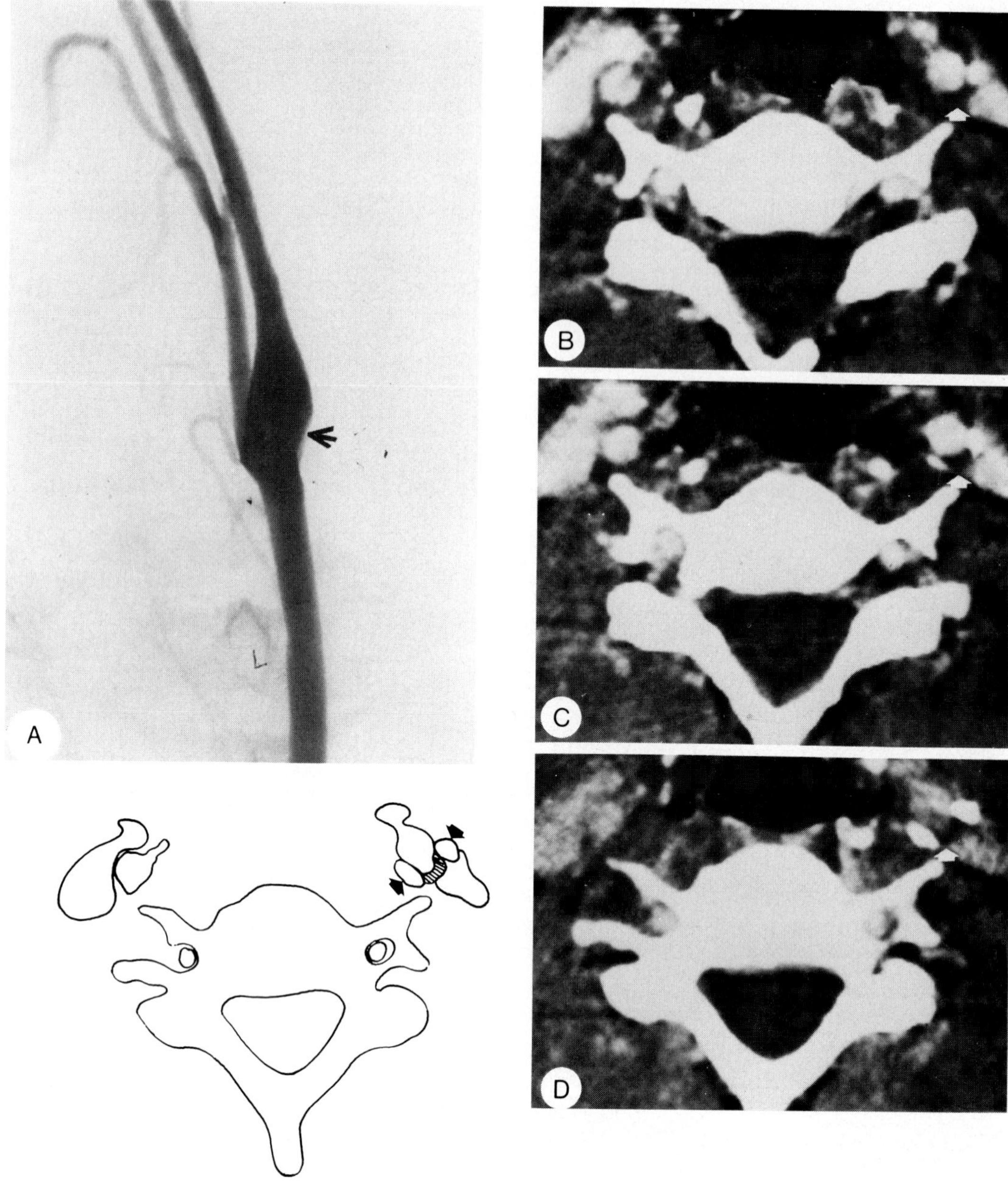

Figure 10–7. A 45-year-old man with left brain TIAs. Angiogram (*A*) shows an intimal defect (1+) on the posterior wall of the internal carotid artery at the bifurcation (arrow). CT (*B*, *C*, and *D*) shows a 2+ change (the CT plaque appears larger than on the angiogram) on the posterior wall of the internal carotid at the bifurcation (solid arrows). Note that there are two areas of calcium deposits within the wall of the artery and not in the atheroma (*C* and *D*). (*E*) Line drawing of *D*, illustrating the posterior wall atheroma (shaded area) and the two areas of calcium deposits in the carotid wall (arrows). (From Heinz, E.R., *et. al.*: Examination of the extracranial carotid bifurcation by thin-section dynamic CT. Direct visualization of intimal atheroma in man (part 2). *Am. J. Neuro. Radiol.* **5**:361–66, 1984a.)

severe pathologic features revealed by CT scanning than by angiography. In four, the pathology was discovered on the side of clinical interest; in two patients, pathology was found on the asymptomatic side (Heinz *et al.*, 1984a).

Computed Tomography of the Carotid Arteries — Discussion

Thin-section CT study of the carotids is the first examination to image carotid atheroma or thrombus in cross-section. Such a study is best done between the unenhanced and the enhanced CT scan when the patient comes to the radiology department for the first examination. The actual picture-taking requires only between 5 and 12 additional minutes and no additional radiological equipment. Direct CT visualization effectively and directly displays the atheroma or thrombus and the remaining lumen and then outlines the arterial wall. It reveals pathology more in depth than standard selective carotid angiography (see Figure 10–8). The examination has shown excellent correlation between the endarterectomy specimens (Heinz *et al.*, 1984b), and these CT images are comparable to the cross-sectional specimens taken at postmortem.

The CT examination overcomes two potential causes of high false-negative findings of carotid angiography. First, the transverse images eliminate the need for multiple radiographic tangential views of the carotid artery for the detection of edge abnormalities. Second, the CT transverse images appear to be better for the evaluation of an atheroma which is hidden by the density of the contrast column on angiography.

That CT examination is limited to 3 to 3.6 cm of the carotid artery may be viewed as a drawback. If, however, the study is done at the time of the original contrast infusion for a new perfusion deficit (TIA or cerebrovascular accident) and it turns out to be negative, the clinician may not want to subject the patient to invasive angiography which still carries a risk in patients with known cerebrovascular disease. If a lesion is seen and no surgery is contemplated, but rather aspirin or dipyridamole therapy is planned, then the patient can be treated in this manner with follow-up studies utilizing CT of the carotid arteries to see whether progression is occurring. Obviously, patients with asymptomatic bruits are ideal candidates for a noninvasive study, such as CT examination of the neck. Leeson and colleagues (in press) also used the CT examination in the neck for known carotid disease. They have shown angiographic internal carotid pseudo-occlusion which was also detected on CT scan (see Figure 10–9). They also demonstrated one patient with thrombus formation in the internal carotid artery (see Figure 10–10) and were able to show significant correlation between size and shape of the specimens found by endarterectomy and the CT examination of the carotid in the neck (Leeson *et al.*, 1985). The same group has described patients with carotid dissection and hemorrhage into atherosclerotic plaque diagnosed by the CT method of examination (see Figure 10–10).

APPLICATION OF COMPUTED TOMOGRAPHY OF THE CAROTID ARTERY IN PSEUDOOCCLUSION, THROMBOTIC OCCLUSION, DISSECTION, AND SHORT-SEGMENT ATHEROSCLEROTIC OCCLUSION

Pseudoocclusion of the Carotid Artery: The "Slim Sign"

Pseudoocclusion of the carotid artery is a near-complete stenosis, followed by a subtle "string" of faintly visualized contrast along the course of the internal carotid artery. It has recently received much attention (Clark *et al.*, 1971; Countee and Vijayanathan, 1979; Gabrielsen *et al.*, 1981) and should alert us to the possibility of a persistent open channel beyond the point of local obstruction. However, when recognizing the presence of the slim sign, one should remember that the ascending pharyngeal artery is one of the main collateral branches from the external carotid and lies almost directly in the course of the internal carotid artery. Filling of the ascending pharyngeal artery should not be confused with the "slim sign." Sometimes the string sign appears to diminish and disappear, and the question arises as to whether the carotid artery is patent all the way to the siphon. Carotid CT, particularly with cursor measurements at the siphon level, can make certain that the artery is truly open. Figure 10–11 shows the CT scan of a patient with a string sign (Cohen *et al.*, 1982).

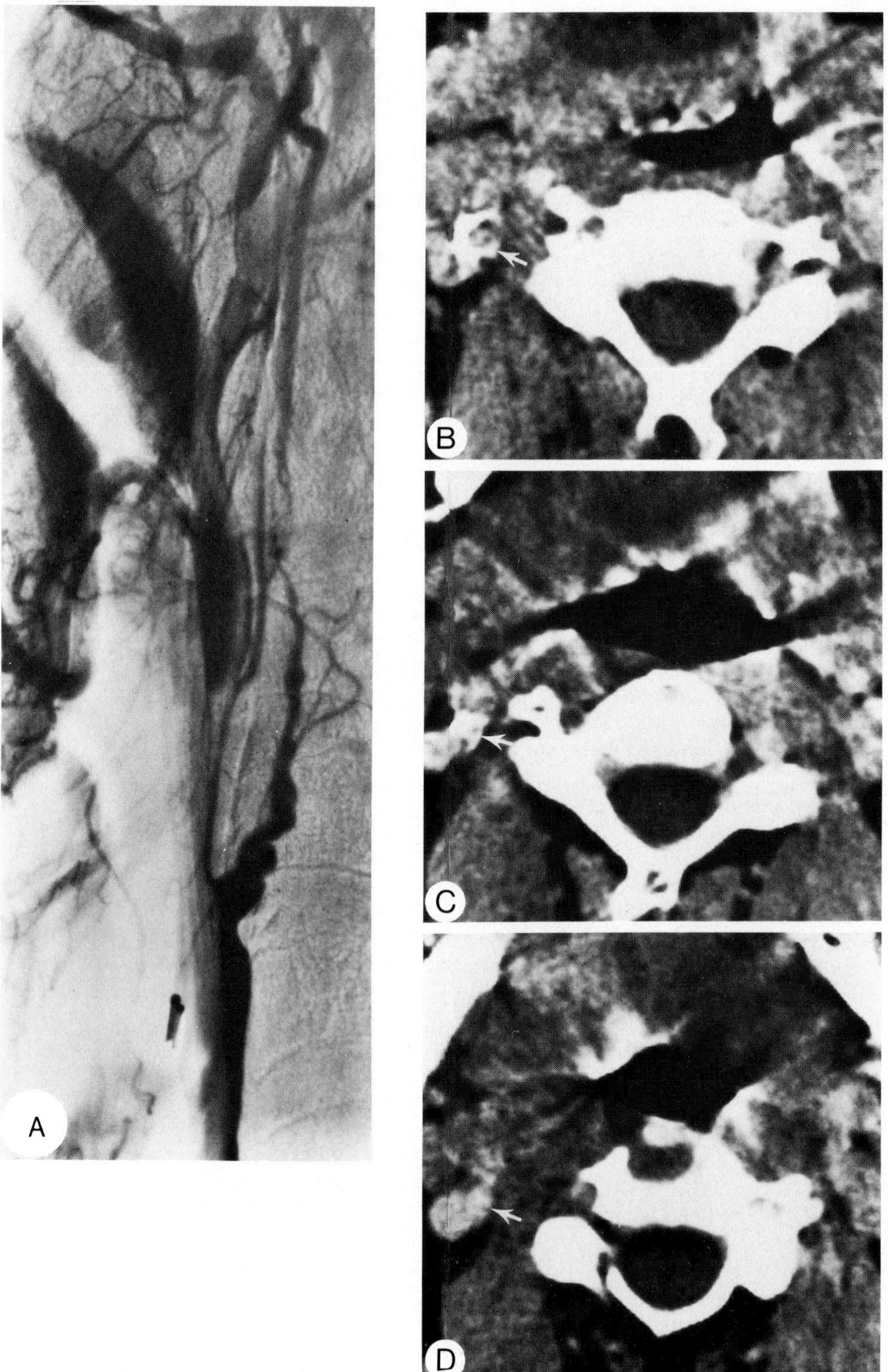
A
B
C
D

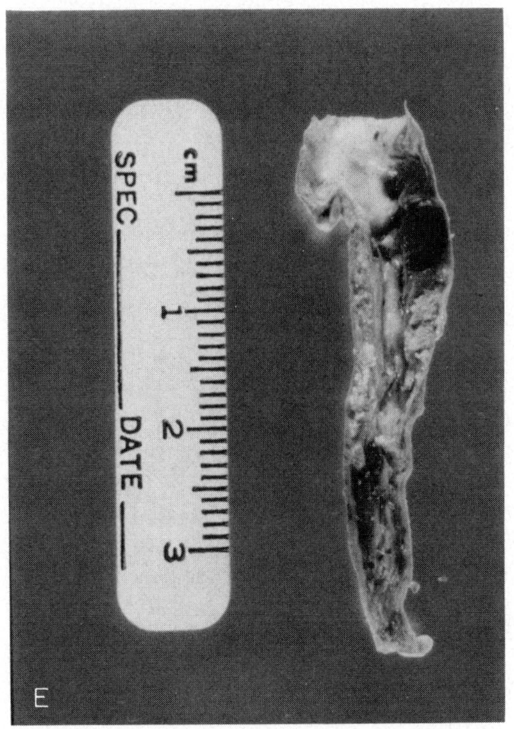

Figure 10–8. A 61-year-old male patient with a history of right hemispheric TIAs. Lateral right common carotid arteriogram (*A*) shows severe irregular narrowing of the proximal right internal carotid artery with a collapsed lumen distally. CT (*B* and *C*) of the proximal right internal carotid artery demonstrates calcified mural thickening and luminal narrowing (arrows). More cephalad CT (*D*) scan reveals patency of the right internal carotid artery (arrow). That there is no significant separation between the internal carotid artery and the internal jugular vein indicates that the internal carotid artery wall is of normal thickness at this level. Plaque removed at endarterectomy (*E*) and sectioned along longitudinal axis shows extensive atheromatous changes with calcification and focal hemorrhage. Courtesy of Mark D. Leeson, M.D., Edwin D. Cacayorian, M.D., and Afif R. Iliya, M.D., Department of Radiology, State University of New York, Upstate Medical Center, Syracuse, New York.

Complete Occlusion Caused by Carotid Thrombus or Embolus

Occasionally, a thrombosis at the bifurcation or just beyond it could cause a high degree of stenosis or complete occlusion. Figure 10–11 is an example of complete carotid occlusion by thrombus as imaged by carotid CT. Note the small trace of contrast material *around* the thrombus (see Figure 10–9). In the slices distal to the thrombus one can readily see reconstitution of the lumen as opacified by contrast material (see Figures 10–9C and D). Such information is not provided by the arteriogram but may be crucial for the diagnosis of pseudo-occlusion and ultimately the decision for endarterectomy rather than external carotid-internal carotid bypass. The characteristic angiographic appearance of carotid occlusion caused by dissection is that of a tapered arterial segment which then terminates completely (see Figure 10–12). Rapid sequential computerized tomography (RSCT) of the carotid arteries distal to this point is quite useful in establishing whether the lumen is truly open so that acute surgical repair may be still possible. Figure 10–10B also shows a dissection; note the CT scans at the level of the pseudo-aneurysm. RSCT scanning can also demonstrate dissection in a vascular segment containing an atherosclerotic plaque. This usually develops underneath the plaque and is frequently associated with hemorrhage into the dissection. The hemorrhage may expand and cause complete compression of the lumen.

Atherosclerotic Occlusion of the Cervical Carotid Artery

Recent reports (Cohen *et al.,* 1982; Yonas and Meyer, 1982) have generated considerable enthusiasm for the use of RSCT in patients with short-segment occlusion of the internal carotid artery because of the possibility of demonstrating the presence of a patent internal carotid artery distal to an angiographically demonstrated occlusion.

It is important to plot the density curves for both the right and left carotid arteries distal to the point of occlusion in the neck as a part of the CT examination. Cohen and associates (1982) have pointed out that RSCT scans taken at the odontoid level first show sparse filling of the distal internal carotid artery, but subsequent scans show good opacification of

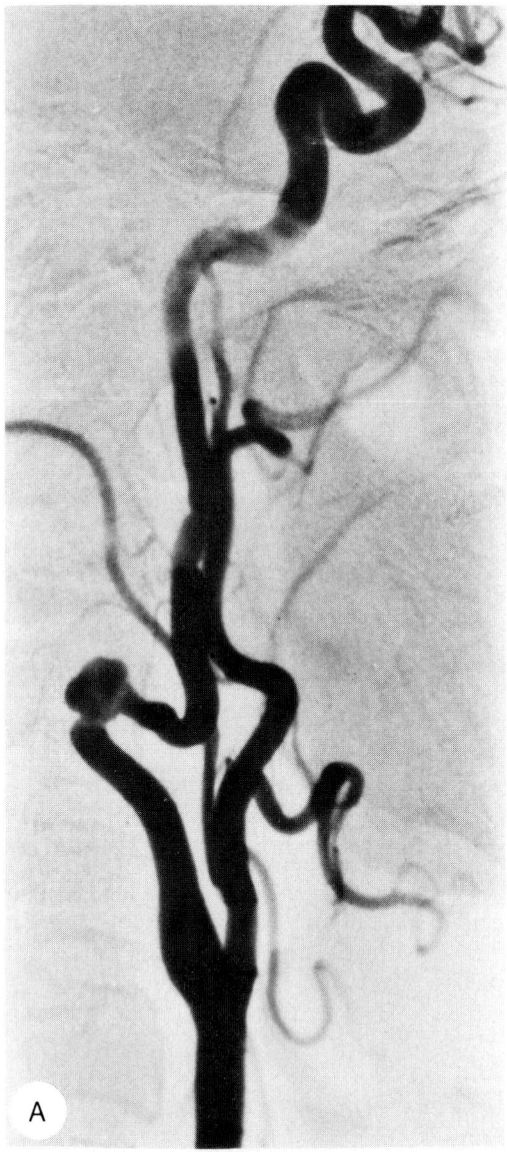

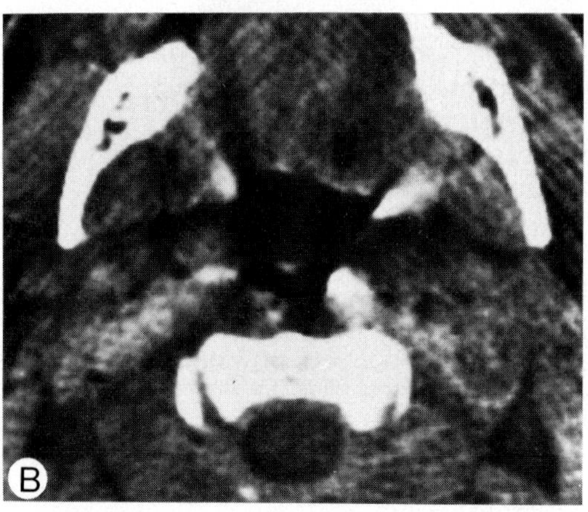

Figure 10–9. A 46-year-old patient who presented with severe left-sided headaches, Horner's syndrome on the left, and left hemispheric TIAs. Lateral arteriogram of the left common carotid (*A*) shows dissecting aneurysm and narrowing of the cervical internal carotid artery. CT section at the level of the aneurysm showing lucency within the aneurysm (*B*). Courtesy of Mark D. Leeson, M.D., Edwin D. Cacayorian, M.D., and Afif R. Iliya, M.D., Department of Radiology, State University of New York, Upstate Medical Center, Syracuse, New York.

the carotids at the skull base (see Figure 10–11). Cursory measurements of the left and right distal internal carotid arteries showed a 69 percent change in density in the right carotid and 65 percent in the left. At surgery, the right internal carotid artery was found to be patent. Preliminary data suggest that there should be at least a 70 percent change in the CT density reading before the internal carotid artery can be called patent (Cohen *et al.,* 1982).

It must be recognized that some opacification of the internal carotid artery may occur via collateral flow from the external carotid artery. These collateral vessels include branches to the carotid bulb and the meningeal branches of the external carotid artery. Therefore, it is also important to take time-density measurements at the C2 level and take CT sections through the internal carotid artery *distal* to the obstruction; otherwise, false-positive RSCT readings are possible. Surgical results may be quite rewarding if the internal carotid artery is found to be patent distal to an occlusion of the common carotid artery or to the origin of the internal carotid artery. Angiography is only of limited value in distinguishing between patients with an occlusion limited to the common carotid and/or short segment of the internal carotid and patients in whom the occlusion extends to the cavernous carotid. In practical terms, this means that if diagnostic studies are limited to angiography alone, surgical exploration is necessary to determine the patency of the internal carotid artery beyond the carotid bifurcation.

Riles and associates (1982) conducted RSCT studies in 15 patients with occluded carotid arteries. No filling of the occluded distal internal carotid artery was seen in 11 patients. In the four remaining patients in whom RSCT scans were positive (that is, the internal carotid artery was shown to be patient), surgical exploration indeed confirmed the patency of that distal internal carotid artery. This allowed

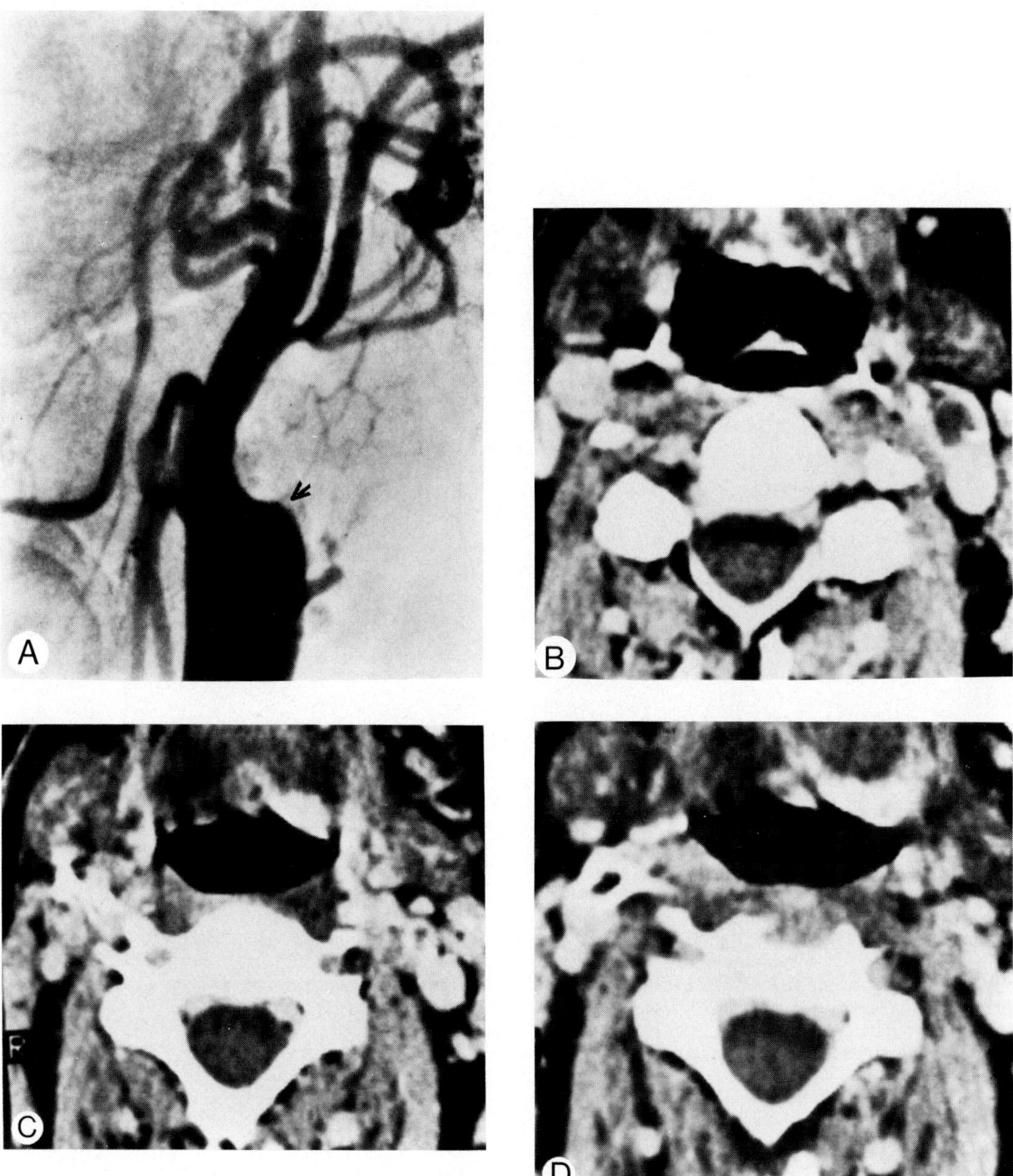

Figure 10–10. A 61-year-old male patient who presented with a left hemispheric stroke. Anteroposterior arteriogram of the left common carotid (*A*) shows complete occlusion of the left internal carotid artery at the origin. CT section at the level of the bifurcation (*B*) shows the origin of the left internal carotid artery consistent with thrombus. More cephalad CT section (*C*) again showing lucency consistent with thrombus in the left internal carotid. The diameter is smaller, suggesting tapering of the thrombus (*C*). CT section taken 1.2 to 1.4 cm above the bifurcation (*D*) shows patency of the lumen of the left internal carotid artery. The patient underwent left superficial temporal artery and middle cerebral artery bypass. Courtesy of Mark D. Leeson, M.D., Edwin D. Cacayorian, M.D., and Afif R. Iliya, M.D., Department of Radiology, State University of New York, Upstate Medical Center, Syracuse, New York.

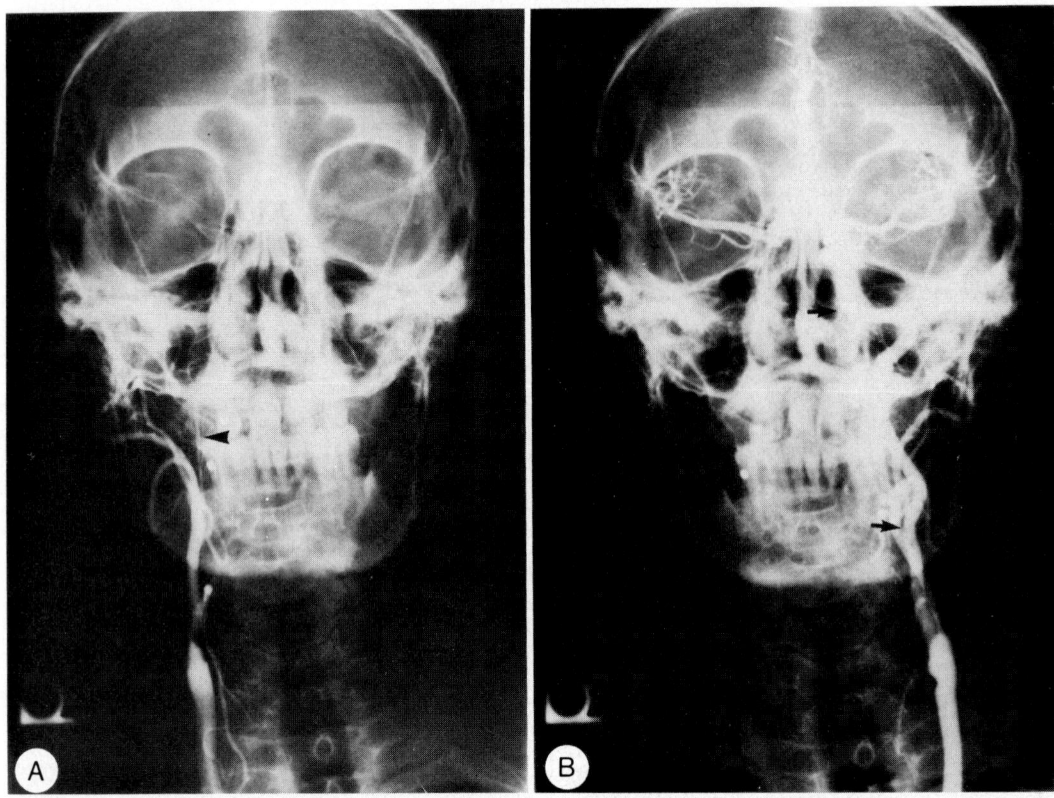

Figure 10–11. Dynamic CT studies performed to evaluate internal carotid artery occlusion (*A*, *B*, and *C* are from a single patient; *D* and *E* are from two different patients). Injection of the right common carotid artery (*A*) shows a small vessel (arrowhead). There is a question whether this is a small, patent right internal carotid artery or a branch of the external carotid artery (arrowhead) (*A*). Injection of the left common carotid artery (*B*) shows filling of the internal carotid artery (arrow) and of both middle cerebral arteries. *C* is a series of dynamic CT scans from the same patient. The right internal carotid artery (arrow) and the left internal carotid artery (arrowhead) are shown on both the initial (top) and maximally filled (bottom) scans. The percentage of change in CT density is 69 percent on the right and 65 percent on the left. The right internal carotid artery was patent at surgery. *D* is a dynamic CT study with analyses. The plotted analysis of the right internal carotid artery (+) is typical for a patent vessel. That from the left internal carotid artery (box) is from an occluded vessel. The peak percentage of change is close to zero. *E* is a dynamic CT study with plotted analysis. Analysis of the left internal carotid artery (+, 2) is again typical of a patent vessel. The analysis of the right internal carotid artery (x, 1) is typical of the group of occluded vessels in which the peak change was from 30 percent to 60 percent (*E*). (From Cohen, W.; Pinto, R.; and Kricheff, L.L.: The value of dynamic scanning. *Radiol. Clin. North. Am.*, **20**:23–35, 1982*b*, with permission.)

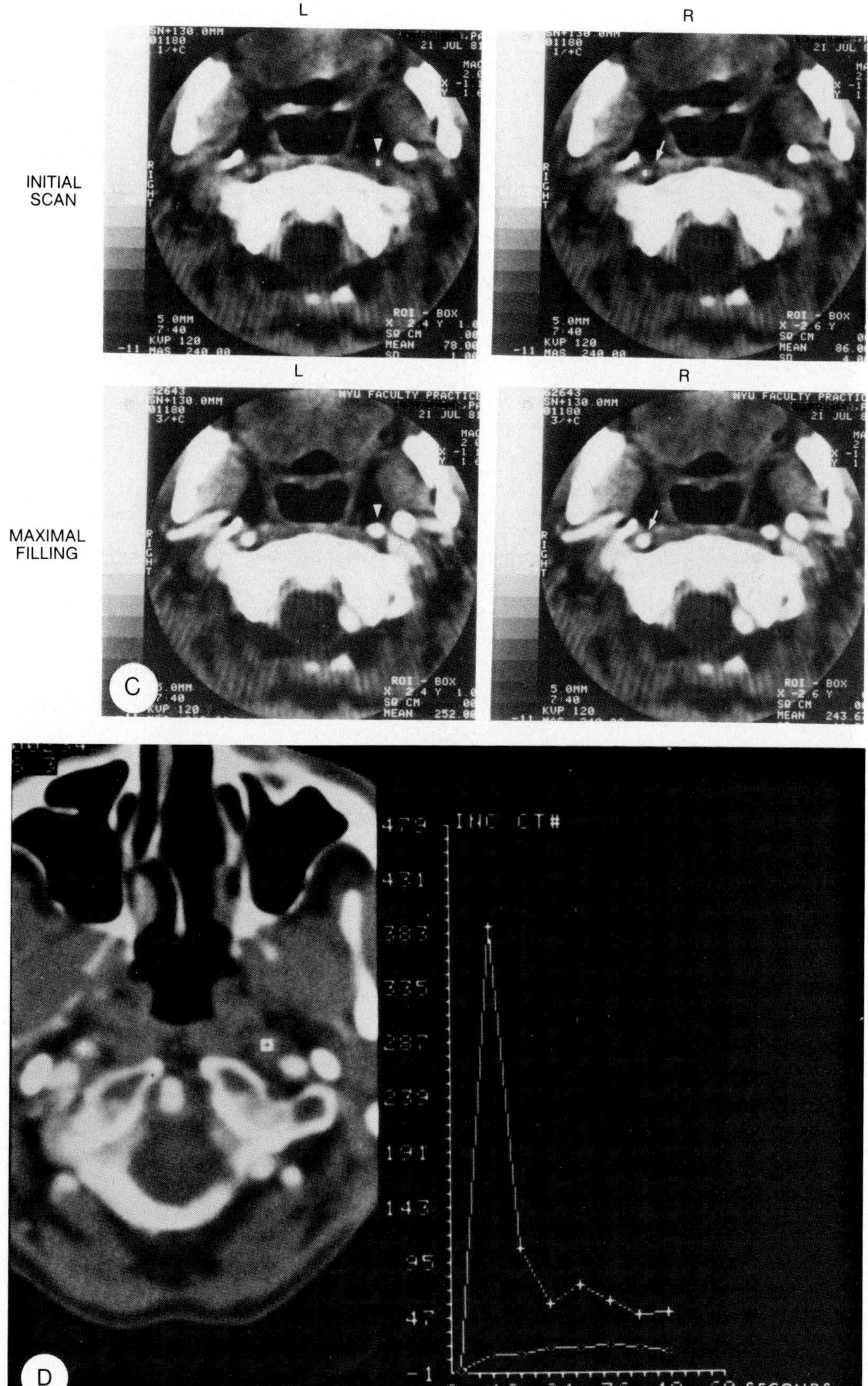

L
R
INITIAL SCAN
L
R
MAXIMAL FILLING
C
D
INC CT#
SECONDS

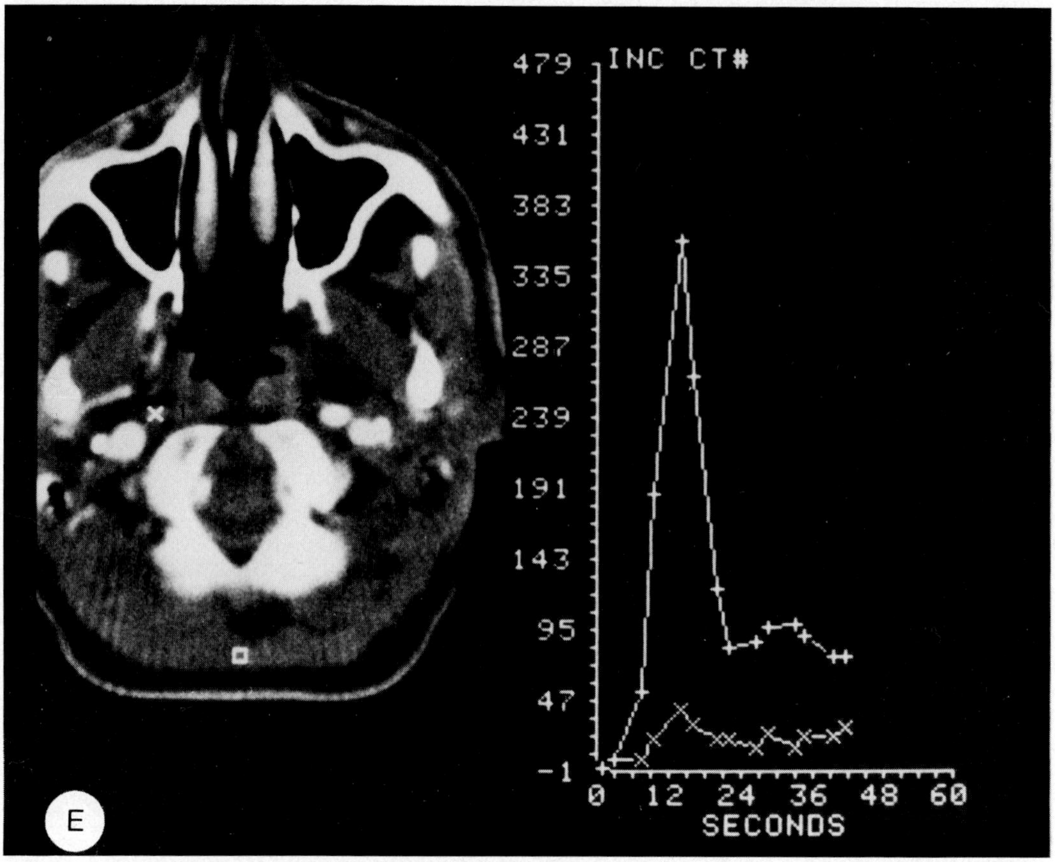

Figure 10–11. (*Continued*) See Legend on page 154.

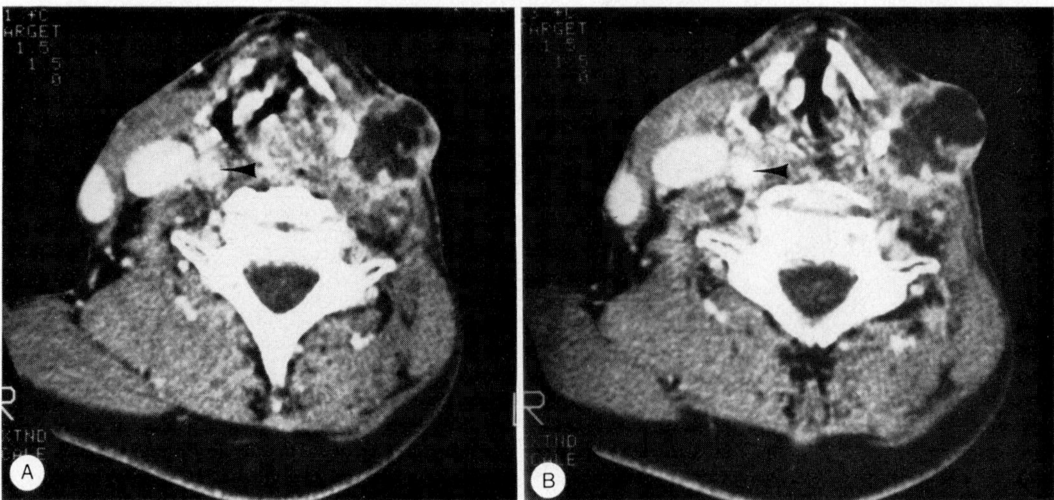

Figure 10–12. CT scans of the neck (*A* and *B*) showing left common carotid artery occlusion by neoplasm. A 60-year-old man with squamous cell carcinoma of the neck with extension to the carotid sheath and occlusion of the left common carotid artery. (Black arrowheads indicate the normal common carotid artery on the *right*). Note that no radiographic contrast material is imaged in the left neck.

endarterectomy or carotid bypass to be performed.

In a later study reviewing 24 patients operated on for carotid occlusions since 1962 (Riles *et al.*, 1984), it was shown that the distal internal or external carotid arteries were visualized in only four (17 percent) of the preoperative angiograms). When all the 24 patients were operated upon, the internal carotid artery was found to be patent in 11 (46 percent) and the external carotid was patent in 15 (62 percent). Of the 15 patients with reconstructions, thromboendarterectomy was performed in six and saphenous vein bypass in nine. Certainly, the high percentage of open internal carotid arteries in this series must raise the question of whether RSCT should not be performed in *all* patients who have angiographic occlusion of the common or internal carotid arteries.

Cervical Carotid Artery Invasion by Tumors

Because the wall of the artery and the surrounding soft tissue can be seen well in CT scanning, carotid involvement can be reasonably well assessed by this technique. Figure 10–12 illustrates a patient with complete common carotid occlusion by squamous cell carcinoma of the neck.

COMPUTED TOMOGRAPHIC BRAIN SCAN AND EXTRACRANIAL VASCULAR DISEASE

CT scanning of the brain is an extremely valuable diagnostic tool in assessing extracranial vascular disease and its effect on the brain. This diagnostic modality has resulted in a highly sensitive yet simple examination that can locate lesions not previously detectable by any other method. Further, it demonstrates small degrees of swelling or edema with extreme sensitivity. CT brain scanning for carotid extracranial disease is particularly useful in either establishing or excluding the presence of cerebral infarction.

While the CT scan may not necessarily show

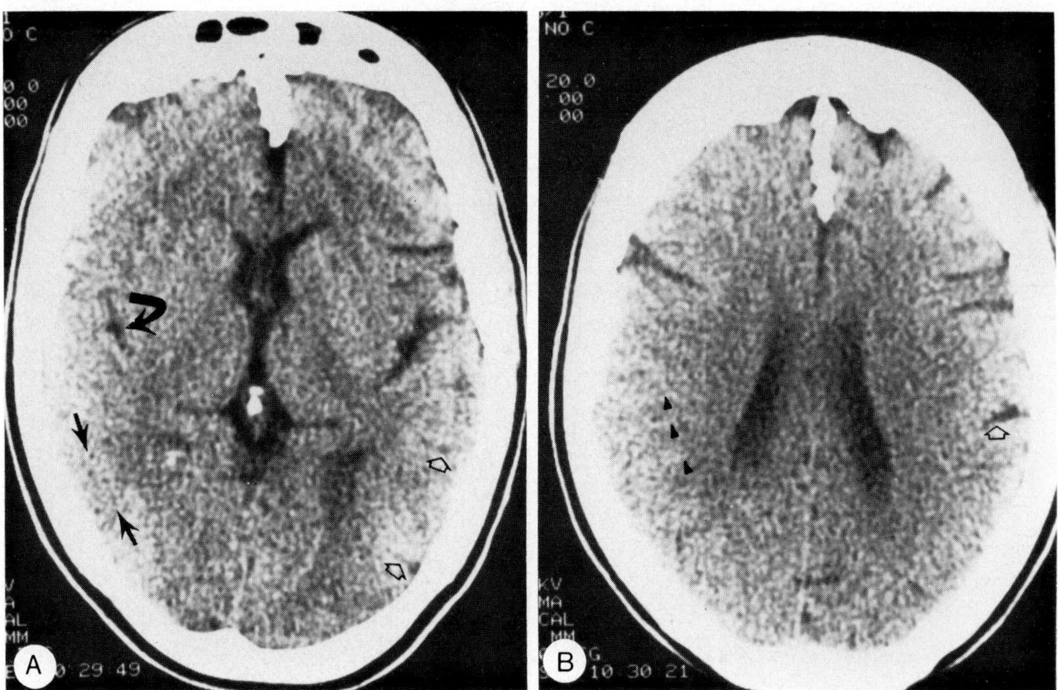

Figure 10–13. CT scans (*A* and *B*) showing earliest signs of a segmental cortical infarct. The new infarction is located in the right middle cerebral artery territory. Segmental loss of cortical density is apparent in the region on observer's left (between two black arrows). Normal cortical sulci fail to visualize on the side of the infarct because the sulci are effaced by local swelling. Normal sulci are seen on the opposite side (open arrows). The third sign of early infarction before segmental hypodensity occurs is effacement of nearby cisterns: the right Sylvian cistern is smaller than the normal left cistern; it has been partly effaced by the swelling (curved arrow). One can sometimes see slight displacement of opacified sulci (small arrowheads). The arrowheads show that the direction of the displacement is anterior.

the infarction within the first 24 hours of its occurrence, the detection rate with CT after the first day is as high as 80 percent (Russell, 1984). The CT brain scan may also give some specific insight into the etiology of the stroke. In embolization, the middle cerebral artery is involved in 90 percent of instances. If the infarct occurs in another cerebral territory, embolization is much less likely. If the CT brain scan shows an infarction in the "watershed" area between the anterior cerebral and the middle cerebral distribution, one is more apt to suspect general circulatory problems as the cause of the infarction. If the infarction does not follow an arterial territory, then venous infarction or the possibility of some totally different etiology should be considered.

Finally, CT of the brain helps to identify hemorrhagic infarctions. This is particularly important when one is assessing the brain before instituting anticoagulant therapy. This aspect will be covered more fully in a later section on therapy.

Cerebral Ischemia

Cerebral ischemia is most commonly manifest clinically as TIAs. Unfortunately, the brain CT scan almost never shows a structural abnormality after a TIA. However, positron emission tomography (PET) studies have shown that there is almost always some irreversible structural damage with each TIA. TIAs are also extremely important warning signals because they may build up in crescendo fashion and terminate in stroke within a matter of hours or days. They may also pass for the moment, then return and leave lasting damage. Siekert and associates (1963) estimated that 30 percent of patients who have TIAs will have a major stroke within five years from the date of onset. Certainly patients who have repeated TIAs in one carotid circulation (which may include episodes of amaurosis fugax) should have detailed carotid artery studies, such as we have outlined for CT examination of the neck in an earlier section. If the TIAs

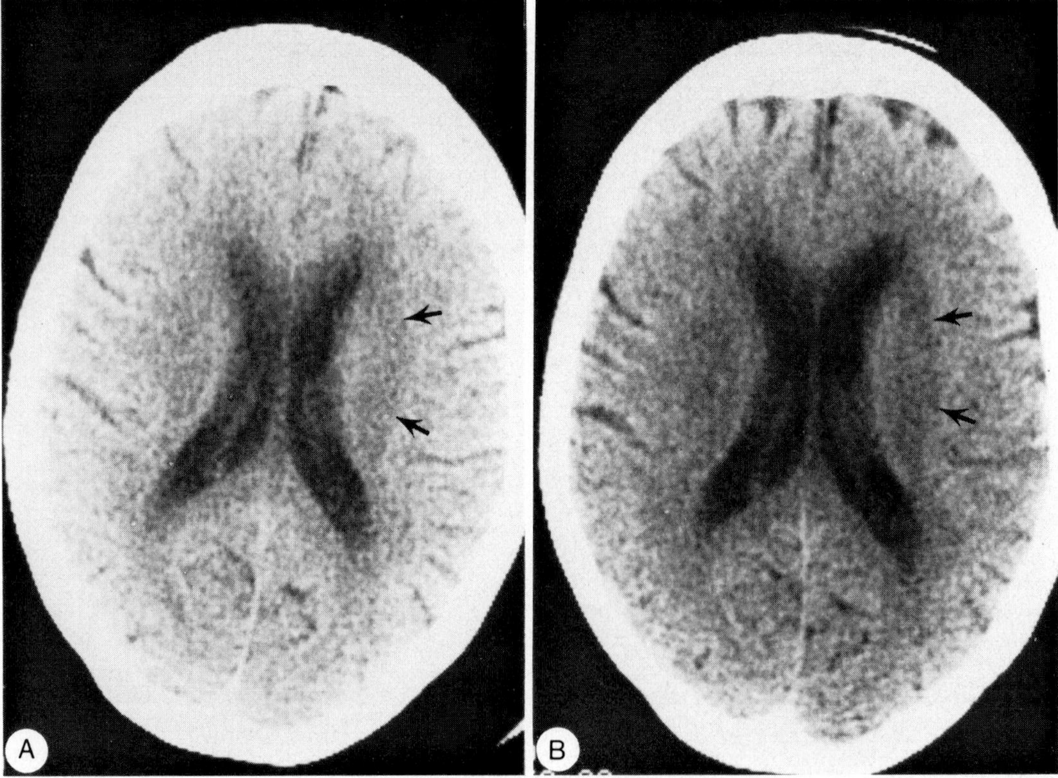

Figure 10–14. Early and later changes in the internal capsule and corona radiata seen on CT after cerebral infarction. At 24 hours postinfarction, the subtle decrease in density in the left corona radiata represents edema secondary to an infarction in the internal capsule, globus pallidus, and corona radiata (arrows) (*A*). Four days later (*B*), CT scan shows a further decrease in density representing persistent edema and a decreased neuronal density.

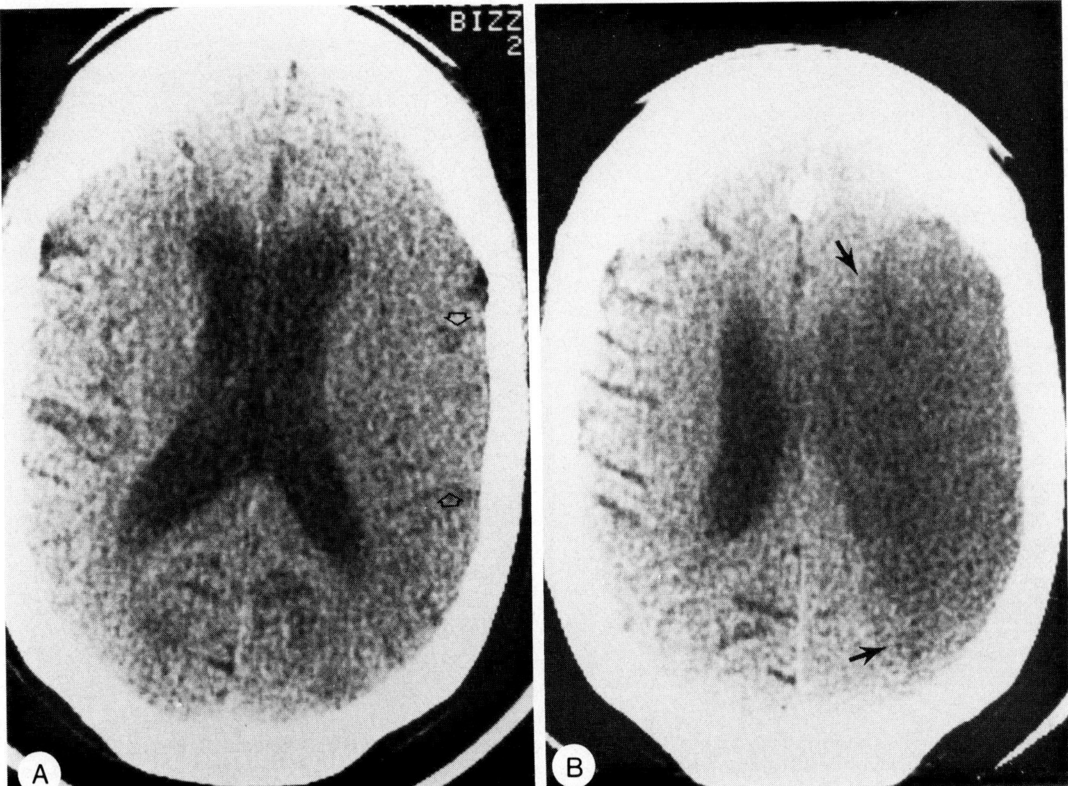

Figure 10–15. An acute infarction of the middle cerebral artery. Within the first 24 hours after infarction, the CT scan may appear almost "negative" on the CT scan (*A*). The infarction is signalled only by a subtle loss of sulci (open arrows) when compared with the opposite hemisphere and loss of cortical density. Four days later (*B*), the infarction is signalled by a significant decrease in density in the left middle cerebral territory (arrow at the margins). The anterior and posterior cerebral territories are spared.

take place in both carotid territories or overlap onto the vertebralbasilar territory, then a central source, such as a myocardial mural thrombus, must be considered.

Cerebral Ischemia and Segmental Infarction

If episodes of cerebral ischemia in the form of TIAs occur and are followed by a local, restricted area of segmental infarction, particularly in the middle cerebral artery territory, one must again strongly consider embolization from the carotid artery. This is particularly true if the episodes always recur in the same carotid distribution.

Hyperperfusion Leading to Infarction

The CT scan without contrast material should be the first diagnostic study performed. Formerly, there was enormous pressure to perform angiography early in patients with stroke. Today, when one obtains a CT scan of the brain and notes cerebral changes related to infarction, there is strong evidence to suggest that angiography should be postponed for at least a week during the period of major blood brain barrier damage. Brian Kendall, of the Queens Square Hospital, has even suggested that a contrast-enhanced CT scan leads to a statistically significantly worsened prognosis; therefore, we have avoided giving contrast whenever possible. Earlier reports on angiography after an acute vascular accident in patients in poor general condition indicated the morbidity rate to increase ten-fold.

Early Changes on Computed Tomography. CT scan of the brain may show even the most subtle signs of infarction in the first three to six hours of onset. These include a local disappearance of cerebral sulci and an absence of cisterns nearby. The cerebral cortex on each side of the brain may show a decrease in the

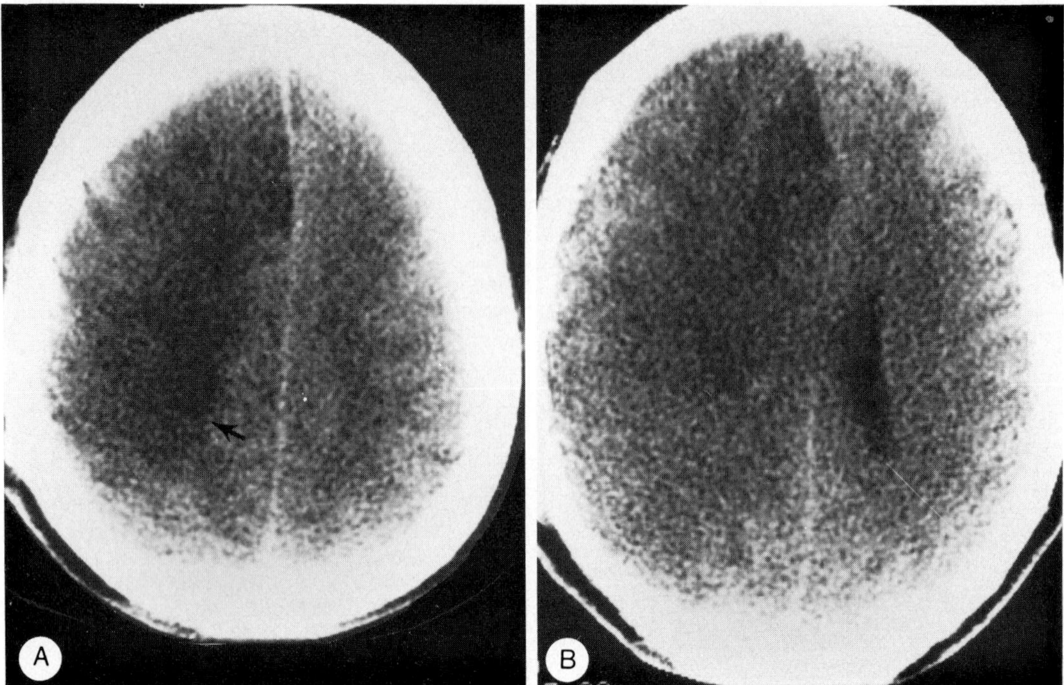

Figure 10–16. CT scans show occlusion of the extracranial carotid artery with infarction of the anterior and middle cerebral arteries. The anatomy of the circle of Willis is normal. Because in such patients the anterior and middle cerebral arteries perfuse from the internal carotid artery, and the posterior cerebral artery is perfused mainly from the vertebral-basilar system, the middle and anterior cerebral artery territory will bear the loss of perfusion with extracranial carotid occlusion. Second day postinfarction, the arrow designates the border of the middle and posterior cerebral territories (*A*). CT scan several days later shows increased swelling of those territories (*B*).

cortical density in the segmental area of the recent infarction. These three signs are frequently positive in CT scans taken during the first 24 hours in cerebral infarction owing to embolus or thrombus. Figure 10–14 shows a patient with a segmental decrease in cortical density and effacement of sulci over the right posterior temporoparietal area. The patient has a segmental infarct; these are the earliest changes visible in such infarctions. Figure 10–15 shows a subtle infarction involving the posterior limb of the internal capsule on Day 1; on Day 4, the completed infarction is much more readily detected. Figure 10–16 shows a CT scan of the brain on the day of a massive left middle cerebral infarction. Note that the rim of cortical density over the temporal lobe is less intense when compared with the other side. Note also the loss of the Sylvian fissure and associated sulci in the left when compared with the right temporal lobe. Four days later, a marked decrease in brain density is seen in the middle cerebral territory. The extensive involvement of the mid- and high convexity of the brain makes one appreciate the size of the middle cerebral artery territory and how small the anterior and posterior cerebral territories are.

Late Changes. There are several predominant patterns involving the arterial territories

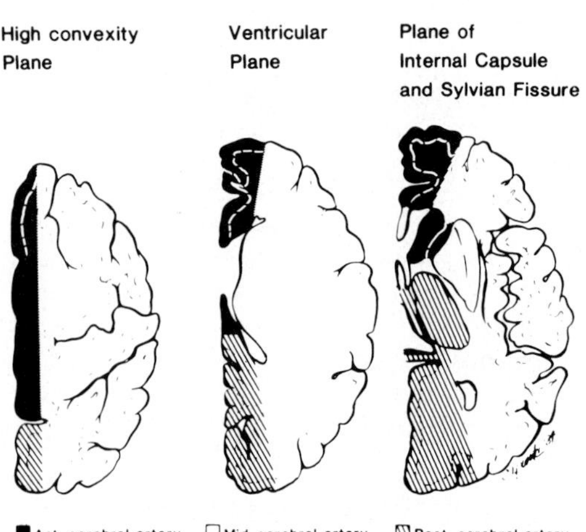

Figure 10–17. A schematic diagram illustrating the territories of the anterior, middle, and posterior cerebral arteries at three different levels of the brain.

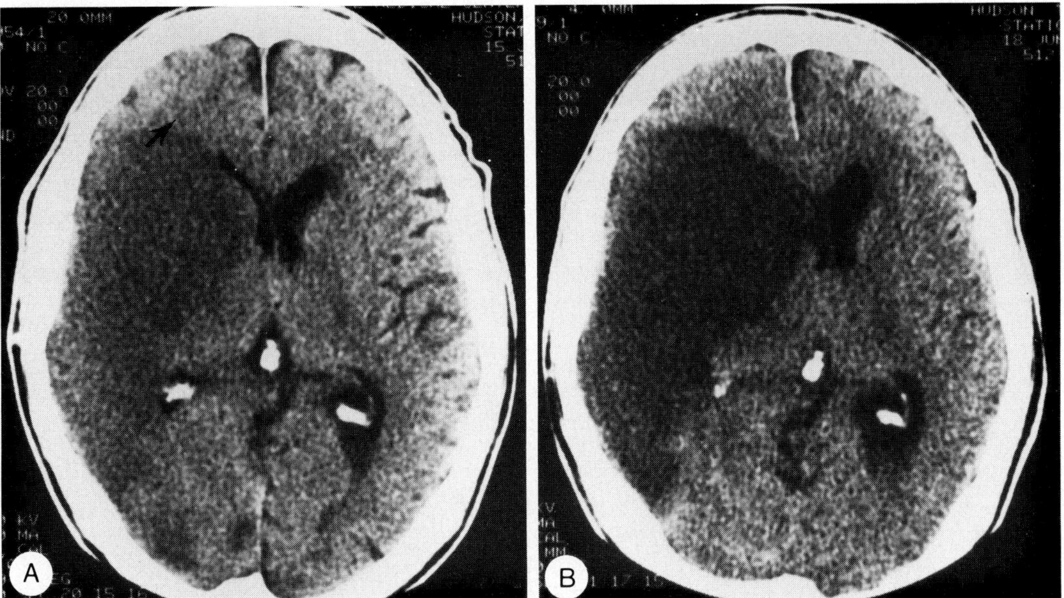

Figure 10 – 18. Extracranial carotid occlusion with middle cerebral artery infarction. Combined middle and anterior cerebral arterial territory infarction usually occurs after carotid occlusion, if, indeed, any infarction occurs. At times, the middle cerebral territory may be the only cerebral territory injured. This phenomenon occurs when the anterior cerebral artery on the side of the carotid occlusion is cross-filled by the contralateral carotid, a variation in the circle of Willis which is seen in 12 percent of patients. Note the sparing of the anterior cerebral artery territory arrow (*A*). Three days later, much more swelling has occurred (*B*).

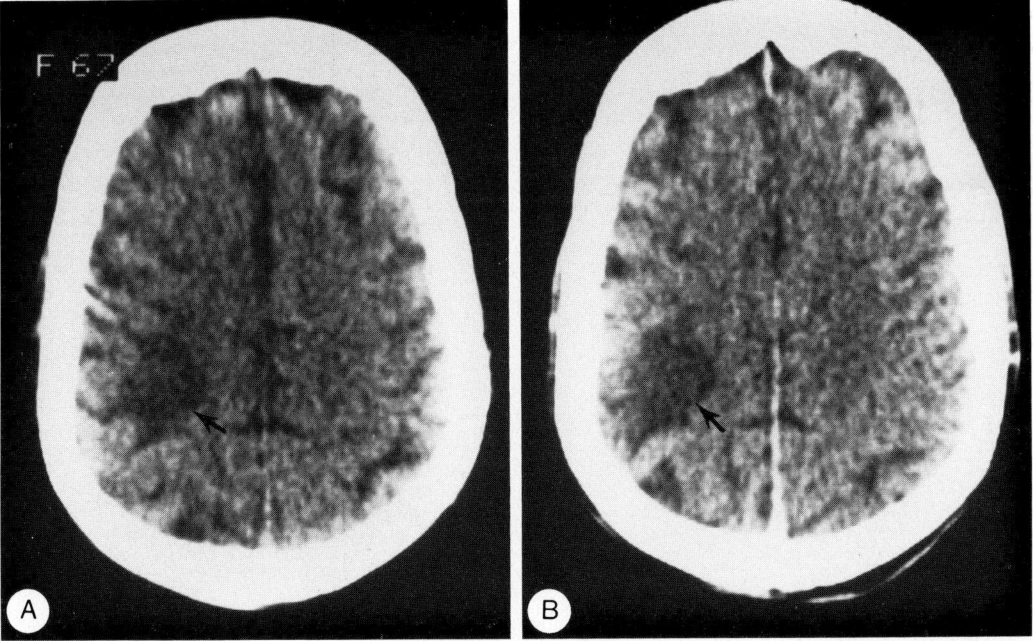

Figure 10 – 19. "Watershed" infarction seen in a 61-year-old woman with two episodes of cardiac arrest after abdominal surgery. Marked hypotension occurred with each episode. *A* and *B*: Note that the large area with decreased density in the right parietal region does not conform to either the middle cerebral or the posterior cerebral artery territory (arrow). Rather, it is precisely between the two territories, or in the "watershed" area less well perfused by each. Therefore, when the cardiac pump fails and the blood pressure falls, these "watershed" zones between anterior, middle, and posterior cerebral artery territories infarct first. The leptomeningeal collaterals are insufficient.

in cerebral infarction. With involvement of the anterior and middle cerebral artery territories (Figure 10–17), always consider a carotid artery occlusion, because both the anterior and the middle cerebral vessels are end-arteries for the internal carotid artery. The brain has only these end-arteries; thus, it must rely on leptomeningeal collaterals from neighboring arterial territories whenever there is an abrupt decrease in arterial pressure in the system. Therefore, it is understandable that cerebral infarction frequently occurs after occlusion in one of the feeding arteries.

Figure 10–18 shows a schematic drawing of the arterial distribution (anterior, middle, and posterior cerebral arteries) for three different levels of the brain.

Middle Cerebral Artery Alone. One may have an isolated infarct in the middle cerebral artery territory when the anterior cerebral artery on the same side is cross-filled from the opposite internal carotid (see Figure 10–19).

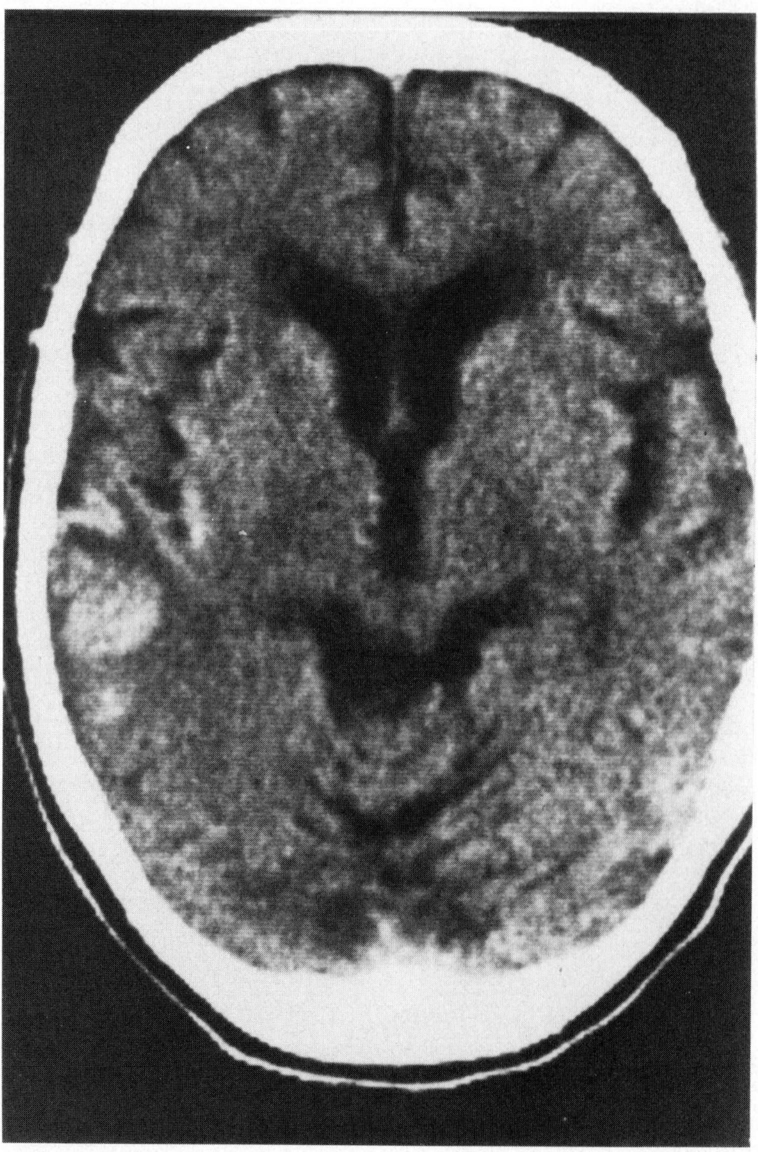

Figure 10–20. A hemorrhagic infarction. None of the preceding CT scans illustrating infarction show any blood. The present example shows a hemorrhagic area within a large middle cerebral infarction. While hemorrhagic infarctions occur in at least 13 percent of all infarctions, CT scans demonstrate hemorrhage only in about 5 percent. This indicates that the CT scan is not sensitive enough to detect many of the areas of hemorrhage, which are often petechial in character.

Because this variation in the circle of Willis occurs in 12 percent of cases, the finding of an isolated middle cerebral artery territory infarction is frequently caused by cervical carotid occlusion. It must not be assumed, though, to be always caused by a large embolus involving the middle cerebral artery alone.

Others. Sometimes the middle cerebral artery and the posterior cerebral artery territories are involved together in internal carotid occlusion. This may occur when the middle cerebral artery and the posterior cerebral artery on the same side are perfused by the internal carotid artery; this includes filling of a large "embryonal" posterior cerebral-posterior communicating artery. In this instance, the proximal posterior cerebral artery from the basilar artery is hypoplastic and all of the blood supply to the posterior cerebral artery comes from the carotid artery, with none from the basilar artery. In these instances, the anterior cerebral artery on the same side almost never fills on angiograms, because it is perfused by the opposite carotid.

"Watershed" infarcts (see Figure 10–20) are identified on CT scans because they typically fall in the transitional zones between the anterior and middle, middle and posterior, and posterior and anterior cerebral arterial territories. They develop because the pressure in the entire circulation drops due to a cardiac event, such as myocardial infarction or arrhythmia, with infarction of the brain tissue at the margins.

CT Scan as a Guide to Therapy

Although hemorrhagic infarction is estimated to occur in 13 percent of all cerebral infarctions, CT scanning can detect diffuse hemorrhage in only 5 percent of all infarctions. In the remaining patients, the quantity of bleeding is scanty, and the blood is scattered through the cortical tissue in an interrupted fashion so that CT scan cannot reliably separate its density from the density of the normal brain. That is why lumbar puncture, which has a high sensitivity for subarachnoid blood, is a very helpful adjunct to CT, when anticoagulation therapy is considered.

REFERENCES

Clark, O.H.; Moore, W.S.; and Hall, A.D.: Radiographically occluded, anatomically patent carotid arteries. *Arch. Surg.* **102**:604–606, 1971.

Cohen, W.A.; Pintos, R.S.; and Kircheff, I.I.: The value of dynamic scanning. *Radiol. Clin. North Am.*, **20**:23–35, 1982.

Countee, R.W., and Vijayanathan, T.: Reconstitution of "totally" occluded internal carotid arteries. *J. Neurosurg.*, **50**:747–57, 1979.

Edwards, J.H.; Kricheff; I.I.; Riles; T.; and Imparato, A.: Angiographically undetected ulceration of the carotid bifurcation as a cause of embolic stroke. *Radiology,* **132**:369–73, 1979.

Gabrielsen, T.I.; Seeger, J.F.; Knake, J.E.; Burke, D.P.; and Stilwill, E.W.: The nearly occluded internal carotid artery: a diagnostic trap. *Radiology,* **138**:611–18, 1981.

Heinz, E.R.; Fuchs, J.; Osborne, D.; Drayer, B.; Yeates, A.; Fuchs, H.; and Pizer, S.: Examination of the carotid bifurcation by thin section dynamic CT: direct visualization of intimal atheroma in man (part 2). *Am. J. Neurol. Radiol.*, **5**:361–66, 1984a.

Heinz, E.R.; Pizer, S.M.; Fuchs, H.; Fram, E.K.; Burger, P.; Drayer, B.P.; and Osborne, D.R.: Examination of the extracranial carotid bifurcation by thin-section dynamic CT: direct visualization of intimal atheroma in man (part 1). *Am. J. Neurol. Radiol.*, **5**:355–59, 1984b.

Leeson, M.D.; Cacayorin, E.D.; Illya, A.R.; Hodge, C.J.; Culebras, A.; Collins, G.H.; and Kieffer, S.A.: Atheromatous extracranial carotid arteries: CT evaluation correlated with arteriography and pathologic examination. *Radiology,* **156**:397–402, 1985.

Riles, R.S.; Imparato, A.M.; Posner, M.P.; and Eikelboom, B.C.: Common carotid occlusion. *Ann. Surg.*, **199**:363–66, 1984.

Riles, R.S.; Posner, M.P.; Cohen, W.A.; Pinto, R; Imparato, A.M.; and Braumann, F.G.: The totally occluded internal carotid artery: preliminary observations using rapid sequential computerized tomographic scanning. *Arch. Surg.*, **117**:1185–88, 1982.

Russell, W.F.: The CT scan in extracranial vascular disease. In *Stroke and the Extracranial Vessels.* Raven Press, New York, 1984.

Siekert, R.G.; Whisnant, J.P.; and Millikan, C.H.: Surgical and anticoagulant therapy of occlusive cerebrovascular disease. *Ann. Intern. Med.*, **58**:637–41, 1963.

Yonas, H., and Meyer, J.: Extreme pseudo-occlusion of the internal carotid artery. *Neurosurgery,* **11**:681–86, 1982.

UNIT III

Management of Diseases of the Carotid Artery

11

Medical Management of Threatened Stroke

ANTHONY J. FURLAN

It has been stated that although more than 80,000 carotid endarterectomies are performed annually in the United States (Dyken and Pokras, 1985), the medical management of risk factors, especially hypertension, rather than surgery appears to be the major reason for the declining stroke rates (Levy, 1979; Whisnant, 1983). Even in patients undergoing cerebrovascular surgery, subsequent medical management is a major determinant of long-term outcome.

The medical management of threatened stroke applies to two broad groups of cerebrovascular patients: those at high risk for future stroke and those with an acute evolving stroke. To date, treatment has been more successful for the former group, but there are several exciting new therapeutic modalities on the horizon for patients with evolving stroke. This chapter reviews some aspects of the medical management of these patients.

IDENTIFYING THE PATIENT AT HIGH RISK FOR STROKE

The cornerstone strategy for lowering the occurrence of stroke is the identification and modification of stroke-risk factors (Wolf *et al.*, 1983), such as age, hypertension, heart disease, and transient ischemic attacks (TIAs). Other risk factors include asymptomatic carotid bruits, hyperlipidemia, diabetes mellitus, and cigarette smoking. Some comments about selected risk factors follow.

Age

Although stroke can occur at any age, the incidence approximately doubles with each decade increased in age.

Cardiac Disease

There is an intricate relationship between cerebrovascular disease and cardiovascular disease. First, about 20 percent of cerebral infarcts are due to cardiac embolism (Barnett, 1983). A cardiac embolic source should be considered in any patient with TIA or cerebral infarction, but especially in those under the age of 50 or in those with any evidence of cardiac disease. The most common cardiac embolic source is chronic, nonvalvular atrial fibrillation (NVAF); others include rheumatic heart disease, myocardial infarction, prosthetic heart valves, and prolapsed mitral valve.

In some patients it may be impossible to tell whether a brain infarct is related to cerebral atherosclerotic disease or to cardiac disease because these often coexist. A common example would be an elderly patient with NVAF and also carotid artery stenosis. It is estimated that 75 percent of cerebral infarcts in patients with NVAF are cardioembolic (Hart *et al.*, 1983), but in the individual patient this may be difficult to determine. In such cases, initial medical management (usually long-term warfarin) is preferable to cerebrovascular surgery unless there is severe, accessible atherosclerotic stenosis in an appropriate vessel.

Aside from the issue of cardioembolic stroke, cardiac disease is the most common cause of long-term mortality in patients with TIA or brain infarction. Hence, knowing the status of the coronary circulation is a critical factor in the management of cerebrovascular patients. Cerebrovascular patients with a significant history of coronary artery disease may require heart catheterization whether or not endarterectomy is planned. In patients who have no history of heart disease, assessment of the coronary circulation through some form of stress testing is probably the prudent approach (Adams *et al.,* 1984).

ASYMPTOMATIC CAROTID BRUITS

There are many causes of neck bruits other than stenosis of the internal carotid artery. In fact, only about 50 percent of cervical bruits are correlated with underlying internal carotid stenosis on angiography. Localized bruits high in the neck near the jaw angle, especially if there is a diastolic component, are best correlated with underlying internal carotid artery stenosis; about 4 percent of the population over age 65 harbors such an asymptomatic bruit (Sandok *et al.,* 1982).

Epidemiologic studies have shown that patients with asymptomatic carotid bruits have an increased risk of stroke, but this applies to all kinds of strokes in all cerebrovascular territories. Hence asymptomatic carotid bruits are best viewed as simply markers of atherosclerotic disease (Heyman *et al.,* 1980; Wolf *et al.,* 1981; Quiñones-Baldrich and Moore 1985; Yatsu and Fields, 1985).

The management of asymptomatic carotid bruits is controversial and requires further study; there is no consensus regarding the evaluation of such patients. There is no randomly controlled evidence proving that repairing an isolated asymptomatic internal carotid artery stenosis, regardless of severity, significantly alters either long-term stroke risk or mortality rates (Mohr, 1982). Because the risk of stroke in patients with asymptomatic bruits is about 2 percent per year (Whisnant, 1983; Mohr, 1982), in my view patients over age 70 with asymptomatic carotid bruits should *not* be investigated with noninvasive tests (NIT) or intravenous digital subtraction angiography (IV-DSA). In younger patients who are in good general medical condition, asymptomatic carotid bruits are often screened for high-grade (80 percent) internal carotid artery stenosis with either NIT or IV-DSA. Patients with significant stenosis can then undergo endarterectomy if there is access to a surgeon who can correct it with an operative morbidity and mortality rate less than 2 percent. Patients with lesser degrees of stenosis and patients over age 70 are managed medically through risk-factor modification, education about TIA, and 5 to 10 gr of aspirin daily. Serial NITs or IV-DSA are done in selected cases at 6 to 12 month intervals. Through observance of these guidelines, the vast majority of patients with asymptomatic carotid bruits can be managed medically.

TRANSIENT ISCHEMIC ATTACKS

TIA is a temporary, *focal* episode of neurologic dysfunction of presumed vascular origin, typically lasting less than five minutes but occasionally as long as 24 hours. TIAs are classified as carotid or vertebral-basilar depending on the vascular territory of the ischemia.

It is important to resist the notion that TIAs are usually or exclusively due to embolization of platelet, fibrin, or atheromatous debris from an atherosclerotic plaque in an extracranial vessel. Although artery-to-artery embolization is an important cause of TIA, up to 50 percent of patients with TIA have normal cerebral angiographic findings (Ramirez-Lassepas *et al.,* 1973). A TIA may reflect arteriolar disease and can herald acute arterial occlusion. Hemodynamic disturbances, such as cardiac dysrhythmia and orthostatic hypotension, are infrequent causes of TIA but occasionally play a contributory role in patients with multiple-vessel occlusions or unilateral high-grade stenosis or occlusion. Embolism from the heart is also an important cause of TIA, especially in patients under age 50. Other possible causes of TIA include nonatherosclerotic arteriopathies and rare hematologic or clotting disorders. Additionally, several neurologic conditions can exactly or closely mimic TIAs. Focal seizures need not alter consciousness, and focal motor or sensory symptoms can occur in migraine in the absence of headache. Occasionally, a cerebral mass lesion presents with a TIA-like episode.

The risk of stroke after TIA depends on a number of variables, including the cause of the attack and the presence of other stroke-risk factors. Among all patients with TIA who do not die of a cause other than stroke, about 33 percent have a stroke within five years of the first attack. Of these, more than 20 percent have strokes within a month and 50 percent within a year of the initial attack (Cartilidge *et al.*, 1977; Whisnant *et al.*, 1973; Whisnant *et al.*, 1983). After the first six months following the onset of TIAs, the incidence of stroke is about 6 percent per year, which is approximately six times the expected rate for a matched normal population. Thus, the duration of TIA is important in predicting the risk of stroke. The number of TIAs and the average duration of an individual TIA are less useful indicators of stroke risk. Many patients have only a single TIA before a stroke, and less than 50 percent of strokes are preceded by a TIA.

When TIAs are due to atherosclerotic disease of the internal carotid system, a decision must be made whether the patient is a candidate for cerebrovascular surgery or for medical therapy. Extracranial-intracranial bypass surgery is ineffective for most patients with occlusion of the internal carotid artery or inaccessible stenosis of the intracranial internal carotid or middle cerebral artery (EC/IC Bypass Study Group, 1985). Carotid endarterectomy has yielded the best results in patients with typical hemispheric carotid TIA or amaurosis fugax who have demonstrable atherosclerosis in the extracranial internal carotid artery on the same side as the symptoms (Robertson, 1983; American Canadian Co-operative Study Group, 1985). Usually stenosis must exceed 50 percent for a patient to qualify for surgery, but endarterectomy is occasionally performed in patients with deep, irregular ulcerations and milder stenosis.

In the best surgical hands, the risk of endarterectomy is from 1 to 10 percent, depending on a number of variables, primarily the medical and neurological condition of the patient (Sundt *et al.*, 1975). In some hospitals, the combined morbidity and mortality rates for carotid endarterectomy may be as high as 21 percent (Easton *et al.*, 1977; Brott and Thalinger, 1985). Thus, in addition to the patient's symptoms, the surgeon's skill and the patient's general condition are critical factors in determining the indication for endarterectomy.

Patients with vertebral-basilar TIAs may have lesions in the vessels feeding the vertebral or basilar arteries. In some instances, these lesions are correctable by endarterectomy or bypass surgery. However, surgically accessible lesions are much less common in these patients than in those with carotid territory TIAs. Hence, patients with vertebral-basilar TIA are usually managed medically. The benefits of carotid endarterectomy for most patients with nonlocalizing symptoms or vertebral-basilar TIAs are doubtful (McNamara *et al.*, 1977; Moufarrij *et al.*, 1984).

Antiplatelet therapy is the preferred form of medical treatment for most patients with TIAs, either as the sole treatment or after cerebrovascular surgery. Warfarin is reserved for patients with cardiac conditions, such as atrial fibrillation or rheumatic heart disease. Sometimes, warfarin is used for two or three months after the onset of TIA, and then the patient is switched to antiplatelet therapy (Sandok *et al.*, 1978). In practice, however, most physicians begin with antiplatelet therapy and consider changing to warfarin if that fails.

The only antiplatelet agent that has been shown to decrease the frequency of TIA and reduce the risk of stroke is aspirin (Dyken, 1983). Aspirin and many nonsteroidal antiinflammatory drugs interfere with platelet aggregation by nonselectively blocking the enzyme cyclo-oxygenase, an important rate-limiting substance in the arachidonic acid cascade. As a result, the formation of thromboxane (a potent platelet aggregant and vasoconstrictor) as well as prostacyclin (an antiaggregant and vasodilator) is inhibited.

In clinical trials, aspirin dosages of from 1,000 to 1,500 mg/day have been used (Dyken, 1983; Canadian Cooperative Study Group, 1978). Considerable in vitro evidence indicates that much lower dosages (i.e., less than 300 mg/day) also inhibit platelet cyclo-oxygenase, the major site of thromboxane formation (Hanley *et al.*, 1981). In theory, lower dosages should not interfere with prostacyclin formation, which occurs in vessel walls. This is a theoretical advantage in patients with cerebral ischemia. However, prescription of so-called minidose (30 mg) aspirin in patients with TIA is premature. The protective action of aspirin may involve pathways other than the arachidonic acid cascade. Also, on the basis of clinical trials many physicians prescribe 300 mg four times a day or 600 mg twice a day. Others advise 300 mg twice a day. If patients have adverse gastrointestinal effects, lower aspirin doses, coated aspirin, or aspirin combined with antacid can be considered.

The other popular available antiplatelet agent is dipyridamole. The usual dosage is 50 mg three times a day or 75 mg twice a day in combination with aspirin. The mechanism by which dipyridamole prevents platelet aggregation is different from that of aspirin. Dipyridamole increases platelet cyclic adenosine monophosphate (CAMP) levels by blocking the enzyme phosphodiesterase; this in turn interferes with platelet calcium release and aggregation. The recently completed aspirin and dipyridamole trial found that the combination of aspirin and dipyridamole was no better in prevention of strokes than aspirin alone (American Canadian Co-operative Study Group, 1985).

Other antiplatelet drugs that selectively block thromboxane synthesis or interfere with platelet function while permitting prostacyclin synthesis are under investigation.

MEDICAL MANAGEMENT OF EVOLVING ATHEROTHROMBOTIC STROKE, PROGRESSING STROKE, AND STROKE-IN-EVOLUTION

If a patient is seen within 24 hours of the sudden onset of a focal neurological deficit and that deficit has not yet resolved, it is uncertain whether it is a TIA, a stroke which may still progress, or a completed infarct. In this situation, the physician must decide whether simply to observe the patient closely or whether to institute immediate medical or surgical therapy in an attempt to prevent further neurological deterioration. Although emergency angiography and endarterectomy are sometimes employed in these patients (Goldstone and Moore, 1978), surgery carries a high risk and is of uncertain benefit in reversing the ischemic process, especially when there has been any lapse of time since the onset. Some of these patients' conditions improve spontaneously. Often, however, the question arises about the efficacy and timing of acute anticoagulant therapy with heparin in an attempt to prevent progressive thrombosis or recurrent embolization in such patients. Unfortunately, a decision regarding therapy in evolving stroke must often be made without precise information regarding the etiology of the stroke or the mechanism of progression. Furthermore, the studies that show a trend favoring heparin therapy for patients with presumed evolving atherothrombotic brain infarction were done before the advent of computed tomography (CT) and have serious methodological flaws (Millikan and McDowell, 1981).

In assessing the efficacy of heparin in a patient with a presumed evolving atherothrombotic brain infarction, an initial evaluation of the severity of the neurologic deficit is made by asking the question: How much neurological function can the patient still lose? Patients with severe deficits or a decrease in level of consciousness should not be given heparin. In patients with milder deficits, acute heparin therapy can be used if no contraindications exist (severe hypertension or active peptic-ulcer disease), and if a reasonable attempt has been made to exclude an intracranial hemorrhage. Intracranial hemorrhage is best excluded by performing a nonenhanced CT scan. If CT scanning is unavailable, lumbar puncture can be performed safely in patients with minor neurological deficits and without evidence of increased intracranial pressure (papilledema, decreased level of consciousness). The absence of grossly bloody spinal fluid provides reasonable, albeit not absolute, evidence against intracranial hemorrhage.

Recommendations regarding heparin dosage and monitoring in patients with evolving atherothrombotic brain infarction derive largely from series of patients with venous thrombosis, pulmonary embolism, or a cardiac embolic source. The optimal dose of heparin to prevent arterial thrombus formation and to minimize the risk of brain hemorrhage in patients with evolving cerebral ischemia has not been well studied. In cerebrovascular patients, in whom the risk of intracranial hemorrhage may be high, it seems safest to use the lowest possible antithrombotic dose of heparin. Bolus injections of heparin should be avoided in these patients, and heparin should be administered by constant infusion. Dosage is usually monitored with the activated partial thromboplastin time, which can be supplemented with various heparin assay systems in high-risk patients. Most patients require 300 to 400 units of heparin kg/24 hours either to keep the activated partial thromboplastin time from 1½ to two times control or to maintain a blood heparin level from 0.2 and 0.5 units/ml (Furlan *et al.,* 1983).

In patients with evolving stroke in the carotid distribution heparin therapy is continued for about 72 hours or until the neurological picture stabilizes. The patient may then undergo angiography, be switched to aspirin or warfarin, or be provided with supportive care depending upon the final neurological outcome. Patients with progressing brain-stem infarction should continue heparin therapy for up to two weeks, at which point the patient is usually prescribed either antiplatelet therapy or long-term warfarin. Low molecular weight dextran, a rheologic agent, has been shown to be of some benefit in patients with acute brain infarction (Wood and Fleischer, 1982). It is also used in patients for whom heparin is contraindicated.

The administration of corticosteroids for acute stroke deserves comment. There is little question that cerebral edema can account for neurological deterioration in some patients after acute brain infarction. Such worsening, which reflects increased intracranial pressure, is generally seen two to four days after the onset of the stroke. Although corticosteroids are very useful for decreasing other forms of cerebral edema, such as that associated with brain tumor, they are of no benefit in reducing edema after brain infarction (Anderson and Cranford, 1979); therefore, they should not be used in the management of acute brain infarction.

Another medical management problem in patients with acute brain infarction is the treatment of hypertension. Although many stroke victims have prior history of hypertension, blood pressure may be acutely and transiently elevated after an infarction even in those persons who previously had normal pressure. Unless this elevation of blood pressure is extreme, a period of bed rest alone is often sufficient to lower the blood pressure to preexisting levels. Cerebral blood flow autoregulation is often impaired in an area of infarction, and some acute stroke victims are passively dependent upon mean arterial pressure to maintain cerebral blood flow. Also, patients with chronic hypertension and atherosclerosis probably require higher than usual mean arterial pressures to maintain normal cerebral blood flow (Strandgaard and Paulson, 1984; Torvik, 1984). Hence, precipitous decreases in blood pressure into the normotensive range should be avoided in patients with acutely evolving strokes. If lowering of the blood pressure is necessary, a graduated decrease into the low or medium hypertensive range is best achieved by using a sodium nitroprusside drip.

Traditional forms of therapy for evolving stroke will probably soon be supplanted by newer treatment modalities based on a better understanding of the pathophysiology of acute focal brain ischemia. Areas currently being explored include opiate antagonists, such as naloxone; free radical scavenger agents; drugs that work through the arachidonic acid cascade, such as prostacyclin infusion; and calcium-entry blockers (Yatsu, 1983; Caplan, 1984; Moncada, 1983). Blood glucose also plays an important role in determining the extent of irreversible brain damage in acute ischemia, probably by influencing brain lactic acid levels (Rehncrona *et al.,* 1980). Evolving brain infarction is such a complex process, however, that it seems doubtful that unimodal therapy will ever be the final answer (Raichle, 1983). The ability to administer these agents within minutes or hours after the onset of ischemia also remains a difficult clinical problem.

MANAGEMENT OF REVERSIBLE ISCHEMIC NEUROLOGIC DEFICITS (RIND)

The timing of angiography and possible endarterectomy after a small completed brain infarction or a so-called reversible ischemic neurologic deficit poses a special problem (Wiebers *et al.,* 1982). If the patient has no or minimal neurologic deficit and an enhanced CT scan is normal, angiography and, if necessary, endarterectomy can be performed during the immediate poststroke period. If there is an infarct on CT, especially on enhanced CT, it is probably safest to defer angiography with possible cerebrovascular surgery for four to six weeks (Robertson, 1983). It may be useful to perform noninvasive tests or an IV-DSA in such patients. If the extracranial vessels are well visualized, the need and urgency of endarterectomy can be better estimated. Also, if surgery is to be postponed, screening tests in the immediate poststroke period can help the physician decide whether or not the patient should be discharged with antiplatelet or anticoagulant therapy depending on the severity of the symptomatic arterial lesion.

REFERENCES

Adams, H.P.; Kassell, N.E.; and Mazuz, H.: The patients with transient ischemic attacks—is this the time for a new therapeutic approach? *Stroke,* **15**:371–75, 1984.

American Canadian Co-operative Study Group: Persantine Aspirin trial in cerebral ischemia. Part II: Endpoint results. *Stroke,* **16**(3):406–15, 1985.

Anderson, D.R., and Cranford, R.E.: Corticosteroids in ischemic stroke. *Stroke,* **10**:68–71, 1979.

Barnett, H.J.M.: Heart in ischemic stroke—a changing emphasis. *Neurol. Clin. North Am.,* **1**:291–315, 1983.

Brott, T., and Thalinger, K.: The practice of carotid endarterectomy in a large metropolitan area. *Stroke,* **15**:950–55, 1985.

Canadian Cooperative Study Group: A randomized trial of aspirin and sulfinpyrazone in threatened stroke. *N. Engl. J. Med.*, **229**(2):53–59, 1978.

Caplan, L.R.: Treatment of cerebral ischemia—where are we headed? *Stroke*, **15**:571–74, 1984.

Cartilidge, N.E.F.; Whisnant, J.P.; and Elveback, L.R.: Carotid and vertebral-basilar transient cerebral ischemic attacks: a community study, Rochester, Minnesota. *Mayo Clin. Proc.*, **52**:117–20, 1977.

Dyken, M.L.: Anticoagulant and platelet-antiaggregation therapy in stroke and threatened stroke. *Neurol. Clin. North Am.*, **1**:223–42, 1983.

Dyken, M.L., and Pokras, R.: The performance of endarterectomy for disease of the extracranial arteries of the head. *Stroke*, **15**:948–50, 1985.

Easton, J.D., and Sherman, D.G.: Stroke and mortality rate in carotid endarterectomy: 228 consecutive operations. *Stroke*, **8**:565–68, 1977.

EC/IC Bypass Study Group: Failure of extracranial–intracranial arterial bypass to reduce the risks of ischemic stroke: Results of an international randomized trial. *N. Engl. J. Med.*, **313**: 1191–1200, 1985.

Furlan, A.J.; Campbell, J.D.; Lucas, F.; *et al.*: Experience with a heparin assay for monitoring heparin therapy in cerebrovascular disease. *Ann. Neurol.*, **14**:129–130, 1983 (Abstract).

Goldstone, J., and Moore, W.S.: A new look at emergency carotid artery operations for the treatment of cerebrovascular insufficiency. *Stroke*, **9**:599–602, 1978.

Hanley, S.P.; Cockbill, S.R.; Bevan, J.; *et al.*: Differential inhibition by low-dose aspirin of human versus prostacyclin synthesis and platelet thromboxane synthesis. *Lancet*, **1**:969–71, 1981.

Hart, R.G.; Sherman, D.G.; Miller, V.T.; and Easton, J.D.: Nonvalvular atrial fibrillation. *Curr. Probl. Cardiol.*, **8**:53–9, 1983.

Heyman, A.; Wilkinson, W.E.; Heyden, S., *et al.*: Risk of stroke in asymptomatic persons with cervical arterial bruits. A population study in Evans County, Georgia. *N. Engl. J. Med.*, **302**:838–41, 1980.

Levy, R.I.: Stroke decline: implications and prospects. *N. Engl. J. Med.*, **300**:490–91, 1979.

McNamara, J.O.; Heyman, A.; Silver, D.; and Mandel, M.E.: The value of carotid endarterectomy in treating transient cerebral ischemia of the posterior circulation. *Neurol. Minneapolis*, **27**:682–84, 1977.

Millikan, C.H., and McDowell, F.H.: Treatment of progressing stroke. *Stroke*, **12**:397–409, 1981.

Mohr, J.P.: Asymptomatic carotid artery disease. *Stroke*, **13**:431–33, 1982.

Moncada, S.: Biology and therapeutic potential of prostacyclin. *Stroke*, **14**:157–68, 1983.

Moufarrij, N.A.; Little, J.R.; Furlan, A.J.; *et al.*: Vertebral artery stenosis: long-term follow-up. *Stroke*, **15**:260–63, 1984.

Quiñones-Baldrich, W.J., and Moore, W.S.: Asymptomatic carotid stenosis. *Arch. Neurol.*, **42**:378–382, 1985.

Raichle, M.E.: The pathophysiology of brain ischemia. *Ann. Neurol.*, **13**:2–10, 1983.

Ramirez-Lassepas, M.; Sandok, B.A.; and Burton, R.C.: Clinical indicators of extracranial carotid artery disease in patients with transient symptoms. *Stroke*, **4**:537–40, 1973.

Rehncrona, S.; Rosen, I.; and Siesjø, B.K.: Excessive cellular acidosis: an important mechanism of neuronal damage in the brain. *Acta Physiol. Scand.*, **110**:435–37, 1980.

Robertson, J.T.: Carotid endarterectomy. *Neurol. Clin. North Am.*, **1**:19–29, 1983.

Sandok, B.A.; Furlan, A.J.; Whisnant, J.P.; and Sundt, T.M.: Guidelines for the management of transient ischemic attacks. *Mayo Clin. Proc.*, **53**:665–74, 1978.

Sandok, B.A.; Whisnant, J.P.; Furlan, A.J.; and Mickell, J.L.: Carotid artery bruits: prevalence survey and differential diagnosis. *Mayo Clin. Proc.*, **57**(4):227–30, 1982.

Strandgaard, S., and Paulson, O.B.: Cerebral autoregulation. *Stroke*, **15**:413–16, 1984.

Sundt, T.M., Jr.; Sandok, B.A.; and Whisnant, J.P.: Carotid endarterectomy: complications and preoperative assessment of risk. *Mayo Clin. Proc.*, **50**:301–6, 1975.

Torvik, A.: The pathogenesis of watershed infarcts in the brain. *Stroke*, **15**:221–23, 1984.

Wiebers, D.O.; Whisnant, J.P., and O'Fallon, W.M.: Reversible ischemic neurologic deficit (RIND) in a community: Rochester, Minnesota, 1955–1974. *Neurology (NY)*, **32**:459–65, 1982.

Whisnant, J.P.: The role of the neurologist in the decline of stroke. *Ann. Neurol.*, **14**:1–7, 1983.

Whisnant, J.P.; Matsumoto, N.; and Elveback, L.R.: Transient cerebral ischemic attacks in a community: Rochester, Minnesota, 1955–1969. *Mayo Clin. Proc.*, **48**:194–98, 1973.

Wolf, P.A.; Kannel, W.B.; Sorlie, P.; and McNamara, P.: Asymptomatic carotid bruit and the risk of stroke. *J.A.M.A.*, **245**:1422–45, 1981.

Wolf, P.A.; Kannel, W.B.; and Verter, J.: Current status of risk factors for stroke. *Neurol. Clin. North Am.*, **1**:317–47, 1983.

Wood, J.H., and Fleischer, A.S.: Observations during hypervolemic hemodilution of patients with acute focal cerebral ischemia. *J.A.M.A.*, **248**:2999–3004, 1982.

Yatsu, F.M.: Pharmacologic protection against ischemic damage. *Neurol. Clin. North Am.*, **1**:37–53, 1983.

Yatsu, F.M., and Fields, W.S.: Asymptomatic carotid bruit, stenosis or ulceration, a conservative approach. *Arch. Neurol.*, **42**:383–85, 1985.

12

Anesthetic Considerations in Carotid Artery Surgery

MICHAEL T. GILLETTE

Since the first carotid reconstruction for occlusive arterial disease in the early 1950s, many anesthetic techniques have been used in the course of this operation. Different drug regimens and various other approaches to cardiovascular and respiratory management have led to greater understanding of the variety of patient responses to the operation. This in turn led to refinement of anesthetic methods. This chapter focuses on current methods of anesthetic management of operations for extracranial occlusions and examines its physiological rationale, its preoperative assessment and preparation, and its intraoperative monitoring and management, and discusses some of the common postoperative problems and their treatment.

PREOPERATIVE ASSESSMENT AND PREPARATION

A patient undergoing surgery for ischemic cerebrovascular disease frequently has multisystem disease and requires a careful and detailed preoperative evaluation. This should include a review of prior anesthetic experience to elicit any problems that may have arisen. The anesthetist should also determine whether the patient has a history of other illnesses or drug allergy and evaluate any medication the patient may be receiving. He should perform a careful review of systems to elicit previously unknown medical problems and should examine the patient for any anatomical problems pertinent to the operation.

Atherosclerosis is a diffuse disease, and a high percentage of patients in need of carotid artery surgery have significant though perhaps asymptomatic coronary artery disease. Up to 30 percent of patients have a history of coronary disease, and a much larger percentage have hypertension. Because many of these patients are unaware of these problems, their signs and symptoms should be sought. Several studies have shown that myocardial infarction is the leading cause of death in the perioperative period (Ennix *et al.*, 1979; Riles *et al.*, 1979; Rubio *et al.*, 1975).

Because cigarette smoking is prominent in the history of these patients, the presence of significant respiratory impairment should be sought. Fortunately, owing to the peripheral nature of carotid surgery, respiratory complications are few; nevertheless, high-risk patients should be identified and prepared appropriately.

Evaluation of the central nervous system should be thorough. The anesthesiologist should be aware of the patient's neurological status and vascular anatomy, since these may have profound effects on the course of the anesthesia. Patients with a stroke in progression or with a completed stroke may be markedly more sensitive to anesthetic and sedative drugs than patients with transient ischemic attacks. In addition, patients with completed strokes may have a significant mass of functionally denervated muscle and may develop life-threatening hyperkalemia if depolarizing muscle relaxants are used. They are also more likely to have cardiovascular lability secondary to the ongoing cerebral process. A knowledge of the patient's vascular anatomy is the key to the anesthesiologist's appreciation of changes related to anesthesia and to carotid cross-clamping. An awareness of the patient's state of consciousness is also important for assessment. Certainly a patient who is drowsy and lethargic preoperatively is likely to remain so in the initial postoperative period.

Many patients may also have some degree of acute or chronic renal failure. Longstanding hypertension or atherosclerotic vascular disease may involve the kidneys to varying degrees, and angiographic dye may cause a further acute worsening. Even patients with end-stage renal disease who are on dialysis and have increased atherogenesis may become candidates for carotid surgery. A careful evaluation of renal function is warranted for appropriate fluid management and drug therapy. Endocrine disease, particularly diabetes, occurs in about 20 percent of patients scheduled for carotid endarterectomy. An understanding of their insulin requirements is crucial for good management.

Most patients who will undergo carotid artery surgery are already receiving one or more drugs. Among the most common are antihypertensives, diuretics, antianginal agents (beta-blockers, calcium-channel blockers, and nitrates), bronchodilators, antiplatelet drugs, anticoagulants, and insulin. Specific concerns and management of those drugs will be discussed later.

In addition to careful review of history, systems, and drug therapy, the anesthesiologist should perform a pertinent physical examination and check for obvious signs of cardiac or respiratory disease. He should observe neck motion which may impair the neurological status because the neck will have to be turned laterally during surgery. He should look closely at airway anatomy to anticipate possible difficulty with intubation and should determine the adequacy of ulnar artery blood flow if insertion of a radial artery monitoring cannula is planned.

Laboratory tests should include a complete blood count with hemoglobin levels, platelet count, electrolytes, blood glucose, blood urea nitrogen (BUN) and creatinine levels, as well as a chest x-ray and electrocardiogram (ECG). Patients with symptoms or history of chronic lung disease may require arterial blood gas analysis and pulmonary function testing. This review of the patient's status permits the anesthesiologist and surgeon to properly evaluate the patient for surgery.

Preoperative preparation for carotid surgery does not differ significantly from that of any other major operation. No patient should undergo elective surgery until significant medical problems are defined and the patient is in the best possible condition.

Cardiovascular disease, especially hypertension and ischemic heart disease, present the greatest threat to the life of the patient. Patients with hypertension are at less risk when their blood pressure is controlled; otherwise, they are likely to have hyper- or hypotension during surgery or in the early postoperative period. This increased lability in blood pressure has been associated with a higher morbidity and mortality rates (Bove *et al.*, 1979; Towne *et al.*, 1980). Antihypertensive medications, except diuretics, should be continued until the time of operation. Oral medications may be taken with small sips of water until surgery. Failure to continue drug therapy until surgery increases the chance of significant hypertension on emergence from anesthesia. Most antihypertensive drugs can be given by either the parenteral or transdermal route if the patient is unable to take oral medication. Hypertensive patients are usually also taking diuretics, many of which deplete potassium. Serum potassium levels should therefore be measured and repleted to normal, especially if the patient is receiving digitalis. Patients receiving diuretics usually have significantly depleted total body potassium levels; thus, serum potassium determinations taken soon after a brief course of potassium replacement may be misleading. The administration of diuretics should cease one to two days before surgery. Patients should not be operated upon when they are in a hypovolemic state because they are difficult to manage from an anesthetic standpoint.

Patients selected for carotid artery surgery frequently have either known or occult concomitant coronary artery disease. Their drug regimen should be continued through surgery. Patients with coronary disease should also have their disease defined and treatment started as necessary before surgery. Those with recent myocardial infarction, unstable or crescendo angina, or severe stable angina with poor exercise tolerance and whose conditions do not improve on medication are candidates for simultaneous coronary artery bypass grafting. When this is not feasible, such patients can benefit from pulmonary artery catheterization and aggressive intraoperative and postoperative hemodynamic control. When it is the surgeon's practice to increase the arterial blood pressure with vasopressors during carotid crossclamping, patients with significant coronary disease should have their pulmonary artery pressure monitored because there is great risk of inducing ischemia (Keats, 1981).

Patients with congestive heart failure should have their blood volume normalized preoperatively and may also require pulmonary pressure monitoring if their circulation is not fully compensated. If they are taking digitalis, its level should be determined. Digitalis should be stopped two days before surgery because it may confound the diagnosis of arrhythmias during surgery. Patients taking digitalis for rhythm control or for poorly compensated congestive heart failure should have the drug continued until surgery.

Most patients with atherosclerotic vascular disease are or have been smokers and may have significant respiratory impairment. Fortunately, because carotid surgery does not cause postoperative costal splinting, respiratory depression associated with the operation is usually brief and can be well controlled by appropriate management. Cases of chronic obstructive lung disease fall into three categories, with some overlap: (1) emphysematous type with destructive airway disease manifested by airtrapping and bronchospasm, (2) asthmatic type with hypertrophic hyperactive airways and bronchospasm, and (3) bronchitic type with heavy sputum production and bronchospasm. Emphysematous patients, though not always responsive to bronchodilators, should have their bronchodilator regimen intensified and continued through surgery. To patients with asthma, steroids may be given preoperatively in an attempt to alleviate bronchospasm which may occur on intubation. Subjects with bronchitis can benefit most from such a preoperative preparation. Patients with acute exacerbations, such as a change in the amount or color of the sputum or decrease in exercise tolerance, should be cleared of infection before surgery. Those with heavy sputum production may benefit from three to five days of preoperative chest physical therapy. Their surgery is best scheduled late morning; thus, with the aid of early-morning chest physical therapy, they have the opportunity to mobilize secretions before the operation. Patients with recent or old neurologic impairment are prone to aspiration and should be cleared of acute respiratory infection when possible.

Certainly, patients who are candidates for carotid artery surgery may have other medical problems, such as renal failure, diabetes, and other endocrine disorders, and should be prepared in the usual fashion.

Premedication for carotid artery surgery should meet requirements for ideal management. If a patient needs to be alert enough to follow commands at the end of the operation for neurological assessment, which is desirable, then obviously he must not be heavily sedated preoperatively. A thorough preoperative visit by the anesthesiologist probably is as effective as premedication in calming the fears of an anxious patient. Light premedication may also be very helpful. Debilitated patients or patients with previous strokes may be especially sensitive to sedatives, which should either be omitted or their dosage reduced. Diazepam in doses of 2 to 10 mg orally two hours before operation usually meets the necessary requirements. Premedication with promethazine, scopolamine, or lorazepam frequently causes excessive sedation and may induce postoperative delirium. We prefer premedicating all patients with cimetidine or ranitidine to reduce the possibility of aspiration.

ANESTHETIC MANAGEMENT

Patients should be brought to the operating room in advance of surgery with adequate time to place appropriate monitoring lines. Routine monitoring on all patients for cerebrovascular surgery should include measurement of the blood pressure both by cuff and by an indwelling arterial cannula, monitoring of the ECG (lead II, V_4 or V_5), and temperature. Carotid surgery is brief and usually does not involve major volume shifts, but patients with a history of myocardial infarctions which have occurred within a year, with unstable angina or resting angina, poor exercise tolerance, poorly compensated congestive heart failure, significant valvular disease, severe chronic obstructive lung disease with pulmonary hypertension, or artificial elevation of blood pressure should also have pulmonary artery pressure monitoring. Atrioventricular sequential pacing catheters are easy to insert, have a greater than 95 percent success rate in atrial or atrioventricular pacing, and may be helpful in managing bradyarrhythmias during surgery as well as postoperatively. Carbon dioxide partial pressure (PCO_2) and/or end-tidal carbon dioxide should be monitored.

With crossclamping and interruption of flow, some brain tissue may become ischemic. Preoperative arteriography may suggest which patients are at high risk, but correlation is far from perfect. Many methods have been used in an attempt to determine adequacy of cerebral circulation during crossclamping, but none has proven absolutely reliable. It is hoped that detection of cerebral hypoxia by newer methods will bring about alteration of surgical and anesthetic management. Monitoring devices currently used to detect cerebral hypoxia include jugular venous saturation measurement, carotid stump pressure, cerebral blood flow, electroencephalogram (EEG), and other related devices, such as compressed spectral array and cerebral function monitors.

Jugular bulb venous oxygen saturation has been applied to assess cerebral function during crossclamping. Early reports suggested that high (greater than 50 percent) saturation is correlated with adequate cerebral circulation. A detailed study by Larson and associates (1967), however, demonstrated that "no reliable relationship could be established between SVO_2 and cerebral function during trial occlusion under local anesthesia." They also had evidence of transient deficits in patients with high saturations.

Measurement of the carotid stump pressure has also been used to assess the adequacy of cerebral perfusion. A carotid stump pressure of 50 torr has been felt to be the critical number below which cerebral ischemia may occur. McKay and associates (1976) proved that stump pressure correlates poorly with cerebral blood flow measurements and EEG changes. In their study, stump pressures were less than 50 torr in 28 percent of patients, while their cerebral blood flow was greater than 24 ml/100 g/min (critical is considered less than 18), and their EEGs were normal. It was further shown that 8 percent of the patients had stump pressures greater than 50 torr while their cerebral blood flow was less than 18 ml/100 g/min and their EEGs indicated cerebral hypoxia.

Cerebral blood flow, as measured by Xenon-133 washout, can be used intraoperatively to assess regional perfusion. The technique, however, is costly and complicated and, therefore, not widely used. The exact amount of reduction in cerebral blood flow that will cause ischemia or infarction is not known, because considerable variation occurs from study to study and patient to patient (McKay *et al.*, 1976; Sundt *et al.*, 1974; Boysen, 1971; Waltz *et al.*, 1972). In general, cerebral blood flow below 15 ml/100 g/min is thought to be associated with ischemia, and below 10 ml/100 g/min is associated with infarction. In the study by Sundt *et al.* (1981), patients with a cerebral blood flow of less than 18 ml/100 g/min responded favorably to temporary indwelling shunting. A more detailed discussion on cerebral blood flow monitoring is given in Chapters 18 and 19.

EEG monitoring may also be used intraoperatively to indirectly assess cerebral perfusion. Full EEG monitoring is believed to reflect changes caused by crossclamping that correlate well with the degree to which cerebral blood flow is reduced (Chiappa *et al.*, 1979; Sundt *et al.*, 1981). Significant EEG changes were observed whenever the cerebral blood flow fell below 15 ml/100 g/min. Significant postoperative neurological deficits were predicted accurately by the EEG, although EEG abnormalities also occurred in patients who had no postoperative neurologic deficits. Full EEG monitoring is, however, time-consuming to set up, cumbersome to handle, and, owing to its complexity, requires active participation and cooperation of a neurologist, anesthetist, and surgeon to interpret changes in light of surgical manipulation and other stimuli as well as those caused by drugs and the depth of anesthesia (Chiappa *et al.*, 1979). Because of the difficulties associated with such an extensive monitoring system, EEG-derived devices gained some popularity. Such cerebral function monitors have a single-lead system and demonstrate power and frequency of electrical activity on each side, which makes changes relatively easy to recognize.

Another derivative of EEG monitoring is the compressed spectral array, a computer-generated display of EEG data which is more easily interpreted than the full EEG. Grundy *et al.* (1981) compared the full EEG, compressed spectral array, and the cerebral function monitor, and found that each reflected appropriate changes in cortical function but that the cerebral function monitor was the most practical for an anesthetist working without the support of an EEG technician and a neurophysiologist.

Although EEG and derived monitors correlate well with changes in cerebral perfusion, their interpretation is confounded by their complexity, the anesthetic drugs used, and surgical manipulation. When anesthesia and surgical personnel are constant and experienced in the use of this equipment, the patients who develop ischemia during carotid crossclamping are clearly identified. However, it is still unclear whether demonstration of decreased perfusion and the use of a shunt based on this information alters the morbidity and mortality rate of the operation. The multiple differences in anesthetic and surgical techniques and patient populations, noted in the literature, make an exact evaluation impossible. It, however, is reasonable to assume that the identification of high-risk patients by either cerebral blood flow measurements (where cerebral blood flow is below 15 to 18 ml/100 g/min) or by EEG changes may guide in the alteration of therapy, either anesthetic or surgical.

Carotid artery surgery may be performed with either local or in general anesthesia. Although local anesthesia has been used successfully in several centers for many years, we see no significant advantage in mortality or morbidity. General anesthesia is better accepted by patients, is equally safe, and may offer some element of cerebral protection. Patients with significant ischemic heart disease also may fare better with general anesthesia, under which heart rate, blood pressure, and oxygenation can be better controlled (see also Chapter 20 on carotid surgery in the awake patient).

The process of anesthesia in the course of a carotid endarterectomy may be divided into five major segments: induction, maintenance, the crossclamping period, the postclamping period, and emergence. Induction is usually accomplished with thiopental sodium often combined with narcotics and xylocaine. This provides a fast, predictable, pleasant induction for the patient. Lightly premedicated patients may arrive in the operating room with elevated blood pressure, which, especially in those with chronic hypertension, may exceed 180/100 mm Hg. The cause of this is complex, with anxiety and endogenous catecholamines playing important roles. After induction, which reduces the stimuli for hypertension, the blood pressure may decrease markedly—occasionally to levels requiring vasopressor support. The myocardial depressant properties of thiopental also may precipitate a decrease in blood pressure. Patients with poorly controlled hypertension are most apt to become hypotensive with induction. Intubation may also cause significant fluctuation in blood pressure which may be prevented by administration of intravenous or topical xylocaine and with narcotics. Significant hypotension may cause myocardial and cerebral ischemia; therefore, it should be treated immediately with an infusion of phenylephrine or other vasopressors. Hypertension and tachycardia from manipulation of the airway in a lightly anesthetized patient could induce myocardial ischemia. Intubation is usually facilitated by muscle relaxants, most commonly succinylcholine. In patients with recent strokes and areas of denervated or partially denervated muscle, succinylcholine may cause an abnormally large release of potassium from muscle, which may be life-threatening. This drug should be avoided in such patients.

Anesthesia may be maintained with barbiturates, inhalation agents, or narcotics with nitrous oxide. Barbiturates offer some cerebral protection secondary to reduced cerebral oxygen consumption, but their usage may be associated with hypotension and delayed awakening. Inhalation agents, such as enflurane, halothane, and isoflurane may also be used. Halothane is a myocardial depressant (which may therefore protect the myocardium) and also a mild vasodilator, usually causing some reduction in blood pressure. It decreases airway reflexes and blunts response to manipulation; therefore, carotid endarterectomy may be performed satisfactorily under light halothane anesthesia without muscle relaxants for maintenance. The low dose of halothane required usually does not cause major hemodynamic imbalance and allows rapid arousal. In addition, it is a potent bronchodilator, which is helpful in chronic smokers and other patients with bronchospastic lung disease. Instead of halothane, enflurane may also be used. However, it does not diminish airway reflexes to the same degree and may also induce seizures at anesthetic concentrations in predisposed patients. Isoflurane does not cause significant myocardial depression but is a marked vasodilator. Hypotension and reflex tachycardia are often associated with isoflurane and it may induce myocardial ischemia. However, it reduces electrical activity and cerebral oxygen consumption and may therefore offer some additional measure of cerebral protection (Newberg *et al.*, 1982). The anesthetic properties of isoflurane permit rapid arousal. Anesthesia may also be maintained with narcotics, or with nitrous oxide and muscle relaxants.

The latter combination probably does not offer the same degree of cerebral protection but provides a better hemodynamic stability and a rapid emergence. It should be emphasized that the minimal surgical stimulus of carotid endarterectomy usually allows the use of a very light plane of anesthesia.

During the maintenance period, blood pressure should be kept in the normal or slightly-above-normal range because autoregulation may not be intact secondary to ischemic disease.

The PCO_2 should be maintained in the normal range. Whereas reducing the PCO_2 increases cerebrovascular resistance and therefore may increase flow to ischemic areas, it may also decrease flow through collateral vessels and thus induce ischemia. Increasing PCO_2 values increases total cerebral blood flow but ischemic areas are probably already maximally dilated; therefore, high PCO_2 levels may cause a steal from ischemic areas. Surgical dissection around the carotid bifurcation may cause bradycardia and hypotension. This may be treated effectively by administering intravenous atropine and/or local injection of one percent xylocaine.

The time of crossclamping the carotid artery is the most critical period of the operation, because cerebral ischemia may occur and become manifest if monitoring is used. Several techniques are used either prophylactically to prevent ischemia, or to treat ischemia if it is detected. These techniques are artificial elevation of blood pressure, application of temporary indwelling shunts, and use of barbiturates or other anesthetics that decrease cerebral oxygen consumption. The value of these techniques is controversial, and each has its own significant risk. Artificial elevation of blood pressure is usually accomplished with the infusion of phenylepinephrine or another vasoconstrictor in an attempt to increase blood supply to poorly perfused areas. The vessels of the poorly perfused areas already being dilated will be affected little by this maneuver; some collateral vessels may be constricted and the flow actually reduced. In patients with ischemic heart disease, profound cardiac ischemia may also develop by this method, and if cardiac output decreases due to ischemia, the cerebral circulation will suffer. An increase in the perioperative myocardial infarction rate, with its associated increased mortality rate, may also occur with this method (Keats, 1981). Patients with known coronary artery disease in whom this technique is planned should have their pulmonary artery occlusion pressures monitored along with their V-5 lead ECG. Myocardial ischemia should be treated promptly. Shunts are used either (1) prophylactically in all patients, (2) in high-risk patients, (3) when ischemia is detected by stump pressure, cerebral blood flow, or EEG, or (4) not at all. The use of shunts is controversial because they require longer crossclamp time and are associated with increased embolism.

Barbiturates may be used to decrease cerebral metabolic rate prophylactically or when ischemia is noted. The benefits of their use is still unclear. Large doses of barbiturates given before clamping will cause marked EEG abnormalities, rendering the EEG ineffective as a monitor of cerebral ischemia. Barbiturates given after clamping may lower blood pressure, thereby worsening ischemia, and may cause delayed awakening from anesthesia.

After the endarterectomy is completed, only the brief period of wound closure time remains. This time is used to lighten anesthesia and to prepare for any sudden change in blood pressure which may occur in the course of awakening. Blood pressure often increases dramatically during emergence owing to surgical denervation of the carotid bulb, which alters the control mechanisms (Lehv *et al.*, 1970; Caplan *et al.*, 1978), and also may be caused by pain from the incision site. Because increased blood pressure may induce myocardial ischemia, bleeding at the operative site, and intracranial hemorrhage (especially if there is a recent stroke) (Caplan *et al.*, 1978), it requires immediate treatment. Sodium nitroprusside should always be available for rapid control. Awakening from anesthesia is usually quick if light premedication and anesthetics have been used. Ideally, the patient should be awake enough to move extremities on command a few minutes after closure of the skin while still in the operating room.

POSTOPERATIVE CONSIDERATIONS

Serious complications that may arise after carotid endarterectomy, especially in the first 24 hours postoperatively, most notably include hypertension, hypotension, stroke, myocardial infarction, and airway obstruction.

Hypertension occurs in a high percentage of patients after carotid endarterectomy, occasionally beginning several hours into the postoperative period. Towne *et al.* (1980), defining hypertension as systolic arterial pressure greater than 200 torr, observed a 19 percent incidence. Lehv *et al.* (1970) reported a 56 percent rate of hypertension using a 15 torr increase as definitive. Both studies suggest that postoperative hypertension is associated with an increase in the number of neurological complications. It is not certain whether the hypertension is the cause or a result of neurological damage. The only factor definitely related to its incidence is preoperative hypertension. Differences in surgical and anesthetic techniques do not seem to be correlated. Multiple factors, such as renin production by the brain (Smith, 1984), may come into play in its genesis. Previously hypertensive patients taking medication often have their medication stopped one or more days before surgery, which may cause rebound or leave them unprotected. Denervation of the carotid sinus may decrease carotid sinus nerve activity with associated hypertension mediated by the medulla. Hypercarbia, though avoided during anesthesia, may develop in the recovery room. Narcotics, muscle relaxants, and increased oxygen concentrations in sensitive patients may also cause carbon dioxide retention and a consequential sympathetic vasoconstrictive response. Subanesthetic concentrations of inhalation anesthetics may, however, block the hypertensive response to hypercarbia. Neurogenic hypertension may also be caused by local or global neurologic injury.

To recognize immediately and treat properly the abnormal fluctuations in blood pressure, continuous indwelling arterial blood pressure monitoring in the operating and recovery rooms is highly advisable and patients should receive antihypertensive agents promptly as required. Control with intravenous sodium nitroprusside is highly effective but it may be associated with marked lability, especially during transport. In a patient in whom hypertension is expected, the careful titration of hydralazine and/or propranolol before awakening may make postoperative hypertension less likely. In general, maintenance of blood pressure at systolic levels below 160 torr with drugs is desirable. The hypertensive response usually lasts less than 12 hours, after which it is possible to resume a normal drug regimen.

Hypotension develops in 28 to 41 percent of all patients after carotid endarterectomy (Bove *et al.*, 1979; Tarlov *et al.*, 1973). It is often associated with bradycardia. The postulated mechanism is that removal of plaque from the artery causes a heightened response of the carotid sinus nerve. This stimulates the medulla to send vagal stimuli to the circulation. Tarlov and associates (1973) found that treatment with colloid plasma expanders before, during, and after surgery reduced the frequency of hypotension. They also found that denervation of the carotid sinus also prevented the hypotensive response that usually persists for only a few hours. Their study antedated the common use of pulmonary artery occlusion pressure and cardiac output monitoring. In a patient so monitored, increased cardiac output along with decreased systemic vascular resistance is observed unless bradycardia is marked. When heart rate is low, treatment with atropine is indicated. In patients with decreased systemic vascular resistance (as is usually the case), infusion of a vasopressor, such as phenylephrine, to maintain blood pressure may be preferable to large amounts of colloid plasma expanders which, when redistributed after vasodilatation abates, may cause cardiac problems in brittle individuals.

Airway problems may also occur after carotid endarterectomy. Hematoma from bleeding at the operative site may obstruct the airway. Laryngeal dysfunction caused by laryngeal nerve injury or postextubation stridor from laryngeal edema could also develop. It may not be easy to exactly define the contribution of these phenomena to postoperative respiratory difficulties. In any event, it is essential to observe respiratory function closely for 18 to 24 hours after surgery when rapid intubation is occasionally required.

Postoperative strokes may be caused by dissection, thrombosis, embolus, hypotension, hypertension with encephalopathy, or hemorrhage and are discussed in Chapter 21. They may cause severe cardiovascular or respiratory dysfunction and need prompt diagnosis and aggressive supportive therapy.

Myocardial infarction has been shown to be the major cause of mortality after carotid artery surgery, occurring in greatest frequency in patients with symptomatic coronary disease (Ennix *et al.*, 1979; Riles *et al.*, 1979; Rubio and Guinn, 1975). Routine postoperative monitoring of the ECG is warranted. Close postoperative control of determinants of myocardial oxygen supply and demand is beneficial, because bradycardia and hypotension or tachycardia and hypertension may well cause myocardial infarction in patients at risk. Because of the cardiovascular lability often seen after carotid endarterectomy, patients with unstable angina, new-onset angina, recent myocardial infarction, angina with poor exercise tolerance, angina of indeterminate nature, nocturnal or resting angina, and angina with congestive heart failure, and asymptomatic patients with known high-risk coronary lesions may benefit from pulmonary artery pressure monitoring in the postoperative period (regarding postoperative complications also see Chapter 21).

In conclusion, anesthetic management of patients undergoing carotid artery surgery has evolved since its beginnings in the 1950s, responding to changes in surgical technique and increased knowledge of the physiologic changes occurring perioperatively. Careful preoperative evaluation focusing on medical problems common to these patients and addressing them intra- and postoperatively has led to the development of anesthetic techniques that allow the safe support of this difficult patient population. The further refinement of anesthetic management, as clinically practical, involves the assessment of determinants of cerebral perfusion and oxygenation, and altering them if necessary and possible.

REFERENCES

Bove, E.; Fry, W.; Gross, W.; and Stanley, J.: Hypotension and hypertension as consequences of baroreceptor dysfunction following carotid endarterectomy. *Surgery,* **85**:633–37, 1979.

Boysen, G.: Cerebral blood flow measurement as a safeguard during carotid endarterectomy. *Stroke,* **2**:1–10, 1971.

Caplan, L.; Skillman, J.; Ojemann, R.; and Fields, W.: Intracerebral hemorrhage following carotid endarterectomy: a hypertensive complication? *Stroke,* **9**:457–60, 1978.

Chiappa, K.; Burke, B., and Young, R.: Results of electroencephalographic monitoring during 367 carotid endarterectomies. *Stroke,* **10**:381–88, 1979.

Ennix, C.; Lawrie, G.; Morris, G.C., Jr.; Crawford, E.S.; Howell, J.F.; Reardon, M.J.; and Weatherford, S.C.: Improved results of carotid endarterectomy in patients with symptomatic coronary disease; an analysis of 1,546 consecutive carotid operations. *Stroke,* **10**:122–25, 1979.

Grundy, B.L.; Webster, M.W.; Nelson, P.; Sanderson, A.C.; Karanjia, P.; and Troost, B.T.: Brain monitoring during carotid endarterectomy. *Anesthesiology,* **55**:A129, 1981.

Keats, A.: Anesthesia for carotid endarterectomy. *Cleve. Clin.,* **48**:68–71, 1981.

Larson, P.; Ehrenfeld, W.; Wade, J.; and Wylie, E.: Jugular venous oxygen saturation as an index of adequacy of cerebral oxygenation. *Surgery,* **62**:31–9, 1967.

Lehv, M.; Salzman, E.; and Silen, W.: Hypertension complicating carotid endarterectomy. *Stroke,* **1**:307–13, 1970.

McKay, R.; Sundt, T.; Michenfelder J.; Gronert, G.; Messick, J.; Sharbrough, F.; and Piepgras, D.: Internal carotid artery stump pressure and cerebral blood flow during carotid endarterectomy: moderation by halothane, enflurane, and Innovar. *Anesthesiology,* **45**:390–99, 1976.

Newberg, L.; Milde, J.; and Michenfelder, J.: Cerebral metabolic effects of isoflurane at and above concentrations which suppress the EEG. *Anesthesiology,* **57**:3, 1982.

Riles, T.; Kopelman, I.; and Imparato, A.: Myocardial infarction following carotid endarterectomy; a review of 683 operations. *Surgery,* **85**:249–52, 1979.

Rubio, P., and Guinn, G.: Myocardial infarction following carotid endarterectomy. *Cardiovasc. Dis. Bull. Texas Heart Inst.,* **2**:402–4, 1975.

Smith, B.L.: Hypertension following carotid endarterectomy: the role of cerebral renin production. *J. Vasc. Surg.,* **1**:623–27, 1984.

Sundt, T.; Sharbrough, F.; Anderson, R.; and Michenfelder, J.: Cerebral blood flow measurements and electroencephalograms during carotid endarterectomy. *J. Neurosurg.,* **41**:310–20, 1974.

Sundt, T.; Sharbrough, F.; Piepgras, D.; Kearns, T.; Messick, J.; and O'Fallon, W.: Correlation of cerebral blood flow and electroencephalographic changes during carotid endarterectomy with results of surgery and hemodynamics of cerebral ischemia. *Mayo Clin. Proc.,* **56**:533–43, 1981.

Tarlov, E.; Schmidek, H.; Scott, R.M.; Wepsic, J.; and Ojemann, R.: Reflex hypotension following carotid endarterectomy: mechanism and management. *J. Neurosurg.,* **39**:323–27, 1973.

Towne, J., and Bernhard, V.: The relationship of postoperative hypertension to complications following carotid endarterectomy. *Surgery,* **88**:575–80, 1980.

Waltz, A.; Sundt, T.; and Michenfelder, J.: Cerebral blood flow during carotid endarterectomy. *Circulation,* **45**:1091–96, 1972.

13

Cerebral Ischemia: Indications for Carotid Endarterectomy

IVAN K. CROSBY and
GEORGE R. HANNA

The evolution of modern surgical techniques has afforded great opportunity for intervention in the usually progressive course of atherosclerotic vascular disease. Removal of a plaque from an artery may reestablish normal, nonturbulent laminar flow, as well as eliminate a potential source of thrombus or embolism. However, the mere opportunity for intervention does not constitute an indication for surgery. The causal mechanisms of cerebral ischemic events are not entirely understood at present. Although survival of the threatened brain cells depends ultimately on receipt of adequate fuel and oxygen, both the delivery and the metabolic system are complex. Failure of either may impair brain function, transiently or permanently. In this chapter, we emphasize mainly the delivery system because it is most amenable to surgical intervention. It is, however, only part of the equation. Although increasing the number of red cells directly improves the ability to carry oxygen, at the same time the increased hematocrit causes an increase in viscosity partly offsetting the gain in oxygenation by slowing delivery. At hematocrit levels above 50 to 55 percent, blood viscosity increases very sharply and may result in a net reduction in tissue oxygenation. Hematocrit and therefore viscosity are transiently increased by dehydration and the use of diuretics. Thus, we are again faced with a paradox: in certain cases minor alterations in the blood may produce a more profcund change in tissue perfusion than major alterations of blood vessels. The relations of viscosity in cerebrovascular disease are reviewed in detail by Thomas (1982).

TRANSIENT ISCHEMIC ATTACKS

A transient cerebral ischemic attack (TIA) is the cessation of function of a localized area of the brain in the distribution of a particular blood vessel, presumably owing to impairment of blood supply to that area. The exact mechanisms remain obscure, but restricted blood flow, intravascular clot formation, and embolization of friable material may all play a role in inducing TIAs. As implied by the word "transient," the attacks are brief, usually lasting only minutes to hours, and are followed by complete recovery of function (see Figure 13–1). A number of distinctive neurological syndromes may occur which are characteristic of the functional neuroanatomy of the ischemic area (see also Chapter 6 on clinical manifestations). The occurrence of a TIA implies that the circulation has been impaired sufficiently to produce failure of neurological function. TIAs are thus regarded as precursors of stroke and warrant a thorough investigation, generally including arteriography (see Figure 13–2). If an isolated plaque is found to be causing stenosis (more than 60 percent in diameter) of the carotid artery on the side appropriate to the TIA, it is usually advisable to remove it by endarterectomy. In cases of severe bilateral stenosis, we recommend operating on the symptomatic side as the primary procedure, fol-

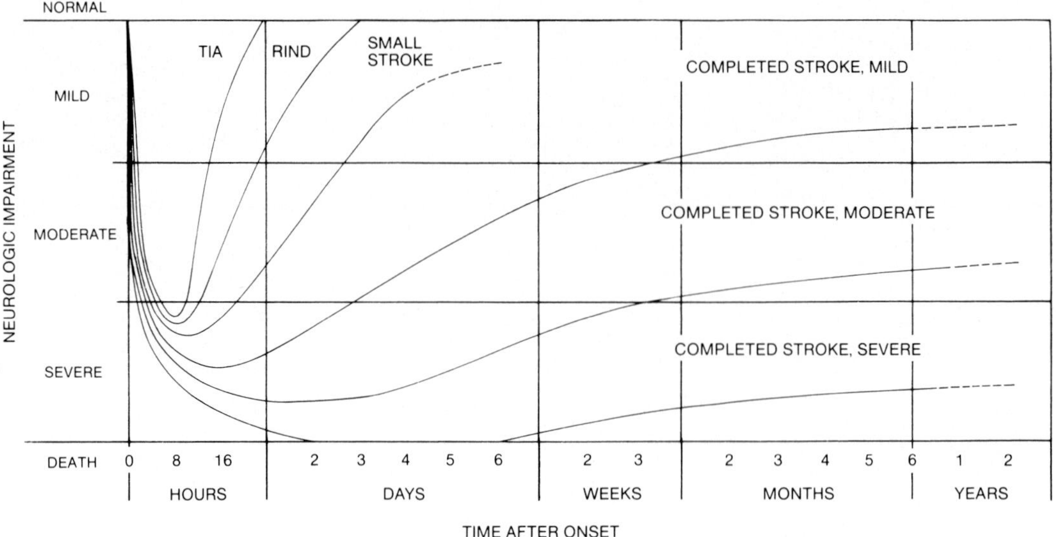

Figure 13–1. Duration of symptoms of cerebrovascular insufficiency correlated with the extent of cortical damage.

lowed by a second-stage operation of the other side after the first has healed. Total occlusion may not be amenable to surgical repair.

Carotid endarterectomy for nonobstructive plaques, or for plaques in locations inappropriate to the neurological syndrome, is a matter of controversy. According to our present understanding of the syndrome, such plaques are probably not responsible for the TIAs. There are a few possible exceptions to this:

1. Plaques containing areas denuded of endothelium and with frank ulceration or cavitation (whether or not they cause stenosis) are thought to be a common source of embolism (see Figure 13–2) either of blood elements (thrombus or platelets) or of detritus from the plaque. The removal of such ulcerated plaques may lessen the risk of further embolism.
2. In those cases in which one internal carotid is totally occluded, the circulation to that hemisphere is supplied mainly by crossflow from the opposite side. In such cases, a plaque in the remaining carotid may be responsible for TIAs in either hemisphere, and its removal is indicated.
3. Similarly, the posterior arterial system may be carotid-dependent, owing to either vertebral arterial disease or anomaly. In such cases, vascular lesions in the carotid artery may give rise to TIA in the posterior circulation.

There are indeed a number of reports of successful correction of posterior circulation TIAs by carotid endarterectomy (e.g., Humphries *et al.,* 1965). Ford and co-workers (1975) and Rosenthal and co-workers (1978) separately conducted retrospective studies of patients with the diagnosis of vertebral-basilar TIA who underwent carotid endarterectomy to relieve the attacks. Both studies included patients having nonlateralized symptoms, as well as those with combined nonlateralized and hemispheric symptoms. It was assumed that relief of carotid stenosis would result in improved general circulation to the brain and, therefore, in relief of the vertebral-basilar TIAs. Although they reviewed a combined total of more than 150 cases and reported excellent improvement in symptoms, it is difficult to analyze these results. The most common symptoms were dizziness, blurred vision, and syncope — not altogether specific for vertebral-basilar ischemia. Nor did improvement correlate well with arteriographic findings or intraoperative vascular pressure studies. Ouriel and co-workers (1984) have attempted to classify such patients further, correlating arteriographic findings of both carotid and vertebral systems with symptoms. They believe that patients with hemodynamically insignificant lesions and/or nonclassic symptoms should be managed nonoperatively. Patients with classic vertebral-basilar insufficiency symptoms and significant stenoses had excellent im-

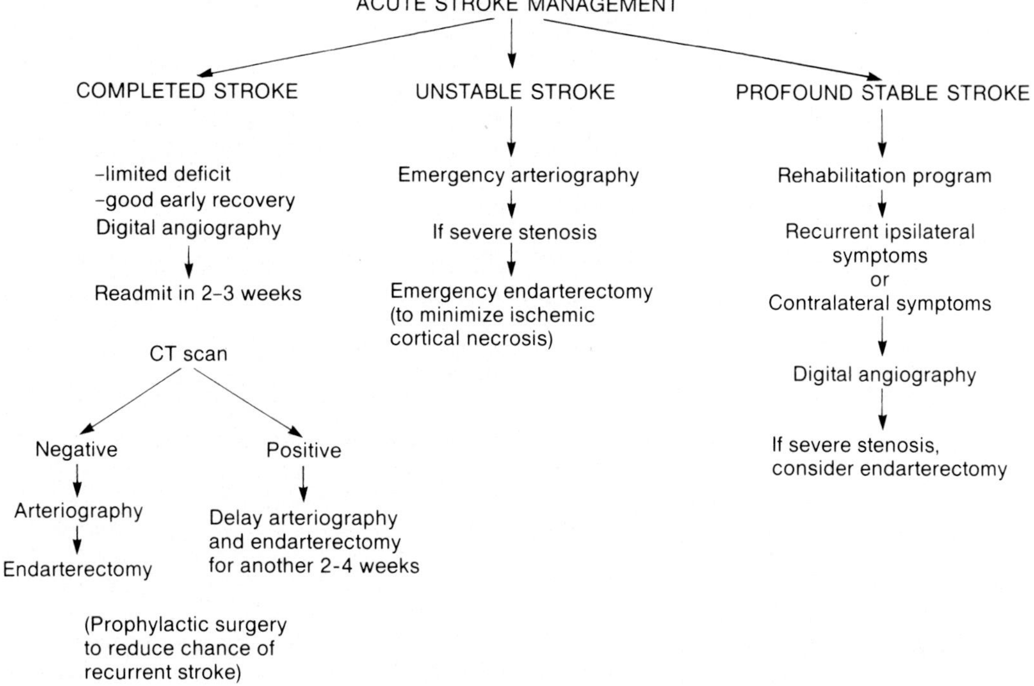

Figure 13–2. Management of patients with acute stroke.

provement with carotid endarterectomy (89 percent asymptomatic at 12 months). It should be remembered that the collateral circulation may be severely deficient in these cases, rendering the operative procedures more hazardous than usual, a factor to be weighed in considering operative intervention (Rosenthal *et al.,* 1978; Imparato *et al.,* 1982). We believe that complete assessment of the status of the blood vessels, including visualization of collateral circulation, is indicated in all cases considered for operation. At present this usually means complete arteriography of the cerebral circulation with intracranial as well as cervical projections.

REVERSIBLE ISCHEMIC NEUROLOGICAL DEFICIT (RIND)

Reversible ischemic neurologic deficit (RIND) is a term used to describe an ischemic episode that is somewhat more than a TIA. It is usually defined as a focal, presumably ischemic, deficit of brain function lasting up to two or three days with full functional recovery. Minimal residua, such as reflex asymmetries without functional impairment, are generally accepted within the definition. Although they are fairly common, whether RINDs are fundamentally different from TIAs other than in degree is not clear. They may be difficult to distinguish from very small infarcts. From a management point of view, we believe that patients having RINDs should be handled similarly to those with TIAs, including evaluation, indications for medical or surgical therapy, and selection of surgical procedure.

SMALL STROKES

By definition, lateralizing neurological deficit that persists for several days and then clears totally or almost totally is not a transient ischemic attack but represents a "small stroke," or a "ministroke." If the patient is neurologically stable, arteriography should be delayed for two weeks and at that stage arteriography should be preceded by computed tomography (CT). If the scan is negative and the arteriogram shows appropriate changes, the patient could undergo elective endarterectomy at that time; if the scan is positive, surgery and in most cases arteriography as well should be delayed for an additional four to six weeks. CT scanning has become helpful in determining the timing of operative intervention, and, in general, if the CT scan is normal, arteriography and endarterectomy can be performed with safety within two or three weeks of the initial neurological insult. Alternatively, because of the reduced morbidity and mortality risks of digital subtraction angiography, it is practical to have this study performed within one or two days of the initial small stroke to delineate the anatomy and simplify the design of the patient management.

COMPLETED STROKES

There is almost universal agreement that patients with recent severe ischemic infarction should not have operative revascularization. Some years ago Wylie (1964) and subsequently Hunter (1965) and Rob (1969) reported high operative mortality rates with revascularization of patients with acute severe strokes. Bauer and co-workers (1969), in a randomized study of 1,225 patients, confirmed these disappointing results after carotid endarterectomy in patients with acute and profound strokes. Despite the improvements in cardiovascular anesthesia and refinements in operative technique, endarterectomy still has little if any role in the management of acute profound strokes. Such patients seem to fare better under careful medical management. Among survivors of strokes, the incidence of a second stroke or extension of the original infarct is much higher than in an age-matched controlled population (Sacco *et al.*, 1982). The ultimate goal of vascular surgery in this subset is stroke prevention, and yet stroke survivors remain a high-risk group of patients. In cases with only mild residua, there is still a great deal left to lose. While we are awaiting stabilization of the original infarction, there is an opportunity to prepare the patient for surgery by treating his heart failure, cardiac arrhythmia, hypertension, ventilatory impairment, hematologic or metabolic disorders, or other risk factors. We believe that under these circumstances, given the proper anatomy of the lesion, operative intervention should be considered as a therapeutic operation. Clearly there is little to be gained by operation when the greater part of the vascular territory has already been infarcted. Severe operative risk factors, such as intractable heart failure or pulmonary disease, also make the option less attractive. The risk of recurrent stroke may be as high as 10 percent per year (Sacco *et al.*, 1982), but may be modified by good medical management—factors to be weighed in the therapeutic consideration. The role of endarterectomy in the treatment of patients with mild strokes remains controversial, due to the marked differences in the reported incidence of operative mortality, morbidity, and the incidence of late recurrent neurological deficits after carotid endarterectomy in stroke patients. Although Bardin *et al.* (1982) reported a 3.7 percent operative mortality and an immediate postoperative deficit of 4.7 percent in patients with neurological deficits, they found a 20 percent five-year incidence of recurrent stroke and concluded that endarterectomy for prevention of recurrent stroke was not superior to nonoperative treatment. The conclusion was based on a comparison made with a natural history series collated from 1968 to 1971. Their high incidence of postoperative stroke death (4.9 percent) and recurrent neurological deficits (17.5 percent) contrasts markedly with the 3.6 percent and 3.8 percent incidence, respectively, reported by Eriksson and co-workers (1981).

Although Thompson (1970) reported similar operative mortality and operative neurological deficits of 3.7 percent and 4.2 percent, his incidence of stroke in long-term follow-up study was only 10 percent. He concluded that in selected patients who had mild strokes and were in stable condition, endarterectomy lowered the incidence of late neurological deficits and resulted in improvement in neurological status beyond that expected based on the natural history of such patients. A study by McCullough *et al.* (1984) involved 118 such patients managed from January 1976 to December 1983. Fifty-nine patients were treated medically, and 59 underwent carotid endarterectomy. The preexisting neurological deficits were classified as mild, moderate, or severe and were the same in both cohorts. The long-term follow-up time in the medical cohort averaged 44.1 months and although there were nine deaths in the medical group, 12 of the 59 nonoperative patients had new neurological deficits; three of these died (at 12, 36, and 48 months) as a result of recurrent stroke. In contrast to this, only two of the 59 surgical patients had new neurological deficits, and there were no stroke-related deaths through an average follow-up time of 41.8 months. When the cumulative probability of remaining free from recurrent deficits was examined in the patients surviving at six years, all of the operative group remained free from recurrent deficits, whereas only 58 percent of the nonoperative patients had no new neurological deficits ($p = 0.02$). These data suggest that stroke patients with fixed mild to moderate neurologic deficits and with "surgical" carotid lesions may be protected from recurrent neurological complications by carotid endarterectomy. With a 1.7 percent hospital mortality rate for stroke patients undergoing carotid endarterectomy, there was a new operative neurological deficit rate of 3.4 percent; an additional 3.4 percent of patients had new neurological deficits in late follow-up study in the McCullough *et al.* series. Their review of the English literature up to the end of 1982 showed that a collective series of 1,572 patients with completed stroke were followed. During the period of follow-up study, 25 percent of the patients had a recurrent fatal stroke, and an additional 35 percent had a recurrent stroke.

UNSTABLE STROKES

In contrast to patients who sustain a major, devastating, acute stroke, a number of stroke patients have only an acute baseline deficit with waxing and waning neurologic signs. This is not to be confused with a progressive inexorable increase in the neurological deficit seen in some patients ("progressive stroke"). The clinical picture is thought to represent a modestly sized cortical defect with an additional zone of brain tissue in jeopardy because of cerebral ischemia. The management of this subgroup of patients with fluctuating neurological signs superimposed on a baseline deficit is still controversial. The goal of aggressive intervention is to restrict the size of the cortical infarct and prevent its further extension with the hope of improving the neurological deficit, even to reach full recovery. The disadvantage of endarterectomy in the acute situation is the possibility of converting an ischemic or white cerebral infarct into a hemorrhagic infarct with worsening of the neurological deficit, even to death. Mentzer *et al.* (1981) found that emergency carotid endarterectomy in 17 patients with an unstable stroke resulted in the death of one patient. Of the remaining 16 patients, none had a worsening of the neurologic deficit, four remained unchanged (24 percent), and 12 (70 percent) either recovered completely or had significant improvement with only a mild residual deficit. Of a contemporary group of patients in Mentzer's study who had unstable strokes and were treated medically, five recovered, all sustaining mild deficits (19 percent); 17 progressed to moderate or severe deficits (66 percent), and four died (15 percent). Thus, emergent carotid endarterectomy in this small subgroup of patients caused a three-fold improvement in neurologic recovery compared with the group not operated upon.

When a patient presents with waxing and waning neurological signs and is thought to have a stroke in evolution, thorough and early angiographic examination of the extracranial and intracranial pathology is important. Emergency carotid endarterectomy performed under optimal circumstances with sophisticated cardiovascular anesthesia and hemodynamic stabilization may result in significant improvement of the neurologic deficit. On the other hand, if the blood pressure is poorly controlled and the patient has a hypertensive crisis, it could result in a hemorrhagic cerebral infarction.

ASYMPTOMATIC STENOSIS

It is debatable whether a patient having only an incidentally discovered carotid bruit without cerebral ischemic symptoms should be subjected to arteriography or surgery if a stenotic lesion is found (Harward *et al.*, 1983). In such patients, the risks of the procedures, although small, may outweigh the risk of stroke. It is sometimes assumed that the degree of stenosis will progress and may cause a permanent stroke as its initial manifestation. Although this undoubtedly may happen at times, the exact occurrence rate of this scenario and the risk factors leading to it are unknown. Stenotic plaques may persist for years without symptoms, but they do tend to become larger and more stenotic with time. Stroke, however, is neither an inevitable nor usually rapid consequence. At arteriography, the finding of an unexpected total occlusion of one internal carotid artery is not rare, and bilateral total occlusions are not unheard of in patients without neurological deficits. It must be presumed that in these patients collateral circulation is adequate to compensate. Furthermore, after successful endarterectomy, plaques recur in a significant number of cases (perhaps 10 percent), sometimes at an alarmingly rapid rate (Bernstein *et al.,* 1983; Salvian *et al.,* 1983; Baker *et al.,* 1983).

The value of surgical intervention in patients with asymptomatic stenoses is debatable. There are, in our view, specific situations in which operation may be definitely justified. As previously mentioned, in cases of severe bilateral stenosis in which only unilateral cerebral symptoms are present, we usually recommend that endarterectomy on the asymptomatic side should be performed later as a second procedure (Thompson, 1979). Asymptomatic stenosis should also be operated upon in patients requiring other surgical procedures which are often associated with hypotension, severe blood loss, or fluctuations in cardiac output. Surgeons are especially concerned about asymptomatic carotid stenosis and the risk of perioperative stroke in patients undergoing major abdominal vascular procedures or cardiac operations (Emery *et al.,* 1983). In the absence of any randomized trial concerning the management of asymptomatic carotid lesions in such patients, there can be no definite consensus. Kartchner (1977) outlined the hemodynamic significance of the carotid artery stenosis in patients with asymptomatic bruits, and Thompson (1980) emphasized the practicality of this approach. In a series of 234 of Kartchner's patients undergoing cardiovascular procedures (including cardiothoracic, abdominal vascular, and peripheral vascular reconstructions), there was a 1 percent stroke rate in 192 patients with normal oculoplethysmograms (OPGs). In 42 patients with abnormal OPGs (moderate to marked carotid flow reduction), there was a 17 percent incidence of operation-related strokes. We believe that this approach is a practical one and can be easily followed. In cardiac surgical patients, who have hemodynamically nonsignificant carotid stenosis of 50 to 80 percent on angiography, the risk of perioperative stroke is probably 1 to 3 percent. Careful stabilization of blood pressure and maintenance of a high perfusion pressure during cardiopulmonary bypass (80 to 100 torrs) will help reduce the incidence of neurological deficits, and the asymptomatic carotid stenosis can be managed in the future on its own merits. In general, the value of carotid endarterectomy in asymptomatic carotid arterial stenosis is doubtful unless the operation and postoperative complications are few. Bardin (1982) stressed that the incidence of operative morality and serious morbidity must be maintained at less than 1 percent.

TOTAL CAROTID OCCLUSION

In most cases, endarterectomy of a chronically occluded internal carotid artery subjects the patient to the risks of anesthesia and surgery with little chance of long-term internal carotid artery patency. In 1980, Hafner (1981) reviewed his experience with thromboendarterectomy performed in 47 patients with total internal carotid artery occlusion. Fifteen patients (32 percent) were considered to have immediate surgical failure; in some of these, the internal carotid was even ligated at the time of endarterectomy. If the endarterectomy produced brisk back-bleeding, the operation was considered a surgical success (32 patients, 68 percent). There was excellent early patency (100 percent) in the 29 patients, studied by either invasive or noninvasive means, after "successful" endarterectomy. If the vessel had been occluded for less than a week, early patency was achieved in 100 percent of the patients. Vessels occluded for 8 to 30 days had a patency rate of 58 to 61 percent and vessels occluded for more than a month had a patency rate of 50 percent. Consideration should certainly be given to endarterectomy of a chronically occluded vessel if angiography of the contralateral carotid system shows delayed filling either in the distal internal carotid artery or in the area of the carotid bifurcation on the occluded side.

If a patient has total occlusion of one carotid artery, has a 50 percent or greater stenosis of the internal carotid artery on the contralateral side, and is having ipsilateral hemispheric symptoms, then endarterectomy of the stenotic contralateral internal carotid artery is indicated. If the contralateral carotid artery is not significantly stenosed, then consideration should be given to the performance of an extracranial-intracranial revascularization procedure on the ipsilateral side.

ACUTE CAROTID OCCLUSION

If the patient is in the hospital undergoing a diagnostic workup of his cerebral ischemic symptoms and the status of his carotid artery changes from a severe stenosis to total occlusion, aggressive intervention should be considered. Sometimes, after arteriography, the shrill, high-pitched bruit of a severe stenosis will disappear and a neurological deficit will develop. The patient may be somewhat obtunded and present some lateralizing signs. Such a scenario is optimal for prompt emergency endarterectomy. Lindberg (1980), Hafner (1981), and Donaldson and Drezner (1983) advocate that endarterectomy be performed within the first several hours after acute occlusion, before large areas of the brain have suffered irreversible damage. However, because of the extent of their collateral circulation, some patients will tolerate acute occlusion superimposed on a critical stenosis without any major neurological deterioration. In such cases we agree with Hafner (1981) that endarterectomy should be performed where possible within the first week after the occlusion. One may expect to obtain an excellent patency rate from this early intervention.

OCCLUSION AFTER CAROTID ENDARTERECTOMY

If a patient undergoes carotid endarterectomy and immediately afterward has no neurological deficits but then, while in the recovery room or intensive-care unit, develops a deficit pertinent to the endarterectomized side, acute operative intervention should be considered because there is a high likelihood that the internal carotid artery has become totally occluded. Some surgeons have OPG equipment available in the recovery room; if this test result is positive, the patient is returned to the operating room for reexploration.

The time needed for a CT scan, digital subtraction angiography, or selective carotid arteriography causes unnecessary delay before restoration of blood flow to the affected hemisphere. Lindberg (1980) in a study of six patients who had acute total occlusion (one after arteriography and five after carotid endarterectomy), noted that three of the patients had complete disappearance of their neurological deficits after emergency surgery and three remained unchanged. There is obvious diagnostic difficulty in differentiating between thrombosis of an endarterectomized vessel and an embolus from an endarterectomized and patent artery. If it is not possible to differentiate with clarity between these two pathological processes, then we agree with Kwaan *et al.* (1979) that emergency surgery should be undertaken, because there is a high likelihood of internal carotid thrombosis.

DIFFUSE BRAIN DYSFUNCTION AND NONLATERALIZED ATTACKS

It is difficult to assess and even more difficult to manage patients with recurring attacks of diffuse or widespread brain dysfunction. The symptoms are impaired consciousness, loss of motor tone, mental aberrations, faintness or dizziness, and a variety of other nonspecific symptoms. If severe, multifocal atherosclerotic vascular disease is found on angiography, it is tempting to assume that operative improvement of the blood supply will result in clinical recovery. Unfortunately, there is little to support this assumption. TIAs of the vertebral-basilar arterial system may present with a variety of symptoms, including loss of consciousness, bilateral loss of motor function, and vertigo. They are often confusing but usually recognizable by the presence of specific deficits referable to a cranial nerve or to cerebellar dysfunction. Clearly defined vertigo with nystagmus is common and must be distinguished from the vague sense of "dizziness" or giddiness. Most cases of vertebral-basilar insufficiency do not readily lend themselves to surgical correction. The vascular lesions are often widespread and surgically inaccessible. Stenosis of a vertebral artery at its origin from the subclavian may be treated by anastomosing it to the nearby carotid artery. Stenosis of the subclavian artery proximal to the vertebral orifice may produce ischemia of the vertebral-basilar territory, the "subclavian-steal" syndrome. Such a situation may be corrected by a variety of anastomotic procedures, if clinically warranted (see also Chapter 29).

Attacks of diffuse or global brain dysfunction are, in our experience, often associated with some systemic disorder, such as hypotension, cardiac arrhythmia, or metabolic derangement. Seizures, sometimes of ischemic cause, may present in this manner rather than as frank convulsions. They are usually detectable by electroencephalographic analysis and are amenable to management with anticonvulsant drugs. Global brain dysfunction with severe, widespread atherosclerosis is not usually treated by carotid endarterectomy, and the operative risk is high owing to the compromise of the collateral blood supply (Imparato *et al.*, 1982).

RECURRENT CAROTID STENOSIS

The same indications for carotid reoperation pertain as in "first-time-around" carotid endarterectomy. Because an interval of some years may have elapsed since the first operation, such patients require thorough reevaluation. A number of other changes in the vascular status are likely to have occurred in the interval, possibly requiring the modification of the therapeutic strategy. The assessment of the degree of restenosis can be obtained by noninvasive hemodynamic studies, digital subtraction angiography, and selective arteriography. If reoperation is to considered, the latter will yield precise knowledge of the limits of the pathological process. Carotid reoperations are slightly more challenging than first-time-around carotid surgery, in that the dissection may be difficult and usually takes longer. Although some investigators advocate repeat endarterectomy, it is often simpler to insert a segmental vein graft with end-to-end anastomosis to the common carotid artery proximally, and the distal end-to-end anastomosis is made to the beveled internal carotid artery. Because the surgical procedure is more time-consuming and the patient may be susceptible to wide swings in blood pressure, hemodynamic monitoring and stabilization of the blood pressure intraoperatively and postoperatively are vital.

In summary, symptoms and signs of cerebral vascular insufficiency range in duration from a few seconds to many months and correlate with the extent of cortical damage (see Figure 13–1). Early after the initial presentation, it may be difficult to distinguish a TIA, a RIND, or a stroke. The use of CT scanning early in the course of the workup of patients with a central nervous system deficit will help delineate the presence or absence of cortical damage.

The management of patients with acute strokes is summarized in Figure 13–2. The goals of surgical intervention are different in patients with a completed stroke, as compared with patients with unstable strokes. In completed stroke patients, delayed endarterectomy is prophylactic and designed to reduce the incidence of subsequent neurological problems; in the unstable stroke patients, it can be instantly therapeutic in that it can minimize the ischemic cortical damage and even cause significant improvement in the presenting neurological deficit. In patients with profound devastating strokes, the initial management is supportive; endarterectomy is indicated only in the period of late follow-up study for the appearance of recurrent ipsilateral symptoms or if contralateral symptoms develop.

REFERENCES

Baker, W.H.; Hayes, A.C.; Mahler, D.; and Littooy, F.N.: Durability of carotid endarterectomy. *Surgery,* **94:**112–15, 1983.

Bardin, J.A.; Bernstein, E.F.; Humber, P.B.; Collins, G.M.; Dilley, R.B.; Devin, J.B.; and Stuart, S.H.: Is carotid endarterectomy beneficial in prevention of recurrent stroke? *Arch. Surg.,* **117:**1401–7, 1982.

Bauer, R.B.,; Meyer, J.S.; Fields, W.S.; Remington, R.; MacDonald, M.C.; and Callen, P.: Joint study of extracranial arterial occlusion. Progress reports of controlled study of long-term survival in patients with and without operation. *J.A.M.A.,* **208:**509–18, 1969.

Bernstein, E.F.; Huber, P.B.; Collins, G.M.; Dilley, R.B.; Devin, J.B.; and Stuart, S.H.: Life expectancy and late stroke following carotid endarterectomy. *Ann. Surg.,* **198:**80–6, 1983.

Donaldson, M.C., and Drezner, A.D.: Surgery for acute carotid occlusion. *Arch. Surg.,* **118:**1266–68, 1983.

Emery, R.W.; Cohn, L.H.; Whittemore, A.D.; Mannick, J.A.; Couch, N.P.; and Collins, J.J., Jr.: Coexistent carotid and coronary artery disease: Surgical management. *Arch. Surg.,* **118:**1035–38, 1983.

Eriksson, S.E.; Link, H.; Alm, A.; Radberg, C.; and Kostulas, V.: Results from 88 consecutive prophylactic carotid endarterectomies in cerebral infarction and transitory ischemic attacks. *Acta Neurol. Scand.,* **63:**209–219, 1981.

Ford, J.J.; Baker, W.H.; and Ehrenhaft, J.L.: Carotid endarterectomy for nonhemispheric transient ischemic attacks. *Arch. Surg.,* **110:**1314–17, 1975.

Hafner, C.D., and Tew, J.M.: Surgical management of the totally occluded internal carotid artery: a 10-year study. *Surgery,* **89:**710–17, 1981.

Harward, T.R.S.; Kroener, J.M.; Wickdom, J.G.; and Bernstein, E.F.: Natural history of asymptomatic ulcerative plaques of the carotid bifurcation. *Am. J. Surg.,* **146:**208–212, 1983.

Humphries, A.W.; Young, J.R.; Beven, E.G.; LeFevre, F.A.; and DeWolfe, V.G.: Relief of vertebrobasilar symptoms by carotid endarterectomy. *Surgery,* **57:**48–52, 1965.

Hunter, J.A.; Julian, O.C.; Dye, W.S.; and Javid, H.: Emergency operation for acute cerebral ischemia due to carotid artery obstruction: Review of 26 cases. *Ann. Surg.,* **162:**901–4, 1965.

Imparato, A.M.; Ramirez, A.; Riles, T.; and Mintzer, R.: Cerebral protection in carotid surgery. *Arch. Surg.,* **117:**1073–78, 1982.

Kartchner, M.M., and McRae, L.P.: Non-invasive evaluation in management of "asymptomatic" carotid bruit. *Surgery,* **82:**840–47, 1977.

Kwaan, J.H.M.; Connolly, J.E.; and Sharefkin, J.B.: Successful management of early stroke after carotid endarterectomy. *Ann. Surg.*, **190**:676–78, 1979.

Lindberg, B.: Acute carotid occlusion: indication for surgery? *J. Cardiovasc. Surg.*, **21**:315–320, 1980.

McCullough, J.L.; Mentzer, R.M., Jr.; Harman, P.K.; Kaiser, D.L.; Kron, I.L.; and Crosby, I.K.: Carotid endarterectomy after a completed stroke: reduction in long-term neurological deterioration. *J. Vasc. Surg.*, **2**:7–14, 1985.

Mentzer, R.M.; Finkelmeier, B.A.; Crosby, I.K.; and Wellons, H.A., Jr.: Emergency carotid endarterectomy for fluctuating neurological deficits. *Surgery*, **89**:60–6, 1981.

Ouriel, K.; May, A.; Ricotta, J.; DeWeese, J.; and Green, R.: Carotid endarterectomy for non-hemispheric symptoms: predictors of success. *J. Vasc. Surg.*, **1**(2):339–45, 1984.

Rob, C.G.: Operation for acute completed stroke due to thrombosis of the internal carotid artery. *Surgery*, **65**:862–65, 1969.

Rosenthal, D.; Cosman, D.; Ledig, B.; and Callow, A.D.: Results of carotid endarterectomy for vertebrobasilar insuffiency. *Surgery*, **113**:1361–64, 1978.

Sacco, R.L.; Wolf, P.A.; Kannel, W.B.; and McNamara, P.M.: Survival and recurrence following stroke: the Framingham study. *Stroke*, **13**:290–95, 1982.

Salvian, A.; Baker, J.D.; Machleder, H.I.; Busuttil, R.W.; Barker, W.F.; and Moore, W.S.: Cause and noninvasive detection of restenosis after carotid endarterectomy. *Am. J. Surg.*, **146**:29–34, 1983.

Thomas, D.J.: Blood viscosity and arterial thromboembolism. In Warlow, C., and Morris, P.J. (eds.): *Transient Ischemic Attacks*. Marcel Dekker, New York, 1982, pages 65–80.

Thompson, J.E.: Discussion of paper by Turnipseed, Birkoff and Belser. *Ann. Surg.*, **192**:368, 1980.

Thompson, J.E.; Austin, D.J.; and Patman, R.D.: Carotid endarterectomy for cerebrovascular insufficiency: long-term results in 592 patients followed up to thirteen years. *Ann. Surg.*, **172**:663–679, 1970.

Thompson, J.E., and Talkington, C.M.: Carotid surgery for cerebral ischemia. *Surg. Clin. North Am.*, **59**:539–553, 1979.

Wylie, E.J.; Hein, M.F.; and Adams, J.E.: Intracranial hemorrhage following surgical revascularization for treatment of acute strokes. *J. Neurosurg.*, **21**:212–15, 1964.

14

Surgical Treatment of Atherosclerotic Occlusive Disease of the Cervical Carotid Artery

FRANCIS ROBICSEK

UNILATERAL INTERNAL CAROTID ARTERY STENOSIS

Atherosclerotic plaque of the carotid bifurcation, the most frequent and most likely cause of cerebral ischemia and infarction, is usually located in the area of the carotid bulb and extends 1 to 2 cm into the internal carotid artery. As the lesion progresses, it involves the orifice of the external carotid artery, and extends higher up into the internal carotid and retrograde into the common carotid. At any stage of the process, thrombosis of the carotid artery may develop.

Restoration of normal blood flow through the stenosed internal carotid artery can be achieved by one or a combination of the following techniques: endarterectomy, thrombectomy, arterioplasty, graft replacement, and bypass.

Exposure of the Carotid Bifurcation

The operation is performed with the patient in the supine posture with the shoulders supported by a rolled-up sheet and the head turned away from the operative site. Care is taken that this final position is not an exaggerated one, capable of producing kinking or exerting undue pressure on the vertebral arteries. Turning the head too far away from the operated side also causes the carotid artery to be covered by the jugular vein and thus be more difficult to dissect. A moderate Trendelenburg position usually further improves the visibility of the operative field.

The exposure of the carotid artery is achieved either through the transverse oblique submandibular approach (see Figure 14–1A) or through a straight or zigzag incision carried along the anterior edge of the sternocleidomastoid muscle (see Figure 14–1B and C). The advantage of the submandibular approach is that it follows the line of the existing skin creases; thus, scar formation is expected to be less unsightly, and is usually hardly noticeable a few months after surgery. The incision is made about a finger's breadth below the angle of the lower jaw and is carried a few centimeters posteriorly and 6 to 8 cm anteriorly parallel with the lower mandibular margin. The disadvantage of this approach is that is necessitates the development of wide skin flaps.

An alternative to the submandibular exposure is the incision which follows the anterior edge of the sternocleidomastoid muscle; its upper end arches slightly toward but stops about 3 cm short of the earlobe (see Figure 14–1B). In determining the length of the incision, it is useful to know the level of the carotid bifurcation as well as the extent and location of the pathological process as reflected by angiography. The advantage of this incision is that it provides an excellent exposure not only to the carotid bifurcation but also to a good portion of the common carotid; if necessary, it can readily be extended both upward toward the mastoid process and downward into the supra-

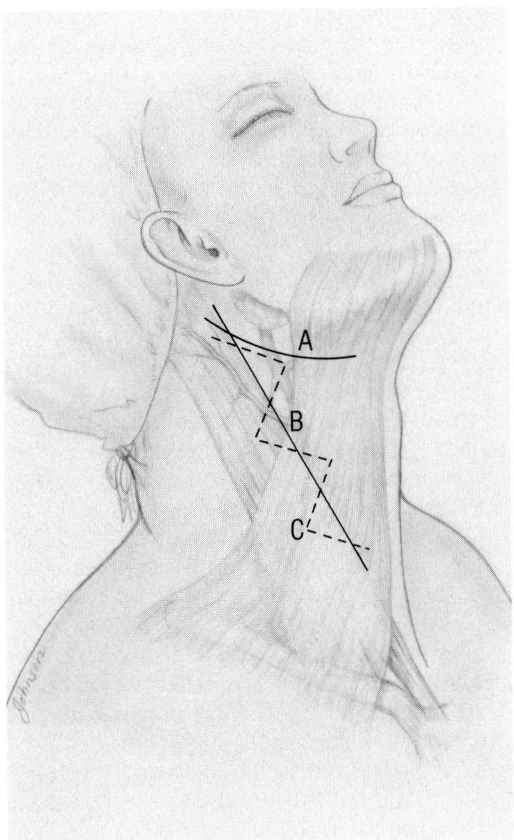

Figure 14–1. Commonly applied incisions to expose the carotid bifurcation. (*A*) Submandibular incision. (*B*) Incision following the anterior edge of the sternocleidomastoid muscle. (*C*) Zigzag exposure.

sternal notch to visualize additional segments of the common, internal, and external carotid arteries. Cicatrix formation in the skin incision may be decreased by a zigzag plastic incision (see Figure 14–1C) and by intracutaneous suture closure.

After sharp division of the subcutaneous tissue and the platysma (see Figure 3–4A), the dissection is carried along the median border of the sternocleidomastoid muscle. A self-retaining retractor may be placed in the incision to provide a convenient exposure through the rest of the operation. Continued sharp dissection is directed toward the palpable common carotid pulse. Lymph nodes are often encountered while the carotid artery is being freed. Here, the proper approach is to dissect the nodes medially and deflect them laterally. The parotid gland can easily be differentiated from subcutaneous fat by its pale color and lobulated structure. Injury to it should be avoided because it may cause postoperative pain associated with salivation or, even worse, produce a salivary fistula see (Figure 3–4B).

To expose the carotid bifurcation, it is necessary to enter the carotid sheath, a fibrous envelope that also surrounds the jugular vein. Within this enclosure, the vein lies anterolaterally and the vagus nerve is usually found behind it (see Figure 3–4C). Next, the internal jugular vein is mobilized by double ligating and dividing some of its medial branches, including the common facial vein. Once the tributaries are divided, the internal jugular vein can be retracted either medially or—as preferred by most surgeons—laterally to allow access to the carotid bifurcation. Occasionally, the hypoglossal nerve is closely attached to the common facial vein, which should be kept in mind when the latter is ligated. After opening the carotid sheath, it is best to mobilize the midportion of the common carotid artery first and then trace it toward its bifurcation as well as upstream far enough to allow sufficient control proximal and distal to the occlusive lesion (see Figure 3–4D). In this area an arterial segment that is least involved in arteriosclerotic changes is selected and encircled with a sling of umbilical tape. The external carotid is freed from its surroundings and a silastic cord is passed around it.

The internal carotid is recognized not only by its posterolateral position but also by what is more characteristic and less variable—its lack of tributaries. The common carotid artery has no branches either; however, in the case of high bifurcation, the superior thyroid or the ascending pharyngeal artery may arise from that vessel. It is important to know that, besides the great vessels, the glossopharyngeal, the vagus, and the spinal accessory nerves also lie within the carotid sheath. Relative to the carotid artery, these nerves occupy a posterior position and are therefore seldom in the way of dissection (see Figure 21–1). Owing to anatomical variations, however, some of them, especially the vagus, may lie more anteriorly and could be injured during exposure of the carotid bifurcation. One must be especially careful in passing tapes around the vessels on the medial and posterior aspect so as not to traumatize the vagus nerve, which lies in close proximity (see Figure 21–2A).

Opinions vary on the degree of dissection necessary to expose the carotid bifurcation. Some surgeons recommend freeing the common carotid and its two branches to obtain control, but also warn that the bifurcation itself should not be dissected circumferentially because this may lead to embolization from plaque or cause injury to adjacent structures, primarily nerves. We have not seen any disadvantages in careful dissection and indeed believe that although it is not an absolute necessity, completely freeing the bifurcation adds to safer control and easier management of the opened carotid.

While isolating the vessels, one should also be careful not to "overclean" them, especially the internal carotid artery, but to leave a healthy layer of adventitia attached to the walls. Otherwise, one may create a situation in which, after the removal of the atheromatous inside layers, there is very little left to suture.

With proximal control obtained, dissection is continued cephalad. To ensure sufficient mobility, the superior thyroid artery may be ligated. In general, care should be taken not to have traction on either the internal or the common carotid while dissection is carried out. Such traction can also be caused inadvertently by an inattentive assistant or simply by having heavy instruments used to "tag" the loops around the arteries hanging over the table. Traction on the carotid bifurcation, however, may be exerted using the vessel loop passed around the external carotid artery. Done properly, this will not occlude the cerebral flow as traction on the internal carotid would. After the carotid bifurcation is freed circumferentially, a silastic cord is also placed around the internal carotid artery. Braided material (tape or suture) is not recommended around the branches of the external carotid because of its "sawing" effect.

Additional exposure and better handling of the internal carotid artery may be obtained by first ligating and then dividing the tissues in the crotch of the carotid bifurcation. This not only facilitates exposure but also prevents annoying oozing into the endarterectomy site from a small artery that occasionally rises at that point.

Some recommend that the crotch of the carotid bifurcation be left alone to avoid damage to the baroreceptor mechanism (Bland *et al.*, 1970), a concern which we did not find justified in our experience. In bilateral operations, however, one may be more careful because some reports (e.g., Wade *et al.*, 1968) indicate that, whereas unilateral carotid surgery does not affect ventilatory control, bilateral carotid endarterectomy may result in loss of carotid body function and cessation of the usual compensatory respiratory and circulating responses to hypoxia.

To prevent the occurrence of bradycardia during surgery, infiltration of the carotid body with 1 percent lidocaine has been recommended (Crawford *et al.*, 1960), a maneuver we seldom found necessary in patients under general anesthesia. The possibility that postoperative transient hypertension—a frequent sequela of carotid surgery—may be blamed on the division of the sinus nerve has been suggested but not proven conclusively.

In the technique of the operation, the level of the carotid bifurcation is of crucial importance. Ideally, it should lie at the limit of the upper and middle third of the incision. Standard anatomy atlases generally place the carotid bifurcation at the height of the upper edge of the thyroid cartilage. In clinical practice, however, this statement does not hold, and the level of the bifurcation may vary significantly within the upper fifth of the area between the inferior margin of the mandible and the upper edge of the clavicle. If the carotid bifurcation is abnormally high or the occlusive atheroma extends distally far into the internal carotid artery, it is necessary to expose the latter for its maximum extracranial length. With proper measures, almost the entire extracranial internal carotid artery can be made available for repair. The once-held view (Blaisdell *et al.*, 1969) that the line drawn between the mastoid process and the caudal mandibular angle on the angiogram also represents the limits of operability is no longer tenable.

The first step in overcoming the difficulties in the exposure is to extend the skin incision, as well as the dissection, toward the mastoid process. In doing so, care should be exerted to mobilize and deflect, but not to injure the tail of the parotid gland. With unusually high carotid bifurcation, it is generally also necessary to dissect the hypoglossal nerve. As the hypoglossal nerve is reflected medially, an arterial branch is seen heading toward the sternocleidomastoid muscle. This fairly constant artery is often accompanied by a vein and occasionally participates in the formation of the so-called carotid sling, which may itself be the cause of internal carotid artery obstruction (see Figure 14–2). This artery is ligated to allow gentle retraction of the hypoglossal nerve medially and upward. In the vicinity of this nerve, blind clamping and the use of cautery should definitely be avoided. An additional

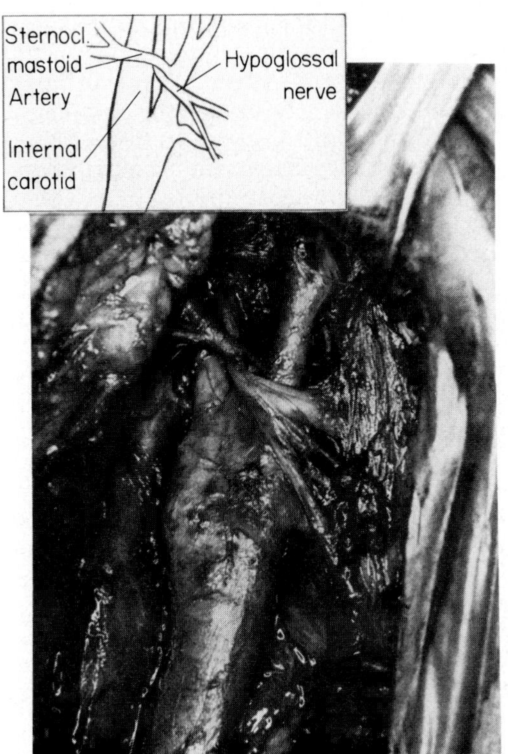

Figure 14–2. The "carotid sling." The internal carotid artery is compressed by both the sternocleidomastoid branch of the external carotid artery and the hypoglossal nerve.

technical maneuver that may alleviate exposure of the distal carotid artery is the division of the ansa hypoglossi. If the digastric and stylohyoid muscles act as obstacles to the exposure of the internal carotid artery, they can also be divided without appreciable clinical consequences. By careful dissection, avoidance of forceful retraction, and division of the sternocleidomastoid artery, the incidence of hypoglossal nerve injury can be avoided.

To obtain better exposure of the most distal portion of the cervical internal carotid artery, it was recommended (Krajicek and Kramer, 1968) that the skin incision should be made along the posterior instead of the anterior border of the sternocleidomastoid muscle and the internal carotid be exposed posteriorly to the internal jugular vein, retracting the vein anteriorly and medially.

If simpler measures fail to provide adequate access to the distal extracranial segment of the internal carotid, consideration should be given to osteotomy of the vertical ramus of the mandible, which is the major obstacle to reaching the most distal cervical portion of the internal carotid artery. The technique of this approach, originally described by Wylie and Ehrenfeld (1970) and later modified by Welsh and associates (1981), is as follows: A transverse submandibular incision is preferred; however, the incision may also be made along the anterior edge of the sternocleidomastoid muscle. In the latter case, it is advisable to extend the incision upward and angle it laterally to the level of the tragus. The main trunk of the facial nerve is identified and dissected free from its bifurcation. The masseter muscle is detached from the mandible and retracted upward. A subperiostial osteotomy is now performed on the vertical ramus of the jaw from the angle to the mandibular notch. The simultaneous rotation of the posterior segment upward and the retraction of the anterior portion forward will allow safe detachment of the digastric muscle from both the mastoid and the styloid process to provide access to the internal carotid artery at its entrance to the skull.

In our own practice we seldom apply these maneuvers. In very difficult cases, however, when access could not be obtained in the usual way, we found that the mobilization and division of the external carotid artery allows further exposure and appropriate access to the most distal subcranial portion of the internal carotid artery. Because in most cases the external carotid artery can be ligated with impunity in the presence of a patent internal carotid, this simple maneuver may "save the day" for the surgeon who struggles to obtain satisfactory exposure.

Once the carotid bifurcation is adequately exposed and sufficiently mobilized, the extent of the occlusive process already demonstrated by preoperative angiography is confirmed by palpation and observation. The most important part of this examination is observance of the color shades of the internal carotid artery. The extent and the location of the atheromatous plaque are usually clearly seen by its yellow tinge shining through the thin vascular wall. Where the atheroma ends, however, the vessel regains the pearl gray-blue color characteristic of the normal internal carotid wall. This observation will become important at a later phase of the operation when the endarterectomy itself is performed and the atheromatous plaque is removed. When the artery retains the pearl gray-blue color above the palpable lesion, one may expect that applying traction of proper strength upon the atheroma will properly "feather it off" where it meets the relatively healthy arterial segment. On the other hand, if the yellow color continues either circumferentially or posteriorly up the internal carotid artery, then it is probable that the distal end of the endarterectomy will create technical problems and require special measures, such as dividing and tucking down the intima with sutures instead of using the simpler "snatch" technique.

It should be kept in mind that every carotid artery may contain loosely attached, potentially stroke-producing thrombi (see Figure 9–20); therefore, its direct manipulation should be minimal (Baker, 1980). Similarly, palpation of the carotid artery should be performed with a very light touch, never by squeezing, because dislodgement of thrombi from atheromatous ulcers is easy and in my opinion occurs more often than is generally believed. A gentle, sensitive finger will usually accurately determine the extent of the occlusive lesion. Combining inspection and palpation with the findings of preoperative arteriography, the surgeon will be able to decide whether it is necessary to expose the artery any further.

Carotid Endarterectomy

Carotid endarterectomy with or without patch angioplasty is the most frequent operation performed in the treatment of cerebral ischemia. Although the operation is limited in anatomical extent and can be performed in a relatively short period, physiological as well as technical problems associated with the procedure are significant and numerous, the margin of technical error is narrow, and irreversible neurological damage can easily develop if any of a number of small and seemingly unimportant details are omitted. The technique described later is that which evolved on our service over the past 30 years, including alternatives occasionally used and approaches recommended by others.

The operation is usually performed under general anesthesia unless the patient has debilitating cardiac or renal disease. An effort is made to perform the operation swiftly, especially if shunts are not used, but also in a deliberate manner, with the aid of a headlight and magnifying loops.

To enter the carotid artery in the area of bifurcation, naturally all incoming and outgoing arteries must be occluded. Because the clamping of these vessels creates a cul-de-sac and a column of stagnating blood in both the internal and common carotid arteries, some recommend systemic heparinization of the patient with planned reversal at the termination of the operation to prevent clotting (Moore, 1983). Some surgeons, including myself, regularly use systemic heparinization in the course of carotid endarterectomies, whereas others do not. If a bypass shunt is not used, some recommend the injection of diluted heparin directly into the proximally occluded internal carotid artery as additional insurance against clot formation (Linton, 1955), a maneuver which we believe to be not only unnecessary but also to have its own inherent risk of embolization.

The amount of heparin given by various surgeons varies from 50 to 100 units/kg. Some surgeons reverse the anticoagulant effects of heparin after the restoration of internal carotid flow to lessen the chances of hematoma formation. Others, believing that heparin will reduce the odds of carotid artery thrombosis, would rather take the chance of hematoma formation in the wound and let the heparin effect wear out rather than neutralize it with protamine sulfate.

In clamping the vessel, one must be aware that even the most carefully constructed vascular clamp is damaging to the arterial wall, especially if the vessel is ravaged by arteriosclerosis. For this reason one should select the least "crushing" instrument suitable for the purpose and avoid repetitious clamping and unclamping as much as possible.

If no shunts are used, the common carotid artery is occluded first, a convenient DeBakey-type curved vascular clamp being applied about 2 cm below the palpated occlusive atheroma. The clamp should be applied horizontally, parallel to the commonly present posterior wall plaque so as to be less traumatic upon the intima, and should not be tightened more than necessary, just enough to prevent bleeding. Completely latched clamps, even those labeled as "noncrushing," can inflict serious damage on the carotid intima. Occlusion of the external carotid may be carried out with either conventional Braimbridge or other "atraumatic" vascular clamps or, preferably, with a Hydrogrip bulldog clamp. The superior thyroid artery, which often rises close to the origin of the internal carotid artery, may be occluded with the same clamp.

Among the vessels one must deal with in the course of carotid endarterectomy, the internal carotid artery is the one most vulnerable to inadvertent intimal damage caused by surgical instruments. Such an injury is especially dangerous because it often occurs in the unopened distal portion of the internal carotid, and, even if it is discovered, it is very difficult to repair. For these reasons we refrain from applying any clamp to the internal carotid artery and control back-bleeding with an internal balloon occluder.

After clamping of the common and external carotid arteries, a longitudinal arteriotomy is made with a No. 11 blade on the anterolateral wall of the common carotid artery proximal to the plaque. The arteriotomy is extended with angled Potts scissors, cutting across the atheroma about 2 to 3 mm beyond the plaque (see Figure 14–3B). Next, the presence or absence of back-bleeding from the internal carotid artery is determined. In patients who have well developed interhemispheric collateral circulation and are thus tolerant of crossclamping, back-bleeding is usually quite brisk. Sparse back-bleeding, however, suggests insufficient collateral circulation and intolerance to crossclamping. The assistant is now requested to gently pinch off the internal carotid artery as distally as possible with a nontraumatic vascular forceps to prevent further blood loss, which would also obscure the operative field. If necessary, the arteriotomy is further extended to permit performance of the endarterectomy in full view, so that the intimal edges either feather off or can be properly tailored. Failure to completely expose the upper end of the plaque predisposes for the development of intimal flap and thrombosis. The minimum length of the arteriotomy is about 3 cm, and on occasion a length of 4 to 6 cm is required.

In the course of the arteriotomy several precautions should be observed:

1. The incision should be carried exactly in the anterior midaxis of the internal carotid well away from the crotch of the bifurcation and never in a meandering manner.
2. The lower jaw of the scissors should follow the natural channel of the remaining lumen.
3. "Picking up" the cut edges of the internal carotid artery at this stage of the operation should generally be avoided, but if it becomes necessary, only wide-grip vascular forceps should be utilized. In retracting the cut arterial wall, the grip on the artery should be broad and the layers held together so as not to separate and break them.

After the arteriotomy is completed, all the blood and loose debris are removed by gentle irrigation with heparinized saline solution, and the interior of the artery is dried. In contrast to suction, which may further dislodge debris and loosen intima, firm compression of the operative field with a 4 × 4 cm sponge dries it immediately. After it is certain that the intraluminal exposure extends well above the upper limit of the occlusive lesion and that the lumen

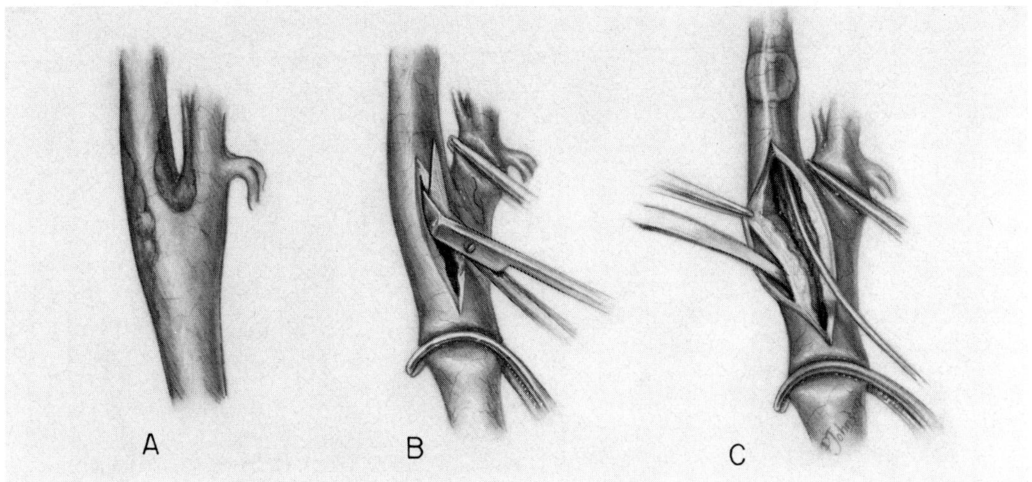

Figure 14–3. Initial steps of carotid endarterectomy. The exposed carotid bifurcation (*A*), extending the arteriotomy using Potts scissors and insertion of the balloon occluder (*C*).

is free of loose debris, an intraluminal balloon occluder is guided carefully up into the internal carotid artery and inflated just enough to stop retrograde seepage of blood (see Figure 14–3C).

The appearance and extent of arteriosclerotic plaques vary considerably. However, in most cases the atheroma begins in the most distal portion of the common carotid artery. It is thickest in the anterolateral part of the sinus, involves the origin of the internal carotid, and gradually thins as it extends upward into the vessel. It usually reaches higher on the posterior than on the anterior aspect. The atheroma can be easily separated from the media at the central part of the lesion, but this becomes more difficult at the thinner ends. The shape of the stricture is usually tubular or hourglass, which on the angiogram appears to place the origin of the internal carotid lower than it is in reality. Less often the stricture is short, ridge-shaped, or even membranous.

If the arteriosclerotic plaque extends very high, it should be approached with great care. After the operative field is dried, cleaned, and carefully inspected, the procedure should be continued without either waste of time or undue haste. The dissection plane for the endarterectomy is developed first, preferably within the common carotid artery, using a Freer elevator (see Figure 14–4). The proper plane of the endarterectomy is usually easy to recognize. Occasionally, however, it is difficult. Dissection between the intimal and medial planes which leaves a thin layer of yellowish media still attached to the wall of the artery is generally preferable though not always possible. When the endarterectomy is completed, it has the advantage of leaving behind a stronger wall which holds sutures reliably and is more resistant to arterial pressure. It can also be expected to create a much smoother separation of the atheroma in the distal internal carotid than when the operator inadvertently or by necessity carries the dissection between the media and the adventitia itself. The latter is indicated by the pink color of the remaining arterial wall. In such a situation

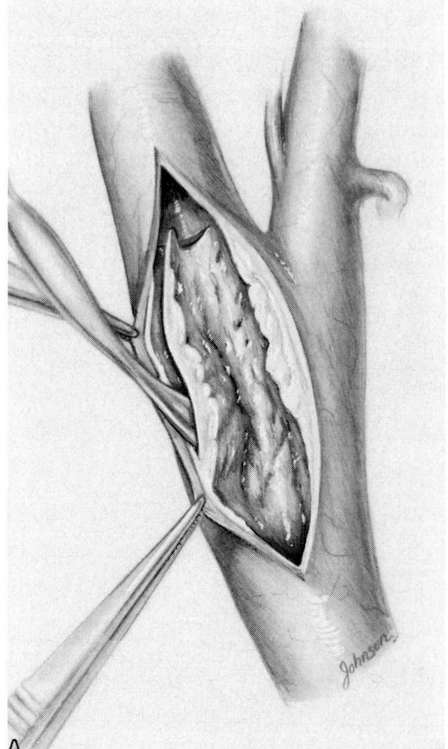

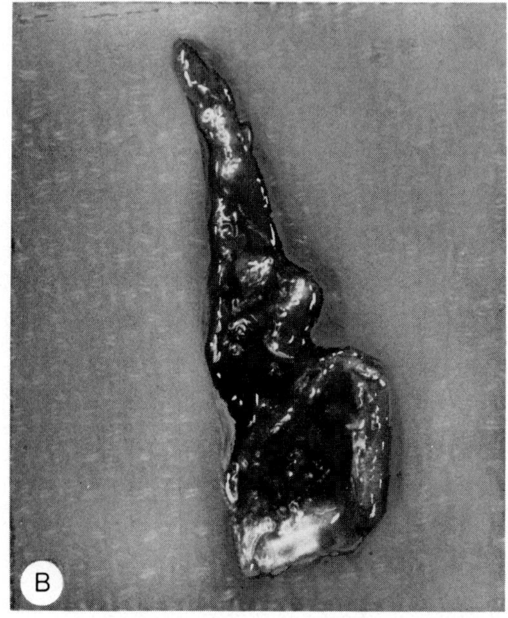

Figure 14–4. Separation of an atheroma. **(A)** Ideally, a thin layer of the media is left attached to the carotid wall. **(B)** Note the "bird beak" tapering of the distal end of this typical endarterectomy specimen that was removed from the bifurcation.

the remaining arterial wall is extremely thin and is more likely to develop tears. Also, although dissection between the media and the adventitial layer is technically easier, it is more difficult to achieve a "clean" break in the distal intima (Moore, 1983).

After the development of the endarterectomy plane, an appropriate instrument—a small, curved hemostat or the elevator itself—is passed under the dissected atheroma, and the core is then divided. In this procedure, care is taken to avoid injury to the remaining arterial wall. The distally still attached atheroma is now elevated, and the dissection is carried upward, while care is exerted to accomplish the separation in a single plane. This is achieved not by merely raising the atheromatous plaque but also by gently pushing the remaining arterial wall off the plaque rather than vice versa. The external carotid may be handled by eversion endarterectomy (see Figure 14-18), during the course of which the atheroma extending into the external carotid artery is separated from the main core, grasped with a forceps, made circumferentially as free as possible, and removed with steady downward traction during which the clamp occluding the external carotid artery is temporarily released to allow the withdrawal of the tongue of the atheroma extending into it. This method of cleaning the external carotid is the easiest; however, it may leave a strictured or even occluded vessel behind. Therefore, it is recommended that, if the external carotid artery is stenosed, it should be handled with the same painstaking technique described here for the internal carotid.

As an alternative to the foregoing method of removal of the atheromatous plaque from the bifurcation, instead of entering the arterial lumen at the beginning of the dissection, the surgeon may initially penetrate only the adventitia and the outer part of the media and then develop a plane of cleavage between the plaque and the remaining vascular wall. The inner layers are divided, and the lumen is entered only after the circumferential separation of the atheroma is completed. This method of core endarterectomy is technically more complicated, and if it has any advantages, I have not yet identified them.

As the dissection approaches the end point of the atheroma in the internal carotid artery, increased attention should be given to even minute technical details to avoid an imperfect terminal cleavage of the endarterectomy plane. To accomplish this, an effort is made to assure that the atheroma thins out distally, even if one has to seek a more superficial plane (Baker, 1980). Before the last 3 to 4 mm are dissected, the surgeon should carefully inspect the upper end of the exposed internal carotid intima. If the top of the yellow atheromatous lesion is clearly distinguishable from the residual normal grayish intima, then the atheroma is teased off with a forceps or a tonsil clamp in a movement that is a combination of traction and eversion but not elevation, while the back wall is pushed away gently with a Freer elevator. If everything goes well, the separation of the atheroma will be sharp between diseased and healthy intima, and the distal end of the removed atheroma will also demonstrate a smoothly tapered, beak-like appearance (see Figure 14-4B). The process in its swiftness and importance can best be compared with the work of a diamond cutter. If the distal margin of the endarterectomy is not discernible through the arteriotomy, the incision is extended upward to allow a more detailed inspection to ensure that the obstructive lesion is indeed eliminated and also that the intimal margin is not detached from the vascular wall.

In the removal of the plaque rents may occur in the remaining vascular wall. This usually happens if the layer of dissection is selected by either choice or necessity in a way which leaves only a very thin wall left to work with. The risk of this is particularly great if the media is markedly calcified. Correction of such tears by direct suturing is usually ineffective because the fragile adventitia that is left holds sutures poorly. Such a situation usually requires the removal of the entire injured vascular segment and replacement with an arterial substitute. The most common cause of tear in the remaining vascular wall is the forceps that holds and exerts tension on the outer layer while the inner core is being removed. It is therefore very important that the surgeon and the assistant use wide-grip vascular pickup forceps and gently hold a large segment of the outer wall instead of using finer instruments that grasp smaller bits of tissue.

If a nonocclusive, smooth intimal plaque extends up beyond safe reach in the internal carotid artery, the surgeon should not attempt the method of traction endarterectomy described previously, but instead should sharply divide the involved intima above the occlusion and tack it down with a vertically placed 7-0 polypropylene running suture. In the course of this procedure, the needle should first be

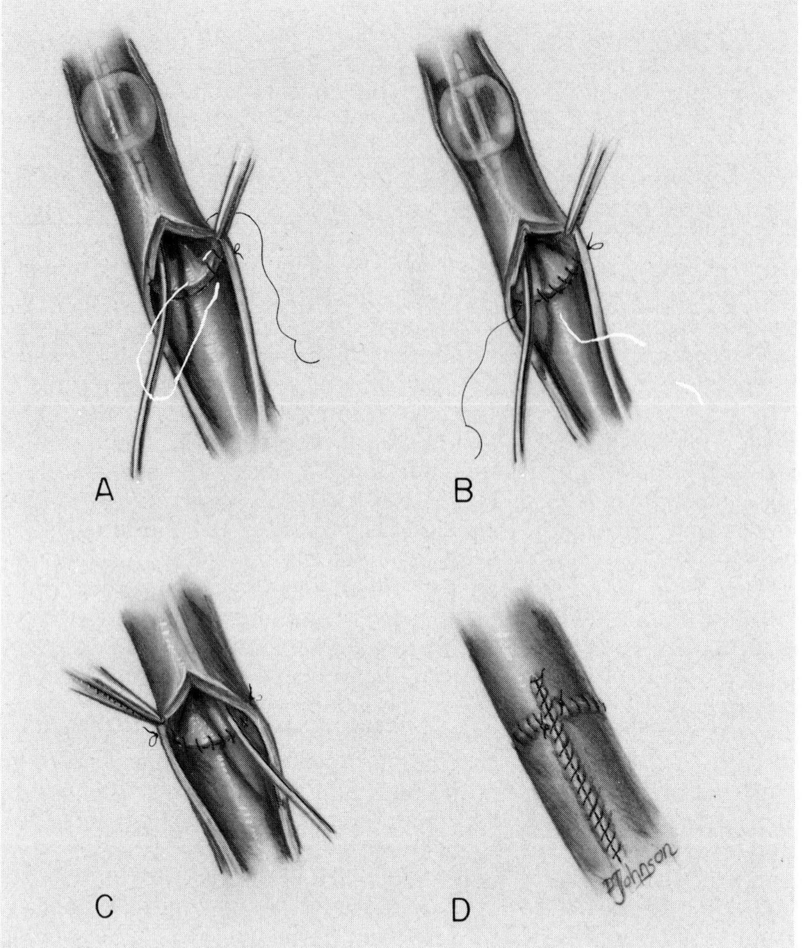

Figure 14–5. The loose distal intimal edge is attached to the carotid wall with an in-and-out continuous suture. Steps of the suture *A–C* and closure of the arteriotomy *D*.

passed from the exterior of the artery into the interior just proximal to the intimal edge (see Figure 14–5A,B), then through the intima and out and continued in this manner for the entire circumference of the artery, and finally tied on the outside (Figure 14–5C and D). Care should be taken to apply just enough tension on the suture line before tying to hold the edge of the divided intima to the rest of the vessel wall but not to "purse-string" the arterial circumference. A similar tacking-down procedure is used if after traction endarterectomy the distal intimal adherence is less than ideal.

After the removal of the distal portion of the atheroma, the smaller proximal part is extracted. Proximal endarterectomy need not be extensive and usually consists only of removal of the intimal layers to a length of a few millimeters. The proximal division of the atheromatous core is performed with scissors turned at a 45 degree angle to ensure a smooth transition (see Figure 14–6). Less than perfect handling of the proximal end of the intima is usually of no serious consequence, but leaving loose flaps may occasionally lead to proximal dissection and occlusion of the common carotid blood flow.

There are rare cases in which the stricture in the internal carotid artery is shelf- or barlike or even membranous. In such instances it may be simply "shaved off" gently with a scalpel or with fine dissecting scissors without disturbing the medial layer of the arterial wall. This technique should be applied only if the remaining interior surface is smooth and firm and shows no threat of ulceration. Because in such cases

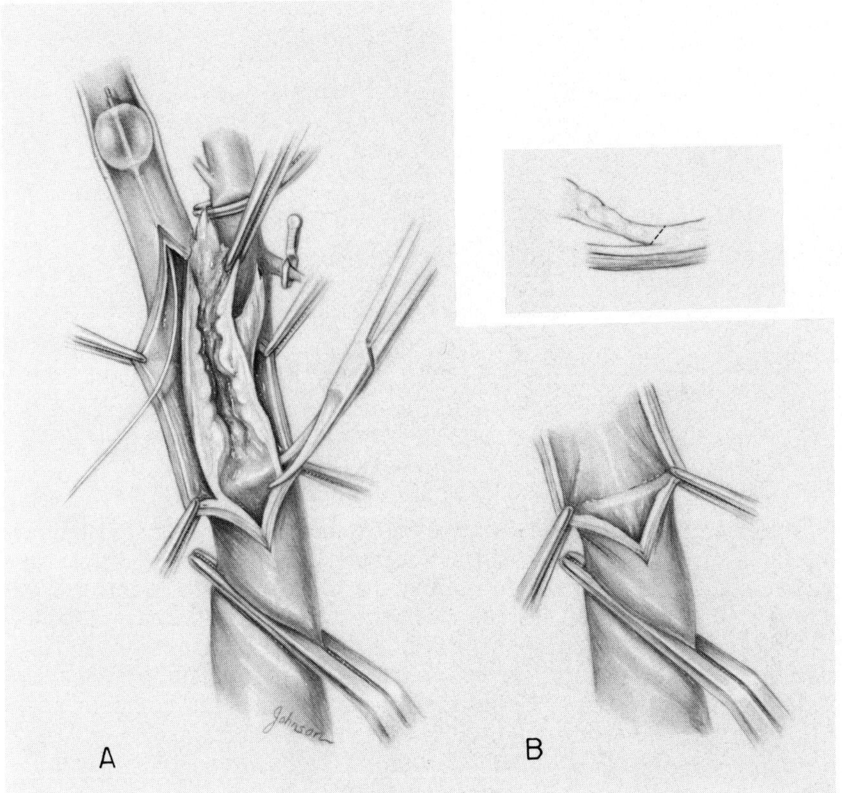

Figure 14-6. The division of the proximal end of the atheroma is performed with scissors held in a slanted position to avoid forming an undermined edge and to provide a smooth intimal transition (*A* and *B*).

the recurrence rate is expected to be high, it is advisable to supplement the removal of the obstruction with patch arterioplasty.

Before closure of the arteriotomy, the interior of the artery should be carefully irrigated with heparinized saline solution and inspected again. Under optimal conditions, removal of the thickened intima leaves a plane with a smooth inner surface and without residual irregularities. If any intimal "tags" remain, they should be removed with a fine hemostat (see Figure 14-7) or with a small pituitary rongeur. Such intimal tags can be more adequately visualized during copious irrigation with heparinized saline solution. A 6-0 polypropylene stay-stitch is placed now in the proximal corner of the arteriotomy, and the incision is closed beginning at the distal end with a 7-0 polypropylene running suture. The stitches are placed through all the remaining layers of the arterial wall just deep enough to prevent cutting through, and not more than 1 mm apart. The upper-corner stitch is critical; if placed improperly, it is the most common cause of postoperative stricture. As the suture line reaches the carotid bulb, it may be tied and changed to a 6-0 polypropylene suture, the surgeon taking deeper "bites" placed at wider intervals. If the endarterectomy has been properly performed and carefully closed, the resulting arterial lumen will be slightly larger than normal. With such judicious technique it is seldom necessary to use a patch to prevent narrowing.

Before the last stitch of the running suture is placed, the stay suture is lifted, and the lower corner of the arteriotomy is made to gape (see Figure 14-8A). The balloon occluder is deflated and withdrawn, and the internal carotid artery is allowed to back-bleed to evacuate air (see Figure 14-8B). This back-bleeding should be allowed to be vigorous but not long-lasting because it further deprives the brain of blood, and by creating a "steal" phenomenon it could cause ischemic damage.

The assistant is now again asked to gently pinch off the internal artery with a vascular forceps this time, however, at its origin so as not to allow entrapment of air in a cul-de-sac

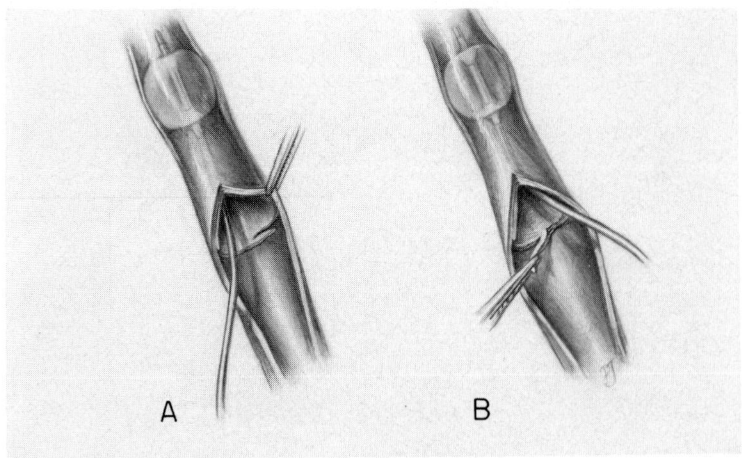

Figure 14–7. Fragile intimal edges are identified (*A*) and handled by gently pulling off the loose twigs in a lateral direction (*B*).

(see Figure 14–8C,D). The external and internal carotid arteries are then released in that order, while the proximal corner of the arteriotomy incision is kept open to evacuate any pockets of air (see Figure 14–8B and C). After the arteriotomy incision is closed, for a short time the blood flow is directed from the common to the external carotid artery to allow any further minute debris that may have been trapped in the artery to be carried into the area supplied by the external rather than the internal carotid artery (see Figures 14–9 and 14–10). After the assistant releases the occlusion of the internal carotid artery, the circulating hep-

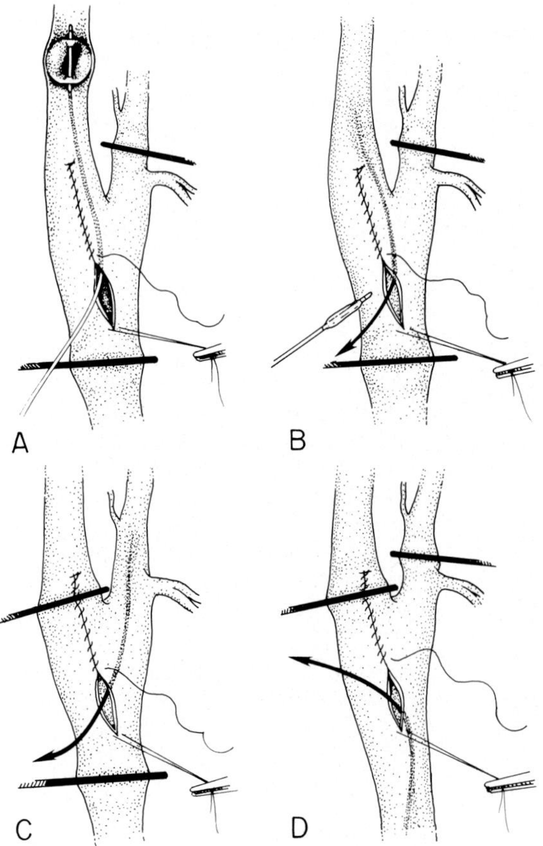

Figure 14–8. The steps for evacuating air and debris by retrograde and anterograde flushing with blood through the arteriotomy incision: The arteriotomy is left to gape (*A*); the internal carotid artery is allowed to "back-bleed" (*B*); the internal carotid artery is pinched off and the external carotid is released (*C*); the external carotid is reclamped and the common carotid artery is flushed (*D*).

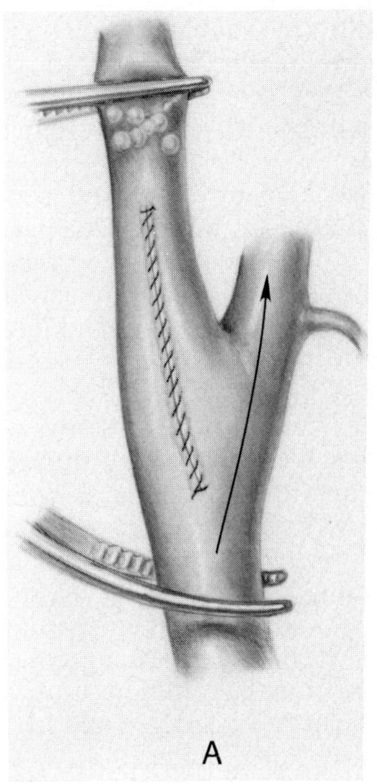

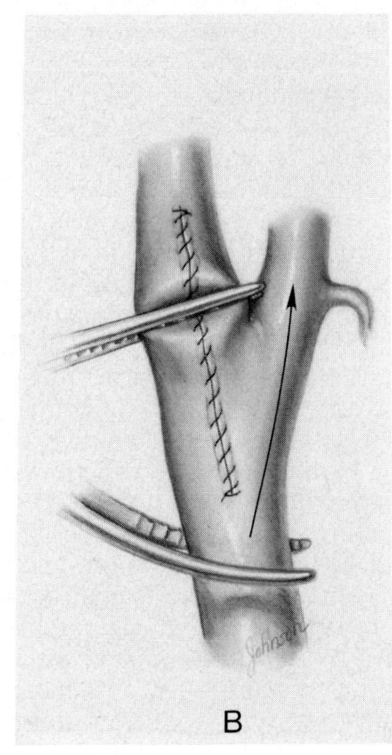

Figure 14–9. After the closure of the endarterectomy, before carotid circulation is restored, the internal carotid artery is pinched off by a hand-held vascular forceps. High application of the forceps (*A*) may lead to entrapment of air bubbles and cerebral embolization. This can be prevented by placing the forceps directly at the level of the origin of the internal carotid (*B*).

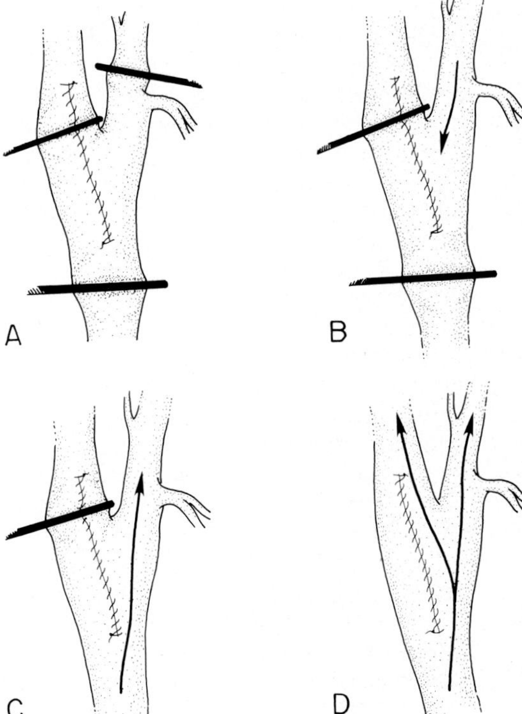

Figure 14–10. Steps for restoring blood flow after closing the arteriotomy. The clamp from the external carotid artery is removed to allow any debris and air still trapped in the bifurcation to be squeezed out through the needle holes and also to reveal any major leaks on the suture line (*A*) and (*B*). The clamp is removed from the common carotid so that any remaining debris can be flushed forward from the bifurcation toward the external carotid rather than into the internal carotid artery (*C*), and as a final step the occlusion of the internal carotid artery is released (*D*).

arin is neutralized with protamine sulfate at the rate of 1 ml for every 1,000 units of heparin. The pulsation of the entire exposed portion of the internal carotid artery is confirmed by palpation and the incision is closed in proper layers. The entire foregoing procedure should take no more than about 1½ hours to perform.

Presence of a palpable thrill after closure of the arteriotomy and reestablishment of blood flow indicates the presence of an intimal flap or a suture-induced stricture, both of which should be rectified immediately by reopening the vessel and removing the flap or by correcting the narrowing with insertion of a diamond-shaped patch.

Some degree of residual narrowing of the internal carotid artery due to leftover stenosis or improper surgical technique has been estimated to be as high as 24 to 30 percent (Blaisdell *et al.,* 1967; Rosental *et al.,* 1973). To be able to recognize and correct such a mishap, Blaisdell recommends the routine use of intraoperative arteriography (Blaisdell *et al.,* 1967). Although the measure is worthy of consideration if doubts exist, we found its routine use unnecessary. We also believe that the arteriogram itself may constitute a hazard because a moderate surgical insult to the brain is inevitable even when the operation is performed with the utmost care and that this insult can be further potentiated by the trauma of an arteriogram performed immediately afterward (See also Chapter 18).

Temporary Shunts. The technique of endarterectomy described previously is modified somewhat if internal shunts are applied.

Among the various shunts available, we feel that the Javid shunt has the best flow characteristics. Before it is inserted, the interior of the shunt should be filled with heparinized saline solution because small air bubbles sometimes adhere to its walls when filled with blood. The proximal end of the Javid shunt is inserted into the common carotid, while the surgeon occludes the latter by pulling the encircling tape against the compressing index finger (see Figure 21–2B). After the proximal end of the shunt is safely in place and held in position by a special ring clamp, blood is allowed to squirt freely from the distal end before the distal end is inserted into the internal carotid, where it is held with a smaller ring clamp. It should be emphasized that the insertion of the distal end of the shunt requires extreme caution to ensure that no atherosclerotic particles are pushed into the internal carotid and from there injected into the cerebral circulation. Similarly, the shunt must be checked and rechecked to be sure that there are no air bubbles in it before the clamp on the shunt is released (see Figure 21–3).

While the endarterectomy is being performed, one must take care that the distal portion of the shunt is not brought into a vertical position because this may cause a T-shaped tear in the upper corner of the endarterectomy which is difficult to repair without causing a stricture (see Figure 21–4).

Another popular shunt is the Pruitt device, which is available in "straight" and Y-shaped varieties (see Figure 19–4). Compared with the Javid shunt, the Pruitt device has the advantage of occluding the vessels with balloons; thus, it is less traumatic than the ring clamps supplied with the Javid shunt. The disadvantages are the smaller lumen and the danger that it may be dislodged from the common carotid.

After completion of the endarterectomy, the arteriotomy is partly closed by starting a running suture of 7-0 polypropylene from the upper end and carrying it down about two-thirds the length of the incision. There the suture is tied, and a new suture line of 6-0 polypropylene is started. Thus, if during the final steps of suturing or tying the knot, which are sometimes carried out in haste, the suture breaks, then the surgeon is not obliged to redo the entire arteriotomy closure, but only its proximal portion. After about two thirds of the incision is closed, a 6-0 polypropylene suture is placed in the proximal end, the shunt is removed, the carotid arteries are occluded, and the arteriotomy suture line is completed and tied to the 6-0 "holding" suture. To decrease cerebral ischemia time, some recommend closing the last part of the arteriotomy with a partially occluding clamp (Thompson and Talkington, 1976). Although this method may shorten carotid crossclamp time by a minute or two, it also makes closure cumbersome and traumatic to the thinned arterial wall. Therefore, in our opinion, unless there are extraordinary reasons for haste, such a clamp should not be applied.

Regarding the use of shunts, surgeons can be divided into three categories: (1) those who always shunt, (2) those who never shunt, (3) those who shunt when they believe that it is specifically indicated in an individual case.

The presumed advantage of the indwelling shunt is theoretical and lies primarily in the following postulates: (1) interruption of the internal carotid flow during carotid endarterectomy may cause severe, even irreversible, cerebral ischemia, and (2) this problem can be prevented by appropriate application of internal shunting. Therefore, the use of a shunt makes no sense unless it is applied within 30 to 45 seconds after the clamping of the carotid artery. To facilitate this, all necessary instruments and shunts should be prepared and made ready before the carotid artery is occluded so as to shorten the period of ischemia.

The disadvantages of the indwelling shunt are technical and believed to be twofold: (1) it increases the danger of cerebral embolization of both air and debris, and (2) because of its position and bulk it makes the technique of endarterectomy more cumbersome. Whereas the first disadvantage is generally acknowledged—even if only to a slight degree—the second is denied by some who maintain that the presence of this firm tube within the fragile endarterectomized vessel has the definite advantage of acting as a stent, aiding significantly in an exact arteriotomy closure. Experience and caution will certainly decrease but not eliminate technical complications caused by the use of indwelling shunts.

Among the various means of assessing the necessity of shunting, the following should be mentioned:

Preoperative data:

1. Arteriographic demonstration of cross-filling from the contralateral hemisphere.
2. Demonstration of a contralateral carotid obstruction.
3. Assessment of neurological status during a trial period of carotid compression.

Intraoperative data:

1. Assessment of neurological data during a trial period of aortic clamping while the patient is under local anesthesia.
2. Electroencephalographic monitoring.
3. Observation of the force and amount of carotid backflow.
4. Measurement of carotid back pressure.

Probably the most important available preoperative data are angiographic findings that indicate impairment of blood flow owing either to poorly developed interhemispheric collaterals or to contralateral carotid artery occlusion, both of which are probably the most clear-cut indications for shunting. We believe that the danger of intraoperative cerebral ischemia is especially high in patients with occluded contralateral carotid arteries, and in these we use temporary indwelling shunts whenever it is technically feasible regardless of physiological indicators.

Crawford and associates (1960) and Dillon and associates (1965) first suggested that the cerebral collateral circulation might be quantitated more accurately by measuring the internal carotid artery back pressure instead of merely estimating the amount of backflow. Moore and Hall (1969) recommended using the same index to determine the tolerance of crossclamping as a means of indicating the need for a temporary indwelling shunt. Back pressure can be obtained through a short 20-gauge needle connected through a fluid-filled flexible extension tube to a strain gauge and oscilloscope, then inserted into the common carotid artery proximal to the stenosing atheroma. After proper position of the needle has been ascertained, the external carotid and the proximal common carotid artery are temporarily clamped. The curve on the oscilloscope at that stage represents the blood pressure in the internal carotid artery which is being fed entirely through collaterals from the contralateral hemisphere and from the vertebral-basilar system. It is believed by those who recommend selective shunting that a back pressure of 50 mm Hg indicates a satisfactory collateral circulation (Wylie, 1980), in the presence of which carotid occlusion of up to 30 minutes can be tolerated well (Hays *et al.*, 1972), and the use of a temporary indwelling shunt is not necessary. Others place the "safe" level of back pressure at a much lower level, such as 40 or even 25 mm Hg (Moore *et al.*, 1967).

Hertzer *et al.* (1978) found that operations performed without shunts in the presence of low carotid back pressure produced a disproportionately high number of permanent strokes (6.9 percent), whereas patients with high back pressure had a low incidence of strokes whether or not shunts were used. Moreover, there was some indication that the use of shunts in the presence of high back pressure increased the occurrence of neurological deficits.

For guidance in our own clinical practice, our group undertook a retrospective study encompassing a total of 281 carotid arterioplasties performed in 265 patients during the period from June 1979 to March 1983 at the Department of Thoracic and Cardiovascular Surgery of the Charlotte Memorial Hospital and Medical Center. The operations were about equally divided among five board-certified surgeons specially trained in vascular surgery, each with more than 10 years' clinical experience and all working in a close clinical partnership. They used comparable surgical techniques; worked with the same neurologic consultants, anesthesiologists, and assistants; and shared the duties of postoperative care. The main—probably the only significant—difference in their methods was that four of the five surgeons (myself among them) routinely used intraoperative shunting unless the anatomical situation made it inadvisable, while the fifth surgeon, somewhat to the disapproval and annoyance of the other four, applied the shunt only in a few cases of severe bilateral disease. There was also some difference among the surgeons regarding the use of heparin during carotid artery occlusion. Carotid artery back pressure, or cerebral function, was not monitored in any of the patients.

The main variables considered in the study were (1) sex of patient, (2) age of patient, (3) surgeon, (4) contralateral disease, (5) heparinization, (6) crossclamping time, (7) simultaneous heart surgery, (8) bilateral surgery, and (9) utilization of temporary shunt.

The answer to the major question of the study is summarized in Table 14-1. That is, there was no statistically significant difference in the outcome of the operation (failure versus success) regardless of whether a shunt was used.

In evaluating the results of our study, we must return to the basic postulate that the ultimate goal of carotid arterioplasty is the prevention of stroke. It is a diabolical paradox that "the condition the operation is designed to prevent is also its most dreaded side effect" (Collins *et al.,* 1978). The divergent opinions on exactly how an intraoperative stroke occurs probably relate to basic theory about why stroke occurs in carotid disease at all. The "ischemists" believe that neurological deficit which may occasionally develop during carotid surgery is the direct consequence of the temporary interruption of the carotid blood flow (Thompson and Talkington, 1976; Thompson, 1979). The "embolists" attribute the cerebral damage to embolization from the operative site. The school to which one belongs may determine the nature of the prevention efforts: the ischemists will try to minimize the time of ischemia and will employ temporary shunts whenever possible as a measure which "often helps and never hurts," whereas the embolists will concentrate on atraumatic technique, will not go out of their way to minimize crossclamp time, but will forgo the use of an indwelling shunt as a measure that may predispose to embolization (see also Chapter 19 on temporary shunts).

Carotid Arterioplasty

If the diameter of the internal carotid artery is very small or if the edges of the arteriotomy hold sutures poorly, a patch arterioplasty may be advisable. Since the introduction of microtechnique and fine monofilament sutures, the lumen of the internal carotid artery is seldom compromised by simple direct closure, and patch angioplasty is utilized less frequently. The disadvantages of patching are that it somewhat prolongs the operative time and that theoretically it may act as a seat for mural thrombus. Reoperations for internal carotid artery stricture almost always require patch arterioplasty. We prefer patch materials that are soft and pliable because they allow the use of fine sutures. The ideal patch material is the patient's own saphenous vein. In our experience, segments of bovine heterograft and Gore-Tex synthetic graft also gave satisfactory results (see Figure 14-11). Patch arterioplasty must be performed carefully because the procedure may offer a false sense of security owing to the appearance of a wide lumen at the center of the graft. However, stenosis can easily occur

Table 14-1. Surgical Outcome (Success or Failure) Comparing Shunt versus No Shunt.

SHUNT/NO SHUNT	DEATH WITH STROKE	+	DEATH WITHOUT STROKE	+	STROKE WITHOUT DEATH	=	TOTAL FAILURE RATE (%)	TOTAL SUCCESSFUL RATE (%)
Shunt	3		2		4		9 (2.9)	299 (97.1)
No shunt	1		2		3		6 (4.7)	122 (95.3)

No significant difference in outcome (success or failure) whether or not a shunt was used ($G = 0.80$, $df = 1$, $p = 0.37$). Note that the failure rate was slightly lower when a shunt was used (2.9 versus 4.7 percent), but this difference could be due to chance. Splitting the failures into (1) deaths with strokes, (2) deaths without strokes, and (3) strokes without deaths reveals no significant trends whether or not a shunt was used.

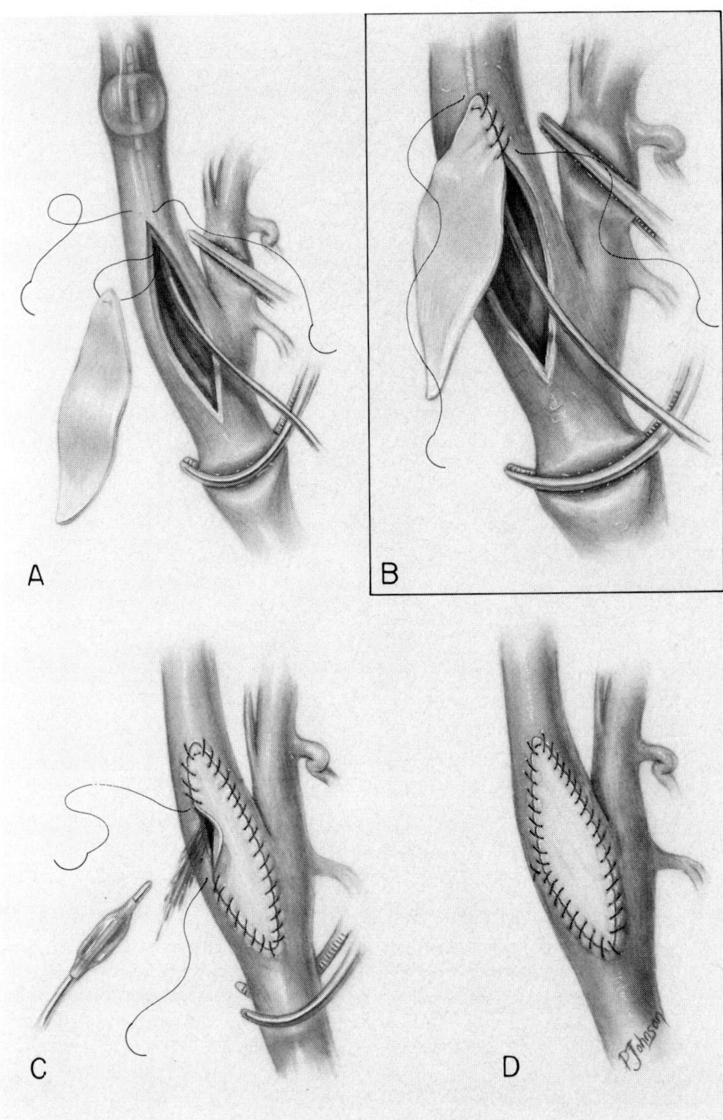

Figure 14–11. Steps in performing a carotid patch arterioplasty. The suturing of the patch begins at the upper corner of the arteriotomy incision (*A*) and continues clockwise (*B*). Before the final stitches, the vessels are flushed both anterograde and retrograde (*C*). The completed patch arterioplasty (*D*).

at the distal end of the patch if the suturing is not performed properly.

An alternative method of enlarging the initial portion of the internal carotid artery is to utilize the adjacent external carotid artery to perform an arterioplasty. This procedure can be performed in two ways; one method sacrifices the external carotid, while the other does not. In the first method, the external carotid artery is dissected free in the necessary length, and the first branches are double-ligated and divided. The common and internal carotid arteries are occluded, the external carotid is divided 2 to 3 cm above its origin, the distal stump is ligated, and the proximal stump is left open. A V-shaped arteriotomy is now performed on the anterior surface of the internal carotid artery, the incision beginning at the appropriate point past the segment to be widened, then curled through the carotid bulb and carried up into the stump of the divided external carotid. After the endarterectomy is completed, the edges of the two branches of the arteriotomy are sutured together in such a way as to apply the proximal external carotid as a live "patch" to the narrowed internal carotid artery (see Figure 14–12A).

Similar results can be obtained but without sacrificing the external carotid by following the more recent "carotid bifurcation advance-

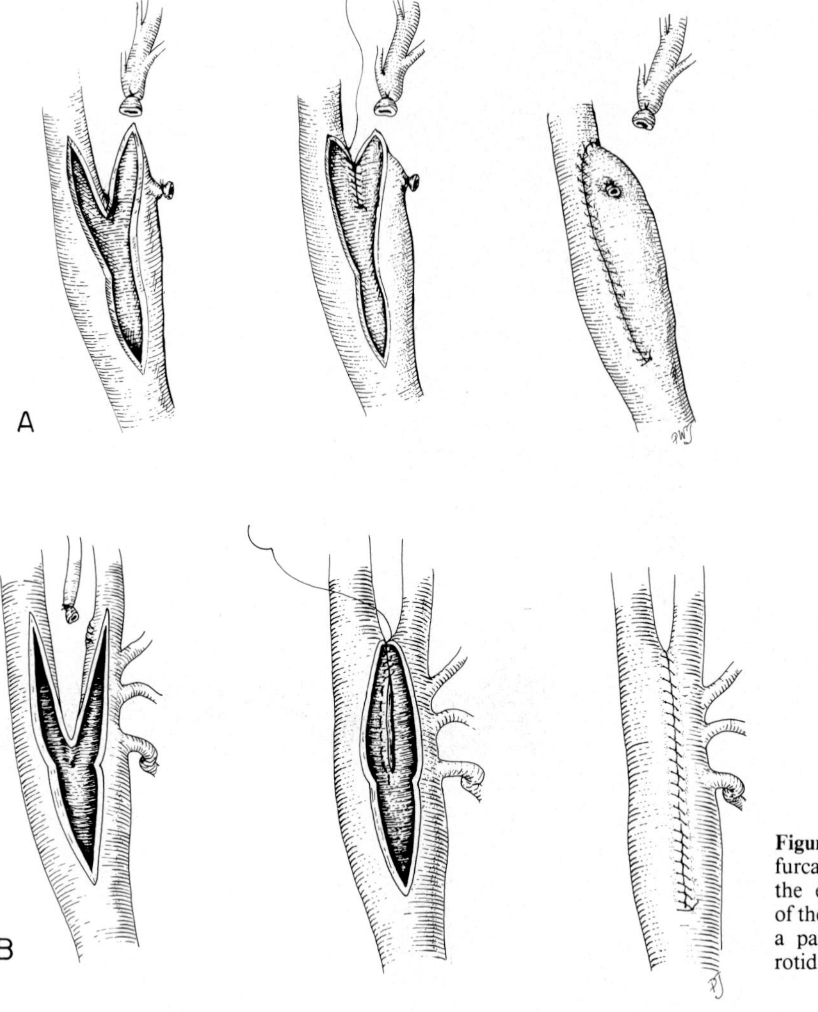

Figure 14–12. **A:** Carotid bifurcation arterioplasty using the endarterectomized stump of the external carotid artery as a patch-in-continuity. **B:** Carotid bifurcation advancement.

ment" procedure of Rosenman and associates (1984). The arteriotomy is performed in the manner described in the preceding paragraph. The external carotid artery, however, is left undivided (see Figure 14–12B).

Graft Replacement

In rare situations, arteriosclerotic damage to the vessels is advanced to such a degree that endarterectomy-even endarterectomy with arterioplasty—will not suffice. Excision of the diseased segment of the internal carotid artery with end-to-end anastomosis is now seldom utilized. Today most such cases are handled by replacement of the internal carotid artery with autogenous saphenous vein or by a synthetic graft. Replacement of the internal carotid artery is seldom required in arteriosclerosis but is more often necessary in fibromuscular hypertrophy or hypoplasia, traumatic lesions, or posttraumatic stenosis.

As stated previously, the ideal graft material for the carotid artery is the autogenous saphenous vein because of its size, pliability, and resistance to infection. If grafting has not been anticipated at the exposure of the artery, however, it is somewhat cumbersome to redrape the patient and expose and remove the saphenous vein. In the carotid area we found Gore-Tex vascular grafts especially useful because they can be handled with ease and anastomosed with very fine suture material even to small, fragile vessels like the internal carotid artery. Other graft materials of the surgeon's preference, such as woven and knitted Dacron grafts, can also be used, especially for larger vessels such as the common carotid artery.

If the carotid bulb is to be preserved, the grafting may be used in a combination of arterial replacement and patch angioplasty. The involved portion of the internal carotid artery is cut off with the carotid bulb in an oblique fashion together with a portion of the carotid bulb itself (see Figure 14–13A). Distally, the internal carotid artery is cut straight across in a fashion to form a "cobra head." The ends of the graft are cut accordingly (see Figure 14–13B), and the anastomoses (the distal first) are made with a 7-0 polypropylene running suture distally and a 6-0 polypropylene running suture proximally (see Figure 14–14C and D). Again, extreme care is exercised to expel air from the graft before the last suture is tied to prevent embolization. Another modality for performing the proximal anastomosis is resection of the carotid bulb, ligation, and division of the external carotid artery, and end-to-end anastomosis between the graft and the common carotid artery.

The radical approach to the management of carotid bifurcation lesions presented by Cormier and Ricco (1983) in some respects returns to the principles of the first operations for carotid occlusion. Because they believe that late embolization may occur from debris at the endarterectomy site or from the site of the endarterectomy, they recommend that the proximal portion of the diseased carotid artery be permanently excluded or removed and the continuity of blood flow to the internal carotid artery reestablished by means of a saphenous vein, anastomosed end to side to both the common and to the divided internal carotid artery. The procedure is as follows:

After the patient is systemically heparinized, the common carotid and its two tributaries are clamped. A suitable site is selected on the anterolateral aspect of the common carotid artery proximal to the atheromatous plaque, and a 3 mm incision is made on the arterial wall with a No. 11 blade. Using a punch, sized appropriately to the caliber of the saphenous vein and inserted through the arteriotomy, a 4 to 5 mm diameter circular hole is cut into the carotid wall. The proximal end of the reversed vein graft is beveled at a 45 degree angle and medially incised to form a "cobra head" and

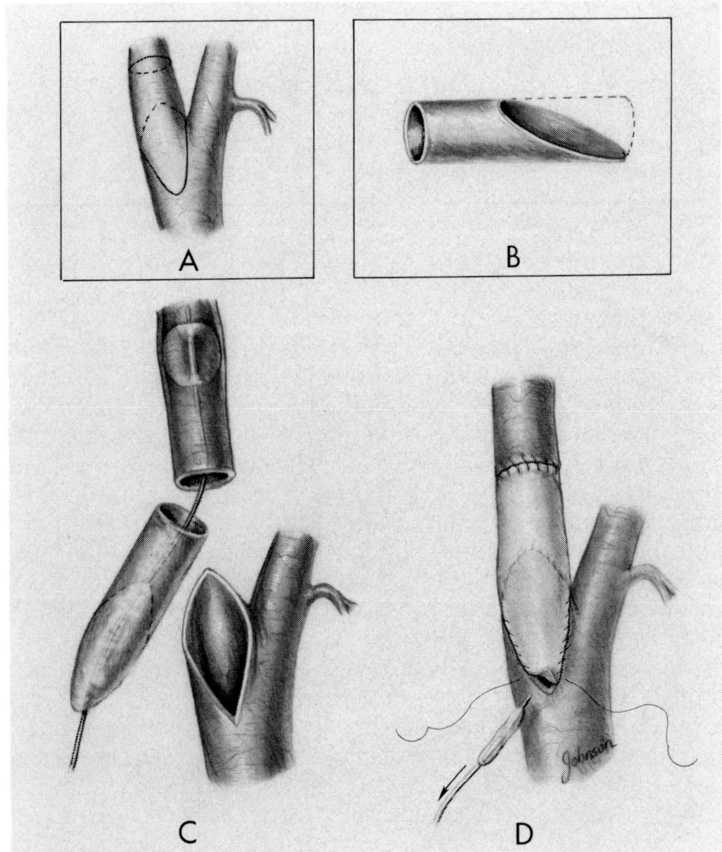

Figure 14–13. Graft placement on the proximal internal carotid artery. The line of arterial resection (*A*), the appropriately tailored graft (*B*) which is positioned through the balloon occluder (*C*). The latter is removed before the final sutures are placed (*D*).

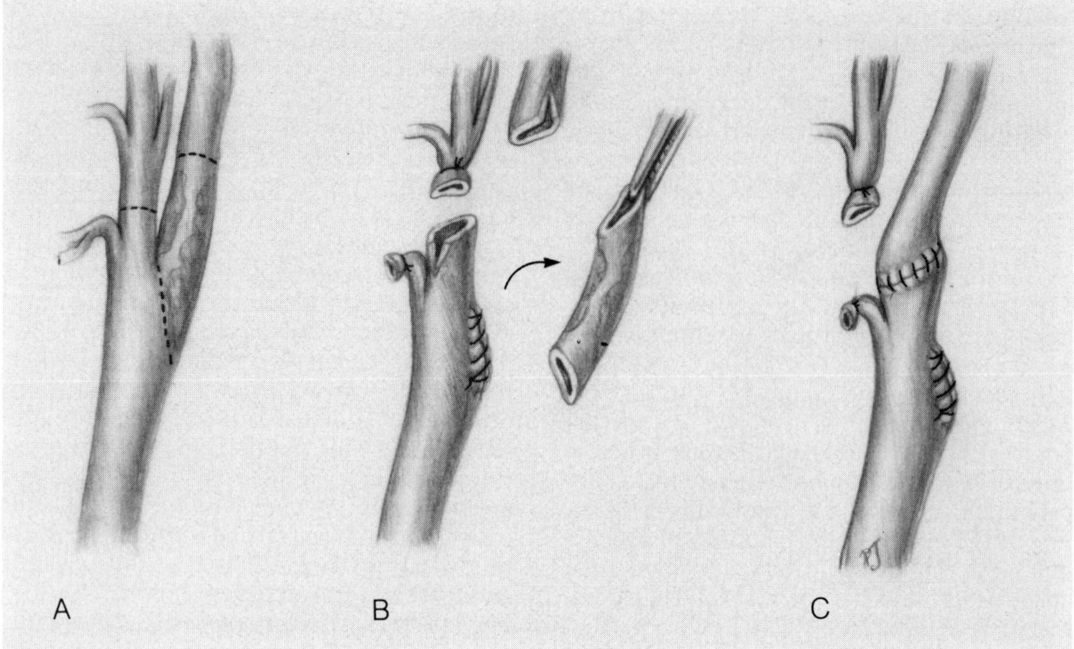

Figure 14–14. The carotid "switch" operation. Outline of the arterial resection (*A*), removal of the diseased segment of the internal carotid artery (*B*) and anastomosis between the proximal stump of the internal and the distal stump of the external carotid arteries (*C*).

then anastomosed end to side to the common carotid artery.

After the anastomosis is completed, all occluding clamps are removed to allow blood flow to the carotids and at the same time to fill the saphenous vein graft and thus facilitate the measurement of its proper length. After this maneuver the clamps are reapplied, and a 5 mm incision is made on the lateral aspect of the internal carotid artery to which the beveled distal end of the vein graft is now anastomosed end to side with a 7-0 running polypropylene suture. Before the final sutures of the anastomosis are taken, the graft as well as the internal carotid artery are flushed first retrograde then anterograde. Before reestablishment of internal carotid flow, the internal carotid artery is permanently occluded at its origin to prevent embolization and propagation of thrombosis from the stenotic plaque. An alternative method to in situ ligation is resection of the involved carotid segment and "flush" through the proximal and distal stumps, as recommended by Cormier and Ricco (1983). If the atheroma extends into the carotid bifurcation, it also should be removed by endarterectomy.

Cormier and Ricco used this procedure in 246 patients with unilateral carotid disease with a neurological complication rate of 0.8 percent. In their complete series, a mortality rate of 0.6 percent and a neurological complication rate of 1.6 percent were reported. The drawbacks to the technique are the prolonged crossclamp time, the necessity for more extensive dissection of the internal carotid artery, and the fact that a vein must be harvested.

Carotid Switch Operation

The first portion of the internal carotid artery may also be replaced with the in situ initial portion of the external carotid. In the course of the operation the proximal portion of the internal carotid artery containing the occlusive lesion is resected. The hole on the carotid bulb is sutured off at an angle to streamline the flow toward the external carotid artery. The distal stump of the internal carotid is held in a Hydrogrip atraumatic vascular clamp. The proximal portion of the external carotid artery is now mobilized in a length corresponding to that of the resected internal carotid segment. Branches rising from this portion are double-ligated and divided. The external carotid is now cross-sectioned at the level of the distal internal carotid stump. The distal end of the divided external carotid artery is ligated and using 7-0 monofilament continuous suture and microsurgical technique an end-to-end anastomosis is performed between the beveled ends of the proximal external and the distal internal carotid arteries (see Figure 14–14).

This procedure has the advantages of eliminating the use of synthetic or vein grafts and requiring only one anastomosis. However, it sacrifices the external carotid, which, in case the internal carotid fails to remain patent, may be a crucial collateral pathway. From a technical standpoint, the operation is rarely feasible because heavy arteriosclerotic changes are seldom limited to the initial portion of the internal carotid only and usually involve the origin of the external carotid artery as well.

BILATERAL INTERNAL CAROTID ARTERY STRICTURE

Bilateral internal carotid artery strictures present their own particular problems. These problems, however, are connected with indication, timing, and risk rather than with the operative technique.

The risk of surgery in a patient with severe bilateral carotid stenosis in terms of postoperative stroke is considerably higher than that in a patient with unilateral lesions (Baker *et al.*, 1977; Collins *et al.*, 1978). The reason is that when one of the internal carotids is temporarily occluded during surgery, because of the contralateral stricture, the collateral flow to the side being operated upon is more likely to be inadequate, and severe ischemia to the corresponding cerebral hemisphere is more likely to develop.

High rates of postoperative problems for bilateral stenoses have been reported by several investigators, stroke being the most frequent complication. Lees and Hertzer (1981), for example, found that the postoperative neurological deficit rate was more than four times greater in patients with bilateral severe carotid artery disease than the rate in those who had unilateral carotid artery stenosis only. Halstuk *et al.* (1984) reported a perioperative stroke rate as high as 8.3 percent. Although opposing views have been expressed by others (Fleming *et al.*, 1977; Moore, 1972; Patterson, 1974; Sundt *et al.*, 1977), common sense dictates that bilateral carotid lesions should be handled especially carefully and that every possible precaution should be taken to avoid an operative disaster. In our patient data we found no statistically significant difference in the occurrence of perioperative strokes in patients with unilateral and bilateral lesions; however, we believe this is because the patients were handled with special care and extraordinary attention. Because the principal danger in the repair of bilateral carotid stenosis is undoubtedly the period of brain ischemia during crossclamping, the application of a temporary indwelling shunt is especially recommended in these cases.

An important question in the management of bilateral strictures is which side should be operated upon first? If the symptoms are hemispheric, most investigators agree that the carotid supplying the involved cerebral area should be operated upon first. If, however, there are symptoms of global ischemia, the proper choice is to address first the side on which the stricture appears on the angiogram to be more severe. If the severity of the stenoses is about the same and the symptoms involve both hemispheres, we recommend operating on the right carotid first in a right-handed person. The reason for this is that in bilateral operations, because of the contralateral stenosis, the first procedure carries a higher risk of intraoperative stroke; if such an event should occur, it would not affect right-hand movement and speech. Naturally, every possible effort should also be made to shorten the time of surgically induced ischemia.

It has also been recommended (Imparato, 1978) that in the order of surgery the dominance of the individual carotid artery, i.e., the carotid artery that supplies the larger areas of brain tissue, should also be considered. According to this principle, it is less dangerous to operate first on the carotid that supplies a lesser area of brain tissue.

The next question is if the symptoms of cerebral ischemia point to only one hemisphere, should the patient undergo unilateral carotid repair on the symptomatic side only, or should both carotid arteries be operated upon? Opinions differ widely on what to do about a contralateral lesion in an asymptomatic patient who has undergone carotid surgery. Older studies limited to a small body of patient data and usually to a short follow-up period (Johnson *et al.*, 1978; Humphries *et al.*, 1976) suggest a relatively low probability that the contralateral asymptomatic lesion will become symptomatic. The more recent and larger series of Thompson *et al.* (1978) and Podore *et al.* (1980), however, seem to indicate that there is a much higher incidence of stroke and transient ischemic attacks attributable to the contralateral lesion and that patients with bilateral carotid artery disease should always be advised to undergo staged carotid endarterectomies. This view has been supported by extensive, long-range observations of Riles *et al.* (1982), who proved that the appearance of late postoperative stroke in carotid disease can be significantly reduced if (1) in single-vessel carotid disease after unilateral endarterectomy the contralateral side is closely monitored and (2) in a case of bilateral disease the stenosis is alleviated on both sides.

The next question that may arise in connection with bilateral carotid endarterectomies is when should the second operation be performed? It is believed (Satiani *et al.*, 1978) that staging of the second endarterectomy one to six weeks after the first procedure is the proper approach to decrease excessive morbidity, such as respiratory problems, severe hypertension, and the increased incidence of neurological deficits that are common after bilateral procedures. This view is generally held by vascular surgeons, despite the fact that in isolated series simultaneous bilateral carotid endarterectomies have been performed with a low rate of neurological complications (Begeant *et al.*, 1975; Clauss *et al.*, 1976). Clauss and associates, for example, reported no mortality or morbidity in a series of eight patients in whom simultaneous surgery for bilateral disease was performed. I am inclined to agree with those who believe that there should be an interval of time between the two operations, but it should not be excessive, and the second procedure should be performed during the same hospitalization period (Bauer *et al.*, 1969), preferably after a four-to five-day interval. In a patient with severe contralateral stenosis, intravenous heparin should be administered in the interim period. Naturally, if there are any complications after the first operation, this time period should be extended as long as the situation dictates.

If there is a possibility that ischemic damage may have occurred during the first operation, this should be evaluated in detail by computed tomography scanning and, if necessary, by angiography. In cases of proven brain injury, the second operation should be delayed four to six weeks. To do otherwise would represent a classic example of "asking for trouble" by creating a situation in which the iatrogenic cerebral insult of the first procedure may be immediately followed and potentiated by the trauma of the second operation. Similarly, peripheral nerve injury, which is a relatively common technical complication, and most of the time merely an annoyance if unilateral, can develop into a full-blown disaster if it occurs bilaterally.

THROMBOSIS OF THE CERVICAL INTERNAL CAROTID ARTERY

Complete occlusion of the internal carotid artery is the most frequent cause of so-called surgical stroke. In 70 to 80 percent of cases it develops from thrombosis superimposed on a carotid bifurcation atheroma (Vollmar, 1966). Besides arteriosclerosis, other conditions may also occasionally induce internal carotid thrombosis, such as trauma, embolus, dissection, aneurysm, arteritis, extrinsic compression, fibromuscular hyperplasia, kinking, and various coagulopathies. Once the thrombosis begins, it usually extends over the next 6 to 24 hours to the level of the first communicating major arterial "pool," the origin of the ophthalmic artery (see Figure 9–31). Later on the clot will organize, and the vessel will either fibrose, or, just the opposite, the distal artery may undergo a partial recanalization. In about one seventh of cases the occlusive plaque is above the level of the bifurcation (see Figure 9–11), usually in the extradural intracranial segment known as the siphon. In such cases the thrombosis will extend retrograde down to the carotid bifurcation (see Figure 14–15).

Indication for surgical management of totally occluded carotid arteries is controversial, and opinions vary from the rigidly conservative to the cautiously radical. Twenty-five years ago, Javid put forward the postulate that complete occlusion of the internal carotid artery is a surgically irreparable lesion (Javid, 1960). Others (Young *et al.*, 1969; Sawyer, 1977), on the other hand, stated that totally occluded internal carotid arteries may be operated upon, but only within the first few hours after occlusion. Still others (Lynch *et al.*, 1981; Thompson *et al.*, 1967) believe that patients with chronic internal carotid occlusion may also be candidates for surgery.

If the internal carotid artery becomes acutely occluded by primary or secondary thrombosis owing to proximal stricture, it can usually be corrected by early surgery involving removal of both the thrombus and the proximal flow-restricting plaque. If, at the comple-

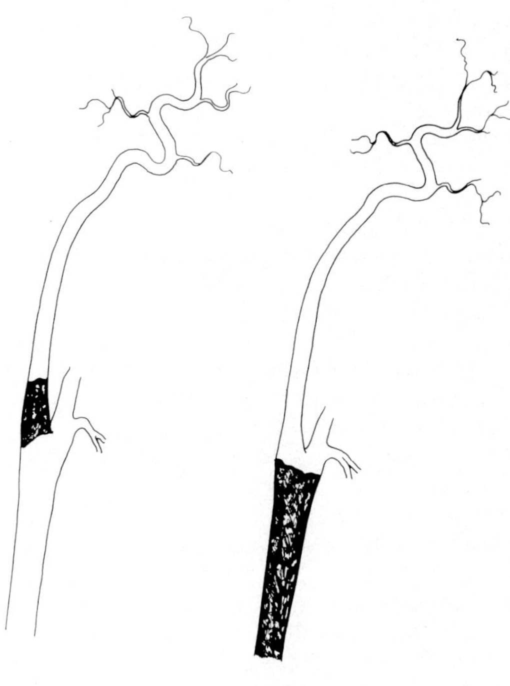

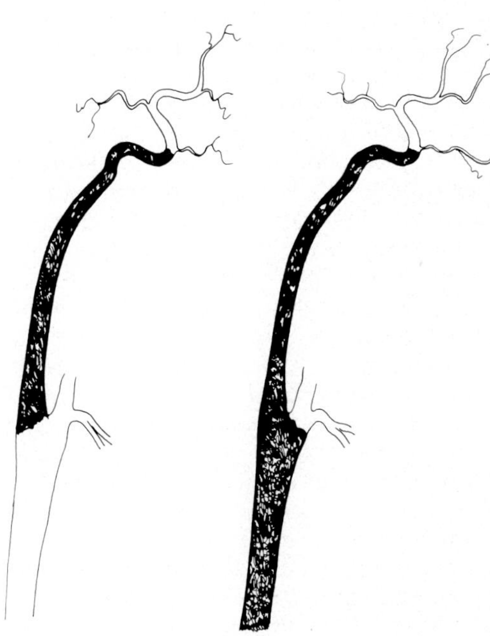

Figure 14-15. The four different types of carotid artery thrombosis.

tion of the procedure, there is satisfactory backflow of blood from the distal internal carotid artery, long-term patency of the vessel can be anticipated. For this reason some surgeons in the 1960s (Hardy *et al.,* 1962; Thompson *et al.,* 1967) recommended early carotid endarterectomy for complete occlusion regardless of the severity of clinical symptoms. Soon, however, it became apparent that in a significant portion of the patients in whom flow had been successfully reestablished severe neurological complications developed. In 1964, Wylie and associates called attention to the alarming fact that patients who undergo restoration of carotid blood flow a few hours or days after the occurrence of a stroke are likely to develop intracranial hemorrhage (Wylie *et al.,* 1964).

Such a hemorrhagic stroke following the restoration of carotid blood flow is generally attributed to the alteration of vascular permeability during the ischemic phase. According to the studies of Millikan (1971), soon after an ischemic infarction severe changes occur in the blood brain barrier which recede gradually over a period of six to 12 weeks. If the blood supply and normal blood pressure in the ischemic area are suddenly restored during this period, worsening and extension of the damage may occur by secondary bleeding into the infarcted area.

Today it is the view of most neurologists and vascular surgeons that the earlier surgery is performed after the occlusion, the higher is the probability of restoring blood flow, but so is the possibility of converting the anemic cerebral infarct into a hemorrhagic one and precipitating the worsening of the neurological status. This is particularly likely to occur in hypertensive patients.

If a brain infarct with a fixed neurologic deficit has already developed, the completely (or even partly) occluded carotid artery should not be operated upon because restoration of flow to the infarcted area may further aggravate the already grave situation. If, however, brain infarct has not yet occurred and the severity of the symptoms fluctuates, one may attempt to restore blood flow to an already occluded internal carotid artery. Most surgeons follow the wise rule laid down by Thompson (1968) that "emergency operations should not be performed on patients with acute profound strokes, rapidly progressing strokes or rapidly improving strokes."If the neurological deficit persists and the patient remains stable, surgery may be reconsidered in four to five weeks, after the chances of hemorrhagic infarction have significantly decreased (see also Chapter 13 on operative indications).

Chronic total occlusion of the internal carotid artery in the absence of symptoms is generally not regarded as an indication for surgery (Thompson, 1968). If, however, the patient has symptoms of intermittent cerebral ischemia, surgical treatment certainly appears to be justified. In this regard the following plan is recommended:

1. Stenotic lesions of the contralateral carotid and/or subclavian steal, if they exist, should be repaired first.
2. If no such lesions are demonstrable or if their correction does not relieve the symptoms of cerebral ischemia, an attempt should be made to restore blood flow through the occluded internal carotid itself. Ipsilateral external carotid artery stenosis, if present, should be repaired concomitantly.
3. If the foregoing efforts fail to relieve the symptoms, extraintracranial bypass may provide the solution (see Figure 9–32).

Of these modalities for treating the completely occluded internal carotid artery, the first solution is undoubtedly the safest and most effective. Whenever the blood flow is also jeopardized through the contralateral carotid or the vertebral vessels by stenotic lesions, the surgeon should concentrate his efforts on reopening those vessels with the hope that by improving the circulation through these vessels enough collateral flow will be delivered to the area of the totally occluded carotid to relieve ischemia. Another important argument for such an approach naturally is the possibility that if the additional vascular occlusions progress, the neurological status of the patient may worsen considerably. A typical example of such a situation is a patient with a completely occluded internal carotid artery on one side and a severely narrowed internal carotid on the other. It has been demonstrated that, even if the symptoms of such a patient point to the occluded side, endarterectomy of the contralateral stenosed artery will produce excellent results in about 80 percent of cases and that the operation can be performed with a relatively low mortality and morbidity rate (Nordhus *et al.*, 1980). Today, the results of carotid endarterectomy in the presence of contralateral total internal carotid occlusion are comparable to those in which the operation is performed for unilateral disease only. Riles *et al.* (1982) followed 146 patients who had unilateral carotid endarterectomy with proven nonstenotic contralateral carotid artery and compared them with 86 patients undergoing the same operation whose contralateral internal carotid was occluded. During the five-year follow-up period, the stroke rates for the two groups were 17.6 and 16.4 percent, respectively.

The outlook for restoring flow in a chronically obstructed carotid artery is dim; only about one of three completely occluded internal carotid arteries can be reopened (Kusunoki *et al.*, 1978; Thompson *et al.*, 1967). Rob and Wheeler (1957) reported 27 patients with symptomatic internal carotid occlusion who underwent direct arterial surgery; a good flow was established in all 11 patients with partial occlusion but in only four of the 16 patients with complete occlusion. In relatively fresh occlusions, the chances of establishing patency are somewhat better (Hunt *et al.*, 1980); in inveterate occlusions they are much worse.

If complete occlusion of the internal carotid artery occurs intracranially, the thrombus will fill the artery retrograde. In such cases removal of the clot only will not eliminate the distal obstacle, and the operation will fail. If, however, as is the case in the great majority of patients, the internal carotid occlusion is caused by a bifurcation atheroma, the situation may be remediable.

The primary factor in predicting success or failure of surgery in such a patient is the presence or absence of filling of the distal internal carotid artery through collaterals. In determining this, one should pay special attention to certain angiographic features that correlate well with the likelihood of a successful operation. Unfortunately, these features are not always readily evident from conventional angiographic techniques. A number of patients who by routine angiography appear to have total internal carotid artery occlusions may actually have extremely severe orifice strictures but patent distal cervical internal carotid arteries. Sometimes these patients can be identified by the so-called slim sign, a trickle of dye passing into the internal carotid artery (see Figure 9–16). This sign was described by Lippman in 1970, and at first it was thought that it represented severe hypoplasia distal to stenotic area. After such patients had been operated upon, however, it became evident that the seemingly small caliber of the vessel was caused not by fibrosis but by layering of the contrast medium passing through the stenosis; the artery itself had a normal diameter distal to the obstruction (Lippman *et al.,* 1970). In cases where the slim sign can be demonstrated, surgical results are usually excellent. In all of Houser's 13 patients with this sign, antero-grade carotid flow resumed postoperatively (Houser *et al.,* 1974). Similar experiences were reported by others (Countee and Vijayan-athan, 1979a).

Even if the cervical segment of the internal carotid artery is completely occluded, in many instances collateral flow will keep the intracranial portion of the internal carotid artery open. In most cases where the intracranial internal carotid artery opacifies through collaterals retrograde to the posterior cavernous sinus, the cervical internal carotid can be reopened by proper instrumentation (Kish *et al.,* 1977). Unfortunately, distal carotid patency cannot always be demonstrated with certainty by routine arteriographic techniques, but high-quality contrast studies or rapid sequential computed tomography may reveal substantial portions of the internal carotid artery to be open indicating feasibility of successful surgical reconstitution (Countee and Vijayanathan, 1979b) (see also Chapter 10 on computerized tomography).

Beside patency of the distal segment, the technical success of reopening the carotid will also be greatly influenced by the degree to which the thrombus is adherent to the intima and by the extent of fibrosis of the arterial wall which regularly accompanies chronic occlusion. The exposure and general technique of reopening the carotid are the same as those described elsewhere for atheromatous carotid stenosis. Before the carotid is opened, the vessel should be carefully examined from the outside. If the internal carotid artery is transformed into a thin fibrous cord up to the base of the skull, further attempts at reconstruction are naturally futile. If, however, the vessel still appears to have an identifiable lumen, then it should be opened and an effort made to clean it out. First, the atheroma, if present, should be removed. Absence of atheroma at the carotid bifurcation is a sign of a poor prognosis because it indicates that the site of primary obstruction lies higher up, intracranially. Under optimal circumstances, the entire plug of red thrombus can be pulled out in one piece by simple traction with a vascular forceps (see Figure 14–28) and brisk back-bleeding will herald the patency of the vessel. If the thrombus breaks up, residual particles can be removed either by inserting a small, soft plastic feeding tube through which suction is applied or by using a small-caliber Fogarty embolectomy catheter (see Figure 14–29). Earlier methods used to removed clots from the internal carotid artery were the "milking technique," retrograde flushing of the artery, and the corkscrew device described by Shaw (1972). Blaisdell *et al.* (1966) recommended saline endarterectomy by injecting normal saline solution under pressure between the occlusive clot and the arterial wall. Of all the methods at the present only two, the application of gentle suction and the use of the Fogarty balloon catheter, are still being used.

Technical manipulations to restore blood flow through a completely occluded carotid artery carry an increased risk of complications. Repeated blind instrumentation may damage the vascular wall or introduce thrombi into the cerebral circulation. Experts in the field especially caution about the use of the Fogarty catheter, which is commonly applied to remove long segments of clots from the internal carotid artery. It should be used with extreme care because of the danger of both perforation of the thin-walled artery and of intracranial embolization. Forceful passage of the catheter or overinflation of the balloon in the cavernous portion of the internal carotid artery can also result in rupture or tear of the arterial wall and the formation of arteriovenous fistulas (see Figure 14–16). Since such an event was first described by Davie and Richardson in 1967, several additional cases have been reported in the literature (Barker *et al.,* 1968; Kakkaseril *et al.,* 1984).

The treatment of these fistulas should be conservative at the beginning because they may close spontaneously. If they persist and the patient is disturbed by the noise caused by the lesion, or exophthalmos or signs of neurological damage appear, then the problem should be handled either by controlled embolization or by ligation of the feeding carotid artery.

Another possible complication of use of the Fogarty balloon catheter is that it may cause dissection of the internal carotid artery. To prevent such a mishap, thrombectomy should be done with extreme caution and with the smallest effective catheter and with a fluid-filled balloon. If instrumental injury of the in-

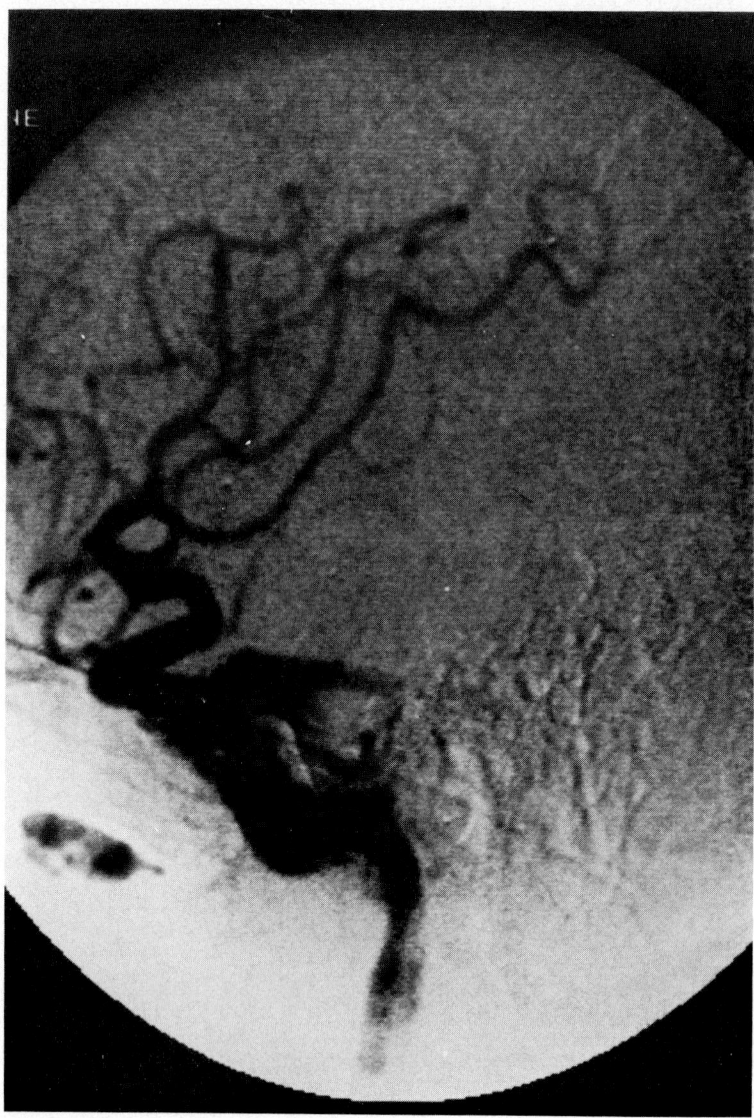

Figure 14–16. Internal carotid-corpus cavernosum fistula caused by injury by Fogarty catheter during clot removal. (From Riles, T.S., *et al*: Comparison of results of bilateral and unilateral carotid endarterectomy five years after surgery. *Surgery*, **91**:258–262, 1982.)

ternal carotid artery is suspected or if slight back-bleeding creates doubt in the mind of the surgeon regarding the distal arterial tree, 10 ml of contrast material should be injected, and an intraoperative angiogram taken to affirm patency. The injection should be done by hand and slowly because contrast material injected under pressure may dislodge thrombi and cause cerebral embolization. If the arteriogram shows injury either to the intracranial carotid or to one of its branches or there is absence of filling of the intracranial carotid, the vessel should be ligated at its origin to prevent further consequences from the vascular injury and to eliminate sources of possible future emboli.

The results of technically successful desobliteration of the chronically obstructed internal carotid artery are encouraging. In the series of patients operated on by Thompson, long-term patency was reestablished in more than a third of the patients, there were no deaths among those with transient symptoms, and all surgical mortalities (5.5 percent) occurred in patients in the completed stroke group (Lynch *et al.*, 1981; Thompson *et al.*, 1967). The other important factor in predicting success is the length of time between occlusion and surgery (Hunt *et al.*, 1980). The passage of time appeared to decrease but did not preclude success. Although the long-range patency rate after surgery for carotid occlusion is lower than that for carotid stenosis (Blaisdell *et al.*, 1969;

Kusunoki *et al.,* 1978), a good share of patients with transient ischemic attacks will have dramatically improved conditions (Hunt *et al.,* 1980).

In bilateral internal total carotid occlusions, Berguer recommends the following surgical tactics (Berguer *et al.,* 1980).

1. If emergency internal carotid thromboendarterectomy can be performed, this should be the first choice in recognizable acute fresh occlusions, unless brain infarction has already occurred.

2. In chronic symptomatic occlusions, subclavian steal should be corrected if present. If there is no steal or if the symptoms persist after its correction, priority should be given to external carotid reconstruction if stenosis is present. With good external carotid inflow, vertebral reconstruction is advised if both vertebrals or the dominant one has stenosis estimated at more than 75 percent.

3. If extracranial reconstruction does not relieve symptoms, consideration should be given to extraintracranial bypass operations.

STENOSIS OF THE EXTERNAL CAROTID ARTERY

Regarding the relative clinical importance of the two tributaries of the common carotid artery, the internal carotid artery is the principal channel supplying the brain with blood. Impairment of blood flow through either of the two internal carotid arteries often leads to serious, even fatal, consequences. In contrast, under normal circumstances the external carotids do not contribute significantly to the cerebral blood supply and may be surgically interrupted with impunity. For this reason, if the flow through the internal carotid artery is unrestricted, stenosis of the external carotid artery has no practical significance. The opposite of this statement is true as well: If the external carotid artery is ligated for technical reasons, it will certainly not increase the cerebral blood flow as has been postulated by some (Bryant, 1974).

The external carotid artery has an incidence of atherosclerotic stenosis and/or ulceration comparable to that of the internal carotid (Martin *et al.,* 1954). In the past, the external carotid was generally regarded as a vessel of secondary importance, the occlusion of which was of no appreciable clinical consequence to either extracranial or intracranial structures. As has been stated, this view may be accurate under normal circumstances, but may not necessarily be true if circulation to the brain is impaired, as is the case in internal carotid occlusion. In such situations the external carotid arteries represent a collateral pathway to the

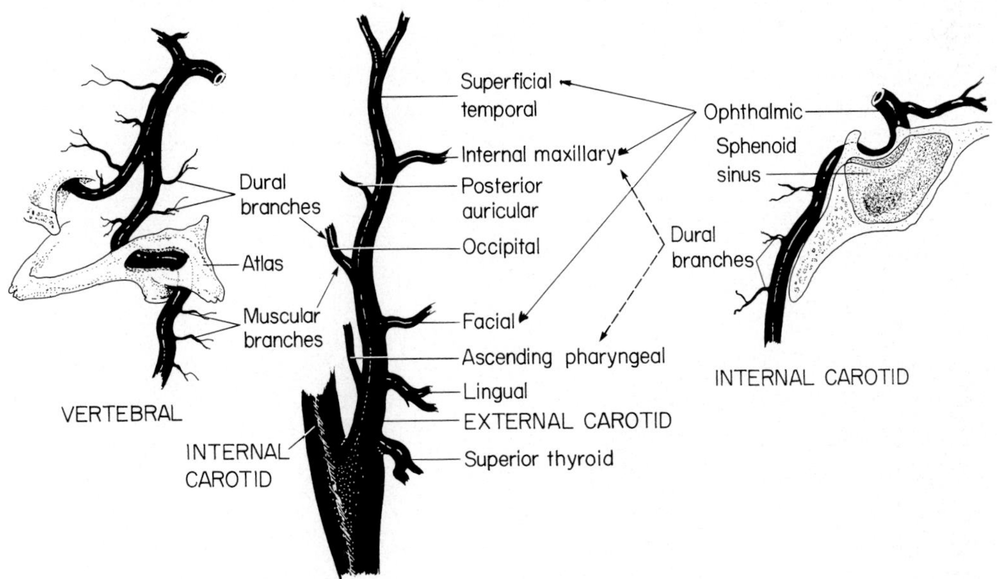

Figure 14–17. The principal tributaries of the external carotid artery and their communications with the vertebral and the internal carotid systems.

brain, the importance of which varies according to the patient's anatomical situation (see Figures 14–17 and 9–31).

The surgeon may encounter stenosis of the external carotid artery in several different clinical situations. The most common of these is stricture of the internal carotid artery associated with external carotid stenosis. When the primary purpose of the surgery is to restore blood flow through the internal carotid artery, some surgeons treat concomitant stenosis of the external carotid artery rather offhandedly and either do nothing about it or perform a so-called eversion endarterectomy. This procedure consists of reaching through the opened carotid bulb arteriotomy into the orifice of the external carotid artery with a curved hemostat, grasping and removing the atheromatous external carotid plug (see Figures 9–33 and 14–18). Because the involvement of the external carotid artery is usually diffuse and severe, it is evident to anyone with appropriate expertise in vascular surgery that after such a maneuver the patient will be left with either a stenosed or occluded external carotid artery.

A departure from this practice was recommended by Karmody *et al.* (1978) who advocate that in the course of a carotid endarterectomy the external carotid artery should receive the same meticulous attention as the internal carotid for the following reasons: (1) if the internal carotid becomes occluded in the postoperative period, the external carotid may serve as an important collateral to the brain and might "save the day;" (2) under the same circumstances patency of the external carotid artery may be essential to the performance of extra- and intracranial bypass operations; (3) carotid bruits originating in the external carotid artery may suggest persisting or recurrent internal carotid artery stricture and could instigate repeated angiographic studies.

For the foregoing reasons Karmody recommends that the blind instrumentation of eversion endarterectomy should be completely abandoned and that the atheroma of the external carotid artery should be removed with the same open technique applied to the internal carotid, if necessary, through a separate arteriotomy, leaving a small bridge between the two incisions (see Figure 14–19).

Another situation in which lesions of the external carotid artery are of clinical importance is embolization to the ipsilateral retina occurring in the absence of common or internal carotid artery disease. In such cases it is logical to conclude that the emboli probably originate from the external carotid artery, and the repair of the latter certainly appears to be justified (Ehrenfeld and Lord, 1969; see Figure 14–20).

Because in cases of total internal carotid artery occlusion, the external carotid artery can provide up to 30 percent of the blood flow to the ipsilateral hemisphere (Fields *et al.*, 1965), if the carotid bifurcation is already being exposed in a patient with the hope of restoring blood flow to a completely occluded internal carotid artery and for technical reasons this proves impossible, the surgeon should definitely perform an ipsilateral external carotid endarterectomy and/or arterioplasty if there is an operable external carotid artery narrowing. This postulate may work in the "opposite" direction as well: When the patient has a completely occluded internal carotid artery and an

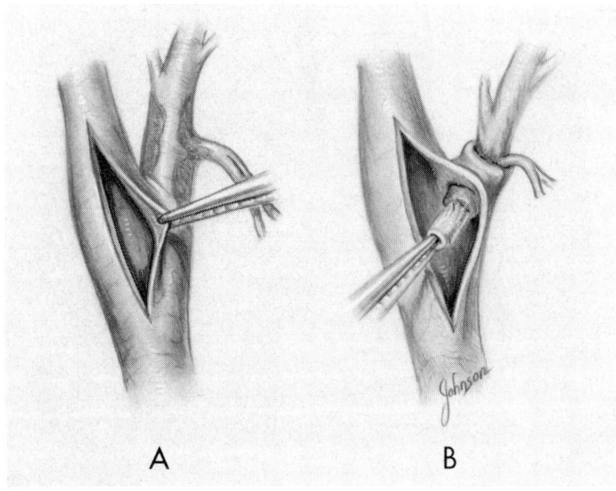

Figure 14–18. Eversion endarterectomy of the external carotid artery. The orifice of the external carotid artery is exposed (*A*) and the atheroma is pulled in the common carotid (*B*).

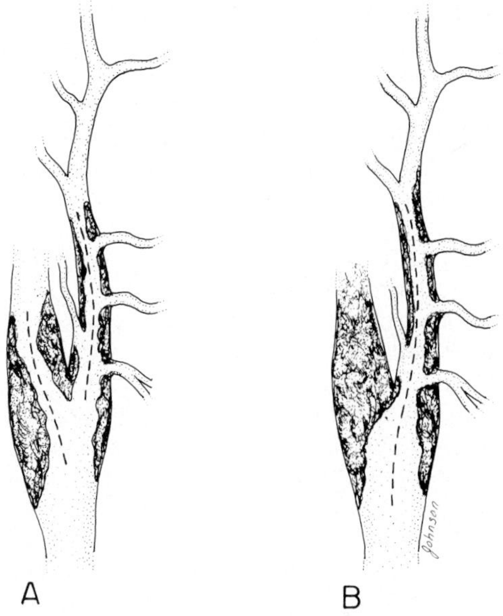

Figure 14–19. Arteriotomy incision for combined internal and external (*A*) and for external only (*B*) carotid endarterectomy. Operative view of combined internal (white arrow) and external (white arrow) endarterectomy and patch graft (*C*).

apparently operable ipsilateral external carotid stricture, the surgeon should be more inclined to explore the internal carotid and attempt to reopen it because if he fails he can still proceed to restore blood flow to the external carotid; thus, the operation is not entirely in vain.

The beneficial effect of external carotid endarterectomy in the presence of a completely occluded internal carotid upon the cerebral blood flow was convincingly proved by Zarins *et al.* (1981), using xenon cerebral blood flow measurements and by Machleder (1973), who demonstrated that the carotid artery back

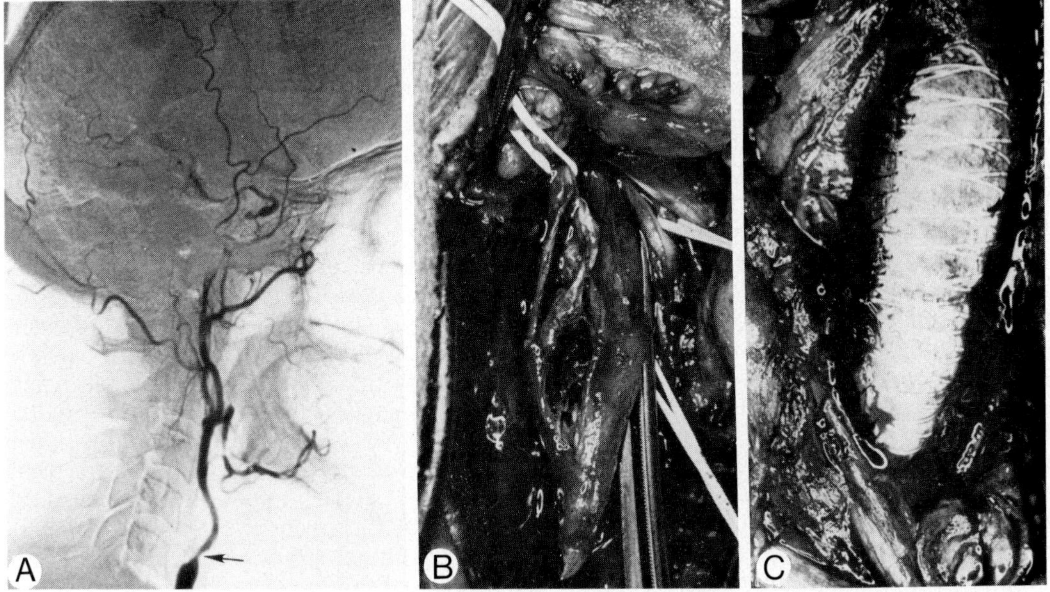

Figure 14–20. Radiogram of complete occlusion of the internal and severe narrowing of the external carotid artery (arrow) in a patient with episodes of transient ischemic attacks and retinal emboli to the ipsilateral eye (*A*). At surgery, a large ulcerated atheroma was found at the orifice of the external carotid artery. After endarterectomy and patch grafting (*B* and *C*), all symptoms ceased.

pressure increases by an average of 21 percent when the external carotid artery on the same side is left open compared with when it is occluded.

Collaterals from the external carotid to the ophthalmic artery, however, are associated with their own hazard too—creating pathways to carry emboli from external carotid atheromas to the retina. In such cases external carotid endarterectomy will eliminate this danger. Good clinical results after external carotid endarterectomies have also been reported in patients with hemispheric symptoms (Berguer and Bauer, 1976; Connolly and Stemmer, 1973), as well as in those with cognitive difficulties (Jacques *et al.*, 1978). Such a favorable outcome of external carotid artery endarterectomy can be expected especially in cases in which an ipsilateral internal carotid artery is occluded and the collateral flow into the distal carotid siphon from branches of the maxillary and superficial temporal arteries passing through the bony orbit exceeds that supplied by the contralateral internal carotid artery through the anterior communicating arteries (Hertzer, 1981). Therefore, in the selection of cases for surgery, careful study of the preoperative angiogram may be very helpful.

Operation on the stenosed external carotid is also necessary whenever ipsilateral superficial temporal artery branch to middle cerebral artery bypass is contemplated. Because the superficial temporal artery is a tributary of the external carotid, occlusion of the latter naturally must be relieved before the temporal artery can be utilized for extraintracranial bypass procedures. Vitek and Morawetz (1982) used the percutaneous balloon technique to dilate lesions at the origin of the external carotid artery as a precursor of later superficial temporal-to-middle cerebral artery anastomosis in three patients. Because there is an excellent chance that the relief of the external carotid stenosis alone may alleviate the symptoms of cerebral ischemia, it is recommended that the performance of extraintracranial bypass should be delayed and the patient reevaluated between the two procedures. Naturally, if the first operation makes the patient asymptomatic, as is often the case, there is no need for the second one (Countee and Vijayanthan, 1979b; Moran *et al.*, 1977).

The surgical technique on the narrowed external carotid artery should be similar to that applied to the internal carotid. As has been stated, eversion external carotid endarterectomy, commonly practiced as a secondary feature if the primary purpose of the operation is to restore internal carotid flow, should not be carried out, especially if the internal carotid artery is permanently occluded, because it will likely leave the intimal edges irregular and ragged, thus predisposing to thrombosis.

The arteriotomy should begin in the common and extend into the external carotid artery. The entire plaque is removed under direct vision, and the first portion of the vessel is enlarged with a patch, if necessary. Some recommend that to obtain a more "streamlined" vascular channel to the reconstructed external carotid, the internal carotid artery, if it is hopelessly occluded, should not be left intact or just simply ligated but be resected "flush" with the bifurcation and its orifice sutured off. This will ensure a smooth, tapering transition from the common to the external carotid. An alternative method of obtaining the same results is the transluminal suture obliteration of the orifice of the internal carotid artery described by Hertzer (1981). Such careful handling of the carotid bifurcation is important because sometimes embolization to the ipsilateral hemisphere continues even after complete occlusion of the internal carotid artery (see Figure 16–3).

Although patch arterioplasty is seldom necessary for the closure of internal carotid endarterectomy, because of the smaller size of the vessel, it is more often needed for external carotid endarterectomy.

Even complete occlusion of the origin of the external carotid does not contraindicate such an operation because collateral flow through several tributaries usually keeps the distal portion of the external carotid patent. If the common carotid is also occluded, revascularization in symptomatic cases can be accomplished by performing a subclavian artery to external carotid artery bypass, preferably using autogenous saphenous vein as a graft. If external carotid endarterectomy does not relieve the symptoms, then extraintracranial bypass from the superficial temporal to the middle cerebral arteries can be carried out. Although the results of external carotid endarterectomy cannot be expected to be as dramatic as those of internal carotid endarterectomy, significant relief of clinical symptoms occurs frequently.

A note of caution regarding external carotid artery revascularization has been sounded by Hollier (1984) who collected several cases of his own and the experiences of others in which total blindness occurred as a complication of external endarterectomy; he attributed this to acute hemorrhage into the previously ischemic retina.

It should also be noted that, contrary to general belief, external carotid endarterectomy is not a simple procedure to be taken lightly. As a matter of fact, because of distal extension of the plaque of the external carotid artery, its removal is technically more difficult than removal of an internal carotid atheroma. Interestingly enough, the rate of postoperative complications and perioperative neurological complications associated with external carotid endarterectomy is also relatively high (Halstuk *et al.,* 1984). This may be due to the fact that in most of these cases the internal carotid arteries are occluded, a condition that places the patients in a high surgical risk category to begin with.

ATHEROSCLEROTIC OCCLUSIVE DISEASE OF THE COMMON CAROTID ARTERY

Patients with completely occluded common carotid arteries constitute a small but important group comprising three to 20 percent of all patients with symptomatic extracranial cerebrovascular lesions. In most cases, atherosclerotic occlusion of the common carotid artery develops from thrombosis superimposed upon an occlusive plaque situated either at the bifurcation (Type I) or at the origin of the artery (Type II; Podore *et al.,* 1981). Regardless of where the primary occlusion occurs, it is inevitably followed by thrombosis of the entire common carotid artery (see Figure 14–21). Common carotid occlusion may also develop from other causes, such as trauma, embolization, aneurysm, or extension of dissection from the aortic arch.

Symptoms of common carotid artery occlusion are largely identical to those described in connection with occlusive internal carotid disease. Patients with interruption of the common carotid blood flow, however, are more likely to have complex clinical problems owing to the fact that they often have associated atherosclerotic lesions in other vessels. If associated lesions are absent and the occlusion occurs gradually, it may remain entirely asymptomatic. In such situations, perfusion to the area previously supplied by the occluded vessel will occur through the bifurcation if spared of occlusion and through the circle of Willis via connections to the contralateral carotid and basilar systems.

Although the *diagnosis* of atherosclerotic common carotid artery occlusion can usually be established with great probability through patient history and physical examination, the single most important symptom being the absence of pulsation of the involved artery, arteriography is recommended for almost every patient with suspected common carotid occlusion. The reasons for this are many: (1) Arteriography will confirm the presence of common carotid artery occlusion and may provide additional clues to its etiology, (2) it will reveal the presence of associated vascular lesions, and (3) it will also supply valuable information regarding the extent of the occlusive process. While we do not advocate that all patients with common carotid occlusion should necessarily be operated upon, it is highly advisable that most of them should be studied arteriographically (see Figure 9–13).

A shortcoming of arteriography is that, although it is always diagnostic as far as the occlusion of the common carotid artery is concerned, it may fail to reveal whether the branches of the carotid bifurcation are open. This is a very important point to keep in mind because the prerequisite of common carotid artery reconstruction is the patency of the "arterial runoff." Therefore, one should not be deterred by nonvisualization of the carotid bifurcation on the arteriogram (see Figure 9–13), but should continue the investigation by specialized radiographic techniques, including dye-enhanced computed tomographic scan, or if the operation is otherwise indicated, should proceed and explore it as the first step of the procedure.

The *operative indication* in symptomatic patients, unless there is some exceptional contraindication, such as terminal cancer, is not especially problematic. The question whether to operate is less certain in a patient with complete common carotid occlusion if symptoms of cerebral ischemia are absent. Because atherosclerosis is always a diffuse and progressive disease, I believe that patients of relatively young and middle ages should have the blood flow reestablished through this very important artery, if possible, even in the absence of pertinent symptoms. In the old or debilitated, however, it may be reasonable to adopt a wait-and-see approach and operate only if symptoms appear. Patients with associated contralateral

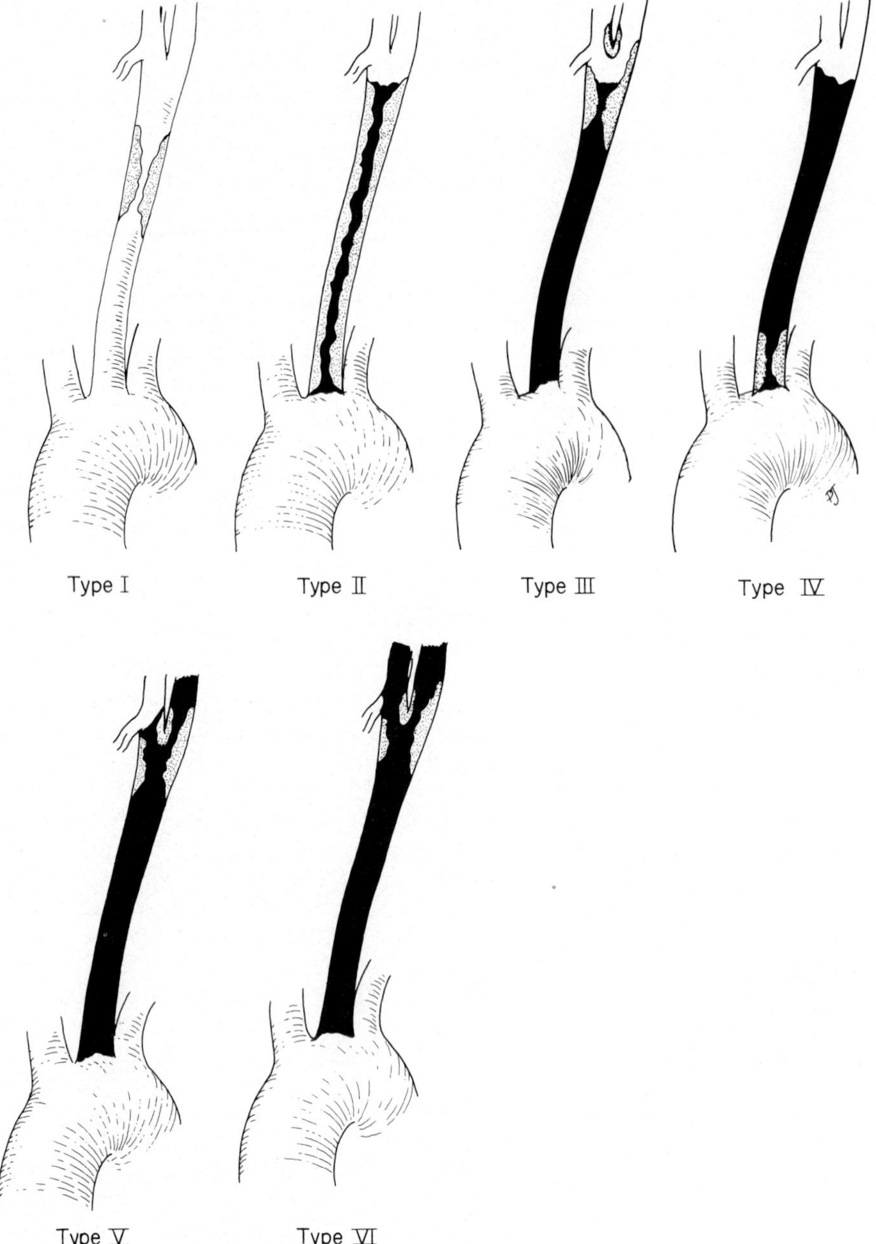

Figure 14–21. The seven different anatomical types of common carotid artery occlusions.

lesions should be treated surgically regardless of age and symptomatology.

Operations designed to restore the blood flow through the common carotid artery occluded by atherosclerotic thrombosis can be divided into three categories: (1) endarterectomy-thrombectomy, (2) grafting of the common carotid artery (with or without distal endarterectomy), and (3) extraanatomical bypass procedures.

The primary determinants in the selection of the appropriate procedure are, in the order of importance: (1) the location of the occlusive plaque, (2) the extent of the thrombosis, (3) the condition of other brachiocephalic arteries, and (4) the preference of the surgeon as dictated by his surgical philosophy.

As far as the location of the plaque and the extent of the thrombosis are concerned, common carotid artery lesions may be divided into the following types (see Figure 14–21): (1) Localized common carotid lesions not involving the bifurcation area (Type I). These are rare, and, unless situated at the origin of the left common carotid artery, are usually treated with endarterectomy or segmental replacement. (2) More extensive lesions of the common carotid (Type II) with or without superimposed thrombosis. (3) Completely occluded carotid arteries caused by either retrograde thrombosis owing to distal (Type III) or proximal atheroma (Type IV) with patent bifurcation are preferably handled with bypass grafting. (4) Bypass grafting may also be applied in patients with occluded common and internal carotids with the external carotid artery still open (Type V). (5) Patients with completely thrombosed cervical carotid systems (Type VI) are seldom candidates for surgery.

In general I believe that bypass grafting or graft replacement of the common carotid artery is preferred to extensive endarterectomy because it is easier to perform, and it assures the absence of residual stenosis. Extraanatomical procedures in general should be reserved for the very few who in this age of modern surgery are unlikely to survive an anterior mediastinotomy. Because the presence of a distal open vessel is a prerequisite of any operation to restore patency regardless of the type of procedure, the involved carotid bifurcation should be carefully inspected. If the carotid bifurcation is hopelessly occluded and flow cannot be established through either of its two tributaries (preferably through the internal carotid, by endarterectomy or other technique), the operation should be aborted.

"ANATOMICAL" PROCEDURES

Endarterectomy of the Common Carotid Artery. Endarterectomy of the common carotid artery may be considered for lesions relatively localized but may also be undertaken for more diffuse atherosclerotic occlusions, including those with superimposed thrombosis. In the latter situation Moore *et al.* (1967) recommended the retrograde "strip" method. The case best suited for this procedure is the one in which carotid occlusion is caused by progression of bifurcation atheroma with retrograde thrombosis (Type III). The procedure is performed as follows.

The carotid bifurcation is exposed, the internal and external carotid arteries are looped, and through a longer-than-usual longitudinal arteriotomy, an appropriate endarterectomy of the carotid bifurcation is carried out in the usual way. A plane of cleavage is now developed retrograde in the common carotid artery between the organized thrombus and the intima; the thrombotic core is divided, and a wire-loop endarterectomy stripper is passed over it. The stripper is then proximally advanced through the entire length of the common carotid into and, if necessary, past its origin into the innominate or the aorta until the entire core is completely detached from the arterial wall. The stripper is now removed, and the organized thrombus is then allowed to be ejected by the upsurging blood, a process facilitated by pulling the core with a clamp or forceps (see Figure 14–22A). If during the process of loop endarterectomy, difficulties are encountered at the proximal end of the common carotid, especially if the operation is performed on the right side, the procedure may be supplemented by sharp division of the core through a separate transverse proximal arteriotomy (see Figure 14–22B).

Although it is described in most textbooks of vascular surgery, retrograde strip-endarterectomy has never been widely performed, and one has the impression that it has been more written about than practiced. This probably is because the procedure cannot be applied in all patients (Moore himself succeeded in only seven of ten cases), and even those cannot be predicted preoperatively. Also, the possibility of incomplete removal or partial dislodgment of the clot carries the risk of both distal embolization and reocclusion.

Grafting of the Common Carotid Artery. An alternative to common carotid endarterectomy is grafting. This can be performed either in the form of replacement or as a bypass. Segmental replacement is seldom utilized in common carotid occlusion but is commonly performed in connection with trauma or aneurysms. Atherosclerotic occlusive conditions usually require complete replacement or a bypass from the aortic arch to the carotid bifurcation (see Figure 14–23).

In the course of bypass operations (see Figure 14–23A,B), the carotid bifurcation is exposed through a separate cervical incision first, to ascertain that it is suitable for receiving the distal end of the graft. Although it has been recommended to split the upper two thirds of the sternum only or to expose the aortic arch through a "trap door" incision or through an anterior right thoracotomy, we found the complete anterior sternotomy approach to

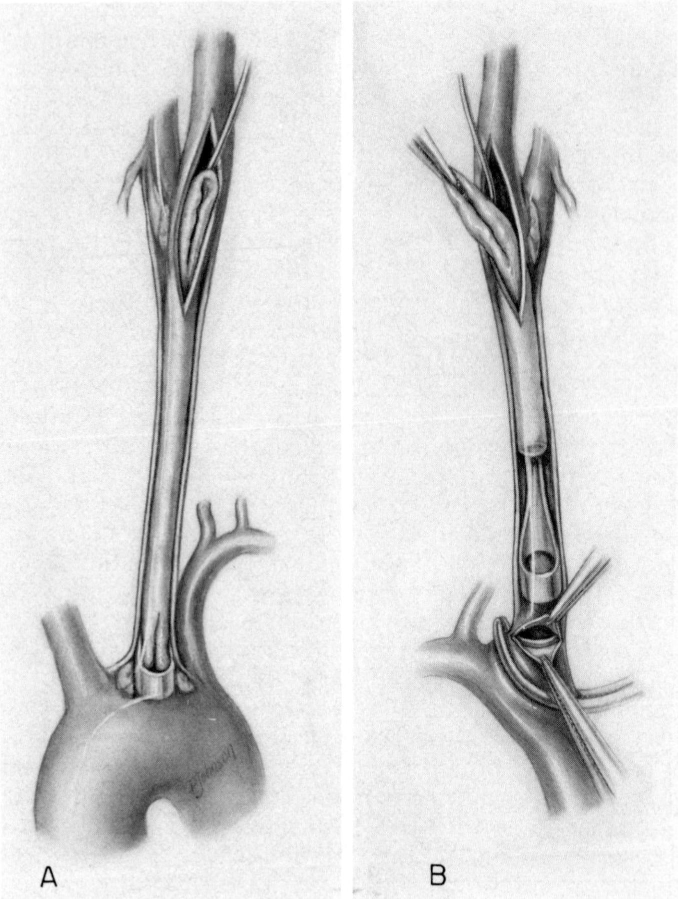

Figure 14–22. Retrograde "strip endarterectomy" of the left (*A*) and right (*B*) common carotid arteries.

provide both a faster and better exposure as well as the potential for a satisfactory closure (see Figure 3–2).

The second incision is made from the sternal notch down to the xyphoid process, and the periosteum is cauterized in the line of the osteotomy (see Figure 14–24). The sternum is then halved in its axis with an oscillating saw or with a Lebsche knife. After the sternal edges are spread with a self-retaining sternal retractor, the remnants of the thymus gland are dissected off up to the innominate vein. The pericardium is opened above the ascending aorta. A partially occluding clamp is applied to the anterior ascending aorta, and a longitudinal incision 1 cm long is made into the excluded aortic segment. The edges of the incision are spread with 6-0 polypropylene retracting sutures and anastomosed to an 8 to 10 mm diameter crimped Dacron prosthetic graft. The anastomosis is made preferably with 4-0 polypropylene running suture buttressed over Teflon felt (see Figure 14–25). After completion of the anastomosis, the clamp is removed, and the very base of the graft is clamped in such a way as not to leave a cul-de-sac where a thrombus might form. The end of the graft is grasped with a long instrument passed from the upper incision down along the carotid artery. The graft is pulled up to the neck and anastomosed end to end with a 4-0 polypropylene running suture to the distal stump of the divided common carotid artery, just below the carotid bifurcation (see Figure 14–25), which, if necessary, was previously endarterectomized. Because of the presence of collateral circulation from the external to the internal carotid, if the anatomical situation allows, these arteries should not be occluded during the performance of the anastomosis, but the common carotid should be clamped and divided just proximal to the carotid bulb. Before the completion of the anastomosis, the air from the arterial stump and the graft should be removed by generous backward and forward flush. The blood flow from the graft is directed

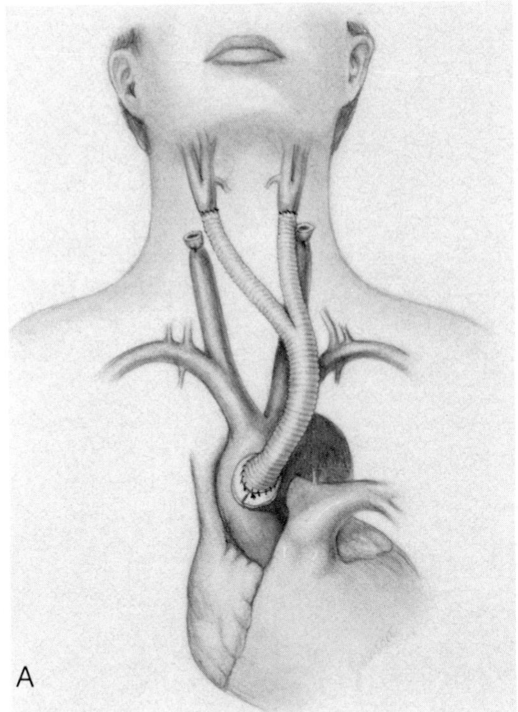

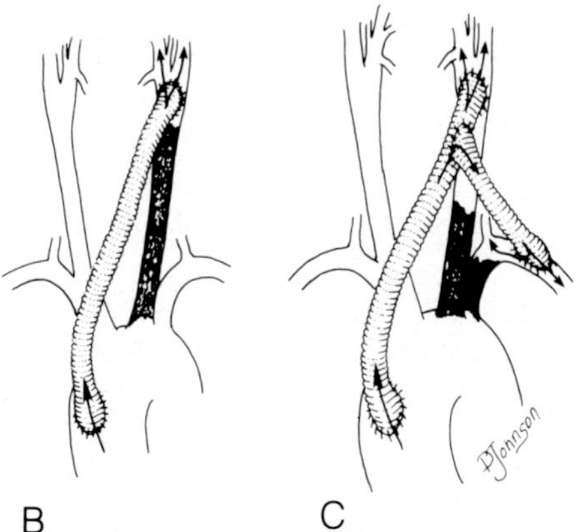

Figure 14-23. Aorta to bilateral common carotid (*A*), aorta to left common carotid (*B*), and aorta to left common carotid to left subclavian artery graft (*C*).

first into the external and then toward the internal carotid to further decrease the possibility of air or debris entering the cerebral circulation. At the termination of the procedure, the divided edges of the sternum are reunited with wire sutures. The pericardial sac is left open, and the mediastinum is drained with a single water-sealed catheter.

In the rare situation in which both common carotid arteries must be replaced with prosthetic grafts, this can be accomplished using a bifurcated prosthesis with a 14 mm diameter body and 8 mm diameter sidearms. To avoid kinking of the limbs of the graft, the body of the graft should be cut short so as not to exceed 2.5 to 3.5 cm in length (see Figure 14-3A) and be appropriately beveled. In patients in whom common carotid artery disease is associated with severe occlusive changes in the carotid bifurcation, the situation may be remedied by aorta-to-internal carotid artery grafting using autogenous saphenous vein as graft material (see Figure 14-26).

Extraanatomical Procedures

Carotid-To-Carotid Bypass Graft. Another type of common carotid artery graft is the extraanatomical carotid-to-carotid bypass shunt which may be used to restore flow to the occluded carotid artery under special circumstances, such as symptomatic innominate artery occlusive disease accompanied by contralateral subclavian artery occlusion. Although, like other extrathoracic-extracranial bypasses, it may spare the patient from a thora-

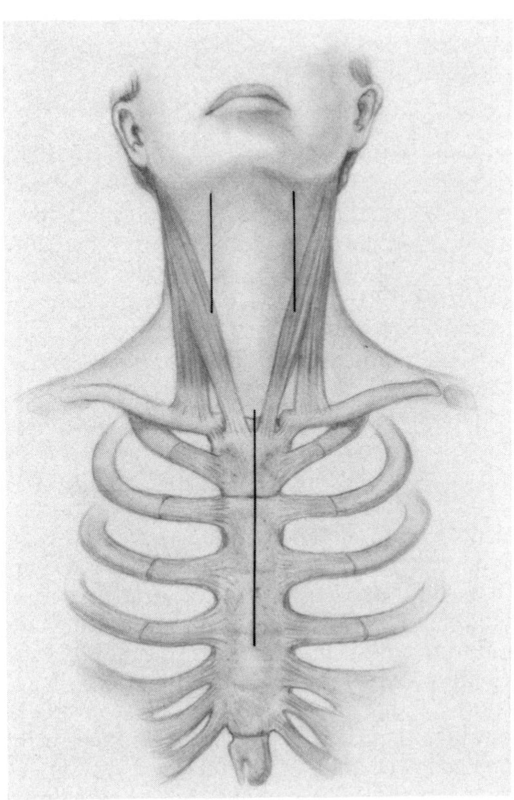

Figure 14-24. Incisions used for simultaneous exposure of the aortic arch and both carotid bifurcations.

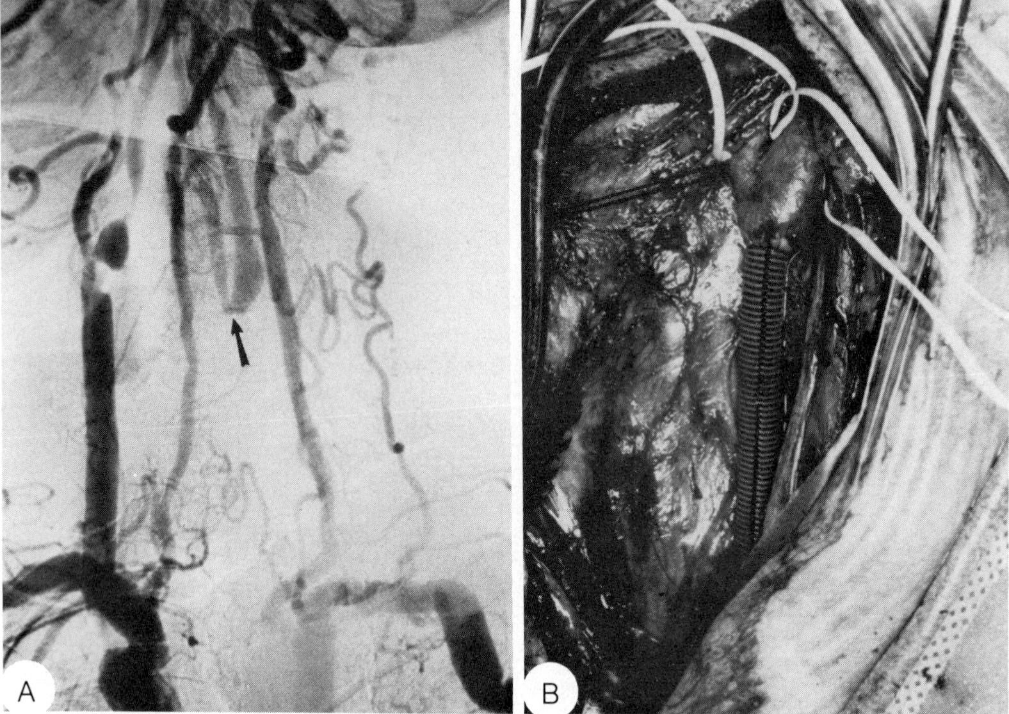

Figure 14-25. Preoperative angiogram (*A*) showing large plaque in the right carotid bifurcation as well as complete occlusion of the left common carotid artery with the left carotid bifurcation (arrow) filling through collaterals. Operative picture (*B*) shows the left common carotid artery replaced with a crimped Dacron prosthesis.

cotomy, it also presents a disadvantage: if the carotid artery is occluded on one side, the surgeon is tampering with the second remaining major vascular channel to the brain, the contralateral carotid artery. Placing the intact carotid and the brain in such jeopardy is seldom justified unless no other donor vessel is available and thoracotomy is definitely contraindicated.

The prerequisites of this operation are (1) stenosis or occlusion near the origin of one of the common carotid arteries, (2) open ipsilateral distal common carotid, and (3) an unobstructed contralateral common carotid artery.

The operation is performed with the patient in a supine position with the head hyperextended. Bilateral incisions, 4 to 5 cm long, are made along the anterior borders of the sternocleidomastoid muscles, and both common carotid arteries are exposed at the level of the omohyoid muscles. The patient is systemically heparinized, and an anastomotic site is selected on the anteromedial aspect of the uninvolved common carotid artery. This artery is now clamped both proximally and distally (to try to use a partially occluded clamp as recommended by some is absolutely futile), and an end-to-side anastomosis is performed between an 8 mm diameter crimped Dacron prosthesis on one end and the common carotid on the other. After the anastomosis is completed, the graft is clamped right at the anastomosis, and the flow through the carotid is restored. The prosthesis is now tunneled in a gentle curve deep to the omohyoid muscles and across to the contralateral (diseased) common carotid artery, where a similar anastomosis is fashioned (see Figure 14-27A). Again, before the last stitches of the anastomosis are placed, bidirectional flushing is carried out to ensure the expulsion of air.

Another variety of carotid-to-carotid bypass employs an autogenous saphenous vein graft anastomosed to the external carotid artery on both sides in a suprahyoid subcutaneous location. This type of bypass is recommended if common carotid artery ligation is necessary because of disruption and hemorrhage owing to infection.

Although carotid-to-carotid artery graft is

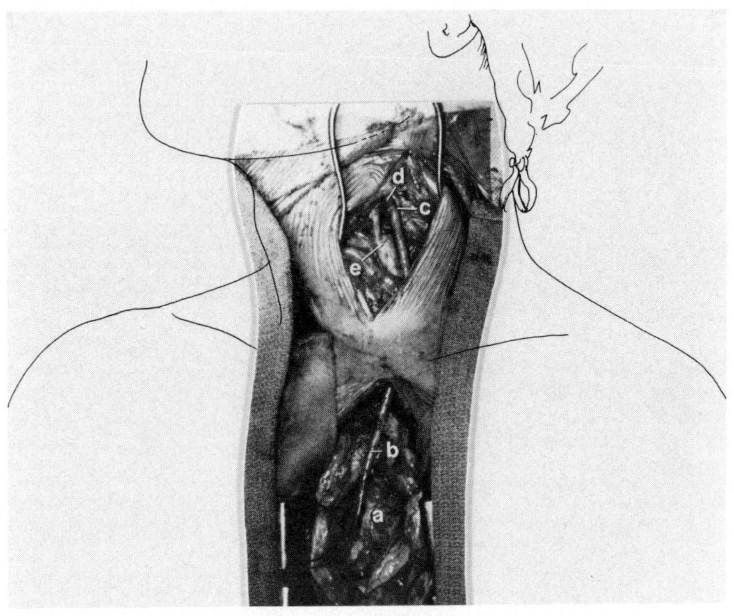

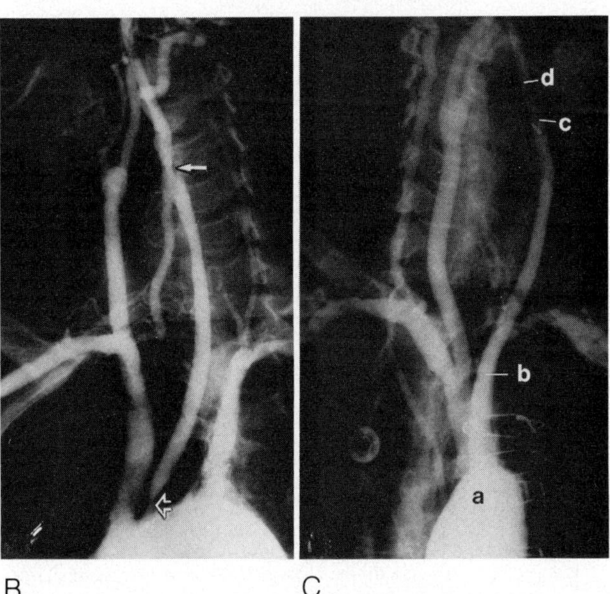

Figure 14–26. Operative picture of aorta-to-left internal carotid artery end-to-end saphenous vein bypass graft performed on a patient with stricture of the origin of the left common carotid and left internal carotid arteries (*A*). Pre (*B*) and postoperative (*C*) angiograms of the same patient. References: aorta *a*, vein graft *b*, graft-to-internal carotid artery anastomisis *c*, internal carotid artery *d* and carotid bifurcation *e*. The open arrow and the white arrow on the preoperative angiogram points to the stricture of the left common and left internal carotid arteries respectively.

simple and effective, it tampers with the contralateral intact carotid artery; therefore, it should be undertaken only when, because of ipsilateral subclavian artery disease, subclavian-to-carotid bypass is not feasible and aorto-to-carotid artery bypass or direct attack on the involved carotid artery itself is contraindicated.

Subclavian Artery-to-Common Carotid Artery Anastomosis. If the stenosis of the common carotid artery is limited to its most proximal segment, restoration of the carotid flow

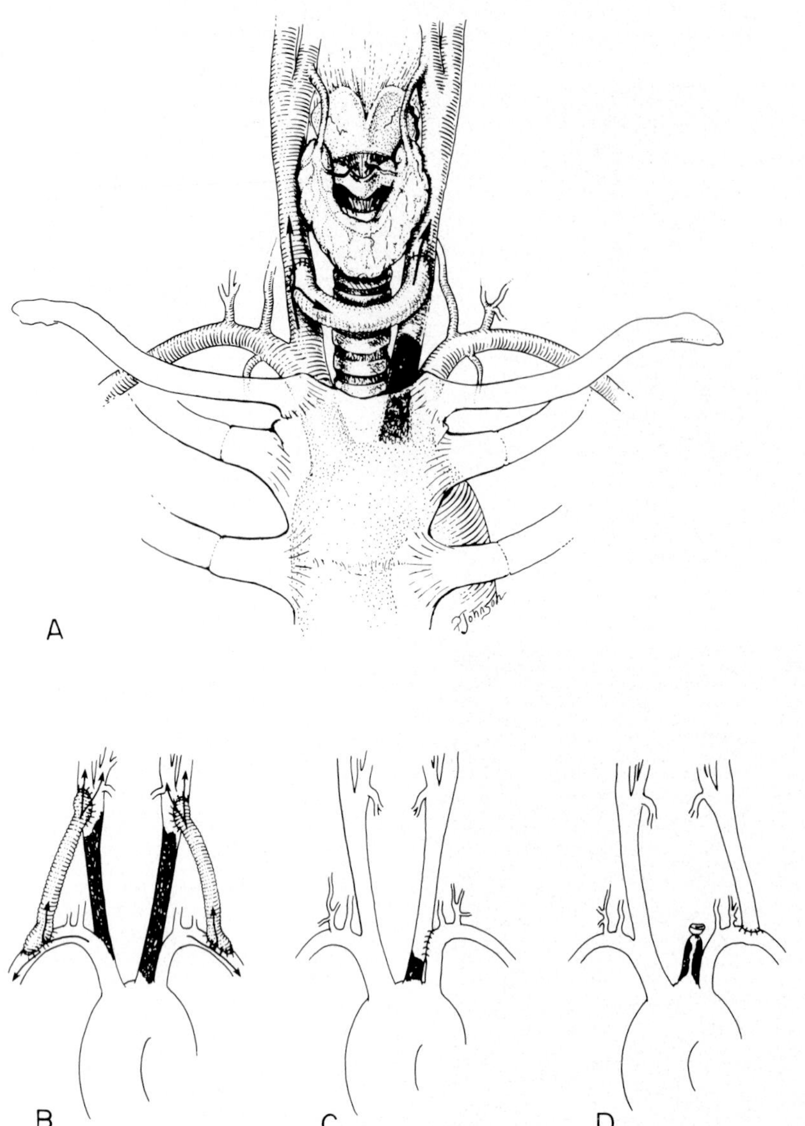

Figure 14–27. Different types of extraanatomical procedures designed to restore blood flow in patients with obstructed common carotid artery: Bilateral subclavian-carotid bypass (*A*). Side-to-side subclavian-to-carotid anastomosis (*B*). Implantation of the carotid in the subclavian artery (*C*). Carotid-to-carotid bypass (*D*).

may also be accomplished either by subclavian-to-common carotid artery bypass graft (see Figure 14–27B), by side-to-side carotid-to-subclavian anastomosis (see Figure 14–27C), or by implanting the common carotid artery end to side into the ipsilateral subclavian artery (see Figure 14–27D). The latter procedures are cumbersome, offer little advantage over the conventional carotid-to-subclavian bypass graft, and therefore are seldom utilized. The technique of inserting a graft between the subclavian and the carotid arteries is described in Chapter 29.

EMBOLIZATION TO THE EXTRACRANIAL CEREBRAL ARTERIES

Most emboli occurring in the extracranial cerebral circulation are situated at the bifurcation of the carotid or, less frequently, of the innominate artery. These clots may come from atherosclerotic ulcers and aneurysms of the proximal arterial tree or from the chambers of the left heart. Because of the suddenness of the circulatory shutdown, the involved vascular bed is unprepared by lack of development of collaterals. Because of this and the accompanying vasospasm, the clinical sequelae of embolic occlusion are more dramatic than those seen in gradually occurring atherosclerotic thrombosis.

The possibility of embolization to the cerebrovascular system should be considered in every patient with rapidly occurring cerebral perfusion deficits, especially in those with known mitral or aortic valvular disease, atrial fibrillation, fresh myocardial infarction, history of peripheral embolization, or aneurysm of the aortic arch or left ventricle. The principal clue to the diagnosis may be the sudden disappearance of carotid pulse, or — if the embolus is lodged in the innominate bifurcation — the cessation of pulsation over both the right carotid and subclavian arteries. When embolization is suspected in a patient with acute cerebral ischemia, an attempt should be made to establish the diagnosis by physical examinations alone and, if it can be performed rapidly enough, by noninvasive studies. Arteriography should be avoided because, besides the time consumed in the procedure, the injection of contrast material may also further aggravate the already critical situation. If everything else fails and surgery is contemplated, exploration of the carotid bifurcation under local anesthesia may be the most appropriate measure to confirm or exclude the diagnosis. The patient in whom symptoms of ischemia are fleeting and the diagnosis and/or localization of the emboli are doubtful should be studied angiographically (see Figure 9–17).

The ideal treatment of acute embolic occlusion of the extracranial cerebral vessels is immediate removal of the clot. Unfortunately, because of the rapidly developing irreversible brain damage, cerebrovascular embolization seldom involves surgical decision making. In rare cases, however, embolectomy may be considered if one of the following conditions can be met: (1) the embolus can be removed within two hours of the occurrence of the vascular occlusion or (2) owing to adequate collateral blood supply or to incomplete occlusion the patient has not developed a "fixed" stroke.

The surgical management of emboli lodged in the extracranial cerebrovascular system is rather simple and consists of exposure and bidirectional control of the embolized artery, arteriotomy, and removal of the thrombus. The opening of the embolized vessel should be performed with caution so as not to squeeze and fragment the occluding clot. If the arteriotomy is performed close to a bifurcation, it should be directed toward the principal "runoff" vessel: the common carotid artery in innominate embolization and the internal carotid when embolization occurs at the carotid bifurcation (see Figure 14–28A). In the course of the procedure, the patient should be fully heparinized, and the heparin should not be neutralized at the completion of the operation.

After the arteriotomy is made, the embolus usually protrudes from the incision. Most of the time it is relatively firm and thus can be easily and completely removed by gentle traction (see Figure 14–28B). This maneuver should be done gingerly so as not to fragment the embolus or lose the in situ-formed "tail" thrombus. If restoration of free lumen is not heralded by brisk forward and back-bleeding, a small Fogarty balloon catheter should be passed into the distal and, if necessary, into the proximal artery to extract residual thrombi (see Figure 14–28C). The maneuver should be repeated until satisfactory backflow and forceful pulsating forward flow are obtained.

Although removal of residual clots with the aid of the Fogarty catheter through the arteriotomy incision can be a very useful adjuvant to the operation, balloon extraction of emboli with the catheter introduced at a remote peripheral site should never be employed as a primary procedure in the extracranial cerebral vessels because it may lead to irretrievable cerebral embolization.

After the operation is completed it is advisable to maintain the patient on long-range anticoagulation to decrease the chances of reembolization. If the source of the emboli can be identified with reasonable certainty, it should be dealt with accordingly: atrial fibrillation should be terminated if possible, proximal thrombi (see Figure 29) or aneurysms should be removed, malfunctioning valve prostheses should be replaced, etc.

If, for various reasons, primarily the passage of time, embolectomy is thought to be inadvisable, the patient should be managed by general supportive measures and with anticoagulants. Before the latter are instituted, however, one must confirm by computed tomography scan

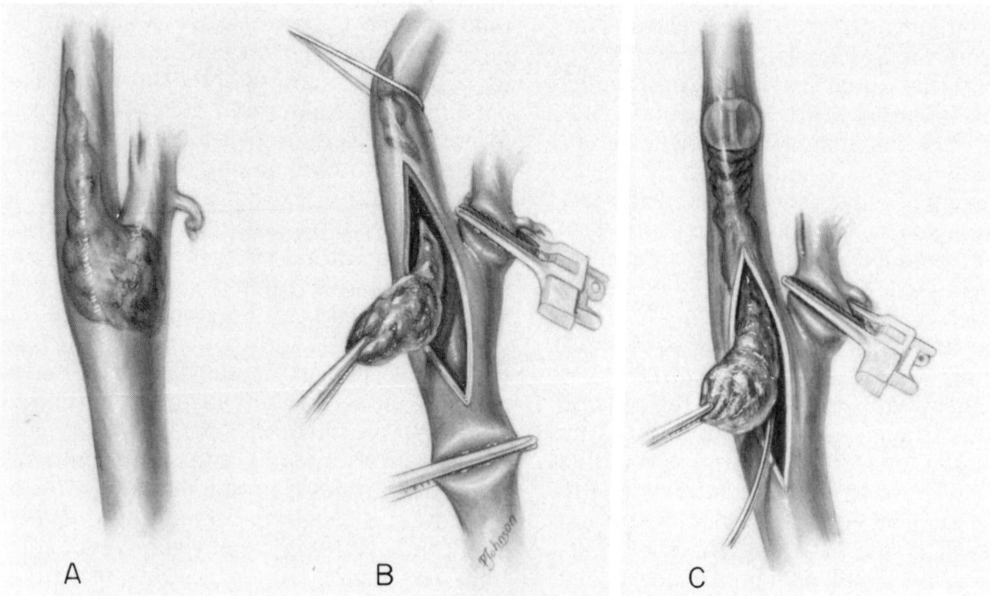

Figure 14–28. The extraction of an embolus lodged in the carotid bifurcation (*A*) by direct extraction (*B*) and by using the Fogarty catheter (*C*).

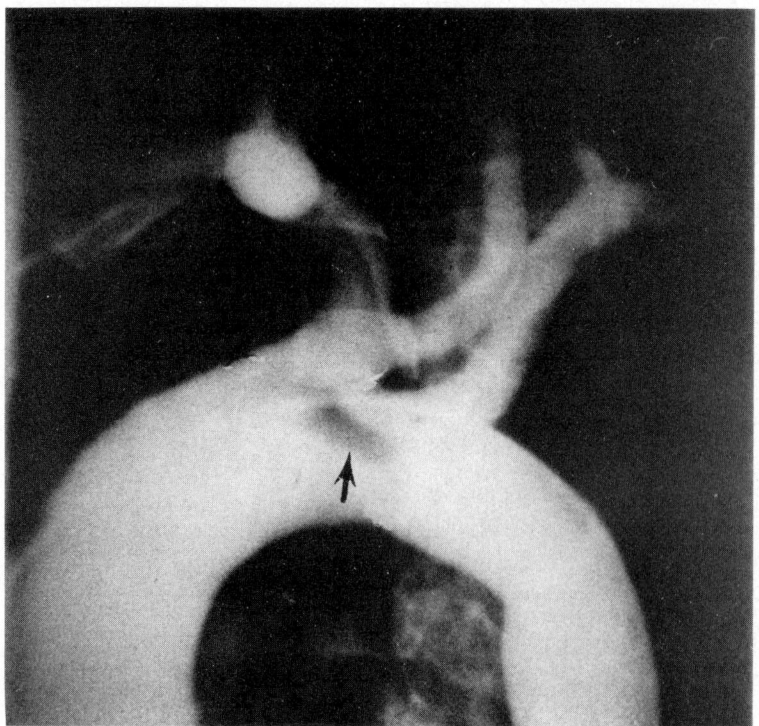

Figure 14–29. Aortogram of a patient with a history of recent repeated cerebral emboli. Note on the aortogram a filling defect (arrow) in the aortic arch representing a large thrombus adherent to an ulcer on the aortic wall.

and by spinal tap studies the absence of hemorrhagic infarction, which may be further extended by anticoagulant therapy.

OPERATION FOR RECURRENT CAROTID STENOSIS

Successful restoration of carotid blood flow can be expected in 98 percent of patients with carotid artery stricture and in 40 percent of patients with totally occluded carotid arteries (Thompson, 1968). There are also many studies indicating that in most cases the endarterectomized carotid artery will remain patent for prolonged periods. A certain number of patients, however, will require reexploration because of recurrence of stenosis at the endarterectomy site. In most recent series, using noninvasive testing, the percentage of restenosis ranged from eight to 12 percent (Baker, 1983; Cantelmo *et al.*, 1981; O'Donnell *et al.*, 1985; Turnipseed *et al.*, 1980; Wylie and Ehrenfeld, 1970). In a report standing alone, Bodily *et al.* (1980) gave a recurrent carotid stenosis rate of 48 percent (see also Chapter 22 on long-term results of carotid endarterectomy).

Before the matter of recurrent carotid stenosis can be addressed in depth, the subject of inadequate primary repair should be discussed. In 1967, Blaisdell, in a prospective intraoperative angiographic study, examined 95 carotid arteriograms performed in the operating room before the closure of the skin incision and found that of those 95, 26 showed either residual or surgery-induced narrowing compromising 30 percent or more of the lumen of the internal carotid artery. Although all of these strictures were corrected, five years later he again discovered two significant stenoses in the 15 patients he had the opportunity to study by angiography or at autopsy (Blaisdell *et al.*, 1967). From this study two important conclusions can be drawn: (1) residual stenosis of the carotid artery is more common than one may expect, and (2) after otherwise successful surgery "true" recurrences do indeed take place.

Residual obstruction of the blood flow in the operated carotid artery detectable in the immediate postoperative period has been attributed to imperfection of the surgical repair (Imparato *et al.*, 1972). Such stenoses may have been either left uncorrected or produced by the use of vascular clamps, intimal shreds, or faulty suturing. To prevent such mishaps, beside intraoperative angiography (Blaisdell *et al.*, 1967), carotid endoscopy (Olinger, 1977) has also been recommended, but neither has been generally accepted by the profession. The best method of prevention of early occlusion is, naturally, thorough technique at the time of the original surgery (see also Chapter 18 on intraoperative evaluation of carotid circulation).

The cause of carotid restenosis that occurs months or years after the operation is more complex; the fate of this denuded layer of media should be studied because it may well explain the occasional (in some series as high as 10 to 12 percent) cases of late recurrence (DeWeese, 1983; Thompson *et al.*, 1970).

The medial layer of a normal extracranial carotid artery is composed of smooth-muscle cells, fibrocytes, and elastic fibers. The latter decrease in number as the artery passes peripherally. Whereas in the common carotid artery elastic elements dominate, the internal carotid changes gradually into a muscular-type vessel with the elastic elements confined to its internal and external elastic lamina (Stehbens, 1972).

Postoperative changes occurring at the endarterectomy site can be grouped in three partly overlapping phases: the acute, the reparative, and the mature phases. The anatomical features of these phases may vary considerably, not only from patient to patient but also in different areas of the same endarterectomy site. In the reparative phase, resolution of the inflammatory response and organization of the mural thrombus to form a neointima will occur. During the mature phase, beginning about a month after surgery, the endarterectomy site is covered with a mature new intima which in its smoothness is indistinguishable from the lining of the rest of the vessel. There is also formation of new elastic tissue (French and Rewcastle, 1974; Gryska, 1959).

The healing of the endarterectomy site was studied in dogs by Dirrenberger and Sundt (1978) by means of angiography as well as with light and electron microscopy. They observed the formation of a thin layer of fibrin and platelet deposits at the site of the stripped endothelium immediately after restoration of blood flow. They also found that unless anticoagulants were given, thrombus developed at the endarterectomy site in 52 percent of the animals while clot formation did not occur if the animals were heparinized. One week later most of the mural thrombus had disappeared, and reendothelialization was well under way.

The smooth healing of the endarterectomy site may be jeopardized by two distinct pathological processes, both leading to carotid restenosis (DeWeese, 1983). The first variety of restenosis was initially described by Cossman *et al.* (1978), who found in a number of cases an excessive myointimal hyperplasia characterized by stellate cells embedded in fibromyxomatous stroma. This in their opinion did not represent true arteriosclerotic changes. Most of these changes occurred in the relatively early postoperative period, none of them later than two years after the initial surgery. Such intimal and neointimal proliferation was also recognized in femoropopliteal reconstructions and was thought to be the reason for about one third of the late occlusions. At the time of reoperation these lesions appear as a pale, firm, homogeneous layer with a smooth, shiny surface (Stoney and String, 1976), occurring primarily in areas where the flow was either very slow or unusually rapid (Imparato *et al.*, 1972). The exact mechanism of this phenomenon is still not completely understood.

Another variety of carotid restenosis is caused by reappearance of the typical atherosclerotic plaque, which commonly occurs late, usually more than two years after the initial surgery (Hertzer *et al.*, 1979; Stoney and String, 1976). Restenosis of the carotid artery after endarterectomy owing to progression of underlying arteriosclerotic disease was documented experimentally in the late 1950s by Gryska (1959), who stripped the intima and part of the media of the aorta of dogs and found that within a few weeks the area was covered with a firm, smooth layer of neointima. If the same animals were fed a high-cholesterol diet and given propylthiouracil, after five months stenosing atheroma developed in the same area. Atherosclerotic restenosis was also documented clinically by several investigators (Kreman *et al.*, 1979; Stoney and String, 1976; Thompson and Talkington, 1976).

In reoperation one should proceed with utmost caution in the dissection of the carotid artery because of adhesions caused by the previous surgery. Unless distal dissection appears to be easy, it is preferable not to ensnare the internal carotid artery but to control backbleeding simply with an internal balloon occluder. In the control of the common and external carotid arteries one should be especially careful to avoid injury not only to the arteries themselves but also to adjacent nerves. In reoperation the danger of peripheral nerve injury, particularly to the hypoglossal nerve, is especially high (Begeant *et al.*, 1975).

In an operation for carotid restenosis, the classic technique of endarterectomy performed in anatomical layers can seldom be followed because the structure of the arterial wall has already been disrupted during the first operation. This is especially true if the restenosis is caused by myointimal thickening where absence of a cleavage plane between the thickened neointimal pad and the rest of the vessel wall renders repeat endarterectomy very difficult, if not impossible. Such cases can be most properly handled by patch arterioplasty. If, on the other hand, restenosis is caused by the progress of the underlying atherosclerosis, a new endarterectomy plane can usually be developed, as was demonstrated in 16 of Stoney and String's 20 cases (1976). Restoration of a proper lumen, however, frequently requires not only removal of the obstructing tissue with sharp dissection but also, more often than not, enlargement of the arterial lumen with a diamond-shaped patch of autogenous vein or synthetic material (see Figure 14-11). In severe cases of arterial or peripheral fibrosis, or if the artery is injured beyond repair in the course of dissection, replacement of the arterial segment may be necessary.

REFERENCES

Bageant, T.E.; Tondini, D.; and Lysons, D.: Bilateral hypoglossal nerve palsy following a second carotid endarterectomy. *Anesthesiology*, **43**:595-96, 1975.

Baker, W.H.; Dorner, D.B.; and Barnes, R.W.: Carotid endarterectomy: is an indwelling shunt necessary? *Surgery*, **82**:321-26, 1977.

Baker, W.H.: Technical advances in carotid surgery. In Bergan, J.F., and Yao, J.S.T. (eds.): *Operative Techniques in Vascular Surgery*. Grune & Stratton, New York, pages 47-52, 1980.

Baker, W.H.; Hayes, A.C.; Mahler, D.; and Littooy, F.N.: Durability of carotid endarterectomy. *Surgery*, **94**:112-15, 1983.

Barker, J.; Harper, A.M.; McDowall, D.G.; Fitch, W.; and Jennett, W.B.: Cerebral blood flow, cerebrospinal fluid pressure and E.E.G. activity during neuroleptanalgesia induced with dehydrobenzperidol and phenoperidine. *Br. J. Anaesth.*, **40**:143-44, 1968.

Bauer, R.B.; Meyer, J.S.; Fields, W.S.; Remington, R.; MacDonald, M.C.; and Callen P.: Joint study of extracranial arterial occlusion: 3. Progress report of controlled study of long-term survival in patients with and without operation. *J.A.M.A.*, **208**:509-18, 1969.

Berguer, R., and Bauer, R.B.: Subclavian artery to external carotid artery bypass graft: improvement of cerebral blood supply. *Arch. Surg.*, **111**:893-96, 1976.

Berguer, R.; McCaffrey, J.F.; and Bauer, R.B.: Bilateral internal carotid artery occlusion: its surgical management. *Arch. Surg.*, **115**:840–43, 1980.

Blaisdell, F.W.; Lim, R.; and Hall, A.D.: Technical result of carotid endarterectomy. *Am. J. Surg.*, **114**:239–46, 1967.

Blaisdell, F.W.; Clauss, R.H.; Galbraith, J.G.; Imparato, A.M.; and Wylie, E.J.: Joint study of extracranial arterial occlusion. 4. Review of surgical considerations. *J.A.M.A.*, **209**:1889–95, 1969.

Blaisdell, F.W.; Hall, A.D.; and Thomas, A.N.: Surgical treatment of chronic internal carotid artery occlusion by saline endarterectomy. *Ann. Surg.*, **163**:103–11, 1966.

Bland, J.E.; Chapman, R.D.; and Wylie, E.J.: Neurological complications of carotid artery surgery. *Ann. Surg.*, **171**:459–64, 1970.

Bodily, K.C.; Aieler, R.W.; Marinelli, M.R.; Thiele, B.L.; Greene, F.M., Jr.; and Strandness, D.E., Jr.: Flow disturbances following carotid endarterectomy. *Surg. Gynecol. Obstet.*, **151**:77–80, 1980.

Bryant, M.F.: Anatomic considerations in carotid endarterectomy. *Surg. Clin. North Am.*, **54**:1291–96, 1974.

Cantelmo, N.L.; Cutler, B.S.; Wheeler, H.B.; Herrmann, J.B.; and Cardullo, P.A.: Non-invasive detection of carotid stenosis following endarterectomy. *Arch. Surg.*, **116**:1005–8, 1981.

Clauss, R.H.; Bole, P.V.; Paredes, M.; Doscer, W.; Adeyemo, A.; and Kremimtzer, M.W.: Simultaneous bilateral carotid endarterectomies. *Arch. Surg.*, **111**: 1304–6, 1976.

Collins, G.J.; Rich, N.M.; Anderson, C.A.; and McDonald, P.T.: Stroke associated with carotid endarterectomy. *Am. J. Surg.*, **135**:221–25, 1978.

Connolly, J.E., and Stemmer, E.A.: Endarterectomy of the external carotid artery: its importance in the surgical management of extracranial cerebrovascular occlusive disease. *Arch. Surg.*, **106**:799–802, 1973.

Cormier, J.M., and Ricco, J.B.: Carotid graft for cerebrovascular insufficiency. In Bergan, J.J., and Yao, J.S.T. (eds.): *Cerebrovascular Insufficiency*. Grune & Stratton, New York, pages 275–307, 1983.

Cossman, D.; Callow, A.D.; Steen, A.; and Matsumoto, G.: Early restenosis after carotid endarterectomy. *Arch. Surg.*, **113**:275–78, 1978.

Countee, R.W. and Vijayanathan, T.: External carotid artery in internal carotid artery occlusion: angiographic, therapeutic, and prognostic considerations. *Stroke*, **10**:450–60, 1979a.

Countee, R.W., and Vijayanathan, T.: Reconstruction of "totally" occluded internal carotid arteries: angiographic and technical considerations. *J. Neurosurg.*, **50**:747–57, 1979b.

Crawford, E.S.; DeBakey, M.E.; Blaisdell, F.W.; Morris, G.C., Jr.; and Fields, W.S.: Hemodynamic alterations in patients with cerebral arterial insufficiency before and after operation. *Surgery*, **48**:76–94, 1960.

Davie, J.C., and Richardson, R.: Distal internal carotid thrombo-embolectomy using a Fogarty catheter in total occlusion. *J. Neurosurg.*, **27**:171–77, 1967.

DeWeese, J.A.: Long-term result of surgery for carotid artery stenosis. In Bergan, J.J., and Yao, J.S.T. (eds.): *Cerebrovascular Insufficiency*. Grune & Stratton, New York, 1983.

Dillon, M.L.; Reeves, J.W.; and Postlethwhait, R.W.: Carotid artery flows and pressures in 22 patients with cerebral vascular insufficiency. *Surgery*, **58**:951–55, 1965.

Dirrenberger, R.A., and Sundt, T.M.: Carotid endarterectomy: temporal profile of the healing process and the effects of anticoagulation therapy. *J. Neurosurg.*, **48**:201–19, 1978.

Ehrenfeld, W.K., and Lord, T.S.A.: Transient monocular blindness through collateral pathways. *Surgery*, **65**:911–15, 1969.

Fields, W.S.; Breutman, M.E.; and Weibel, J.: Collateral circulation of the brain. *Monogr. Surg. Sci.*, **2**:183–259, 1965.

Fleming, R.; Griesdale, D.; Schutz, H.; and Hogan, M.: Carotid endarterectomy: factors contributing to changing morbidity and mortality. Presented at the Forty-fifth Meeting of the American Association of Neurological Surgeons, Toronto, Ontario, April 25, 1977.

French, B.N., and Rewcastle, N.B.: Sequential morphological changes at the site of carotid endarterectomy. *J. Neurosurg.*, **41**:745–54, 1974.

Gryska, P.F.: The development of atheroma in arteries subjected to experimental thromboendarterectomy. *Surgery*, **45**:655–60, 1959.

Halstuk, K.S.; Baker, W.H.; and Littooy, F.N.: External carotid endarterectomy. *J. Vasc. Surg.*, **1**:398–402, 1984.

Hardy, W.G.; Lindner, D.W.; Thomas, L.M.; and Gurdjian, E.S.: Anticipated clinical course in carotid artery occlusion. *Arch. Neurol.*, **6**:138–50, 1962.

Hays, R.J.; Levinson, S.A., and Wylie, E.J.: Intraoperative measurement of carotid back pressure as a guide to operative management for carotid endarterectomy. *Surgery*, **72**:953–60, 1972.

Hertzer, N.R.; Beven, E.G.; Greenstreet, R.L; and Humphries, A.W.: Internal carotid back pressure, intraoperative shunting, ulcerated atheromata, and the incidence of stroke during carotid endarterectomy. *Surgery*, **83**:306–12, 1978.

Hertzer, N.R.; Martinez, B.D.; and Beven, E.C.: Recurrent stenosis after carotid endarterectomy. *Surg. Gynecol. Obstet.*, **149**:360–64, 1979.

Hertzer, N.R.: External carotid endarterectomy. *Surg. Gynecol. Obstet.*, **153**:186–90, 1981.

Hollier, L.H.: Discussion in the *Proceedings of the Southern Association of Vascular Surgeons*, St.Thomas, V.I., January 18–21, 1984.

Houser, O.W.; Sundt, T.M., Jr.; Holman, C.B.; Sandok, B.A.; and Burton, R.C.: Atheromatous disease of the carotid artery: correlation of angiographic, clinical, and surgical findings. *J. Neurosurg.*, **41**:321–31, 1974.

Humphries, A.W.; Young, J.R.; Santilli, P.H.; Beven, E.G.; and deWolfe, V.G.: Unoperated, asymptomatic significant internal carotid artery stenosis: a review of 182 instances. *Surgery*, **80**:695–98, 1976.

Hunt, D.G.; Wheeler, C.G.; Bukhari, H.I.; and Hempel, G.K.: Surgical management of total carotid artery occlusion: an update. *Am. J. Surg.*, **139**:700–3, 1980.

Imparato, A.M.: Discussion of Santiani, B.; Liapis, C; Pflug, B.; Vasko, J.S.; and Evans, W.E.: Role of staging in bilateral carotid endarterectomy. *Surgery*, **84**:784–92, 1978.

Imparato, A.M; Bracco, A.; Kim, G.E.; and Bergmann, L: The hypoglossal nerve in carotid arterial reconstructions. *Stroke*, **3**:576–78, 1972.

Jacques, S.; Garner, J.T.; Tager, R.; Rosenstock, J.; and Fields, T.: Improved cognition after external carotid endarterectomy. *Surg. Neurol.*, **10**:223–25, 1978.

Javid, H.: Surgical management of cerebral vascular insufficiency. *Arch. Surg.*, **80**:883–89, 1960.

Johnson, N.; Burnham, S.J.; Flanigan, P.; Goodreau, J.J.; Yao, J.S.T.; and Bergan, J.J.: Carotid endarterectomy: a follow-up study of the contralateral non-operated carotid artery. *Ann. Surg.*, **188**:748–52, 1978.

Karmody, A.M.; Shah, D.M.; Monoce, V.J.; and Leather, R.R.: On surgical reconstruction of the external carotid artery. *Am. J. Surg.*, **136**:176–80, 1978.

Kakkaseril, J.S.; Tomsick, T.A.; Arbough, J.A.; and Conley, J.J.: Carotid cavernous fistula following Fogarty catheter thrombectomy. *Arch. Surg.*, **119**:1095–96, 1984.

Kish, G.F.; Adkins, P.C.; and Slovin, A.J.: The totally occluded internal carotid artery: indications for surgery. *Am. J. Surg.*, **134**:288–92, 1977.

Krajicek, M., and Kramar, M.: The lateral approach to the extracranial segment of the carotid artery. *J. Cardiovasc. Surg.*, **9**:302–4, 1968.

Kremen, J.E.; Gee, W.; Kaupp; H.A.; and McDonald, K.M.: Restenosis or occlusion after carotid endarterectomy: a survey with ocular pneumoplethysmography. *Arch. Surg.*, **114**:608–10, 1979.

Kusunoki, T.; Rowed, D.W.; Tator, C.H.; and Lougheed, W.M.: Thromboendarterectomy for total occlusion of the internal carotid artery: a reappraisal of risks, success rate, and potential benefits. *Stroke*, **9**:34–8, 1978.

Lees, C.D., and Hertzer, N.R.: Postoperative stroke and late neurologic complications after carotid endarterectomy. *Arch. Surg.*, **116**:1561–68, 1981.

Linton, R.R.: Some practical considerations in the surgery of blood vessel grafts. *Surgery*, **38**:817–34, 1955.

Lippman, H.H.; Sundt, T.M., Jr.; and Holman, C.B.: The poststenotic carotid slim sign: spurious internal carotid hypoplasia. *Mayo Clin. Proc.*, **45**:762–67, 1970.

Lynch, T.G.; Wright, C.B.; Miller, E.V.; and Slaymaker, R.N.: Evaluation of cerebrovascular Doppler examination and oculopneumoplethysmography in a clinical perspective. *Stroke*, **12**:325–30, 1981.

Machleder, H.I.: Evaluation of patients with cerebral disease using the Doppler ophthalmic test. *Angiology*, **24**:374–81, 1973.

Martin, F.P.; Lukeman, J.M; Ranson, R.F.; and Geppert, L.J.: Mucormycosis of the central nervous system associated with thrombosis of the internal carotid artery. *J. Pediatr.*, **44**:437–42, 1954.

Millikan, C.H.: Reassessment of anticoagulant therapy in various types of occlusive cerebrovascular disease. *Stroke*, **2**:201–8, 1971.

Moore, W.J.: Discussion of Hays, R.J.; Levinson, S.A.; and Wylie, E.J.: Intraoperative measurement of carotid back pressure as a guide to operative management for carotid endarterectomy. *Surgery*, **72**:953–60, 1972.

Moore, W.S.; Blaisdell, F.W.; and Hall, A.D.: Retrograde thrombectomy for chronic occlusion of the common carotid artery. *Arch. Surg.*, **95**:664–73, 1967.

Moore, W.S., and Hall, A.D.: Carotid artery back pressure: a test of cerebral tolerance to temporary carotid occlusion. *Arch. Surg.*, **99**:702–10, 1969.

Moore, W.S.: *Vascular Surgery: A Comprehensive Review.* Grune & Stratton, New York, 1983.

Moran, J.M.; Reichman, H.; and Baker, W.H.: Staged intracranial and extracranial revascularization. *Arch. Surg.*, **112**:1424–28, 1977.

Nordhus, D.; Ekestrom, S.; and Lillequist, L.: Unusual indications for carotid artery surgery. *Acta Chir. Scand.*, **146**:5–8, 1980.

O'Donnell, T.F.; Callow, A.D.; Scott, G.; Shepard, A.D.; Heggerick, P.; and Millackey, W.C.: Ultrasound characteristics of recurrent carotid disease: hypothesis explaining the low incidence of symptomatic recurrence. *J. Vasc. Surg.*, **2**:26–41, 1985.

Olinger, C.P.: Carotid artery endoscopy (autopsy). *Surg. Neurol.*, **7**:7–13, 1977.

Patterson, R.H.: Risk of carotid surgery with occlusion of the contralateral carotid artery. *Arch. Neurol.*, **30**:188–89, 1974.

Podore, P.C.; DeWeese, J.A.; May, A.G.; and Rob, C.G.: The asymptomatic contralateral carotid artery stenosis: a five-year follow-up study following carotid endarterectomy. Presented at the Society for Vascular Surgery, Chicago, June, 1980.

Podore, P.C.; Rob, C.G.; DeWeese, J.A.; and Green, R.M.: Chronic common carotid occlusion. *Stroke*, **12**:98–100, 1981.

Riles, R.S.; Imparato, A.M.; Mintzer, B.S.; and Baumann, F.G.: Comparison of results of bilateral and unilateral carotid endarterectomy five years after surgery. *Surgery*, **91**:258–62, 1982.

Rob, C., and Wheeler, E.B.: Thrombosis of internal carotid artery created by arterial surgery. *Br. Med. J.*, **2**:264–66, 1957.

Rosenman, J.; Edwards, W.S.; Robillard, D.; and Geary, G: Carotid arterial bifurcation advancement. *Surg. Gynecol. Obstet.*, **159**:260–64, 1984.

Rosenthal, J.J.; Gaspar, M.R.; and Movius, H.J.: Intraöperative arteriography in carotid thromboendarterectomy. *Arch. Surg.*,**106**:806–08, 1973.

Satiani, B.; Liapis, C.L.; Pflug, B.; Vasko, J.S.; and Evans, W.E.: Role of staging in bilateral carotid endarterectomy. *Surgery*, **84**:784–92, 1978.

Sawyer, P.N.: Questions and answers section. *J.A.M.A.*, **238**:1566, 1977.

Shaw, D.A.: Investigation of stroke. *Br. Med. J.*, **1**:91–3, 1972.

Stehbens, W.E.: *Pathology of the Cerebral Blood Vessels.* C.V. Mosby, Saint Louis, Missouri, 1972.

Stoney, R.J., and String, S.T.: Recurrent carotid stenosis. *Surgery*, **80**:705–10, 1976.

Sundt, T.M., Jr.; Houser, O.W.; and Sharbrough, F.W.: Carotid endarterectomy: results, complications, and monitoring techniques. *Adv. Neurol.*, **16**:97–119, 1977.

Thompson, J.E.: *Surgery for Cerebrovascular Insufficiency (Stroke) with Special Emphasis on Carotid Endarterectomy.* Charles C. Thomas, Springfield, Illinois, 1968.

Thompson, J.E.: Carotid surgery for cerebral ischemia. *Surg. Clin. North. Am.*, **59**:539–53, 1979.

Thompson, J.E; Austin, D.J.; and Patman, R.D.: Endarterectomy of the totally occluded carotid artery for stroke. *Arch. Surg.*, **95**:791–801, 1967.

Thompson, J.E.; Austin, D.J.; and Patman, R.D.: Carotid endarterectomy for cerebrovascular insufficiency: long-term results in 592 patients followed up to thirteen years. *Ann. Surg.*, **172**:663–79, 1970.

Thompson, J.E.; Patman, R.D.; and Talkington, C.M.: Management of asymptomatic carotid bruit. Long-term outcome of patients having endarterectomy compared with unoperated controls. *Ann. Surg.*, **188**:308–16, 1978.

Thompson, J.E., and Talkington, C.M.: Carotid endarterectomy: surgical progress. *Ann. Surg.*, **184**:1–15, 1976.

Turnipseed, W.D.; Berkoff, H.A.; and Crummy, A.: Postoperative occlusion after carotid endarterectomy. *Arch. Surg.*, **115**:573–74, 1980.

Vitek, J.J., and Morawetz, R.B.: Percutaneous transluminal angioplasty of the external carotid artery. *Am. J. Neuroradiol.*, **3**:541–46, 1982.

Vollmar, J.: Die chirurgische Prophylaxe des Schlanganfalls. *Fortschr. Med.*, **84**:857, 1966.

Wade, J.G.; Larson, C.P.; Hickey, R.F.; and Ehrenfeld, W.K.: Effect of carotid endarterectomy on chemoreceptor and baroreceptor function. *Surg. Forum,* **19**:144–45, 1968.

Welsh, P.; Pradier, R.; and Repetto, R.: Fibromuscular dysplasia of the distal cervical internal carotid artery. *J. Cardiovasc. Surg.,* **22**:321–26, 1981.

Wylie, E.J.; Hein, M.F.; and Adams, J.E.: Intracranial hemorrhage following surgical revascularization for treatment of acute strokes. *J. Neurosurg.,* **21**:212–15, 1964.

Wylie, E.J., and Ehrenfeld, W.K.: *Extracranial Occlusive Cerebrovascular Disease: Diagnosis and Management.* W.B. Saunders, Philadelphia, Pennsylvania, page 27, 1970.

Wylie, E.J.: Vascular surgery: reflections of the past three decades: presidential address. *Surgery,* **88**:743–47, 1980.

Wylie, E.J., and Ehrenfeld, W.K.: *Extracranial Occlusive Cerebrovascular Disease: Diagnosis and Management.* W.B. Saunders, Philadelphia, Pennsylvania, 1970.

Young, J.G.; Humphries, A.W.; Beven, E.G.; and de-Wolfe, V.G.: Carotid endarterectomy without a shunt. *Arch. Surg.,* **99**:293–97, 1969.

Zarins, C.K.; Del Baccaro, E.J.; Johns, L.; Turcotte, J.K.; and Dohrmann, G.J.: Increased cerebral blood flow after external carotid artery revascularization. *Surgery,* **89**:730–34, 1981.

15

Extracranial-Intracranial Arterial Bypass for Internal Carotid Artery Occlusion

DUKE S. SAMSON

SUPERFICIAL TEMPORAL TO MIDDLE CEREBRAL ARTERY BYPASS

Symptomatic cerebral ischemia may occur in the territory of any of the terminal branches of the internal carotid artery or may affect neural structures normally supplied by the end-arteries of the vertebral-basilar system. In clinical practice, however, the overwhelming preponderance of ischemic cerebral vascular disease occurs in the distribution of the principal division of the internal carotid artery — the middle cerebral artery, which irrigates the bulk of the cortical aspects of frontal, parietal, and temporal lobes and also major portions of the deep cerebral white matter and basal ganglia. Patients undergoing angiographic investigation for middle cerebral artery ischemic episodes will usually be found to have ulcerated or stenotic lesions of the cervical carotid artery which are suitable for classic extracranial revascularization procedures. In 15 to 20 percent of such patients, however, the angiographic lesions thought responsible for the patients' symptoms will be of a nature or location not amenable to treatment by cervical carotid endarterectomy.

In order of frequency, these unique lesions include complete internal carotid artery occlusion, internal carotid artery stenosis (siphonous carotid), middle cerebral artery stenosis or occlusion, and, least frequently, complete common carotid artery occlusion. Cerebral ischemia in the presence of such angiographic findings generally represents the failure of the collateral hemispheral circulation to compensate for the impaired flow to blood through the carotid-middle cerebral channel. The circle of Willis, a most effective anastomotic vascular arrangement at the base of the brain, theoretically allows blood from either of the two carotid arteries or the basilar artery to be shunted into the terminal segments of either carotid or basilar distribution in response to decrease in flow and in resistance in these vascular networks. Although anatomically complete in only about 50 percent of the population, this anastomotic system represents a most important source of potential collateral flow (contralateral carotid and vertebral-basilar) in cases of carotid occlusion and is frequently adequate to sustain normal cerebral perfusion in the presence of ipsilateral internal carotid artery occlusion by retrograde flow through the ophthalmic artery to the intracranial internal carotid artery (Toole and Patel, 1974). Extracranial-intracranial arterial bypass is in essence an attempt to surgically augment the external carotid artery component of this collateral flow system by creating a direct connection between the external carotid artery system and a cortical branch of the underperfused middle cerebral artery distribution.

Rationale

Normal internal carotid artery flow, measured either at the most distal point in the neck or proximal to the internal carotid artery bifurcation intracranially, is roughly 300 ml/min and flow in the main trunk of the middle cerebral artery is in the neighborhood of 150 to 175 ml/mm (Nornes and Wikeby, 1977). In the healthy adult these flow rates produce a normal regional cerebral blood flow in the middle cerebral distribution of roughly 55 ml per 100 g of brain tissue per minute (55 ml/100 g/min; Lassen and Ingvar, 1963; Samson *et al.*, 1981). Laboratory and clinical studies have demonstrated that symptomatic cerebral ischemia does not occur until cerebral blood flow drops to the level of about 20 ml/100 g/min. Furthermore, true neuronal death or infarction occurs only when focal regional cerebral blood flow drops to levels below 12 ml/100 g/min (Sundt *et al.*, 1969; Sundt *et al.*, 1971). These values demonstrate the significant safety factor built into the autoregulatory mechanisms of the cerebral circulation and indicate that relatively small increases in collateral flow will alter regional cerebral blood flow enough to avert the onset of cerebral ischemia or infarction (Fein and Molinari, 1974; Heilbrun *et al.*, 1975; Marzewsky *et al.*, 1982).

Normal flow in the external carotid branches most frequently employed in extracranial-intracranial bypass surgery averages 25 to 30 ml/min and, as such, theoretically represents the possibility of acute augmentation of middle cerebral artery flow by 15 to 20 percent (Heilbrun *et al.*, 1975; Samson and Boone, 1978). Studies of chronic cases have demonstrated that such a donor external carotid branch when diverted from the low-flow, high resistance field of the distal external carotid artery to the low resistance vascular bed of the middle cerebral territory will undergo prompt and progressive increases in diameter. This angiographically demonstrable dilatation signals impressive increases in overall collateral blood flow (flow being proportional to the fourth power of the radius), so that ultimate flow through the anastomotic channel may in some cases approach 100 ml/min (Samson and Boone, 1978).

Surgical Technique

Extracranial-intracranial arterial bypass in its simplest version, that is, the superficial temporal-middle cerebral cortical branch anastomosis, is a routine, straightforward microsurgical procedure, initially designed and performed by Yasargil (1969) and R.P. Donaghy (1972). Its goal is the construction of a microsurgical anastomosis between a branch of the superficial temporal artery and a cortical branch of the symptomatic middle cerebral distribution (Chater *et al.*, 1975; Donaghy, 1972; Samson and Boone, 1978). In the course of the operation, a linear incision is made over the posterior branch of the superficial temporal artery and extended posteriorly to form a small skin flap centered 6 to 7 cm superior to the external auditory meatus (see Figure 15–1) (Chater *et al.*, 1976). The underlying temporalis muscle is incised in a stellate fashion and a small 3 to 4 cm diameter free craniotomy flap centered on the posterior aspect of the sylvian fissure is fashioned. After dural opening, the cortex is inspected for an appropriate recipient vessel.

After a middle cerebral cortical branch greater than 1 mm has been identified, its

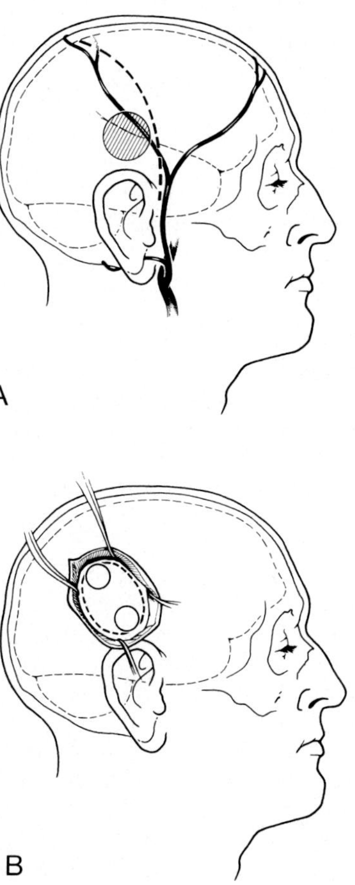

Figure 15–1. Exposure of the superficial temporal artery. The part to be exposed is marked with the shaded circle. The dotted line indicates the skin incision (*A*). Outline of the burr-holes and craniotomy to prepare the transfer of the superficial temporal artery into the skull cavity (*B*).

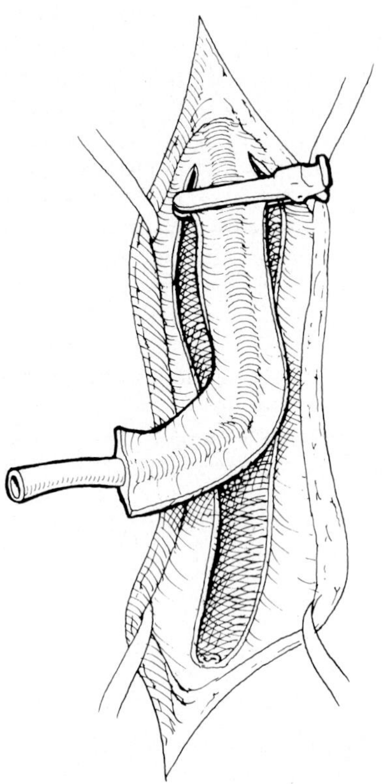

Figure 15-2. Preparation of the superficial temporal artery pedicle.

overlying arachnoid membrane is opened under magnified vision, and the cortical vessel is freed from small perforating arteries and isolated from the cortex by a small underlying rubber dam. The posterior branch of the superficial temporal artery is then dissected free from its attachments to the galea and scalp and occluded by a temporary vascular clip at its origin (see Figure 15-2). After being cut to an appropriate length, it is irrigated with heparinized saline solution and its distal tip is beveled at approximately 45 degrees. The recipient cortical vessel is isolated between fine clips, and a generous (3 to 4 mm long) linear or ellipsoid arteriotomy is performed (see Figure 15-3). The recipient vessel is then washed with heparinized saline solution, and an end-to-side anastomosis is performed between the donor superficial temporal artery and the recipient cortical artery. The anastomosis is done under 25 to 40X magnification using a 10 degree Nylon or prolene suture in either an interrupted or a running fashion (see Figure 15-4). The time from middle cerebral branch occlusion to restoration of focal flow should not exceed 30 to 45 minutes. After clip removal and routine hemostasis, the bone flap is resutured in place after a small bony tunnel is left open for passage of the donor artery.

This relatively simple technical procedure requires none of the usual extensive and potentially hazardous physiological and pharmacological manipulations common to many neurosurgical operative procedures. Brain tissue is not subjected to retraction; as a matter of fact, the cortex is almost never touched by the surgeon. Systematic hypotension and induced hypocapnia are avoided. Osmotic diuretics and cerebral spinal fluid drainage are not required for reduction of intracranial volume, and anticoagulants are not used. These important factors contribute to the low mortality and morbidity rates associated with this procedure. In the appropriate clinical and radiographic situations it is a reasonable therapeutic alternative even in patients with significant systematic and cardiovascular disease.

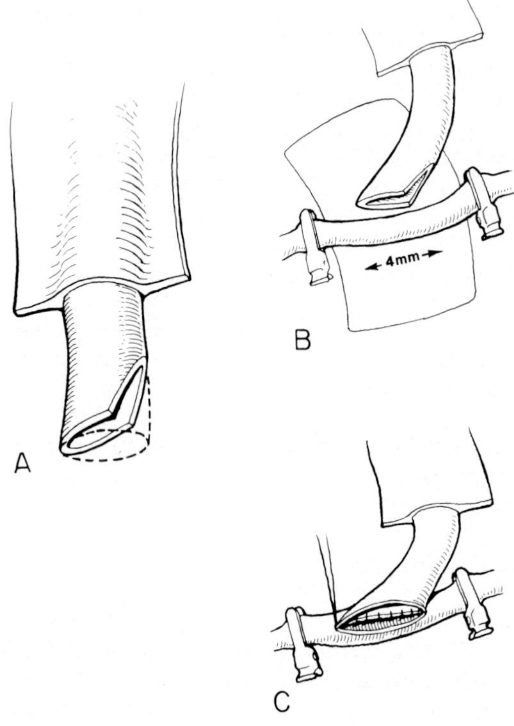

Figure 15-3. Preparation of the superficial temporal artery (*A*) and its approximation (*B*) and anastomosis (*C*) to the middle cerebral artery.

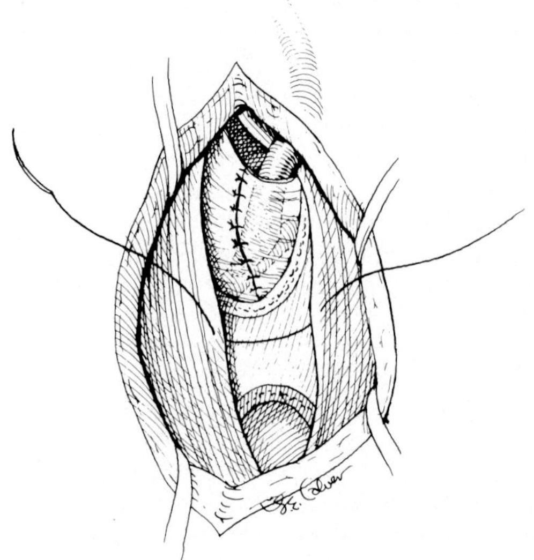

Figure 15–4. Closure of the incision after superficial temporal-to-middle cerebral artery anastomosis.

Results

Since the introduction of this technique in 1969, an estimated 7,000 such operations have been performed worldwide. While accurate evaluation of the procedure's efficacy and place in the treatment of cerebral ischemia as compared to the use of platelet suppressive agents must await the results of a randomized international cooperative study begun in 1977 (Barnett and Peerless, 1981), copious data concerning individual results are available (Chater, 1983, Medhorn *et al.,* 1979; Samson and Boone, 1978). In the hands of experienced microvascular surgeons, patency rates of the routine superficial temporal-middle cerebral anastomotic procedure as verified by routine postoperative angiography should approach 95 percent (see Figure 9-32).

Perioperative mortality and morbidity figures relate to and reflect the nature and severity of the ischemic event for which the bypass procedure is performed. Those figures are lowest in patients operated on for transient ischemic deficits and markedly higher in those undergoing revascularization for acute stroke or stroke-in-evolution (Samson and Boone, 1978). Patients with normal baseline neurological function who have transient ischemic events due to a completely occluded internal carotid artery should undergo revascularization with an operative mortality of about 2 percent and significant perioperative morbidity rates not exceeding 4 percent (Chater, 1983; Medhorn *et al.,* 1979; Samson *et al.,* 1979). Acute cerebral revascularization procedures performed in the face of significant neurological deficit of recent onset or progression, however, are attended by a relatively high incidence of either neurological deterioration or death. The principal cause of perioperative mortality in most series has been hemorrhagic cerebral infarction in surgical patients with acute neurological deficits and cardiac complications in patients undergoing surgery for transient ischemic episodes (Samson and Boone, 1978).

As mentioned previously, the long-term neurological consequences of extracranial intracranial arterial bypass have yet to be definitively established. We expect that the results of a randomized international study comparing the merits of this surgical procedure with platelet suppression agents in the treatment of a variety of forms of acute and chronic cerebral ischemic states will supply important additional data on the subject (Barnett and Peerless, 1981). In the selected surgical series reported to date, 80 to 85 percent of patients with transient ischemic episodes in the middle cerebral distribution who have undergone extracranial-intracranial bypass have reported cessation of their ischemic events (Chater, 1983; Medhorn *et al.,* 1979; Samson and Boone, 1978). An additional 10 percent continued to have ischemic events for a brief time after surgery only. Transient ischemic attacks have remained unchanged in roughly 5 percent. Four to 5 percent of patients who undergo a successful bypass procedure will subsequently have a completed stroke, roughly half of those strokes being in the distribution of the bypass procedure (Chater, 1983; Medhorn *et al.,* 1979; Samson and Boone, 1978). Although these preliminary results are definitely encouraging, especially in light of the high incidence of graft patency and relatively low surgical mortality and morbidity rates, adequate data to support the use of extracranial-intracranial bypass in all transient ischemic attack patients with carotid occlusion are not yet available.

Extracranial-intracranial bypass, when used in the treatment of patients with stroke-in-evolution, partial nonprogressive strokes, or so-called "stutter" strokes, produces less favorable neurological result than the same procedure in patients with transient ischemic attack. The several small series reported to date demonstrate resolution of neurological deficit in roughly 30 percent of the patients, arrest of neurological deficit in an additional 30 percent, and a progression or worsening of neurological deficit subsequent to the surgery in roughly 40 percent of the patients (Chater and Popp, 1976; Reichman, 1976; Samson and Boone, 1978; Yasargil and Yonekawa, 1977). As mentioned previously, it is in this group of patients with acute cerebral ischemia that the bypass procedure, like carotid endarterectomy, carries the highest mortality and morbidity risk.

A third group of patients, those with completed strokes and fixed, stable neurologic deficits, have also been subjected to cerebral revascularization but in relatively small numbers. Fifteen to 20 percent of completed-stroke patients can be demonstrated to have some degree (usually slight) of objective and subjective improvement after extracranial-intracranial bypass (Sundt *et al.*, 1976; Yasargil and Yonekawa, 1977). However, no important neurologic recovery occurs in the overwhelming majority (70 percent), and some degree of neurological deterioration will be seen in 5 to 10 percent of patients with fixed neurological deficits after extracranial-intracranial bypass. A subsequent second stroke in the area of the bypass procedure has been reported in about 3 percent of the patients with completed stroke who have undergone the bypass procedure. This figure may be of importance, because natural-history studies suggest the incidence of second "same-territory" stroke may be as high as 20 percent (Hutchinson and Atkinson, 1975). Extracranial-intracranial bypass may theoretically be of benefit in selected patients with completed strokes who have a good neurological recovery and critically compromised collateral flow. In such patients, extraintracranial bypass may decrease risk of a subsequent potentially catastrophic infarction.

OTHER EXTRAINCRANIAL BYPASS PROCEDURES

Since the development of extraintracranial bypass procedures, a significant number of patients have come to medical attention who theoretically and angiographically might benefit from augmentation of external carotid collateral circulation to the middle cerebral distribution but are not candidates for the routine superficial temporal-middle cerebral artery bypass procedure. In certain patients, donor branches of the external carotid artery are absent or inadequate for congenital or traumatic reasons. In others, clinical findings and investigative studies may demonstrate an acute need for higher volume of collateral flow, as in patients with acute carotid or middle cerebral artery occlusion secondary to trauma or to surgical maneuvers necessary to exclude a difficult intracranial aneurysm or facilitate intracranial or cervicofacial tumor removal (Samson *et al.*, 1981). In such situations, several innovative alternatives to the routine bypass procedure (superficial temporal-middle cerebral bypass) have been developed over the past 12 years. The first of these represents only a slight modification of the original superficial temporal-to-middle cerebral anastomosis by using a branch of the occipital artery as the donor vessel (Spetzler and Chater, 1976). This procedure is most often used when the branches of the superficial temporal artery are not suitable for anastomosis. It requires a somewhat more posteriorly placed skin and bone incision and is a slightly more difficult technical procedure because of the nature and course of the occipital artery.

The rest of the extraintracranial revascularization procedures require interposition vessel grafting and at least two anastomoses (Samson *et al.*, 1981). Short grafts have frequently been used to connect the proximal superficial temporal or occipital arteries with the cortical branch of the middle cerebral artery when distal branches were of insufficient caliber. In general these procedures employ a small-diameter vein or arterial graft connected proximally to an external carotid branch by an end-to-end anastomosis and distally to the cortical recipient by an end-to-side anastomosis. Such operations are performed in much the same fashion as the routine bypass procedures and, aside from the necessity of graft harvest, pose no new or unusual technical demands over those routinely encountered in the classic operation. Longer interposition grafts, reaching from the area of the carotid bifurcation or from the subclavian artery to the symptomatic middle cerebral distribution, have also been used with increasing frequency in recent years in specific situations, such as traumatic internal carotid injuries or common carotid occlusion (Chater, 1983; Cote *et al.*, 1983; Furlan *et al.*, 1980; Marzewsky *et al.*, 1982). Interposition conduits have included autogenous venous grafts, free arterial grafts, and certain synthetic materials, such as Gore-Tex. These procedures are obviously more ambitious and complicated than a routine extracranial-intracranial bypass and require, in addition to graft harvest, rather extensive cervical dissections, a large proximal anastomosis, and construction of a soft-tissue tunnel from the proximal to the distal anastomotic sites. Systemic anticoagulation is advisable at least during the proximal anastomosis, and significant dissection may be required in the sylvian fissure to identify an appropriate recipient vessel.

In light of the increased complexity and technical demands of such procedures it would be expected that the overall surgical results would perhaps be less encouraging than those experienced with the routine extracranial-intracranial bypass procedure. Long-term patency rates in most series have ranged from 75 to 80 percent with a relatively high frequency of early graft closure related principally to technical problems and to disparity between donor-recipient vessels (Samson *et al.*, 1981). Furthermore, because blood volume initially passing through the vein graft can be as high as 100 to 120 ml/min, there is an increased incidence of perioperative intracerebral hemorrhage, especially early in the postoperative periods. The largest series published to date suggests that up to 20 percent of the patients undergoing such a procedure may fall victim to this complication (Samson *et al.*, 1981). Intraparenchymal hemorrhage in such cases may relate not only to reperfusion of the infarcted brain tissue but also to sudden exposure of the chronically ischemic, maximally dilated, low resistance cerebral vascular network to the unregulated high pressure flow of the systemic circulation. Surprisingly, once past the initial postoperative period, long-term neurologic outcome is encouraging with significant reductions in subsequent ischemic events paralleling the results seen with the conventional bypass procedure (Samson *et al.*, 1981).

Long-term follow-up studies demonstrate with increasing frequency that internal carotid artery occlusion (Cote *et al.*, 1983; Furlan *et al.*, 1980) and high-grade intracranial carotid stenosis (Craig *et al.*, 1982; Marzewsky *et al.*, 1982) are not benign conditions, with subsequent 5 to 15 percent per year stroke rates in the affected hemisphere. In these patients, multiple therapeutic options are available including platelet suppression, systemic anticoagulation, external carotid endarterectomy, internal carotid "stumpectomy," contralateral internal carotid endarterectomy, and extracranial-intracranial arterial bypass. No single approach is adequate, much less ideal, for every patient. The therapeutic alternatives must be tailored to the individual clinical and radiologic situation without regard to disciplinary borderlines. Careful evaluation of patient symptoms, potential risk factors, and initial response to platelet suppressive therapy must be considered and noninvasive screening tests liberally employed when appropriate. Initial radiographic investigation must detail the nature and configuration of the carotid occlusion and fully outline the available sources of collateral supply and the presence or absence of other cervical and intracranial vascular lesions. Preoperative computed tomography scanning is essential, and, when available, cerebral blood-flow measurements should be obtained in all patients undergoing evaluation. Only from such a broad data base is the clinician able to select for each patient the therapeutic approach which will provide a maximal opportunity to avoid subsequent and perhaps disabling cerebral ischemic episodes.

REFERENCES

Barnett, H.J.M., and Peerless, S.J.: Collaborative EC/IC bypass study: the rationale and a progress report. In Moosy, J., and Reinmuth, O.M. (eds.): *Cerebrovascular Diseases*. Raven Press, New York, 1981.

Chater, N., and Popp, J.: Microsurgical vascular bypass for occlusive cerebrovascular disease: review of 100 cases. *Surg. Neurol.*, **6**:115–8, 1976.

Chater, N.; Spetzler, R.; and Mani, J.: The spectrum of cerebrovascular occlusive disease suitable for microvascular bypass surgery. *Angiology*, **26**:235–51, 1975.

Chater, N.; Spetzler, R.; Tonnemacher, K.; and Wilson, C.B.: Microvascular bypass surgery. Part 1. Anatomical studies. *J. Neurosurg.*, **44**:712–4, 1976.

Chater, N.N.: Results of neurosurgical microvascular extracranial-intracranial bypass for stroke: a decade of experience. *West. J. Med.*, **138**:531–3, 1983.

Cote, R.; Barnett, H.J.M.; and Taylor, D.W.: Internal carotid occlusion: a prospective study. *Stroke*, **14**:898–902, 1983.

Craig, D.R.; Meguro, K.; Watridge, C.; Robertson J.T.; Barnett, H.J.; and Fox, A.J.: Intracranial internal carotid artery stenosis. *Stroke*, **13**:825–8, 1982.

Donaghy, R.M.P.: Neurologic surgery. *Surg. Gynecol. Obstet.*, **134**:269–71, 1972.

Fein, J.M., and Molinari, G.: Experimental augmentation of regional cerebral blood flow by microvascular anastomosis. *J. Neurosurg.*, **41**:421–6, 1974.

Furlan, A.J.; Whisnant, J.P.; and Baker, H.L., Jr.: Long term prognosis after carotid artery occlusion. *Neurology*, **30**:986–8, 1980.

Heilbrun, M.P.; Reichman, O.H.; Anderson, R.E.; and Roberts, T.S.: Regional cerebral blood flow studies following superficial temporal-middle cerebral artery anastomosis. *J. Neurosurg.,* **43**:706-16, 1975.

Hutchinson, E.C., and Atkinson, E.I.: *Strokes: Natural History, Pathology and Surgical Treatment.* London, W.B. Saunders Co., 1975.

Lassen, N.A., and Ingvar, D.H.: Regional cerebral blood flow measurement in man: a review. *Arch. Neurol.,* **9**:615-22, 1963.

Marzewski, D.S.; Furlan, A.J.; St. Louis, P.; Little, J.R.; Modie, W.T.; and Williams, G.: Intracranial internal carotid artery stenosis: long term prognosis. *Stroke,* **13**:821-4, 1982.

Medhorn, L.T.M.; Hoffman, W.F.; and Chater, N.C.: Microvascular neurosurgical arterial bypass for cerebral ischemia: a decade of development. *World J. Surg.,* **3**:197-206, 1979.

Nornes, H., and Wikeby, P.: Cerebral arterial blood flow and aneurysm surgery. Part 1. Local arterial flow dynamics. *J. Neurosurg.,* **47**:810-8, 1977.

Reichman, O.H.: Complications of cerebral revascularization. *Clin. Neurosurg.,* **23**:318-35, 1976.

Samson, D.; Hodosh, R.M.; and Clark, W.K.: Microsurgical treatment of transient cerebral ischemia: preliminary results in 50 cases. *J.A.M.A.,* **241**:376-78, 1979.

Samson, D.S., and Boone, S.: Extracranial-intracranial (EC-IC) arterial bypass: past performance and current concepts. *Neurosurgery,* **3**:79-86, 1978.

Samson, D.S.; Gewertz, B.L.; Beyer, C.W.; and Hodosh, R.M.: Saphenous vein interposition grafts in the microsurgical treatment of cerebral ischemia. *Arch. Surg.,* **116**:1578-82, 1981.

Spetzler, R., and Chater, N.: Microvascular bypass surgery. Part 2. Physiological studies. *J. Neurosurg.,* **45**:508-13, 1976.

Sundt, T.M., Jr.; Grant, W.C.; and Garcia, J.H.: Restoration of middle cerebral artery flow in experimental infarction. *J. Neurosurg.,* **31**:311-21, 1969.

Sundt, T.M., Jr.; Siekert, R.G.; Piepgras, D.G.; Sharbrough, F.W.; and Houser, O.W.: Bypass surgery for vascular disease of the carotid system. *Mayo Clin. Proc.,* **51**:677-92, 1976.

Sundt, T.M., Jr., and Waltz, A.G.: Cerebral ischemia and reactive hyperemia: studies of cortical blood flow and microcirculation before, during, and after temporary occlusion of middle cerebral artery of squirrel monkeys. *Cir. Res.,* **28**:426-33, 1971.

Toole, J.F., and Patel, A.W.: *Cerebrovascular Disorders,* 2nd ed. McGraw-Hill, New York, pages 187-214, 1974.

Yasargil, M.G.: Anastomosis between the superficial temporal artery and a branch of the middle cerebral artery. In Yasargil, M.G. (ed.): *Microsurgery Applied to Neurosurgery.* George Thieme Verlag, Stuttgart, 1969.

Yasargil, M.G., and Yonekawa, Y.: Results of microsurgical extra-intracranial arterial bypass in the treatment of cerebral ischemia. *Neurosurgery,* **1**:22-4, 1977.

16

The Management of Nonobstructive Ulcerated Plaques of the Carotid Bifurcation

JOSEPH W. COOK

HISTORY AND EVOLUTION OF CONCEPTS

Mechanisms proposed to explain the clinical picture of transient episodic neurological deficits that may lead to a permanent defect include vasospasm, transient systemic hypotension, carotid artery kinking, polycythemia, anemia, transient shunts, peripheral emboli, and reduction of blood flow by arterial stenosis. Clinical experience indicates that symptoms caused by carotid artery kinking, polycythemia, and anemia are relatively rare. Similarly, vasospasm is unlikely to occur in a localized area to produce related similar ischemic attacks, because carbon dioxide and other intracerebral vasodilators do not relieve transient ischemic attacks (Eastcott *et al.,* 1954; Millikan, 1965). Abnormal shunting may be seen in conditions such as the subclavian steal syndrome but again they do not explain the symptoms of most patients.

Mechanical obstruction to flow was and still is widely accepted as an important factor in the development of cerebral ischemia. To explain the intermittent nature of the attacks, this concept was coupled with the suggestion that transient episodes of systemic hypotension could trigger the intermittent episodes of cerebral ischemia in the presence of highly stenotic carotid arteries (Denny-Brown, 1960). The validity of this postulate has been challenged by numerous observations because transient ischemic attacks (TIAs) cannot be induced with the deliberate production of systemic hypotension (Kendall and Marshall, 1963). To undermine further the role of transient systemic hypotension, ophthalmic artery pressures were found to remain constant during ischemic attacks (Russell and Cranstone, 1961). Furthermore, in the presence of tight bifurcation lesions, total cerebral blood flow has been measured as being normal; it did not increase after endarterectomy. Sundt, in carefully conducted studies, has shown no decrease in cerebral blood flow until the internal carotid lumen is reduced to 1 mm in diameter (90 percent stenosis (Sundt *et al.,* 1981). Yet many patients have been relieved of TIAs by surgical removal of less stenotic plaques. It is also notable that TIAs have ceased in many patients after the carotid artery lesion has progressed to total occlusion (Drake and Drake, 1968). This lack of confirmation of the hemodynamic theory has led to a more general acceptance of the role of emboli as the link between carotid bifurcation lesions and cerebral dysfunction.

At the turn of the century Chiari (1905) suggested that carotid lesions are a potential source of cerebral emboli. Further corroboration to the embolus theory was added when Millikan and associates (1955) and Fisher (1958) demonstrated the relief of TIAs by anticoagulants. If a simple hemodynamic mechanism were operative, then neither anticoagulants nor total occlusion could relieve intermittent ischemia, whereas both would reduce the incidence of emboli. The observation by Hollenhorst (1961) of "yellow and white inclusions," presumably cholesterol emboli in retinal arterioles, was a major contribution to understanding embolic processes. Such emboli were found in 9.5 percent of 235 patients with extracranial arterial lesions. Microemboli were also demonstrated histologically in a patient with monocular blindness (McBrien *et al.,* 1963). In 1963, Julian and associates reported a series of patients in whom ulceration was observed in carotid plaques removed at endarterectomy. Because in some instances thrombus was seen attached to the ulcer, he suggested that such thrombus might embolize. Moore and Hall (1968) reported a series of carotid endarterectomies of nonstenotic (50 percent) ulcerated carotid plaques which resulted in complete relief of transient ischemic episodes. The fact that relief was obtained by removal of nonstenotic ulcers implies that the beneficial effect of most carotid endarterectomies is due to elimination of the source of emboli. Kishore and associates (1971) found an increased incidence of middle cerebral artery occlusions in a series of patients with ulcerated or irregular carotid plaques, suggesting an embolic source.

PATHOLOGY AND DYNAMICS

Symptoms of cerebral ischemia may be produced by embolization of platelet aggregates, thrombus, or cholesterol emboli (see Figure 16–1). The type of embolus will largely depend on flow dynamics and plaque morphology.

Although the exact series of events leading to atheroma formation has not been defined, much evidence has accumulated to suggest that the initiating factor is endothelial injury (Ross *et al.,* 1980) caused by turbulence at the orifices of arterial branches and that systemic events, such as hypertension and diabetes, may also play a contributing role. When endothelium is damaged, platelets adhere to the denuded vessel wall, and this promotes thrombus formation. Lipid may accumulate by entering the wall from the serum and also by in situ smooth muscle cell synthesis (Goldstein and Brown, 1977) (see also Chapter 3 on the carotid plaque).

Once a plaque is formed, secondary changes usually occur. Imparato and associates (1983) and Lusby and coworkers (1982) have independently reported series of surgically removed specimens showing frequent hemorrhage into the atheroma. Such hemorrhage may be related to the proliferation of small vessels observed in the base of some plaques. A plaque hematoma will result in acute reduction of the lumen of the vessel and may cause rupture of the plaque with consequent release of atheromatous material and clot (see Figure 16–2). Lusby reported fresh intraplaque hemorrhage in 92.5 percent of atheromas removed from symptomatic patients and in 27 percent of plaques removed from asymptomatic patients. He suggests that the development of intraplaque hemorrhage is the event that triggers the onset of symptoms.

An atheroma that is low in collagen is soft,

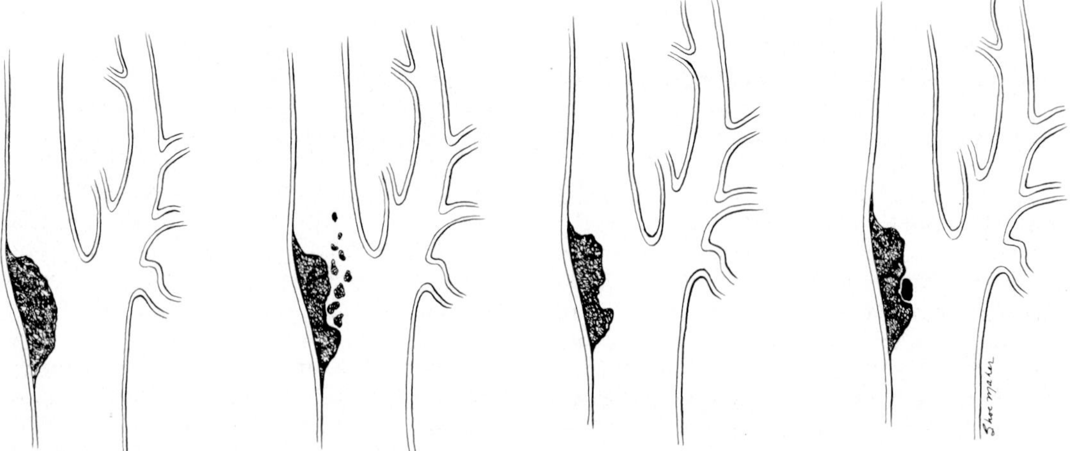

Figure 16–1. Rupture of the carotid bifurcation plaque causes embolization of atheromatous debris leaving an ulcer. The ulcer then acts as a site for the formation of further thrombi.

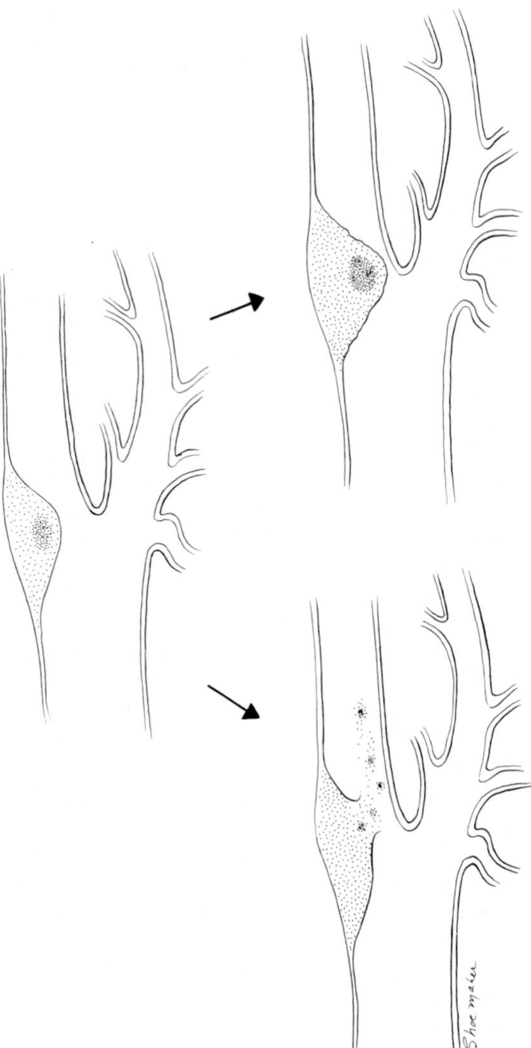

Figure 16–2. Illustration of the possible consequences of an intraplaque hemorrhage. The plaque may expand (upper arrow) causing acute obstruction of the internal carotid and/or rupture (lower arrow), inducing embolization of plaque contents including clot from the hematoma.

friable, and rich in lipids. Trauma and expansion of such a plaque may easily lead to rupture, atheromatous embolization, and the formation of a surface crater, which is a further nidus to platelet thrombi formation that may then embolize. The incidence of microscopic ulceration in carotid plaques has been reported to vary from 50 to 60 percent (Blaisdell *et al.*, 1974; Bartynski *et al.*, 1981). Hertzer and associates (1977) observed small ulcers in up to 25 percent of plaques. With the scanning electron microscope, intimal disruptions with adherent platelets and fibrin were reported in all of eight plaques examined (Hertzer *et al.*, 1977). The investigators suggest that ulcerations and thrombi from 100 to 600 μm are large enough in size to produce symptoms because the diameter of the central retinal artery is about 250 μm. Such ulcerations are consistent with the "response to injury" theory of plaque formation discussed previously.

The tendency of patients to have similar recurrent neurological defects during TIAs suggests that emboli may repeatedly travel to the same destination. Millikan demonstrated this fact in monkeys by injecting metal beads at the same point in the carotid artery, all of which traveled to the same intracranial artery. He concluded that flow will float emboli from a point source (ulcer) to the same terminal branch by selective streaming.

Sources for emboli may include the aorta, the innominate, and the vertebral systems, as well as the carotid bifurcation. On rare occasions, TIAs may occur in the presence of a completely occluded internal carotid artery. Barnett and associates (1978) studied a series of nine such patients and identified the stump of the internal carotid artery as the source of thrombi. Such thrombi may then embolize through the external carotid artery and lodge in retinal or intracranial arteries (see Figure 16–3). Such attacks were relieved by resection of the stump (see Figure 14–20).

DIAGNOSIS

The preoperative diagnosis of carotid artery ulceration depends on its radiographic demonstration. Blaisdell and associates (1974) defined radiographic criteria for ulceration as (1) a penetrating niche, (2) irregularity in the silhouette of the artery, (3) delayed washout of contrast in areas of stenosis, and (4) a double density superimposed on the artery. The accuracy of radiographic diagnosis of ulceration is reported to range from 50 to 86 percent (Blaisdell *et al.*, 1974; Bartynski *et al.*, 1981). This low rate of accuracy is related to several factors including the small size of some ulcers. The angiographic projection must also show the ulcer in profile, and if the ulcer is filled with thrombus, it will not be seen at all. Compounding these difficulties are superficial ulcers which may give rise to symptom-producing emboli but are too shallow to be recognized radiographically. This lack of accuracy

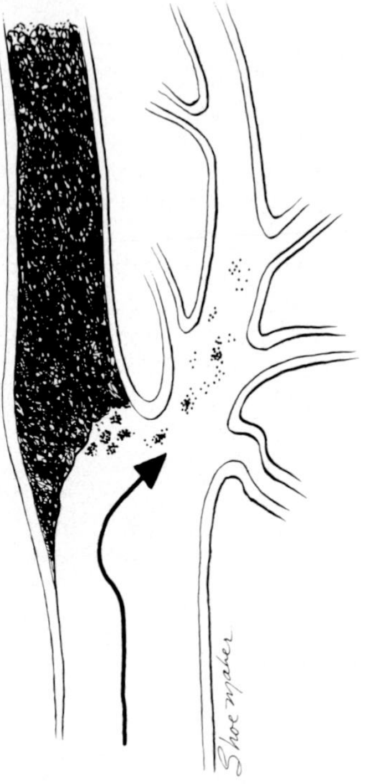

Figure 16-3. Embolization of material into the external carotid artery from the stump of a totally occluded internal carotid artery.

of angiographic demonstration of carotid ulcers has markedly retarded the delineation and understanding of the natural history of this condition (see Figures 9-18 and 19).

Moore and associates (1978) proposed a classification of carotid bifurcation ulcers based on size and shape. Type A ulcers are small, Type B ulcers are large, and Type C ulcers are even larger with multiple craters. Moore's correlation between ulcer type and prognosis is discussed later.

Although noninvasive carotid studies, including M-mode imaging, have achieved reasonable accurate assessment of the degree of carotid stenosis, the resolution of scanning has not yet reached levels where nonstenotic ulcers can be accurately diagnosed (see also Chapter 6 on clinical manifestations of carotid disease).

CLINICAL MANAGEMENT

In order to define the appropriate management of ulcerated carotid plaques, the natural history of such lesions must be studied. Unfortunately, there is a lack of large well-controlled prospective series on this subject. Dixon and associates (1982) studied a group of patients with nonstenotic asymptomatic carotid ulcers. Patients with small ulcers (Type A) had a 0.9 percent annual stroke rate. Patients with larger ulcers (Type B) and multiple ulcers (Type C) had annual stroke rates of 4.5 and 7.5 percent, respectively. Dixon and colleagues recommend prophylactic endarterectomy in Types B and C. There were no antecedent warning TIAs in this group of patients, a finding that differs from other reports. Harward and associates (1983) studied a similar group with nonstenotic Type A and B ulcers and found a benign prognosis for both groups. Grotta and associates (1984) concluded that the arteriographically proven presence of an ulcer did not influence prognosis in symptomatic or asymptomatic patients unless there was associated stenosis of more than 50 percent. In no study was the use of platelet antagonists or other anticoagulants controlled.

The role of anticoagulation in the treatment of ulcerated plaques has not been adequately evaluated. Although the Canadian Cooperative Study Group (1978) found that aspirin decreased the incidence of neurological events in males with extracranial vascular disease, it failed to analyze the effect of aspirin on patients with proven ulcerated plaques. Fields and associates (1978) also reported the benefit of aspirin in patients who were not operated upon and in endarterectomized patients. Dipyridamole and sulfinpyrazone have also been shown effective in preventing platelet aggregation in vitro but have not been proven useful in patients with cerebrovascular disease (Canadian Cooperative Study Group, 1978; Acheson *et al.*, 1969). Anticoagulants in patients with ulcerated carotid plaques could also mask the occurrence of warning TIAs while the plaque progresses to the point of occlusion. Anticoagulants are also a possible cause of occlusion by promoting hemorrhage into the plaque. The probability of these mechanisms, however, is entirely speculative and is yet to be supported by appropriate clinical trials (see also Chapter 11 on medical management of carotid disease).

When confronted with the management of a patient with a carotid lesion, the clinician has two basic choices: (1) carotid endarterectomy, or (2) observation with or without anticoagulation. In the case of ulcerated plaques, the decision cannot be rigidly based on data because of the absence of large prospective studies. Consideration must also be given to the expected results of endarterectomy, to patient compliance, and to the feasibility of careful follow up. With these variations in mind, our practice for treating these patients is as follows.

If a patient presents with a hemispheric TIA and only a small nonstenotic ulcer is found on angiography (Type A or B), we treat the patient with aspirin and dipyridamole. The same regimen is prescribed for patients with small asymptomatic ulcers fortuitously discovered at arteriography. Such patients have been found in two prospective studies to have a benign prognosis (Dixon *et al.*, 1982; Harward *et al.*, 1983). Although similar data are not available for the symptomatic group, it seems logical that if these patients can be made asymptomatic with a low risk platelet antagonist regimen their prognosis will remain good. Education is crucial, and the patient and his/her family must report any symptom of transient neurological dysfunction which would prompt immediate reconsideration for surgery. Equally important, we feel, is the regular follow up of these patients with noninvasive studies, because most of these plaques steadily increase in size (Javid *et al.*, 1970). A reassessment is mandatory if the lesions become significantly stenotic or TIAs recur despite well-controlled medical management.

In patients with compound or cavernous ulcers, endarterectomy is indicated irrespective of symptoms. Although these lesions are relatively rare, our experience is that at surgery they are soft and friable and portions of the plaque itself are probably embolizing. Anticoagulation will not retard this process. The lesions have an annual stroke rate of 7.5 percent (Dixon *et al.*, 1982), which seems to justify this aggressive approach (see also Chapter 13 on surgical indications in carotid artery disease).

Regardless of the presence or absence of symptoms we recommend carotid endarterectomy for ulcerated plaques large enough to cause greater than 50 percent stenosis. Two series (Grotta *et al.*, 1984; Dorazio *et al.*, 1980) have noted a poor prognosis for this group if the patients are not operated upon. If the thesis is correct that most TIAs result from emboli originating from ulcerations, then it is interesting to speculate on how the presence of stenosis increases the frequency of these events. One possibility, noted previously, is that hemorrhage into a plaque may be the cause of the acute onset of symptoms and anticoagulation may lead to or worsen this process. Because hemorrhage into a large stenotic plaque is more likely to cause complete arterial occlusion than if the plaque were small, it seems reasonable to recommend endarterectomy for patients harboring large plaques. If carotid endarterectomy can be performed with low mortality and morbidity, then this would be our choice for these lesions. The surgical technique of carotid endarterectomy is discussed elsewhere in this book (See Chapter 14). When surgery is performed for a known ulcerated plaque, the fact that a thrombus loosely adherent to the plaque may be present must be constantly borne in mind. This possibility should prompt strict avoidance of manipulation of the carotid bifurcation before clamping the internal carotid. If a shunt is used, then it should be inserted very carefully under visual control, the surgeon being sure that the arteriotomy extends well proximal and distal to the lesion.

REFERENCES

Acheson, J.; Danta, G.; and Hutchinson, E.C.: Controlled trial of dipyridamole in cerebral vascular disease. *Br. Med. J.*, **1**:614–15, 1969.

Barnett, H.J.M.; Peerless, S.J.; and Kaufman, J.C.E.: "Stump" of the internal carotid artery—a source for further cerebral embolic ischemia. *Stroke*, **9**:448–56, 1978.

Bartynski, W.S.; Darbouze, P.; and Nemir, P., Jr.: Significance of ulcerated plaque in transient cerebral ischemia. *Am. J. Surg.*, **141**:353–57, 1981.

Blaisdell, F.W.; Glickman, M.; and Trunkey, D.D.: Ulcerated atheroma of the carotid artery. *Arch. Surg.*, **108**:491–96, 1974.

Canadian Cooperative Study Group: A randomized trial of aspirin and sulfinpyrazone in threatened stroke. *N. Engl. J. Med.*, **299**:53–9, 1978.

Chiari, H.: Ueber das Verhalten des Teilungswinkels der Carotis communis bei der Endarteritis chronica deformans. *Verh. Dtsch. Ges. Pathol.*, **9**:326–30, 1905.

Denny-Brown, D.: Recurrent cerebrovascular episodes. *Arch. Neurol.*, **2**:194–210, 1960.

Dixon, S.; Pais, S.P.; Raviola, C.; Gomes, A.; Machleder, H.I.; Baker, J.D.; Busuttil, R.W.; Barker, W.F., and Moore, W.S.: Natural history of nonstenotic asymptomatic ulcerative lesions of the carotid artery. *Arch. Surg.*, **117**:1493–98, 1982.

Dorazio, R.A.; Ezzet, F.; and Nesbitt, N.J.: Long-term follow-up of asymptomatic carotid bruits. *Am. J. Surg.*, **140**:212–13, 1980.

Drake, W.E., Jr., and Drake, M.A.L.: Clinical and angiographic correlates of cerebrovascular insufficiency. *Am. J. Med.*, **45**:253–70, 1968.

Eastcott, H.H.G.; Pickering, G.W.; and Rob, C.G.: Reconstruction of internal carotid artery in a patient with intermittent attacks of hemiplegia. *Lancet*, **2**:994–96, 1954.

Fields, W.S.; Lemak, N.A.; Frankowski, R.F.; and Hardy,

R.J.: Controlled trial of aspirin in cerebral ischemia. Part 2. Surgical group. *Stroke,* **9**:309–19, 1978.

Fisher, C.M.: The use of anticoagulants in cerebral thrombosis. *Neurology,* **8**:311–32, 1958.

Goldstein, J.L., and Brown, M.S.: The low density lipoprotein pathway and its relationship to atherosclerosis. *Annu. Rev. Biochem.,* **46**:897–930, 1977.

Grotta, J.C.U.; Bigelow, R.H.; Hankins, L.; and Fields, W.S.: The significance of carotid stenosis or ulceration. *Neurology,* **34**:437–42, 1984.

Harward, T.R.S.; Kroener, J.M.; Wickbom, I.G.; and Bernstein, E.F.: Natural history of asymptomatic ulcerative plaques of the carotid bifurcation. *Am. J. Surg.,* **146**:208–12, 1983.

Hertzer, N.R.; Beven, E.G.; and Benjamin, S.P.: Ultramicroscopic ulcerations and thrombi of the carotid bifurcation. *Arch. Surg.,* **112**:1394–1402, 1977.

Hollenhorst, R.W.: Significance of bright plaques in the retinal arterioles. *J.A.M.A.,* **178**:23–29, 1961.

Imparato, A.M.; Riles, T.S.; Mintzer, R.; and Bauman, F.G.: The importance of hemorrhage in the relationship between gross morphologic characteristics and cerebral symptoms in 376 carotid artery plaques. *Ann. Surg.,* **197**(2):195–203, 1983.

Javid, H.; Ostermiller, W.E.; Hengesh, J.W.; Dye, W.S.; Hunter, J.A.; Najafi, H.; and Julian, D.C.: Natural history of carotid bifurcation atheroma. *Surgery,* **67**:80–86, 1970.

Julian, O.C.; Dye, W.S.; Javid, H.; and Hunter, J.A.: Ulcerative lesions of the carotid artery bifurcation. *Arch. Surg.,* **86**:803–89, 1963.

Kendall, R.E., and Marshall, J.: Role of hypotension in the genesis of transient focal cerebral ischemic attacks. *Br. Med. J.,* **2**:344–48, 1963.

Kishore, P.R.S.; Chase, N.E.; and Kricheff, I.I.: Carotid stenosis and intracranial emboli. *Radiology,* **100**:351–56, 1971.

Lusby, R.J.; Ferrell, L.D.; Ehrenfeld, W.K.; Stoney, R.J.; and Wylie, E.J.: Carotid plaque hemorrhage: its role in production of cerebral ischemia. *Arch. Surg.,* **117**(11):1479–88, 1982.

McBrien, D.J.; Bradley, R.D.; and Ashton, N.: The nature of retinal emboli in stenosis of the internal carotid artery. *Lancet,* **1**:697–99, 1963.

Millikan, C.H.: The pathogenesis of transient focal cerebral ischemia. *Circulation,* **32**:438–50, 1965.

Millikan, C.H.; Siekert, R.G.; and Shick, R.M.: Studies in cerebrovascular disease. 5. The use of anticoagulant drugs in the treatment of intermittent insufficiency of the internal carotid arterial system. *Proc. Staff Mtg. Mayo Clin.,* **30**:578, 1955.

Moore, W.S., and Hall, A.D.: Ulcerated atheroma of the carotid artery: a cause of transient cerebral ischemia. *Am. J. Surg.,* **116**:237–42, 1968.

Moore, W.S.; Boren, C.; Malone, J.M.; Roon, A.J.; Eisenberg, R.; Goldstone, J.; and Mani, R.: Natural history of nonstenotic asymptomatic ulcerative lesions of the carotid artery. *Arch. Surg.,* **113**:1352–59, 1978.

Ross, R.; Vogel, A.; Raines, E.; and Kariya, B.: The platelet derived growth factor. In Grotto, A.M.; Smith, L.C., and Allen, B.B. (eds.): *Atherosclerosis V: Proceedings of Fifth International Symposium.* Springer-Verlag, New York, pages 442–49, 1980.

Russel, R.W., and Cronstone, W.I.: Ophthalmodynamometry in carotid artery disease. *J. Neurol. Neurosurg. Psychiatry* **24**: 281, 1961.

Sundt, T.M., Jr.; Sharbrough, F.W.; Piepgras, D.G.; Kearns, T.P.; Messick, J.M., Jr.; and O'Fallon, W.M.: Correlation of cerebral blood flow and electroencephalographic changes during carotid endarterectomy: with results of surgery and hemodynamics of cerebral ischemia. *Mayo Clin. Proc.,* **56**(9):533–43, 1981.

17

Positional Obstruction of the Carotid Arteries. Fibromuscular Dysplasia

FRANCIS ROBICSEK

POSITIONAL OBSTRUCTION OF THE CAROTID ARTERIES

Embryologically, the internal carotid artery is a derivate of the dorsal aorta and the third branchial arch. It runs a tortuous course which gradually straightens as the fetal heart and large vessels recede into the mediastinum. Inordinate differential growth, however, may disrupt this process and cause persistence of the embryonic arterial bend and also produce different degrees of undulations and loops which may be observed in fetuses as well as in young children.

Another much more common mechanism by which these and similar changes may be produced is normal arterial aging. As a person grows older, muscle cells in the vessel wall degenerate, elastic fibers fragment, collagen and ground substances aggregate. As a result of this process, to which the carotid appears to be especially susceptible, the arterial diameter as well as length may increase, and vessels may become redundant. These events may be enhanced by associated hypertension or fibromuscular hyperplasia.

Tortuosity of the carotid arteries is a common phenomenon. The first accurate anatomical description of internal carotid tortuosity comes from the pen of G.H. Edington, of Glasgow, who during an anatomic dissection found that both internal carotid arteries were significantly elongated and made several "sudden turns" before entering the bony canal. He speculated that the condition "may be associated with the arteritis of chronic nephritis, . . . but its occurrence in a young subject may be explained by abnormal persistence of portions of the embryonic arches" (Edington, 1901).

Deterling in 1952 reported 81 cases of carotid tortuosity published in the literature and 21 cases of his own. In a large series of unselected arteriograms, some degree of redundance was found in 5 to 15 percent of the patients (Cioffi *et al.*, 1975; Najafi *et al.*, 1964). In cases with diagnosed arteriosclerosis of the carotid arteries, this number increased to 24 percent (Bauer *et al.*, 1961). Because of the tendency of the human body to maintain elongated vessels in a gently curved rather than in an angulated position, most of these persons go through life without symptoms of cerebral ischemia. Under certain conditions, however, carotid tortuosity can become clinically manifest and require surgical correction.

Morphologically, carotid tortuosity can be divided into two principal varieties: coils and kinks. The degree of coiling may vary from gentle C- or S-shaped elongation to a full 360 degree loop, which may occur at any segment of the internal or common carotid artery. In contrast to coils, kinks are sharp angulations usually found where the internal carotid artery bows at fixed points at the base of the skull. Whereas coils are often congenital and usually asymptomatic, kinks are commonly associated with arteriosclerosis and with subinti-

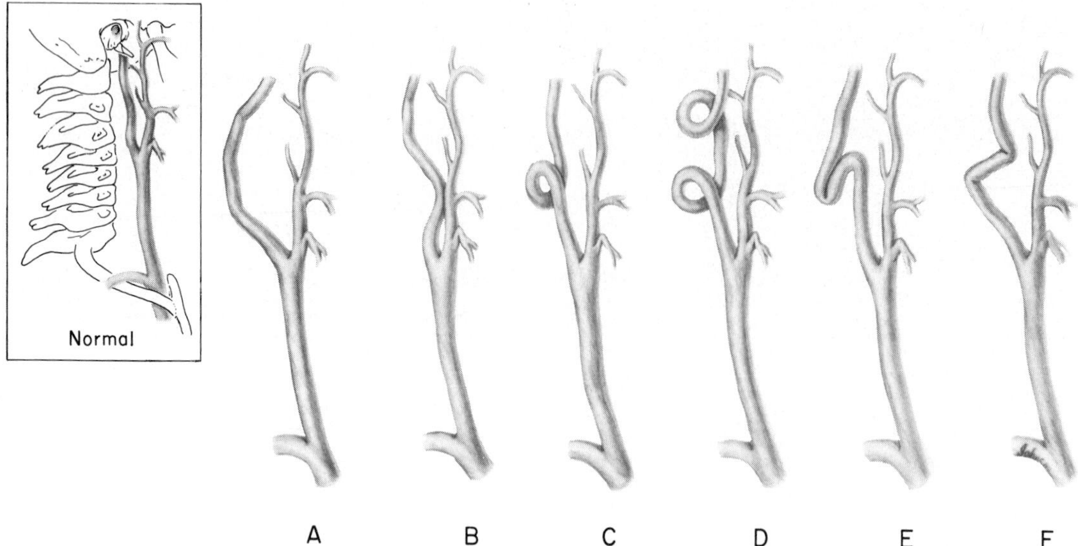

Figure 17–1. Different types of internal carotid elongation and tortuosity: C-shaped elongation, (*A*); S-shaped elongation (*B*); coil (*C*); double coil (*D*); buckle (*E*); and kink (*F*).

mal atheromatous deposits and more often cause symptoms of cerebral ischemia (see Figures 17–1 and 9–5).

The hemodynamic obstacle created by carotid kinks was analyzed in the in-depth study of Eichhorn and Schlicht (1969), who found that carotid angulations are primarily systolic obstructions, maximal in systole and least significant in diastole; therefore, their degree is related to both the height and the duration of the systolic pulse wave. From their study, it is also evident that tachycardia, in which the diastolic time decreases, unfavorably influences flow through kinked carotid arteries.

A particular form of carotid elongation is that which becomes manifest during operations performed on the carotid for other reasons, such as atherosclerotic stricture or ulceration. In the course of such procedures, the abnormally long internal carotid artery, heretofore kept in a gently curved posture by attachments of connective tissue, may be mobilized to such a degree that it coils or kinks (see Figure 17–2). Both spontaneous and surgically induced buckling must be corrected if it appears to impair the blood supply to the brain.

In a discussion of anatomical and clinical carotid elongation and angulation, it should be emphasized that there are other extrinsic causes of carotid obstruction which may cause the same or similar symptoms. A kink may also occur at a single point and may develop without the presence of elongation or tortuosity (Carney and Anderson, 1981). An example of the latter is compression of the internal carotid artery by inflammatory lymph nodes.

The diagnosis of carotid artery angulation is almost always made by angiography performed either incidentally or in search of occlusive lesions. Clinical history seldom contributes to the recognition of this disease because any symptoms that may be present are indistinguishable from those caused by intrinsic carotid lesions. Carotid elongation and angulation may produce symptoms by several mechanisms, e.g., embolization of fibrin or, more commonly, by reduction of flow. The latter may be exaggerated by ipsi- or contralateral rotation, flexion, or extension of the neck. In the most typical cases of symptomatic carotid tortuosities, episodes of cerebral ischemia may be triggered by postural changes of the head, especially by rotating the head toward the affected side. By exaggerating the already existing angulation, this maneuver may produce complete obstruction to the carotid blood flow. Such a mechanism was suggested by Gegenbauer (1899) and was confirmed angiographically by Bauer and associates (1961), who found that in all cases they studied in which buckling was demonstrated with the head in neutral position, the condition was made worse by rotation of the head.

Stanton and associates (1978) studied the

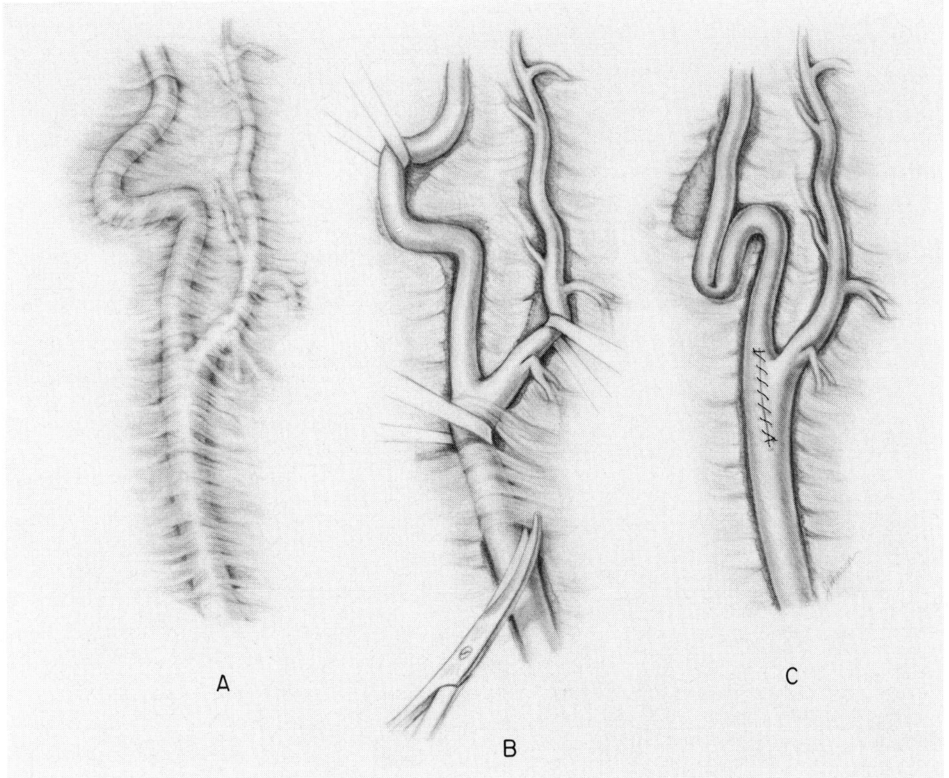

Figure 17–2. S-shaped nonocclusive tortuosity of the internal carotid artery (*A*). By dissecting the artery free in the course of carotid endarterectomy (*B*), the tortuosity may be converted into occlusive buckling (*C*).

effects of postural change upon the blood flow through buckled carotid arteries before, during, and after angioplasty. Correlating preoperative data obtained by noninvasive oculoplethysmography and with intraoperative electromagnetic flow measurements, they reported a reduction in flow of 30 to 80 percent in positional testing during operations in all patients who had similar response preoperatively. Furthermore, surgical correction of the tortuosity eliminated the effects of posture upon the internal carotid artery flow (Stanton *et al.,* 1978). These findings were similar to those of Herrschaft *et al.,* who in 1975 documented an average decrease in blood flow of 38 percent in the kinked carotid artery and return to near normal after surgical correction.

In the pathophysiology of symptomatic carotid tortuosity, the syndrome called *hypoglossal carotid entrapment* (Carney and Anderson, 1982) deserves special attention. This condition, which is often, though not always, associated with elongation of the carotid artery, is usually caused by infections of the respiratory tract. Inflammations of the nasopharynx, usually occurring during childhood, may fuse lymph nodes around the external and internal carotid arteries and the hypoglossal nerve into a rigid structural relationship which makes the vessels especially vulnerable both to compression by lymph nodes and to postural changes. Furthermore, the stretched hypoglossal nerve may also cut deeply into the carotid artery.

In positional obstructions of the internal carotid artery, the styloid process and the styloid ligament have also been implicated. The syndrome which has been described by Eagle (1979) (hence the name "Eagle syndrome") is thought to be caused by pressure on the internal and external carotid artery by the elongated and/or deviated styloid process, causing diminution of the arterial lumen. Symptoms of this disease, such as unilateral headache, facial pain, and swallowing difficulties, may reflect the impediment of blood flow through the internal carotid artery or may be caused by the stretching of the hypoglossal nerve.

Although demonstrating the presence of ca-

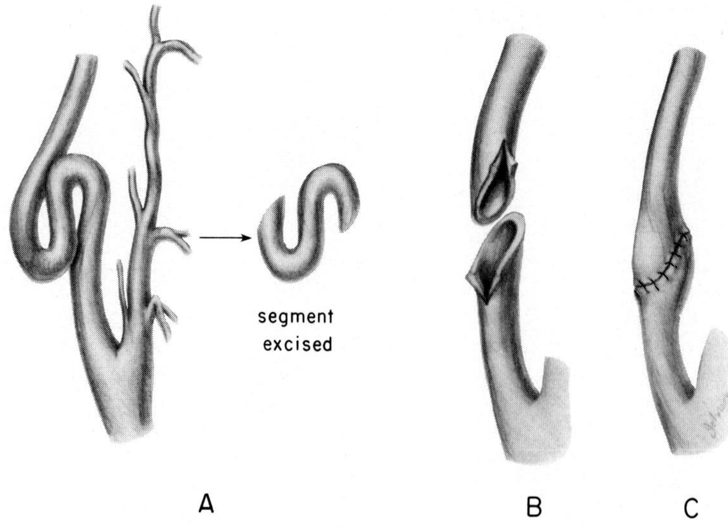

Figure 17–3. Surgical treatment of the buckled internal carotid artery (*A*) by resection (*B*) and end-to-end anastomosis (*C*).

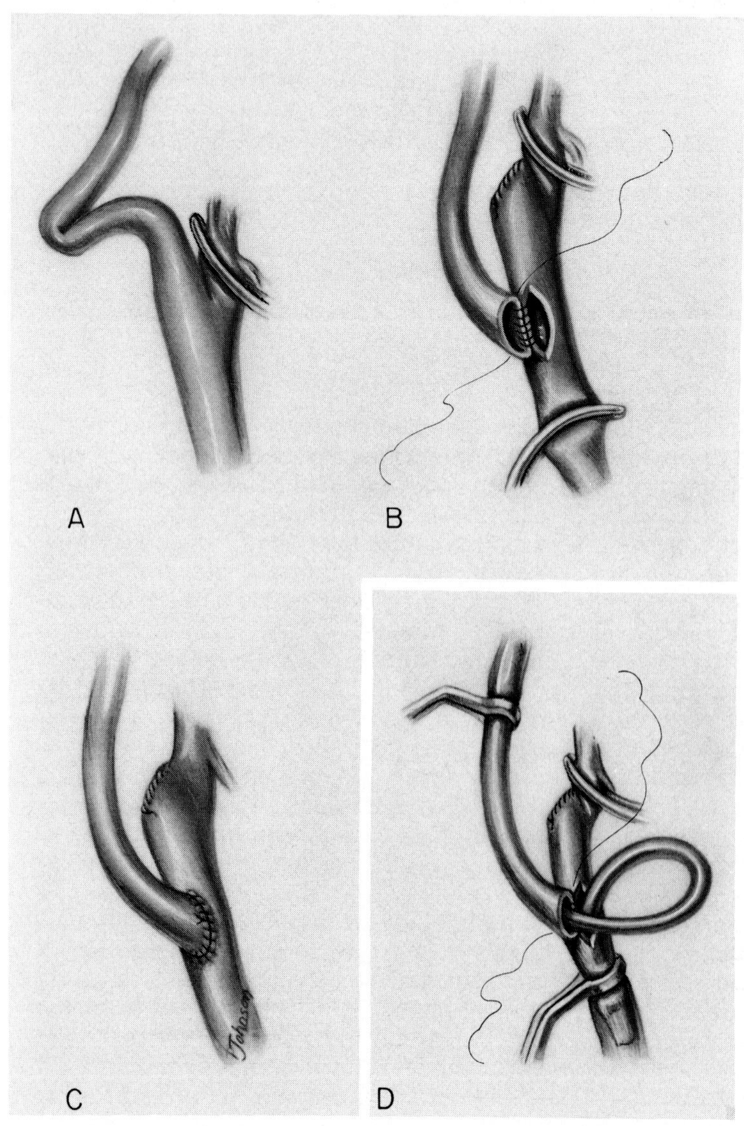

Figure 17–4. Proximal transposition of the origin of the elongated internal carotid artery (*A*–*C*). The same procedure using temporary indwelling shunting (*D*).

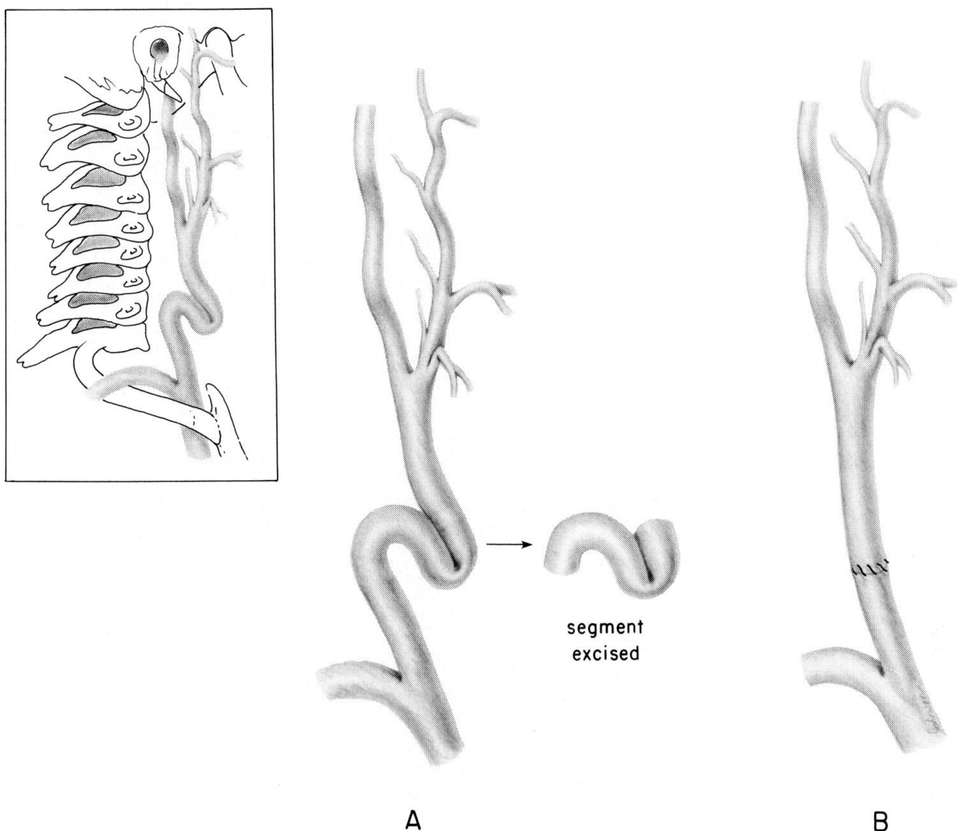

Figure 17–5. Correction of elongation and buckling of the common carotid artery (*A*) by resection and end-to-end anastomosis (*B*).

rotid buckling by angiography is easy, the establishment of operative indication is difficult. Because of a lack of in-depth studies on a large clinical sample which would demonstrate a clear correlation between stroke and carotid tortuosity, the possible significance of carotid coils and kinks is not fully appreciated by the medical profession.

Because the first symptom of carotid insufficiency may be a full-blown stroke, we believe that severe cases of carotid angulation should be surgically treated even if they do not cause any symptoms. Similarly, buckles that become manifest in the course of carotid endarterectomies should be concomitantly corrected.

The indication for surgery, however, is far from clear if the angulation appears to be significant but not very severe. If asymptomatic, the patient should be warned of possible future signs of cerebral ischemia and followed closely, but not be operated upon. If, on the other hand, neurological symptoms seem to implicate the involved artery and there is no other apparent lesion that can be held responsible, operative correction of the kink or coil is proper. The most problematic cases are those in which angulation is of appreciable degree but the symptoms indicate diffuse rather than hemispheric perfusion deficit. In such patients, one should proceed with extreme caution and with deliberation in which the neurologist should certainly participate. Moderate tortuosities with no hemodynamic significance should not be operated upon.

Although tortuosity of the carotid arteries was already referred to in the mid-nineteenth century (Coulson, 1852), its possible role in cerebrovascular insufficiency was not appreciated until 1951, when Riser performed the first surgical procedure to correct the anomaly (Riser *et al.*, 1951). The operation consisted of straightening the course of the internal carotid artery by suturing it to the underside of the sternocleidomastoid muscle. This procedure and other palliative closed operations using muscle interposition or suspension are now

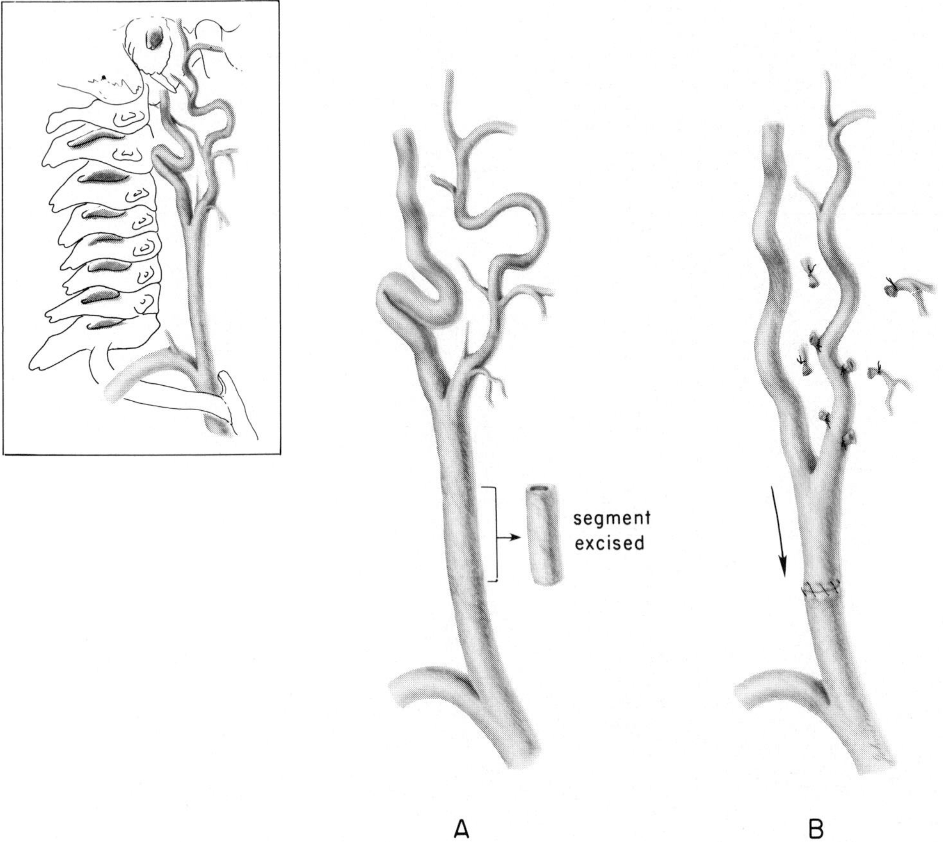

Figure 17-6. Schematic presentation (*A* and *B*) and operative photographs (*C*–*H*) of internal carotid artery tortuosity and buckling associated with external carotid artery elongation.

considered to be of only historical interest, primarily because they do not permit intraluminal inspection and do not eliminate the basic pathogenetic factor, the elongation of the artery.

The first patients in whom angulation of the internal carotid artery was successfully treated by resection was reported by Gass in 1958. He presented seven patients with cerebrovascular insufficiency believed to be caused by elongation and buckling of the internal carotid artery. In one of the seven cases, the redundant coil of the internal carotid artery was excised and an end-to-end anastomosis was performed (see Figure 17–3). The patient became asymptomatic; however, angiography performed three months later demonstrated thrombotic occlusion of the anastomosis.

The case reported by Gass was important for two reasons: (1) it demonstrated the unreliability of clinical symptoms both in indication for surgery and in evaluation of postoperative results, a problem that still plagues clinical investigation of carotid angulations, and (2) it called attention to the technical difficulties that may be encountered in anastomosing the divided internal carotid artery, the stumps of which often have "markedly different calibers at the two ends" (Gass, 1958).

The latter difficulty was eliminated by the method successfully introduced by Quattlebaum and associates (1959), who corrected kinking of the internal carotid artery by resecting a 2 cm segment of the common carotid. Since these first successful operations Quattlebaum and associates (1973) and others have presented a large number of patients with angulation of the internal carotid artery operated upon with a variety of techniques, including the following:

1. Resection of the internal carotid artery and end-to-end anastomosis (see Figure 17–3).

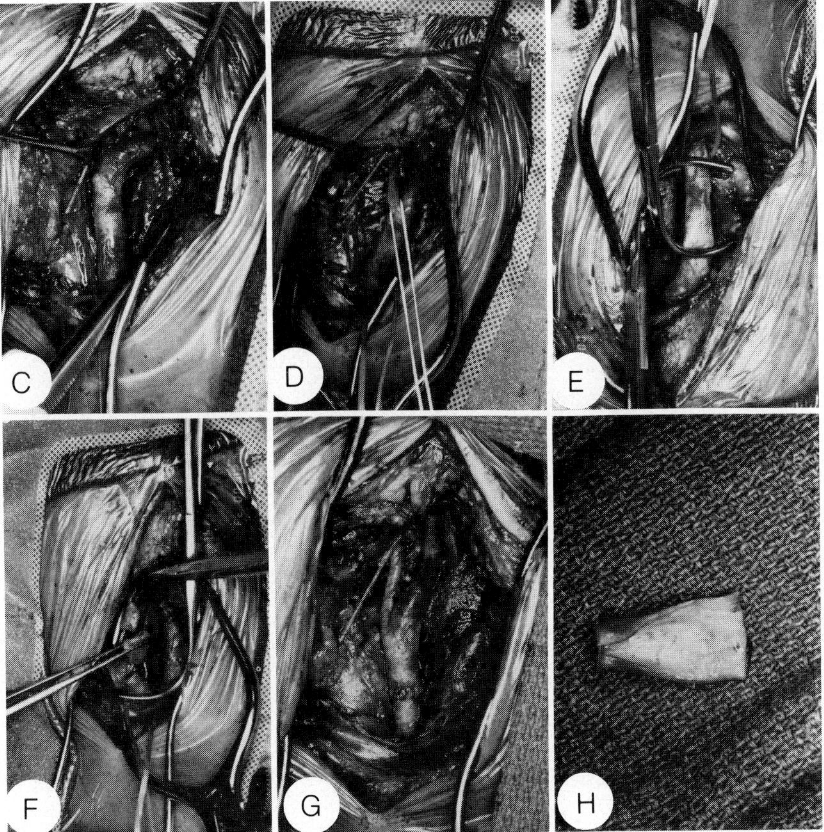

Figure 17–6 (continued). On the operative photographs: (*C*) the exposed buckle on the internal carotid artery; (*D*) mobilization of the external carotid; (*E* and *F*) resection of the common carotid and (*G*) end-to-end anastomosis of the same; and (*H*) the resected specimen (portion of the common carotid artery).

2. Partial or total resection of the carotid bifurcation with end-to-end anastomosis between the internal and common carotid arteries.
3. Resection of the common carotid artery and end-to-end anastomosis.
4. Transplantation of the origin of the internal carotid artery end-to-side into the proximal common carotid (see Figure 17–4).

Some of these operations were performed with additional modifications to remove arteriosclerotic plaques, or to dilate vessels intrinsically narrowed by fibromuscular hyperplasia. The surgeons were divided on whether or not to use shunts during the period of carotid occlusion.

Our own experience (Robicsek *et al.*, 1965; Sanger *et al.*, 1965; Robicsek *et al.*, 1967; and Robicsek and Daugherty, 1970) consists of 46 patients operated upon over a period of two decades. We found a modification of the technique described by Quattlebaum and associates (1959, 1973) to be the most rewarding. Quattlebaum's postulate is that, whereas the internal carotid because of its size and location is difficult to anastomose, the common carotid is easy to expose, mobilize, resect, and anastomose. He recommended that in patients with internal carotid elongation, coils, and kinks the common rather than the internal carotid should be shortened with the usual exposure of the involved carotid arteries through an incision carried along the anterior border of the sternocleidomastoid muscle. The distal two thirds of the common carotid, the extracranial portion of the internal, and the proximal part of the external carotid arteries are meticulously dissected free. Special attention is given to severing all the connective tissue attachments to the internal carotid artery. The superior thyroid artery and the carotid sinus nerve are divided. The rest of the operation is carried out according to the pathology of the particular patient and may also be modified depending on the surgeon's decision whether or not to use a temporary bypass shunt during the period of carotid crossclamping.

In our patients we utilize the following techniques, based on the "Quattlebaum principle":

1. *Kinking of the common carotid artery.* Although elongation and tortuosity of the common carotid artery are common among the elderly, especially if they also have hypertension, buckling of the common carotid which may potentially endanger blood flow is extremely rare (occurring only once in our experience). The surgical management of the condition is simple, and consists of the resection of an appropriate length and end-to-end anastomosis of the common carotid artery (see Figure 17–5).
2. *Elongation of both the internal and external carotid arteries with coiling or kinking of the internal carotid.* In such a situation special care is taken that beside the internal carotid a comparable length of the external carotid artery is also adequately mobilized. The latter requires the division of not only the superior thyroid but also the lingual and external maxillary branches. This is followed by segmental resection of the common carotid artery, a maneuver that displaces the carotid bifurcation downward, thus straightening the course of the internal carotid (see Figure 17–6).
3. *Elongation and kinking or buckling of the internal carotid only.* This is the most common form of carotid artery kinking, occurring in about two thirds of our patients. If, in such a case, the external carotid artery is not elongated, it should be divided to allow the downward displace-

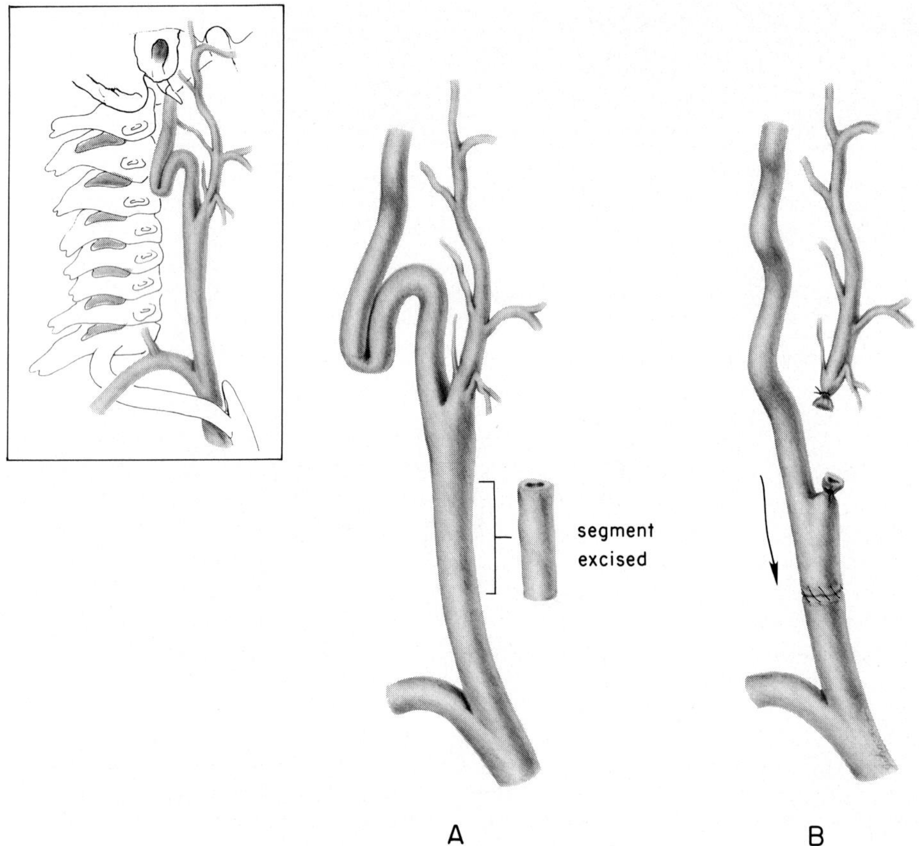

Figure 17–7. Management of buckling of the internal carotid artery (*A*) by division of the external carotid artery and resection of the common carotid artery (*B*).

ment of the carotid bifurcation. This move creates a "single-course" vessel of the internal and common carotid arteries, which can then be easily shortened and straightened by segmental resection of the latter (see Figure 17–7).

This maneuver, i.e., double ligation and division of the external carotid, may also be very useful in routine carotid endarterectomies when the carotid bifurcation is abnormally high, because it allows a much more favorable exposure of the internal carotid artery. Although it has the theoretical disadvantage of possibly decreasing the periorbital collateral circulation to the brain, we do not believe that this is significant unless one or both of the internal carotid arteries are also occluded.

4. *Buckling of the carotid arteries associated with intrinsic arteriosclerotic occlusive disease.* As already mentioned, there are two forms of this condition: (1) the patient presents preoperatively with *both* buckling and intrinsic occlusive disease, or (2) buckling develops in the course of surgical dissection during carotid endarterectomy. In the latter case, the surgeon may realize at the termination of the procedure that he started out with a carotid artery occluded by a plaque and ended with a carotid artery narrowed by elongation and kinking. In either case the elongation should be corrected concomitantly with the endarterectomy. (See Figures 17–8 to 11).
5. *Fibroelastosis of the internal carotid artery associated with kinking of the same vessel.* Although we have no knowledge that simultaneous fibroelastosis and primary buckling of the carotid artery have ever been observed, the weakening of the wall of the internal carotid artery caused by fibroelastosis not infrequently leads to kinking. Attempts to eliminate the kink by resection and/or grafting of the internal carotid itself may produce disastrous results because of the fragility of the wall and the difficulties that may be caused in exposure. The situation can usually be easily corrected by careful instrumental

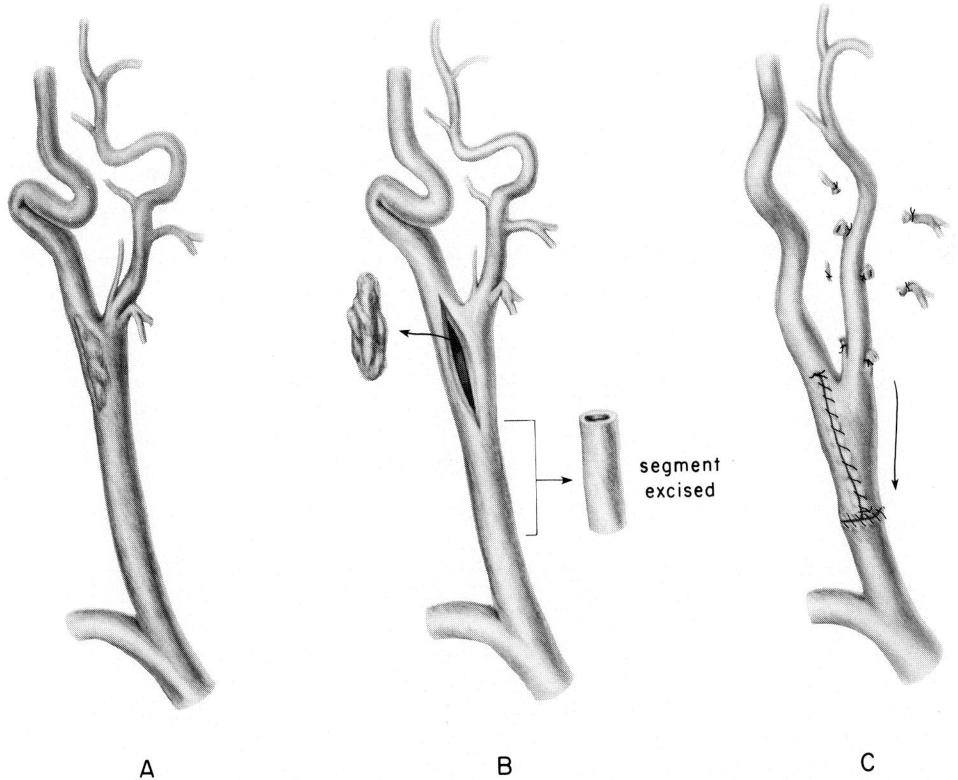

Figure 17–8. Treatment of carotid bifurcation atheroma associated with elongation of both internal and external carotid arteries and buckling of the internal carotid (*A*). After endarterectomy, the carotid bifurcation is transposed caudally by mobilization of both the internal and external carotid arteries, and resecting a segment of the common carotid (*B* and *C*).

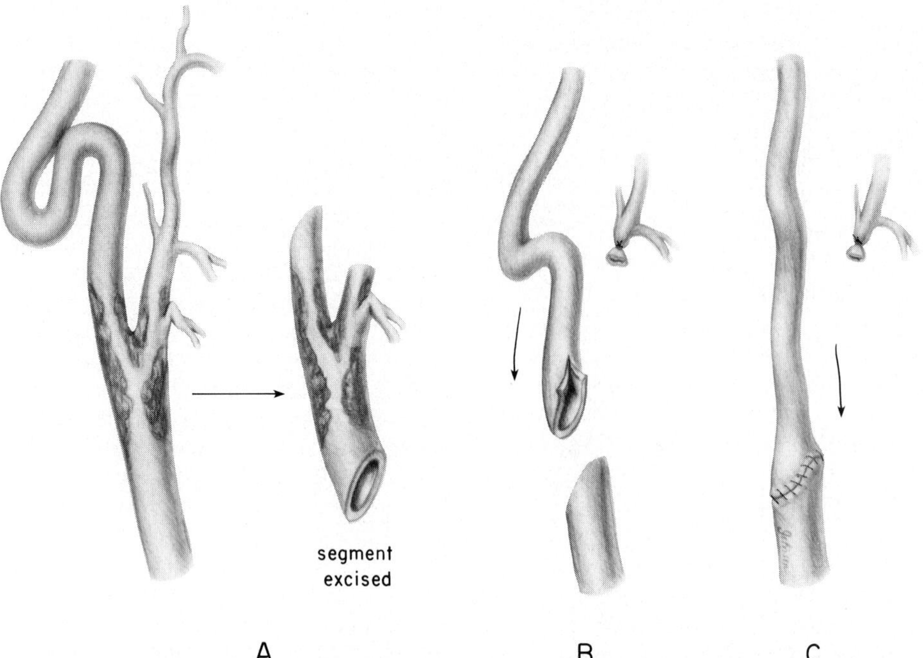

Figure 17–9. Treatment of severe arteriosclerotic stricture of the carotid bifurcation and the internal carotid artery combined with elongation and buckling (*A*) by bifurcation resection (*B*) and end-to-end anastomosis between the common and internal carotid arteries (*C*).

dilatation of the internal carotid artery with graduated Bakes dilators as recommended by Morris and associates (1968), followed by segmental resection of the common carotid (see Figure 17–12).

6. *Hypoglossal carotid entrapment syndrome.* Surgical correction of the hypoglossal carotid entrapment syndrome involves the separation of the vascular structure from the hypoglossal nerve by careful dissection, in the course of which involved lymph nodes are removed and the descending branch of the nerve and the sternocleidomastoid branch of the external carotid may need to be divided. It is especially important to dissect the internal carotid artery in its entire length. If, after it is freed, the vessel appears to be unduly elongated, which is the case more often than not, its course should be straightened, preferably by shortening the common carotid. On rare occasions, the nerve may cut into the internal carotid artery deeply enough to damage the intima to such a degree that, in addition to external constriction and kinking, intrinsic stricture also occurs. If this is suspected, the lumen of the internal carotid artery should be mensurated with dilators, and, if necessary, the stricture should be excised (see Figure 17–13).

Using the foregoing techniques, correction of carotid elongation and angulation can be performed safely with low surgical risk. It should also be emphasized, however, that the cause-and-consequence relation between carotid angulation and clinical symptoms is less certain than that between intrinsic carotid lesions and symptoms of cerebral ischemia. Therefore, the matter of surgical indication should be approached very carefully and individualized for every patient.

FIBROMUSCULAR DYSPLASIA OF THE EXTRACRANIAL CAROTID ARTERIES

Fibromuscular dysplasia of the extracranial carotid arteries is a relatively rare segmental disease of unknown cause. Even its exact pathologic definition is uncertain, and most authors refer to it by defining what it is not rather than what it is, i.e., "nonatherosclerotic." Harrington and associates (1970) and Houser and associates (1971), in two separate studies en-

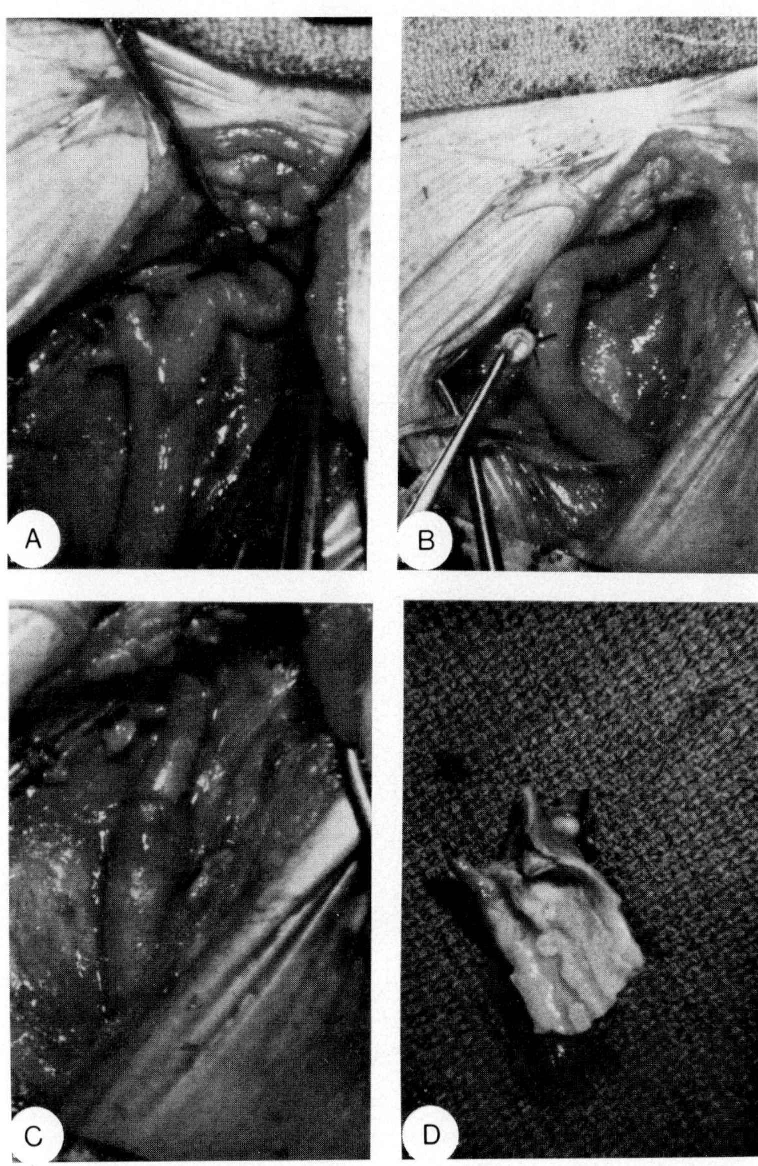

Figure 17–10. Correction of severe arteriosclerotic stricture of the carotid bifurcation associated with elongation and buckling of the internal carotid artery by division of the external carotid (*A*). Resection of the carotid bifurcation (*B*). End-to-end anastomosis between the common and internal carotid arteries (*C*). The resected specimen (*D*).

compassing a total of 9,500 carotid angiograms, found fibromuscular dysplasia of the cervical internal carotid arteries in 0.25 and 0.68 percent of patients, respectively.

The morphological diagnosis of fibromuscular dysplasia depends on the characteristic "beaded" or "corkscrew" appearance of the artery (see Figure 9–23). This alternating constriction and dilatation of the normally smooth arterial outline, affecting the middle 2 to 3 cm length of the cervical internal carotid artery at the level of the second cervical vertebra, an area of the vessel that is usually spared arteriosclerosis, is pathognomic.

Elongation is also a common feature of fibromuscular dysplasia. The relationship of elongation and positional obstruction to fibromuscular dysplasia of the cervical carotid artery is most interesting. Undoubtedly, fibromuscular dysplasia can be the cause of and coexist with carotid elongation and tortuosity.

Histologically, there are three types of fibromuscular dysplasia: Type I, intimal fibroplasia; Type II, medial or fibromuscular stenosis, which is characterized by hyperplasia of the medial muscular layer, disruption of the internal elastic membranes, and focal or tubular microaneurysms; and Type III, subadventitial

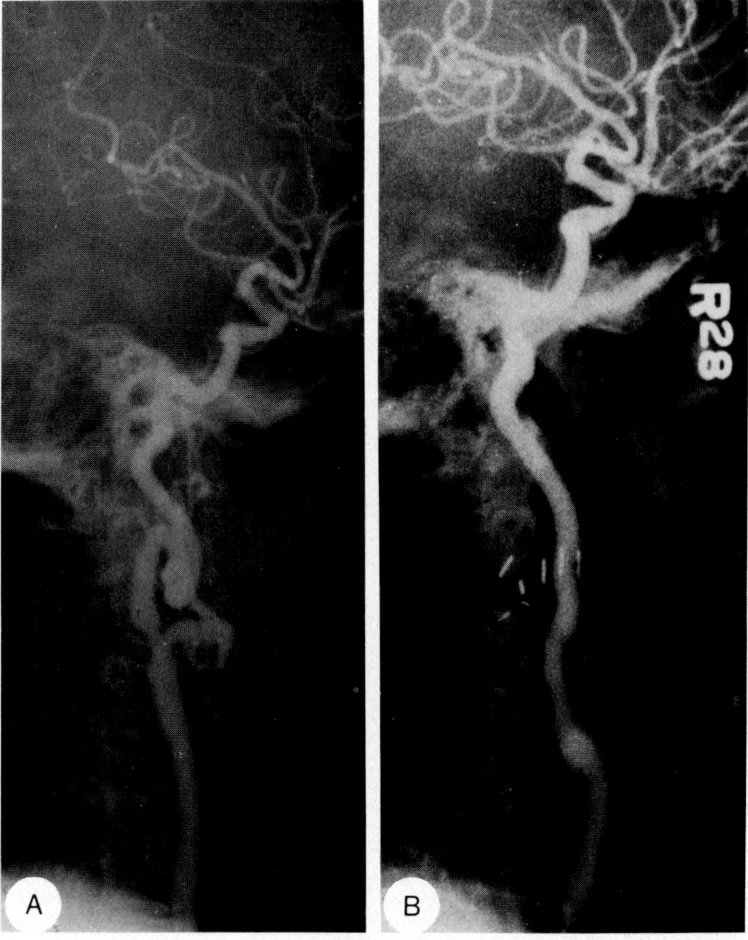

Figure 17–11. Preoperative (*A*) and postoperative (*B*) angiograms of the case shown in Figure 17–10.

fibroplasia, in which stenoses are produced by periarterial fibrosis. Various combinations of these three patterns may occur in the same patient.

From a clinical viewpoint, the term *fibromuscular dysplasia* generally refers to Type II (see Figure 17–14). This disease not only causes stenosis by hyperplasia of some elements of the vascular wall but also induces defects in the elastic layers of the media. The latter predisposes to outpouching and eventually may proceed to full-fledged large saccular aneurysms. Dissection may also be a common complication of the disease.

Fibromuscular dysplasia was first recognized in the renal arteries by Leadbetter and Burkland (1938), and initially was believed to be a lesion particular to those vessels. It is not surprising, therefore, that in earlier years most studies of the disease dealt with its relation to renal hypertension. The first reported occurrence of extrarenal fibromuscular dysplasia, that of the celiac artery, was described by Palubinskas and Ripley in 1964. Since then the disease has been recognized with increasing frequency not only in the renal, splanchnic, carotid, subclavian, coronary, and vertebral arteries, but even in some of the visceral veins as well.

The clinical significance of fibromuscular dysplasia varies and depends mainly upon which artery is involved and to what degree. It appears to be most serious when the internal carotid and renal arteries are diseased, although significant symptoms caused by involvement of other arteries also occurs. Only sporadic cases of intracranial fibromuscular dysplasia have been observed, most of them involving the intrapetrosal segment of the carotid siphon (Bergan and MacDonald, 1969).

Interestingly enough, although true intracranial fibromuscular dysplasia is rare, both solitary and multiple intracranial berry-type aneurysms occur frequently in patients with

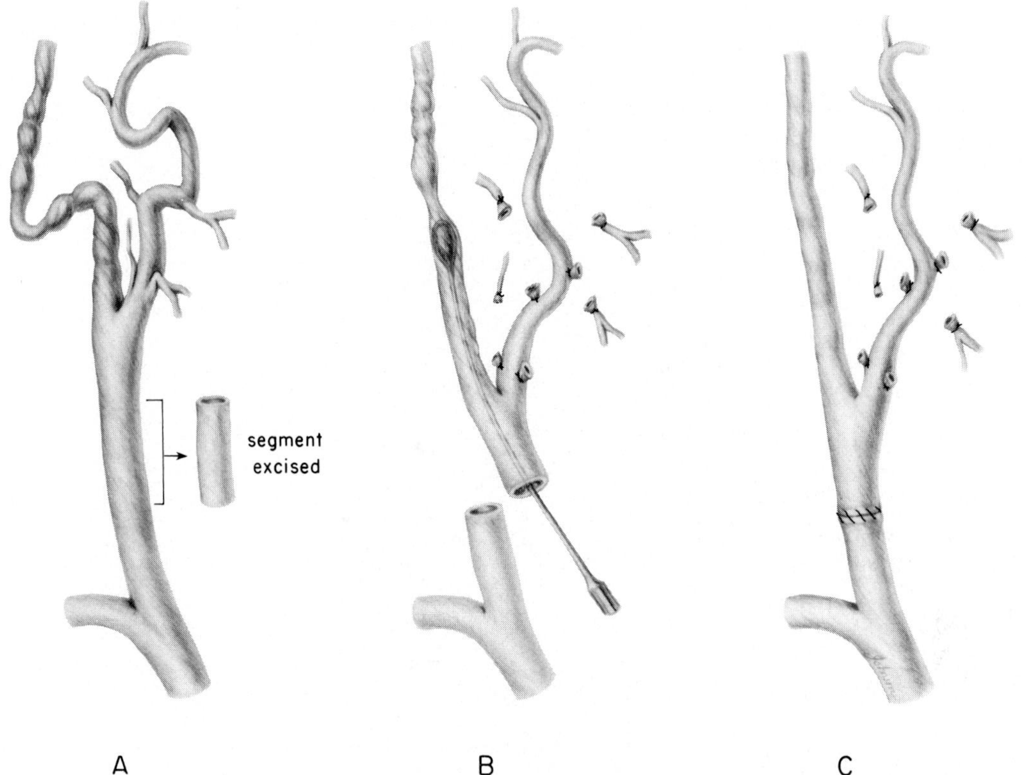

Figure 17–12. The management of multiple fibromuscular strictures of the internal carotid artery associated with internal and external elongation and tortuosity. The procedure includes (*A*) segmental resection of the common carotid, (*B*) transluminal dilatation, and (*C*) caudal transposition of the mobilized carotid bifurcation.

fibromuscular dysplastic disease of the renal (Wylie *et al.*, 1962) and cervical internal carotid arteries, as was the case in seven of Stanley's 14 patients (Stanley *et al.*, 1975). The exact relationship between these berry-type aneurysms and fibromuscular dysplasia is unknown; however, some histological similarities have been recognized (Stanley *et al.*, 1975).

The presence of fibromuscular dysplasia in the cervical internal carotid artery was first diagnosed angiographically by Palubinskas and Ripley in 1964. A detailed histological study of the condition was reported by Connett and Lansche (1965), who also performed the first operation for this disease.

The disease most commonly occurs in females (60 to 80 percent of all cases reported; Stanley *et al.*, 1975). The average age of patients is 57.7 years, about ten years younger than those with arteriosclerotic strictures observed in the same age group. Ochsner and associates (1977) described the disease in three children under ten years of age. Of the 138 patients collected in the literature by Stanley, 64 percent had bilateral disease (Stanley *et al.*, 1975). Such bilateral lesions are especially common in young women.

As for the origin of this disease, its topical occurrence in the carotid artery is both interesting and puzzling. The frequent coincidence with elongation lends support to the theory of Stanley, who believes that abnormal stresses are acting on segments of the arterial wall which is partly deprived of its blood supply from the vasa vasorum. In an appropriate hormonal milieu, these events may lead to ischemic damage to the media and disruption of the elastic layer (Stanley *et al.*, 1975). Into which histologic type the disease may progress will largely depend on the location, length, and diameter of the involved vessel, as well as on the degree of the medial injury and the presence or absence of reparative processes. The importance of genetic factors in the development of fibromuscular dysplasia is suggested by the fact that similar lesions frequently occur simultaneously in different parts of the body.

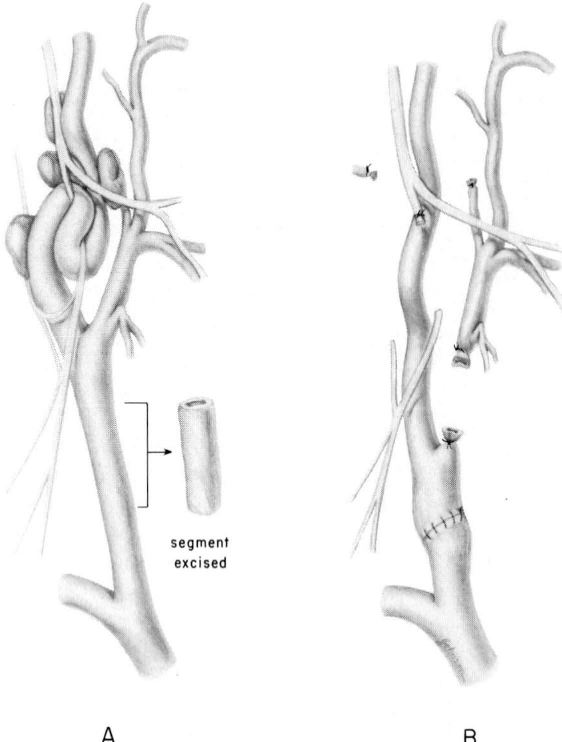

Figure 17–13. Carotid artery entrapment by inflammatory lymph nodes and by the hypoglossal nerve (*A*). Treatment by ligation and division of the external carotid and the sternocleidomastoid artery, division of the ansa hypoglossi, removal of the inflammatory lymph nodes, and caudal transposition of the bifurcation (*B*).

Paulson hypothesized that the disease is the result of inappropriate multiplication of cells in certain muscular arteries and that such proliferation may be enhanced by antiovulants. He also postulated that ergot preparations commonly used for migraine headaches also predispose to fibroelastic muscular degeneration (Paulson *et al.,* 1978). A similar theory is the monoclonal concept, according to which certain mutant cells associated with arteriosclerotic plaques may be stimulated into neoplastic proliferation by certain toxins, hormones, ischemia, or by stretching of the vascular wall.

Earlier investigators regarded fibromuscular dysplasia of the extracranial cerebral arteries as merely an incidental angiographic finding. Now it is evident that this disease is often associated with cerebrovascular symptoms (Bergan and MacDonald, 1969) attributable to hypoperfusion of the brain; such symptoms may be caused either by a single area of severe stricture or by a series of subcritical stenoses. Some believe that they may also be instigated by repeated episodes of embolization of platelet aggregates and clusters of fibrin formed on the irregular intimal ridges which, like arteriosclerotic plaques, tend to reduce internal carotid flow and create niches with eddy currents. Here, thrombi may form and emboli emanate, in some cases leading to complete thrombotic occlusion. Beside embolization and thrombosis, dissection, kinking, and aneurysmal rupture constitute additional hazards of the disease. Any or all of these conditions may cause vertigo, motor weakness, headaches, blackout episodes, focal seizures, dizziness, or frank stroke.

The only physical findings that may be present in an asymptomatic case are bruits, which are heard in only one fourth of the patients (Effeney *et al.,* 1979). Hypertension is not uncommon, occurring in one third of the cases.

The diagnosis of fibromuscular hyperplasia is usually established by angiography. Because of the common association of contralateral cervical carotid, vertebral, and intracranial vascular disease, the angiographic workup should include a complete four-vessel extraintracranial visualization. If, as is commonly done, the angiography is performed by the transfemoral catheter approach, the renal vessels should be visualized as well, especially if the patient is hypertensive, because the renal arteries are also affected in about half of the

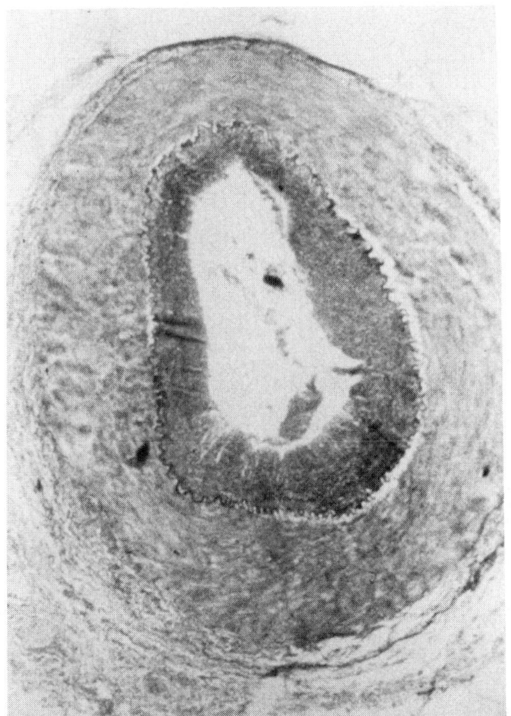

Figure 17–14. Microscopic picture of fibromuscular arterial dysplasia.

patients. Angiographic patterns of fibromuscular dysplasia of the internal carotid artery vary from the well-known classic beaded appearance to more isolated stenotic lesions. Osborne and Anderson (1977) list three angiographic patterns characteristic of cephalic fibromuscular dysplasia which loosely correspond to the histological groups previously described: (1) isolated, usually membranous stenosis, (2) the typical "string-of-beads" appearance of multiple occlusive ridges alternating with moderately dilated segments, and (3) tubular stenosis of varying lengths. Beside these forms, atypical cases characterized by saccular aneurysms, buckling, or kinking may also occur (see Figures 9–23 and 24).

The most common type is undoubtedly the so-called "pearl necklace" or "string-of-beads" appearance present in approximately 80 percent of patients (Osborne and Anderson, 1977). Such a radiographic picture is created by a line of alternating normal and dilated arterial segments separated by irregularly spaced membranous or semimembranous ridges. This type of angiographic manifestation usually corresponds to histologic Type II. A less common radiologic manifestation is concentric tubular stenosis, which may be associated with any of the three histological groups and also with a number of other conditions, such as various types of arteritis or arteriosclerosis. The "giveaway" sign in the differential diagnosis of fibrodysplastic and atherosclerotic lesions is their location. Wheras arteriosclerotic lesions usually involve the most proximal segment of the internal carotid artery, that area is usually spared by fibrodysplasia.

Care must be taken in the angiographic evaluation of fibromuscular dysplasia because in rare instances angiographic flow patterns called "stationary waves," which occur in anatomically normal carotid arteries, may closely mimic the typical string-of-beads appearance (see also Chapter 9 on arteriographic diagnosis).

Because fibromuscular dysplasia is one of the most common causes of sudden unexplained occlusions of the internal carotid artery in children and young adults, incidentally diagnosed severe lesions, even if asymptomatic, should be operated upon. Similarly, although dissection caused by fibromuscular dysplasia may or may not create a serious obstacle to the blood flow and symptoms of cerebral ischemia, because of the ever-present danger of an acute thrombosis, it should be surgically corrected, preferably by excision and replacement with an autogenous saphenous vein graft. Naturally, any symptoms or signs referable to cerebral ischemia and/or embolization are significant and indicate that the patient with fibromuscular dysplasia of the carotid artery is a potential candidate for surgery.

Because of the fragility of the internal carotid artery afflicted with this disease, the planning for the operation should be careful and the technique painstaking. Methods applied in the surgical correction of fibromuscular dysplasia of the internal carotid artery differ from those applied in atheromatous strictures. In the latter, surgery deals primarily with orifice lesions of the carotid bifurcation and the operation usually consists of removal of plaques that extend only a short distance into the internal carotid artery. Procedures for treating fibromuscular dysplasia, however, must cope with lesions that involve primarily the middle third of the internal carotid but that often extend as high as the base of the skull.

At the present time several types of operations are recommended, but there is no single procedure that is universally accepted as the

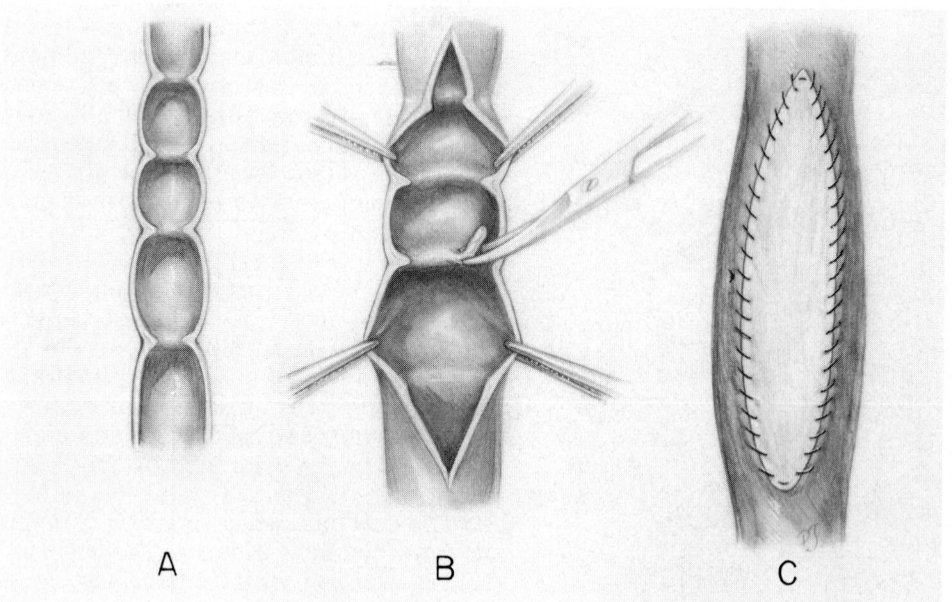

Figure 17-15. Treatment of fibromuscular dysplasia (*A*) of the internal carotid artery by direct excision of the occlusive "bridges," (*B*) and patch arterioplasty (*C*).

preferred method. The first operation to correct fibromuscular dysplasia of the internal carotid artery was performed by Connett in 1965 (Connett and Lansche, 1965). The early procedures, which consisted of resection of the involved segment usually followed by end-to-end anastomosis, are still considered acceptable, especially if the lesion is short and/or the artery is significantly elongated. In general, however, I do not recommend this procedure because of the danger of localized anastomotic stricture. If resection is contemplated, it is preferable to combine it with graft replacement with autogenous saphenous vein, which allows more versatility and precision in the anastomotic technique. Whenever a vein-to-internal carotid artery anastomosis is performed, it is advisable to spatulate it in such a way that the circumference of the anastomosis is about 2.5 times that of the internal carotid artery.

Patch angioplasty with or without the excision of the dysplastic intimal "rings" has also been described for the treatment of carotid fibromuscular dysplasia (Lamis *et al.,* 1971). In this technique the arteriotomy is extended from the carotid sinus in the anterior midaxis up into the internal carotid artery a few millimeters above the level of the most distal obstructive intimal ridge. The cut edges of the artery are retracted with 7-0 polypropylene holding sutures so that the tubular intimal surface is changed into a flat plate. With fine-curved dissecting scissors or a very sharp small pituitary forceps, the intimal ridges are removed one by one. Extreme caution should be used not to cut off the ridges too close to their base because if the outermost layers of the media are removed, the thin adventitia may not hold arterial pressure, and the vessel may rupture when blood flow is restored. For the same reason one should avoid lifting and "puckering" the intimal ridges, which can also lead to injury to the outside layers (see Figure 17-15).

After the ridges are removed, the surgeon should pause and reevaluate the situation. If the caliber of the internal carotid artery is large, then the vessel may be closed with a single row of 7-0 continuous polypropylene sutures. If, however, there is a question that the lumen of the internal carotid may not be large enough, the artery should be closed with a diamond-shaped patch. Because of the extreme fragility of the diseased carotid artery, only very fine sutures and soft, easy-to-sew patch material—preferably autogenous saphenous vein—should be used. If the elongation is significant, especially if it is associated with kinking or buckling, the shortening of the course of the carotid is mandatory to ensure the success of the operation. Whenever fibromuscular dysplasia of the midportion of the cervical internal carotid artery is associated with atheromatous stricture, endarterectomy should be added to whatever procedure is used to relieve the dysplastic stenosis (see Figure 17–12).

An alternative method to excision of dysplastic intimal ridges under direct vision has been presented by Balaji and DeWeese (1980). They accomplished not only the fracture but also extraction of intimal rings by means of a balloon embolectomy catheter. Although this technique may work under special circumstances, I do not believe that it provides either the assurance of success or the safety of direct excision.

Morris (1968) recommends intraluminal graded dilatation for the treatment of fibromuscular dysplasia. During the operation, a linear arteriotomy 2 to 3 cm long is made on the right anterolateral aspect of the carotid sinus. The course of the incision is directed toward the rise of the internal carotid artery. If external inspection of the internal carotid artery reveals yellow discoloration, indicating associated arterioscleratic changes, or if the palpating finger feels hardened areas in the arterial wall, the arteriotomy is extended into the internal carotid artery, and lesions are dealt with under direct vision. If no associated arteriosclerotic changes are detected, the arteriotomy is limited to the carotid sinus alone.

First, the presence of a patent distal artery is confirmed by allowing blood to bleed back from the distal carotid. After patency of the internal carotid artery is proved by backflush of blood, its lumen is gently enlarged by breaking the intimal membranes one by one, using Bakes-type coronary dilators of increasing diameters from 1 to 3 to 4 mm. Successful dilatation is indicated by the feel of the dilator to overcome the resistance while "popping" through the stricture and by the easy reinsertion of the instrument after the initial passage (see Figure 17–16).

When the surgeon is not sure that the dilator has been advanced to the base of the skull, Moore (1983) recommends obtaining a plain x-ray film with a dilator in place and comparing it with the preoperative angiogram to ensure that the dilator has passed the distal end of the involved segment. Between dilatations the artery is allowed to bleed back freely to flush out loose debris. The dilatation should progress to the bony foramen. Use of dilators larger than 4 mm in diameter is not recommended because of the danger of suture stenosis owing to overstretching.

During the dilatation longitudinal tears in the intima may occur, and if they do, they will inevitably lead to dissection and intra- or postoperative thrombosis with all of its potentially disastrous consequences. To prevent such mishaps, it is important to moisten the dilator before using it to make it more slippery and to see that the internal carotid artery is straightened by freeing both the internal and the external carotids from their investing tissue and pulling the bifurcation downward (Ehrenfeld and Wylie, 1974) before dilatation is undertaken (see Figure 17–17). If injury is suspected, all further efforts at dilatation should cease, and the internal carotid artery should be opened. If the damage to the artery is irreparable, the vessel should be replaced. The usual technique of carotid dilatation precludes the use of a shunt (Effeney *et al.,* 1979).

After demonstrations that satisfactory results can be obtained with Morris's less radical operation, it became widely accepted as the procedure of choice. In the late 1970s, however, direct procedures made somewhat of a comeback; it is now recommended by some that correction of fibromuscular dysplasia should always be performed under direct vision and should include resection of the involved segment and its replacement with autogenous saphenous vein. Because such an operation usually requires exposure of the entire length of the cervical internal carotid artery, it may become necessary to resect part of the vertical ramus of the mandible to gain satisfactory access.

Graduated dilation of fibromuscular stricture of the carotid artery with a Fogarty balloon catheter introduced into the surgically exposed carotid artery instead of Bakes-type dilators was recommended by Upson and Raza (1976) and was a forerunner of percutaneous carotid balloon dilatation. This alternative to open graduated dilatation of the fibrodysplastic internal carotid artery has been offered in the form of percutaneous transluminal balloon angioplasty, which achieves gradual dilatation without direct exposure of the vessel (Belain *et al.,* 1982; Dublin *et al.,* 1983). The advantages of percutaneous versus

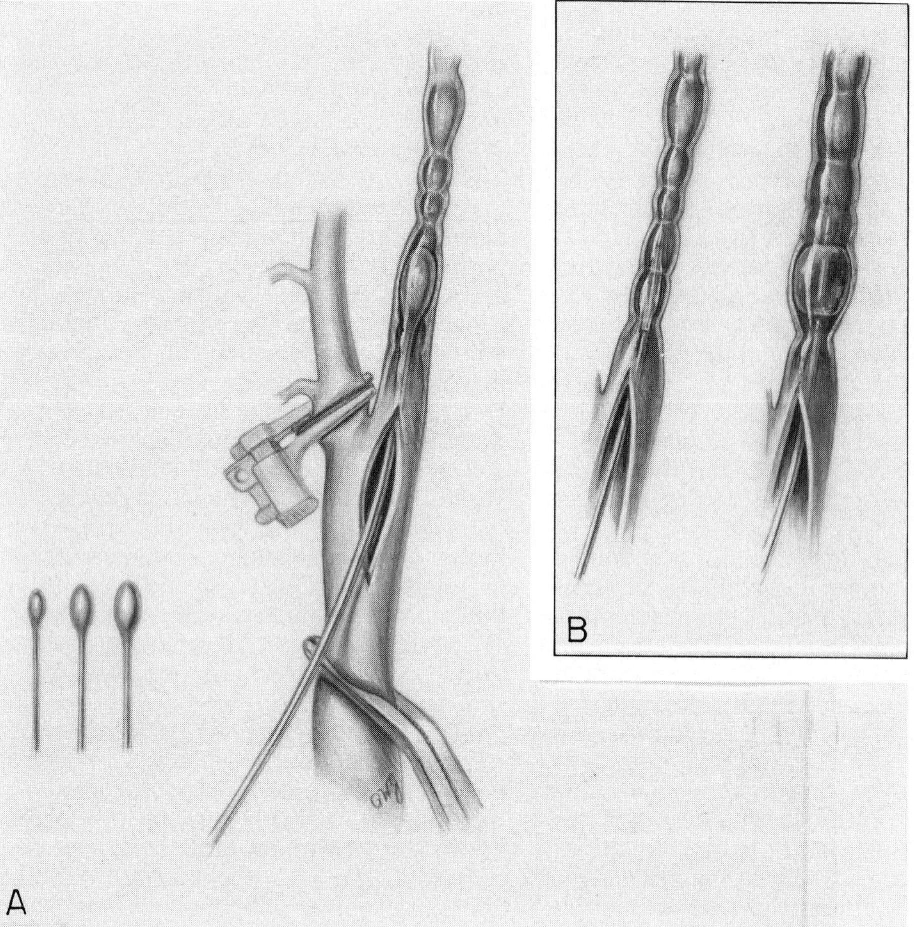

Figure 17–16. Transluminal dilatation of fibromuscular strictures of the internal carotid artery using graduated Baker-type dilators (*A*) and balloon catheter (*B*).

open dilatation are listed by Dublin as follows: continuous fluoroscopic observation, absence of an incision, and an awake patient under local anesthetic control only (Dublin *et al.*, 1983).

The results of Saddekin and associates (1980) indicate that, while some fibromuscular dysplastic strictures may be amenable to percutaneous balloon dilatation, the results will largely depend on the histologic type. In the "medial type" (Type III), the stricture appears to dilate most easily by concentric stretching and some shearing of the fibrous tissue, which then heals in its dilated state. Such concentric stretching may not be possible in Types I and II, in which fibroplasia may be eccentric. Dilatation is also ineffective in the presence of kinking or buckling induced by elongation and/or perivascular fibrosis. The method of percutaneous balloon dilatation has been successfully applied in a limited number of cases of internal and external carotid artery stricture of dysplastic origin (Belain *et al.*, 1982; Hasso *et al.*, 1981). Proper angiographic workup (Dublin *et al.*, 1983) and systematic heparinization (Hasso *et al.*, 1981) during the procedure are measures recommended to prevent cerebral embolization. Although the long-range results of percutaneous dilatation of fibrodysplastic carotid lesions are yet unknown, it is suggested that satisfactory, lasting results similar to those demonstrated in the same disease of the renal arteries will be demonstrated (Dublin *et al.*, 1983; Saddekin *et al.*, 1980).

Despite the technical ease with which some cases of fibromuscular dysplasia of the internal carotid artery can be handled with percutane-

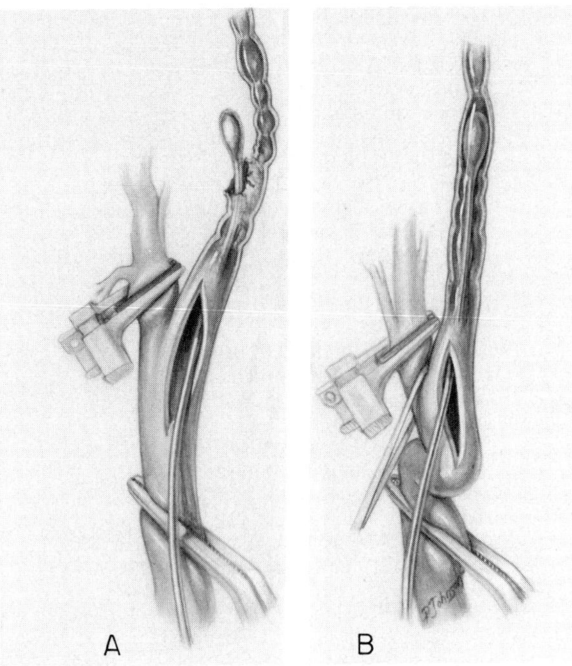

Figure 17-17. Perforation of the wall of the internal carotid artery in the course of dilatation (*A*) may be prevented by pulling down its origin, thus straightening its course (*B*).

ous dilation, the method also has shortcomings. Beside the already discussed possibility of serious injury to the arterial wall, the procedure is also unsuitable for cases in which there are saccular aneurysms or partial or total thrombosis, and it could be very dangerous if dissection is present. Dissections owing to balloon overdistention or to faulty insertion of the catheter have also been described as complications of this procedure (Pollock and Jackson, 1971).

REFERENCES

Balaji, M.R., and DeWeese, J.A.: Fibromuscular dysplasia of the internal carotid artery. *Arch. Surg.*, **115**:984-86, 1980.

Bauer, R.; Sheehan, S.; and Meyer, J.S.: Arteriographic study of cerebrovascular disease II. Cerebral symptoms due to kinking, tortuosity, and compression of the carotid and vertebral arteries in the neck. *Arch. Neurol.*, **4**:119-31, 1961.

Belain, A.; Vesela, M.; Vanek, I.; and Peregrin, T.H.: Percutaneous fibromuscular dysplasia of the internal carotid artery. *Cardiovasc. Interven. Radiol.*, **5**:79-81, 1982.

Bergan, J.J., and MacDonald, J.R.: Recognition of cerebrovascular fibromuscular hyperplasia. *Arch. Surg.*, **98**:332-35, 1969.

Carney, A.L., and Anderson, E.M.: Hypoglossal carotid entrapment syndrome. *Advances in Neurology*. **30**:223-47, 1981.

Cioffi, F.A.; Meduri, M.; Tomosello, F.; Bonavita, V.; and Corforti, P.: Kinking and coiling of the internal carotid artery: clinical-statistical observations and surgical perspectives. *J. Neurosurg. Sci.*, **19**:15-22, 1975.

Connett, M.C., and Lansche, K.M.: Fibromuscular hyperplasia of internal carotid artery: report of a case. *Ann. Surg.*, **162**:59-62, 1965.

Coulson, C.: Peculiar disposition of the large vessels, producing a tumour of the root of the neck. *Trans. Pathol. Soc. (Lond.)*, **3**:302, 1852.

Deterling, R.A.: Tortuous right common carotid artery simulating aneurysm. *Angiology*, **3**:483-92, 1952.

Dublin, A.B.; Baltaxe, H.H.; and Cully, A.C.: Percutaneous transluminal carotid angioplasty in fibromuscular dysplasia. *J. Neurosurg.*, **59**:162-65, 1983.

Eagle, W.W.: Symptomatic elongated styloid process. *Arch. Otolaryngol.*, **49**:490-503, 1949.

Edington, G.H.: Tortuosity of both internal carotid arteries. *Br. Med. J.*, **2**:1526, 1901.

Effeney, D.J.; Ehrenfeld, W.K.; Stoney, R.J.; and Wylie, E.J.: Fibromuscular dyplasia of the internal carotid artery. *World J. Surg.*, **3**:179-86, 1979.

Ehrenfeld, W.K.; Stoney, R. J.; and Wylie, E.J.: Fibromuscular hyperplasia of the internal carotid artery. *Arch. Surg.*, **95**:284-87, 1967.

Ehrenfeld, W.L., and Wylie, E.J.: Fibromuscular dysplasia of the internal carotid artery: surgical management. *Arch. Surg.*, **109**:676-81, 1974.

Eichhorn, O., and Schlicht, L.: The importance of hydraulic principles in the regulations of cerebral blood flow. In Meyer, J.S.; Lechner, H., and Eichorn, O. (eds.): *Re-*

search on the Cerebral Circulation. Charles C Thomas, Springfield, Illinois, pages 332–46, 1969.

Gass, H.H.: Kinks and coils of the cervical carotid artery. *Surg. Forum,* **9**:721–24, 1958.

Gegenbauer, C.: *Lehrbuch der Anatomie und Physiologie des Menschen,* 7th ed. W. Schwabe, Munich, page 255, 1899.

Harrington, O.B.; Crosby, V.G.; and Nicholas, L.: Fibromuscular hyperplasia of the internal carotid artery. *Ann. Thorac. Surg.,* **9**:516–24, 1970.

Hasso, A.N.; Bird, C.R.; Zinke, D.E.; and Thompson, J.R.: Fibromuscular dysplasia of the internal carotid artery: percutaneous transluminal angioplasty. *A.J.R.,* **136**:955–60, 1981.

Herrschaft, P.; Duus, P.; Gleim, F.; and Ungehauer, G.: Preoperative cerebral blood flow in patients with carotid artery stenosis. In Langfett, T.W. (ed.): *Cerebral Circulation and Metabolism.* Springer Verlag, New York, pages 276–82, 1975.

Houser, O.W.; Baker, H.J.; Sandok, B.A.; and Holley, K.E.: Cephalic arterial fibromuscular dysplasia. *Radiology,* **101**:605–11, 1971.

Hsu, I., and Kistin, A.D.: Buckling of the great vessels: a clinical and angiocardiographic study. *Arch. Intern. Med.,* **98**:712–19, 1956.

Lamis, P.A.; Carson, W.P.; Wilson, J.P.; and Letton, A.H.: Recognition and treatment of fibromuscular hyperplasia of the internal carotid artery. *Surgery,* **69**:498–503, 1971.

Leadbetter, W.F., and Burkland, C.E.: Hypertension in unilateral renal disease. *J. Urol.,* **39**:611–26, 1938.

Moore, S.W.: *Vascular Surgery: A Comprehensive Review.* Grune & Stratton, New York, 1983.

Morris, G.C., Jr.; Lechter, A.; and DeBakey, M.E.: Surgical treatment of fibromuscular disease of the carotid arteries. *Arch. Surg.,* **96**:636–42, 1968.

Najafi, H.; Javid, H.; Dye, W.S.; Hunter, J.A.; and Julian, O.C.: Kinked internal carotid artery: clinical evaluation and surgical correction. *Arch. Surg.,* **89**:134–43, 1964.

Ochsner, J.L.; Hughes, J.P.; Leonard, G.L.; and Mills, N.L.: Elastic tissue dysplasia of the internal carotid artery. *Ann. Surg.,* **185**:684–92, 1977.

Osborne, A.C., and Anderson, R.E.: Angiographic spectrum of cervical and intracranial fibromuscular dysplasia. *Stroke,* **8**:617–26, 1977.

Palubinskas, A.J., and Ripley, H.R.: Fibromuscular hyperplasia in extrarenal arteries. *Radiology,* **82**:451–55, 1964.

Paulson, W.G.; Boesel, C.P.; and Evans, W.E.: Fibromuscular dysplasia. *Arch. Neurol.,* **35**:287–90, 1978.

Pollock, M., and Jackson, B.M.: Fibromuscular dysplasia of the carotid arteries. *Neurology,* **21**:1226–30, 1971.

Quattlebaum, J.K., Jr.; Upson, E.T.; and Neville, R.L.: Stroke associated with elongation and kinking of the internal carotid artery: report of three cases treated by segmental resection of the carotid artery. *Ann. Surg.,* **150**:824–32, 1959.

Quattlebaum, J.K., Jr; Wade, J.S.; and Whiddon, C.M.: Stroke associated with elongation and kinking of the carotid artery: long-term follow up. *Ann. Surg.,* **177**:572, 1973.

Riser, M.; Geraud, J.; Ducoudray, J.; and Ribaut, L.: Dolichocarotide interne avec syndrome vertigineux, *Rev. Neurol.* **85**:145–47, 1951.

Robicsek, F.; Alexander, J.P.; Sanger, P.W.; Taylor, F.H.; and Gallucci, V.: Intermittent occlusion of the internal carotid artery by detached intima. *Angiology.* **16**:18–20, 1965.

Robicsek, F., and Daugherty, H.K.: Redundancy of the carotid artery combined with intrinsic occlusion. A radical surgical approach. *Vascular Surgery.* **4**:101–5, 1970.

Saddekin, S.; Sniderman, K.W.; Hilton, S.; and Sos, T.A.: Percutaneous transluminal angioplasty of nonatherosclerotic lesions. *A.J.R.,* **135**:975–82, 1980.

Sanger, P.W.; Robicsek, F.; Pritchard, W.L.; Daugherty, H.K.; and Gallucci, V.: Cerebral ischemia caused by kinking of the carotid artery. *N.C. Med. J.,* **26**:542–47, 1965.

Sanger, P.W.; Robicsek, F.; and Ibrahim, K.: Aneurysm of the left ventricle with peripheral embolization. *N.C. Med. J.* **27**:67–70, 1966.

Stanley, J.C.; Gewertz, B.L.; Bove, E.L.; Sottiura, V.; and Fry, W.J.: Arterial fibrodysplasia: histopathologic character and current etiologic concepts. *Arch. Surg.,* **110**:561–66, 1975.

Stanton, P.E., Jr.; McClusky, D.A., Jr.; and Lamis, P.A.: Hemodynamic assessment and surgical correction of kinking of the internal carotid artery. *Surgery,* **84**:793–801, 1978.

Toole, J.F., and Tucker, S.H.: Influence of head position upon cerebral circulation: studies on blood flow in cadavers. *Arch. Neurol.,* **2**:616–23, 1960.

Upson, J., and Raza, S.T.: Fibromuscular dysplasia of internal carotid arteries. *N.Y. State J. Med.,* **76**:972–74, 1976.

Wylie, E.J.; Perloff, D.; and Wellington, D.J.: Fibromuscular hyperplasia of the renal arteries. *Ann. Surg.,* **156**:592–609, 1962.

18

Intraoperative Evaluation of the Carotid Circulation

STEWART M. SCOTT

According to the report of the Inter-Society Commission, the incidence of perioperative stroke after carotid endarterectomy is expected to be less than 2 percent (DeWeese *et al.*, 1976). To achieve these results, not only is good surgical technique necessary, but patient selection is also important. Patients who have residual neurological deficit before carotid endarterectomy have a ten-times-greater incidence of both death and stroke postoperatively than patients free of preoperative neurological damage. Such perioperative stroke may be caused by (1) cerebral ischemia occurring during temporary carotid artery occlusion, (2) embolization of air, atheroma, or thrombus into the cerebral circulation, or (3) the formation of an intimal flap during endarterectomy. Ischemia can be avoided by routine or selective shunting. Emboli can be prevented by careful dissection and cautious use of intraluminal shunts. Intimal flaps and stenosis, however, can be recognized and corrected only if intraoperative or postoperative angiography is performed.

According to published data, such unexpected defects may be found in 10 to 25 percent of patients if intraoperative carotid arteriograms are done (DeWeese *et al.*, 1976). These defects may or may not be associated with clinical symptoms or neurological sequelae. Indeed, complete occlusion of the carotid artery may occur in the asymptomatic postoperative patients (see Figure 18–1). The incidence of recurrent stenosis in the symptomatic patient after carotid endarterectomy is 1 to 5 percent (Stoney and String, 1976; Turnipseed *et al.*, 1980; Zierler *et al.*, 1982). An additional 8 percent of patients without symptoms can be shown to have restenosis (Kremen *et al.*, 1979). It has been observed that intraoperative arteriography can reduce the incidence of perioperative stroke (Scott *et al.*, 1982). It is possible that some of these "recurrent" stenoses are in reality residual defects unrecognized during surgery, and it is even likely that some of the "restenoses" are not true recurrences but simply obstructions created by the surgical intervention itself. Therefore, it is possible that intraoperative arteriography can decrease the incidence of carotid artery restenosis. However, intraoperative arteriography is time-consuming and even hazardous, especially if performed by an inexperienced surgical team. For these reasons, other ways to assess the cerebral circulation during surgery have been sought. They have included the use of radioisotopes to measure blood flow, electroencephalography, square-wave electromagnetic flowmeters, Doppler flowmeters, ultrasound imaging, and even vascular endoscopy. Although eventually there may be satisfactory alternatives to arteriography, at the present time the intraoperative anteriogram is the most reliable way to assess the carotid circulation during surgery.

INTRAOPERATIVE CAROTID ARTERIOGRAPHY

Blaisdell and associates (1967) observed that a satisfactory clinical response after carotid endarterectomy does not always indicate a

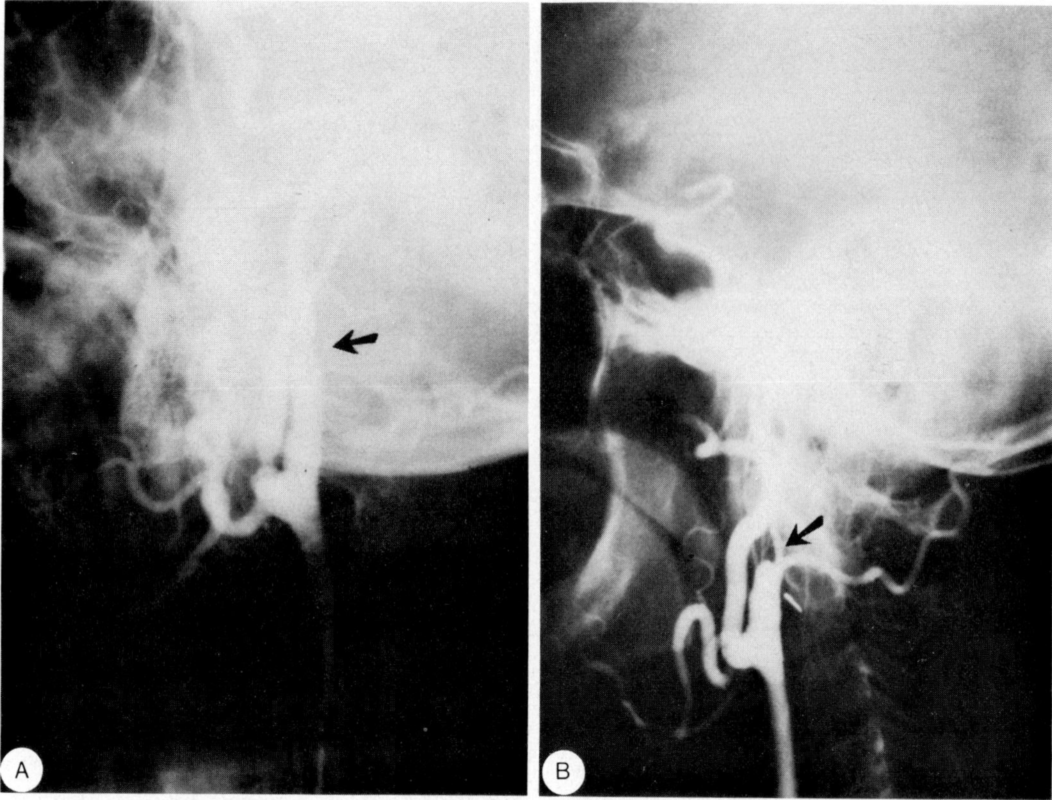

Figure 18-1. Intraoperative carotid arteriogram showing a defect in the internal carotid artery *(A)*. The defect was not repaired. A postoperative arteriogram in the same patient who was completely asymptomatic. The internal carotid artery is now totally occluded *(B)*. From Scott, S. M.; Sethi, G. K.; Bridgman, A. H.: Perioperative stroke during carotid endarterectomy: the value of intraoperative angiography. *J. Cardiovasc. Surg.*, **23**:353-58, 1982, with permission.

good technical result. Blaisdell performed intraoperative carotid arteriograms in 100 consecutive patients and found 26 unsuspected intraluminal defects. From this experience, he recommended that intraoperative arteriography be performed routinely after carotid endarterectomy. This opinion was shared by Rosenthal, who found unacceptable defects in 8 percent of 260 consecutive patients who had intraoperative arteriography after carotid endarterectomy (Rosenthal *et al.*, 1973). In 1975, Hobson and associates reviewed 50 intraoperative carotid arteriograms performed at the Walter Reed Army Medical Center and found defects in two internal (4 percent) and in three external (6 percent) carotid arteries (Hobson *et al.*, 1975). These investigators also recommended routine use of intraoperative carotid arteriography. Three years later, Andersen and associates again reviewed the Walter Reed Army Medical Center experience (Andersen *et al.*, 1978). In 131 consecutive arteriograms, unacceptable defects were found in seven patients (5.3 percent). Subintimal extravasation of dye occurred in two patients during arteriography, and in one of these patients, permanent hemiparesis developed. Noting that their intraoperative carotid anteriograms were frequently of poor quality and that the procedure was at times hazardous, it was their conclusion that intraoperative arteriography should not be performed routinely but should be reserved for (1) patients in whom difficulty is encountered in passing a shunt, suggesting the possibility of intimal injury, (2) instances in which a distal intimal flap is suspected, (3) evaluation of an apparent stricture, and (4) assessment of a technically difficult procedure. Routine intraoperative arteriography may not be necessary for most surgeons, but Blaisdell recommends that if neurological complications after carotid endarterectomy are excessive — that is, greater than 2 percent — routine intraoperative carotid arteriography should be used to eliminate the technical complications that can account for many postoperative neurologic problems (Blaisdell, 1978). This has also been true in our experience (Scott *et al.*, 1982). We reviewed our results in 283 patients; routine intraoperative arteriography was associated with a reduction in operative mortality owing to stroke from 2.7 to 0.7 percent and with a reduction of perioperative stroke from 4.1 to 0.7 percent. (see Figure 18–1).

For the experienced surgeon, routine intraoperative carotid arteriography may be a necessity, but the value of this procedure should not be overlooked. It should be utilized at least selectively as recommended by Andersen (1978).

Technique of Intraoperative Arteriography

The patient is positioned on a radiolucent operating table while being prepared for surgery. An X-ray cassette with film is properly aligned at this time. On completing the endarterectomy, a small metal clip is applied to the adventitia of the internal carotid artery to identify the distal end of the arteriotomy on the arteriogram. We use OL-1 X-ray film or its equivalent in a grid cassette and a three-phase portable X-ray unit. Care is taken that the cassette is perpendicular to the X-ray tube to prevent grid distortion and that the distance from the tube to the patient is maximal. The X-ray field is coned to cover a 14 × 17 in cassette. The optimal X-ray exposure is determined for the equipment being used. The films are processed immediately after exposure and examined. An experienced X-ray technician is essential.

A 19-gauge needle is inserted into the common carotid artery with the tip pointed proximally. One should be careful to ensure that the needle is free within the lumen of the vessel. If the needle is pointed distally, the dye can stream selectively into either the internal or the external carotid artery, resulting in incomplete visualization (see Figure 18–2). Should subin-

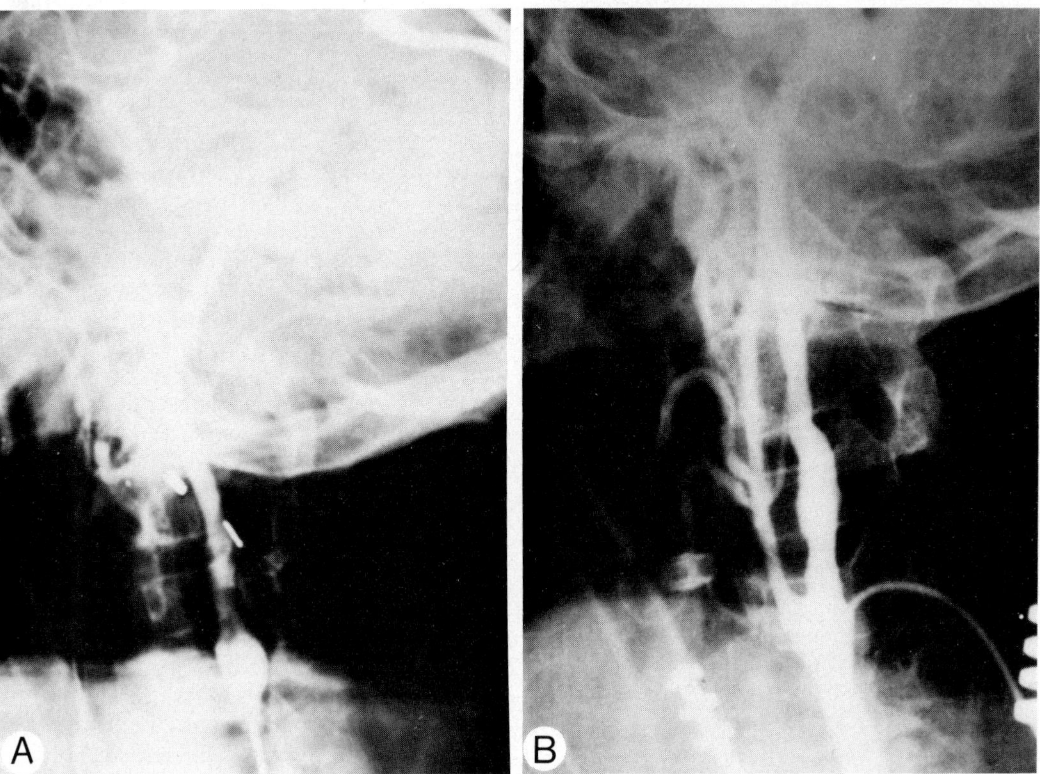

Figure 18–2. An intraoperative carotid arteriogram. The needle through which the contrast material is injected is pointed distally. The contrast material is selectively delivered into the internal carotid artery *(A)*. The arteriogram is repeated with the needle pointed proximally. There is good visualization of the common carotid artery, the bifurcation, and both branches *(B)*.

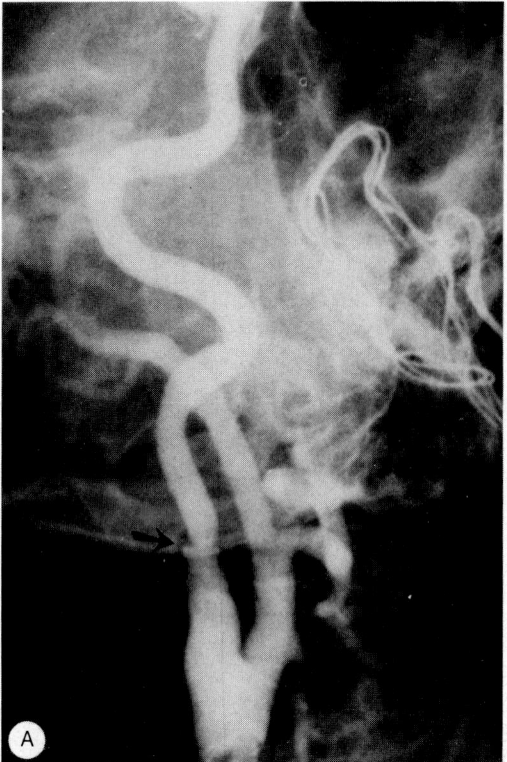

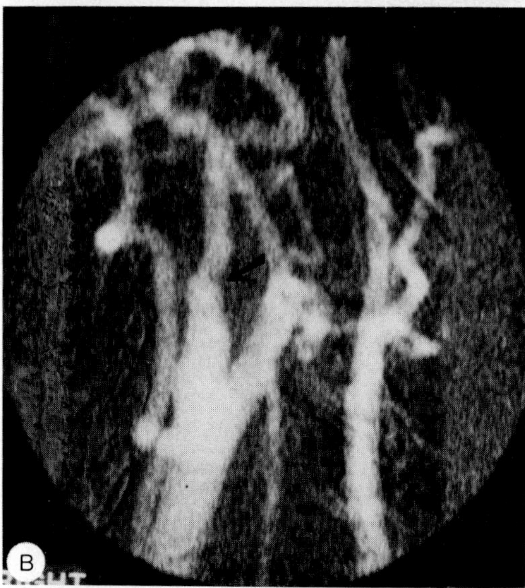

Figure 18–3. An intraoperative carotid arteriogram showing an irregularity in the wall of the internal carotid artery *(A)*. A postoperative digital subtraction angiogram demonstrates persistence of the irregularity but no evidence of obstruction or stenosis *(B)*.

timal extravasation occur, dissection or an intimal flap is less likely to result if the needle is pointed proximally against the flow of blood. Ten ml of 65 percent contrast material is injected rapidly with a small caliber syringe with a 15 or 20 ml capacity. The X-ray film is exposed when 7 or 8 ml of contrast material have been injected. If the injection is stopped too soon, the contrast material may be washed away before the film is exposed.

Results of Angiography

With experience, good arteriograms can always be obtained. Unsatisfactory arteriograms may be repeated, but preferably only once to avoid the administration of an excessive amount of contrast material and to avoid prolonging anesthesia time. The freshly endarterectomized carotid artery usually has a slightly irregular appearance (see Figure 18–3). Smooth areas of narrowing suggesting spasm may be present where occluding vascular clamps or tapes were used (see Figure 18–4). These must be distinguished from intraluminal lesions and narrowings of the suture lines. The radiopaque marker identifying the limits of the arteriotomy will help make this distinction.

As previously noted, the incidence of reported technical defects varies from 5 to 25 percent. We reviewed 107 consecutive intraoperative arteriograms performed at our hospital and found 29 defects in internal carotid arteries. There were 16 areas of stenosis, 12 intimal flaps, and one complete occlusion. Twelve of the defects required revision and were subsequently satisfactorily repaired (see Figure 18–5). Of the 27 defects found in the external carotid arteries, six were repaired (see Figure 18–6). Defects judged to be either insignificant or not amenable to repair were not corrected.

To determine whether or not intraoperative carotid arteriography was of value in preventing neurological injury, we compared the results obtained in a series of patients in whom we used intraoperative arteriography at first selectively and later routinely with results from an earlier group of patients in whom intraoperative arteriography was not used (see Table 18–1). The number of perioperative strokes resulting in permanent injury or death was reduced from 4.1 percent in the earlier group of patients to 0.7 percent in the later group in whom we used intraoperative arteriography.

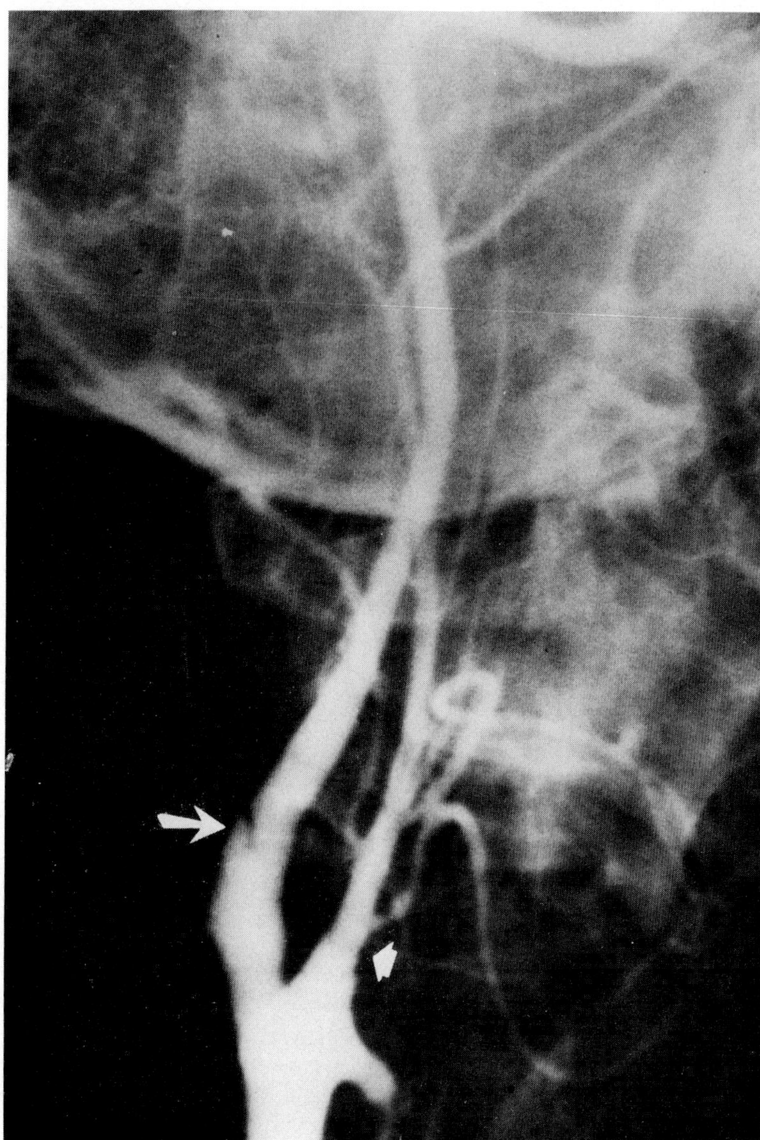

Figure 18–4. An intraoperative carotid arteriogram shows a thin symmetric intimal flap in the internal carotid artery (arrow). Note the area of narrowing presumably owing to a vascular clamp (arrowhead). From: Scott, S.M.; Sethi, G.K.; and Bridgman, A.H.: Perioperative stroke during carotid endarterectomy: the value of intraoperative angiography. *J. Cardiovascular Surg.* (Torino), **23**:353–58, 1982, with permission.

Complications of Intraoperative Arteriography

As already noted, intraoperative arteriography is not without hazards. However, the risks are few, and they can be reduced by simple precautions. Air embolism is avoided by carefully excluding air bubbles from the syringe, the tubing, and the needle. Subintimal extravasation is prevented by assuring that the needle is positioned properly within the lumen of the artery and that the syringe aspirates freely. One should always check the container from which the contrast material is withdrawn to be certain that the proper dye is used and that it is of the desired concentration. A too concentrated solution or an excessive amount of dye may not be tolerated by the patient. A history of dye sensitivity ought to be noted before surgery, and in such a case one may elect to omit arteriography.

ALTERNATE METHODS OF INTRAOPERATIVE ASSESSMENT OF CAROTID FLOW AFTER VASCULAR RECONSTRUCTION

Because intraoperative carotid arteriography extends anesthesia time and causes addi-

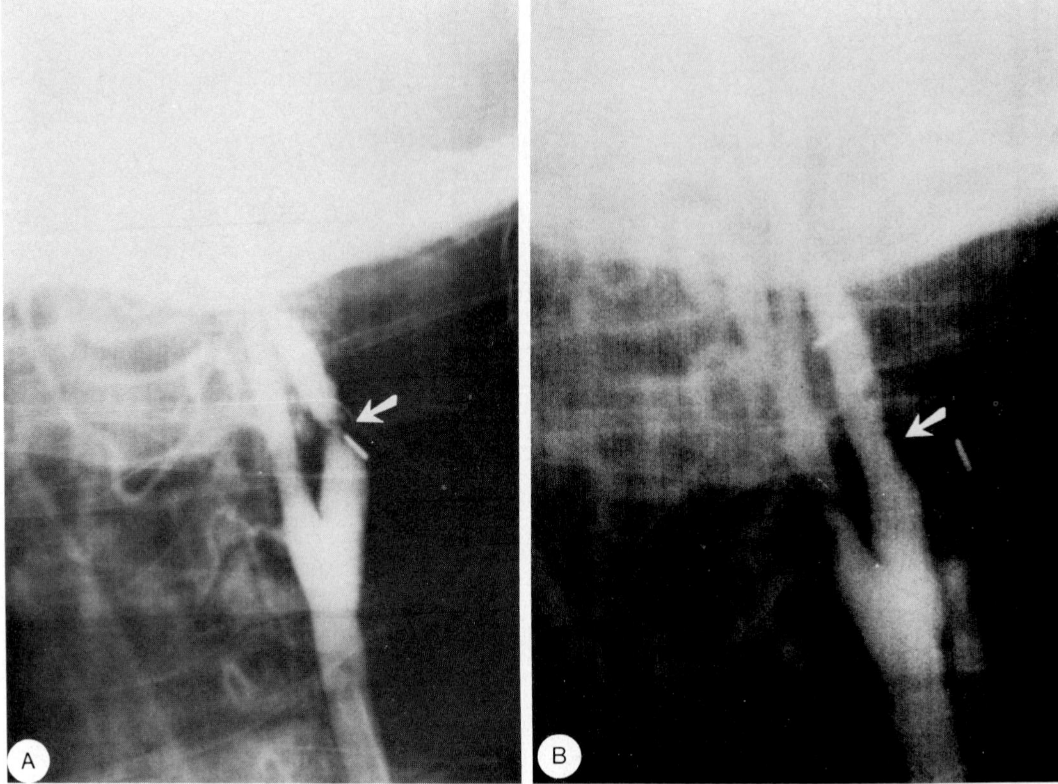

Figure 18-5. An intraoperative carotid arteriogram showing stenosis of the internal carotid artery after endarterectomy *(A)*. A repeat arteriogram after satisfactory revision of the area of stenosis *(B)*.

tional risk of injury to the patient, more rapid and less invasive methods of assessing the carotid circulation after endarterectomy have been sought.

Regional Anesthesia

Perhaps the earliest method of assessing the carotid circulation at surgery was to operate with local anesthesia and to monitor the awake patient (Blaisdell, 1978; Rich and Hobson, 1975). This technique is used primarily to determine whether or not the patient can tolerate carotid artery occlusion. Regional or local anesthesia allows the surgeon to observe whether or not the patient is neurologically intact as soon as the endarterectomy is completed (see also Chapter 20). Now that there are other means of monitoring and assessing cerebral blood flow, most surgeons prefer general anesthesia because it is more comfortable for the patient and allows the surgeon to operate without haste or compromise.

Electroencephalography

For some surgeons, the electroencephalogram (EEG) provides a reliable way of monitoring blood flow to the cerebral cortex. Sundt and his associates at the Mayo Clinic used a

Table 18-1. Carotid Endarterectomy with and without Intraoperative Arteriography

	ENDARTERECTOMIES N	DEATHS FROM STROKES N (%)	STROKES WITH RESIDUAL (%) N (%)	DEATHS AND STROKES WITH RESIDUAL N (%)
With arteriograms	137	1 (0.7)	0	1 (0.7)
Without arteriograms	146	4 (2.7)	2 (1.4)	6 (4.1)

From: S.M. Scott, G.K. Sethi; and A.H. Bridgman: Perioperative stroke during carotid endarterectomy: the value of intraoperative angiography. *J. Cardiovasc. Surg. (Torino)* **23**:353-58, 1982, with permission.

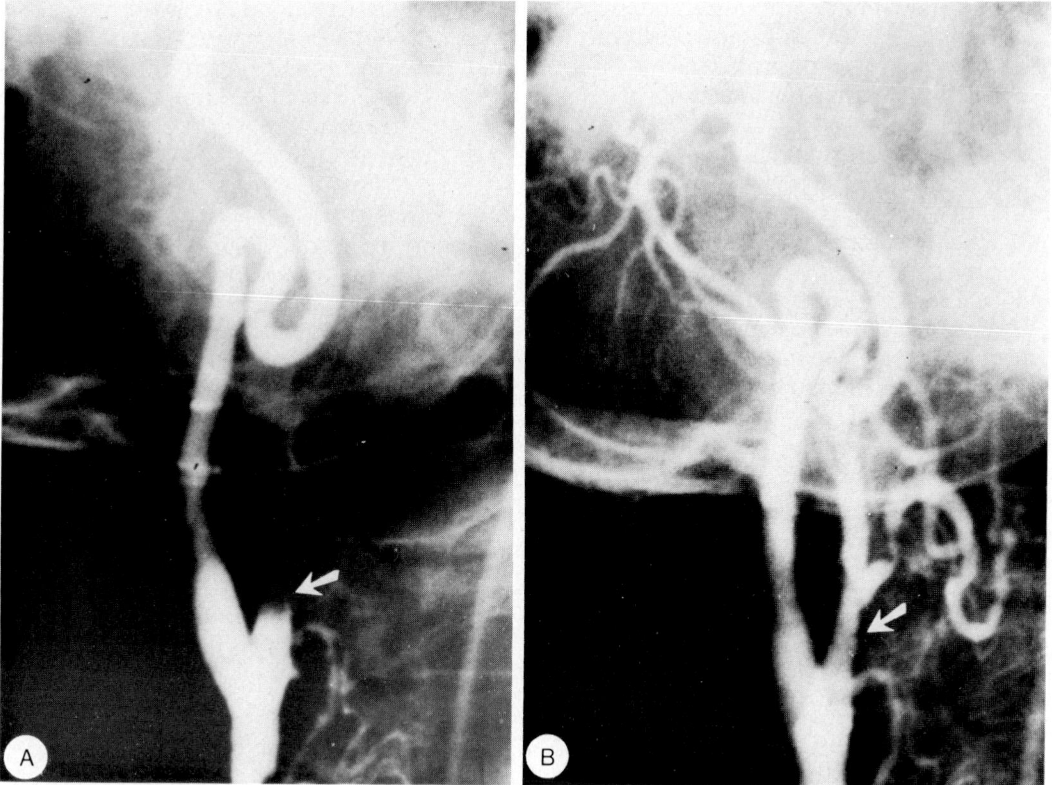

Figure 18–6. An intraoperative carotid arteriogram showing occlusion of the external carotid artery *(A)*. An intraoperative arteriogram showing a patent external carotid artery after repair of the defect *(B)*.

continuous 16-channel EEG tracing in the operating room (Sundt *et al.*, 1981). According to their report, they have never observed a patient emerging from anesthesia with a new neurological deficit that was not predicted by changes in the EEG. In 1,145 patients operated on in whom intraoperative EEG was used to monitor cerebral ischemia, focal changes occurred in 321. The EEG reverted to baseline in 319 of these patients when a shunt was inserted. Skill is needed to interpret the intraoperative EEG. Changes can result not only from ischemia owing to carotid artery occlusion or emboli but also from excessive depth of anesthesia (see also Chapter 12).

Cerebral Blood Flow

Blood flow to the brain has been measured by means of radioisotopes, square-wave electomagnetic flowmeters, and Doppler ultrasound. Cerebral blood flow can be determined by injecting Xenon 133 into the internal carotid artery. Clearance of the Xenon 133 is measured with a scintillation detector positioned over the region of the brain in the distribution of the middle cerebral artery (Waltz *et al.,* 1972). Close correlation between blood flow measured in this manner and changes noted on the EEG has been found (Sundt, 1983). Rapid EEG changes occur at measured flows of less than 10 ml/100 mg; the patient with a flow less than this when the carotid artery is occluded should be shunted. Increases in blood flow after endarterectomy, when measured with Xenon 133, are usually very modest.

Blood flow within the carotid artery can also be measured before and after carotid endarterectomy with a square-wave electromagnetic flowmeter (Hobson *et al.*, 1975; Dillon *et al.*, 1965). Flow can also be measured during endarterectomy by use of an electromagnetic flowmeter attached to an indwelling shunt (Ekestrom, 1968). If a shunt is poorly placed or kinked, the diminished flow through the shunt can be detected with the flowmeter. Carotid artery flow may be modified not only by any stenosis that may be present but also by peripheral arterial resistance and arterial pressure.

Therefore, flow before and after endarterectomy is somewhat variable. However, detecting changes in flow within the carotid artery may be helpful in assessing the results of a surgical procedure.

The Doppler ultrasound flowmeter has been used by a number of surgeons to evaluate their results after various procedures, including carotid endarterectomy (Keitzer *et al.,* 1972; Mozersky *et al.,* 1973). The output of the Doppler flowmeter is an audible signal, and both experience and subjective interpretation are required to use the instrument reliably. If the signals from the Doppler are either low-pitched and damped or high-pitched and continuous, there is probably residual narrowing of the reconstructed artery. Narrowing causes an increase in the velocity of blood flow through the artery, which results in a high frequency or high-pitched sound from the Doppler.

It is sometimes difficult for a surgeon to interpret Doppler sounds that result from various degrees of deformity of reconstructed arteries. Hearing perception certainly is not uniform in all of us. Indeed, some persons may have a very limited hearing range. It is very helpful, therefore, to be able to visualize the audible signal. This is accomplished by displaying the frequencies of the sound signal in real-time on a cathode-ray tube or television screen. This technique is known as *spectral analysis.* Both continuous signals (Spencer and Reid, 1979) and pulsed Doppler signals (Blackshear *et al.,* 1980) have been used with the spectum analyzer, which displays the frequencies as an amplitude wave form (see Figure 18–7). Frequency analysis used intraoperatively has been found to be a sensitive predictor of arterial stenosis. The velocity of blood flow increases with stenosis, resulting in high-peaked frequencies during the systolic portion of the frequency wave form. The maximum or peak frequency is proportional to the degree of stenosis. Mean frequency throughout the cardiac cycle does not correlate as well as peak frequency with the degree of stenosis, but in the presence of stenosis and turbulent flow the shape of the curve is broadened as a result of the higher frequencies present in the diastolic portion of the wave form.

Zierler and associates (1983) reported their experience with real-time spectral analysis to detect defects after carotid endarterectomy. They used a pulsed Doppler in preference to the continuous-wave Doppler because the latter derives its signal from the entire arterial blood-flow profile and includes velocity gradients normally present near the arterial wall. Their probe, a small ultrasonic transducer mounted on a 16 gauge needle, is a direction-sensitive 20 MHz pulsed Doppler velocimeter

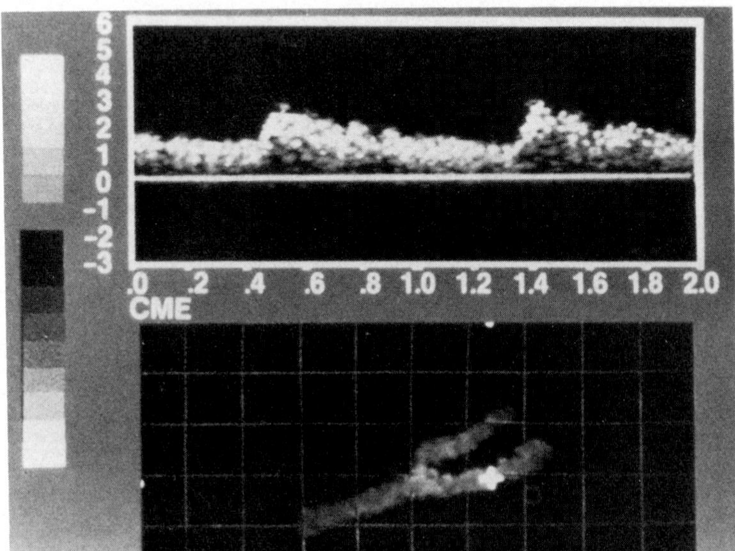

Figure 18–7. Transcutaneous ultrasound with spectral analysis. Displayed is the sound spectrum from a 5 MHz probe placed directly over a normal internal carotid artery. The Doppler delivers a continuous-wave signal. The frequency of the signal is displayed as an amplitude curve. The loudness of the signal determines the color of the display, red indicating maximum intensity. Reproduction courtesy Carolina Medical Electronics, King, North Carolina.

capable of measuring a sample of volume 0.2 mm^3 at any point between 1.3 and 11.5 mm from the end of the probe. The transducer is placed directly on the surface of the artery at a 60 degree angle and is acoustically coupled with saline solution. The diameter of the artery is measured so that the depth of the signal can be positioned in the center of the artery with a range control.

This instrument was used before and after carotid endarterectomy in 50 patients who also had intraoperative arteriography (Zierler *et al.*, 1984). Technical errors requiring correction were identified in two patients. False-positive findings were present in five patients, and there were no false-negative results. Zierler concluded that this is a very sensitive procedure which can be used to screen for patients who should have intraoperative arteriography.

We have used intraoperatively a continuous-wave Doppler with a 10 MHz probe and a spectrum analyzer to assess carotid endarterectomy (see Figure 18–8). This system is very sensitive to turbulent flow and has not been successful in our experience in eliminating the need for intraoperative arteriography after carotid endarterectomy.

Real-Time B-Mode Imaging

Real-time B-mode ultrasound has been used to image arteries during surgery (Lane and Appleberg, 1982; Sigel *et al.*, 1982). Sigel in

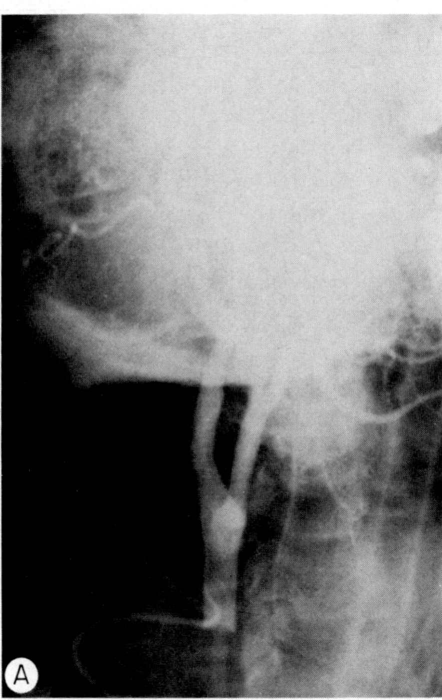

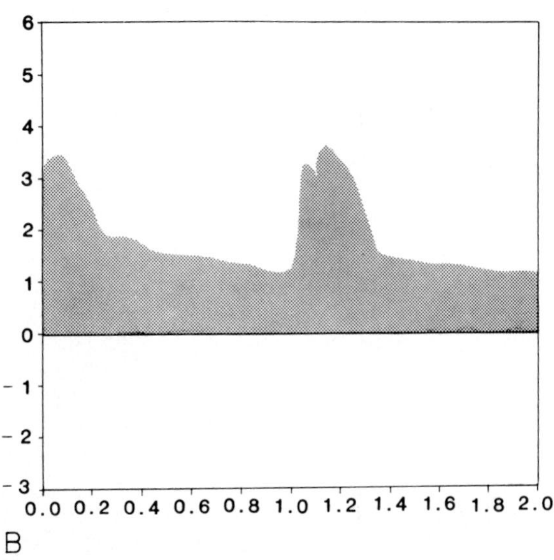

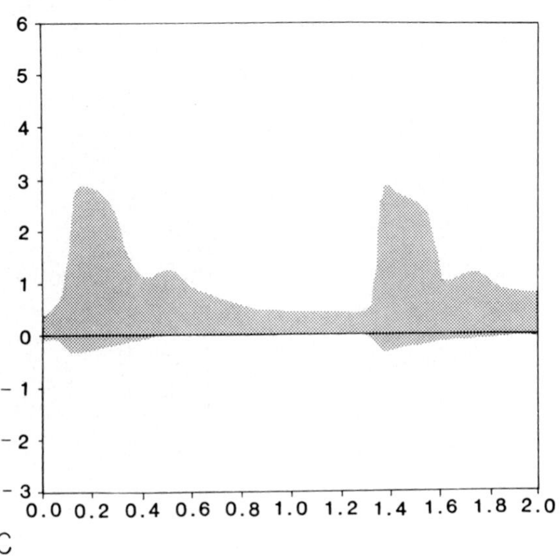

Figure 18–8. A normal intraoperative carotid arteriogram after carotid endarterectomy *(A)*. Intraoperative Doppler (ultrasound with frequency analysis) of the internal carotid artery *(B)*. Intraoperative Doppler of the external carotid artey *(C)*. All curves have low peak frequencies, implying low velocity blood flow and no stenosis.

particular has utilized a small sector-scanning transducer to detect arterial strictures, thrombi, and intimal flaps (see Figure 18–9). When ultrasound imaging was compared with arteriography in experimental animals, ultrasound was found to be significantly more sensitive in identifying intimal flaps and thombi (Coelho *et al.,* 1981). In 70 patients requiring various vascular operations in which intraoperative ultrasound evaluation was used, Sigel identified 15 defects in 14 of these patients (Sigel, 1982). Only one defect was considered significant enough to require revision. Lane and Appleberg (1982) report a similar experience with 60 intraoperative scans after carotid endarterectomy. They detected nine abnormalities (15 percent), four of which required revision.

Real-time B-mode ultrasound imaging is a procedure that the experienced surgeon can perform easily and rapidly. The ultrasound transducer is positioned directly on the surface of the surgically exposed artery. This allows a high focus, high frequency transducer to be used. High frequency transducers give better resolution than the low frequency transducers that must be used in transcutaneous studies to obtain the depth of penetration required. By varying the position of the transducer, an artery can be scanned in cross section, longitudinally, and in multiple planes. Arteriography is usually limited to a single plane.

It requires training and experience to learn the technique of B-mode ultrasound imaging and to interpret the results. This technique will not always identify fresh clot (Anderson *et al.,* 1979) Stasis of unclotted blood, as in a clamped artery, produces internal echoes that obscure the vessel walls. Some prosthetic materials that might be used in vascular reconstruction are also echogenic (Sigel, 1982). In some instances, ultrasound is too sensitive and may exaggerate the presence of minor defects. The greatest disadvantage of ultrasound, however, is the high cost of the instrument. Some of the newer commercially available instruments have remarkable resolution and utilize transducers with side ports to make intraoperative manipulation easier, as well as traditional transducers with end apertures. It is entirely

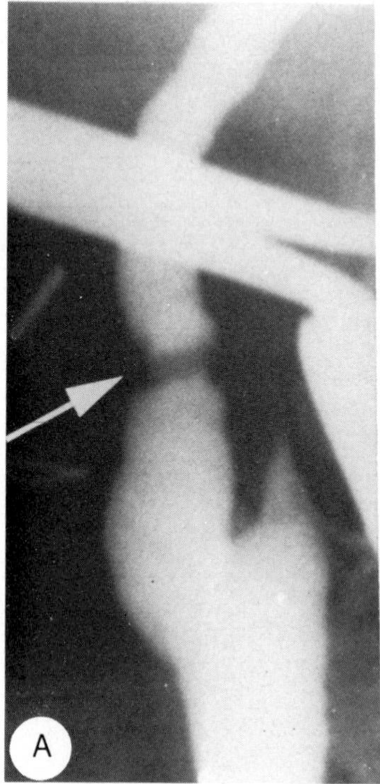

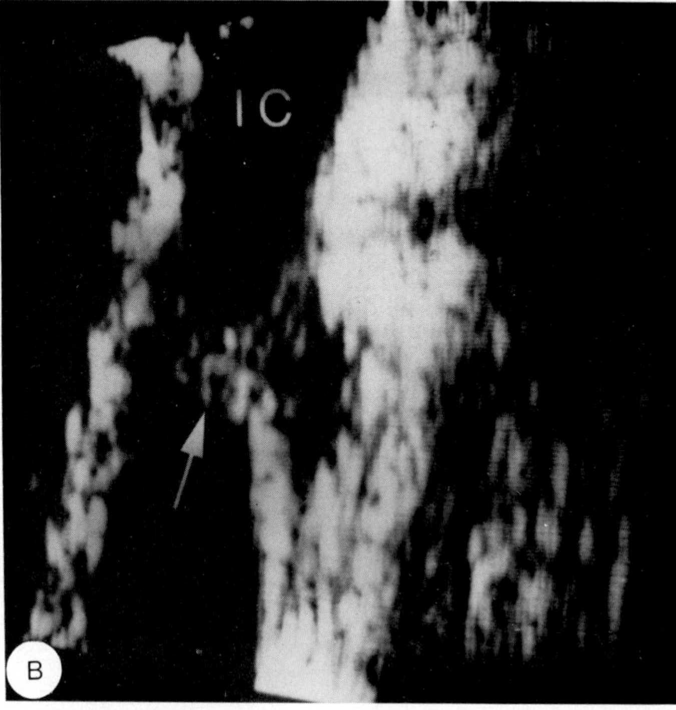

Figure 18–9. Intraoperative arteriogram *(A)* and real-time B-mode ultrasound image *(B)* of the internal carotid artery (IC) obtained after carotid endarterectomy. A 5 mm intimal flap (arrow) is present. The artery was reexplored, and the flap was removed. From Sigel, B. S.: Imaging ultrasound in the intraoperative diagnosis of vascular defects. *J. Ultrasound Med.,* **2**:337–43, 1983, with permission.

possible that B-mode ultrasound may someday replace the intraoperative carotid arteriogram.

VASCULAR ENDOSCOPY

Although operative endoscopy has been useful in many urological, biliary, and orthopedic procedures, it has had very limited application in vascular surgery. Towne and Bernhard (1977) have reported using the choledochoscope and arthroscope to visualize the luminal surface of the internal carotid artery after carotid endarterectomy. The procedure was attempted in 35 patients but could not be completed in eight with the instruments available. Thirteen internal carotid arteries were examined, and atheromatous shreds were seen in the lumens of two. It remains to be seen whether this procedure will prove to be a useful adjunct for intraoperative assessment.

REFERENCES

Andersen, C.A.; Collins, G.J.; and Rich, N.M.: Routine operative anteriography during carotid endarterectomy: a reassessment. *Surgery,* **83**:67–71, 1978.

Anderson, J.C.; Baltaxe, H.A.; and Wolf, G.L.: Inability to show clot: one limitation of ultrasonography of the abdominal aorta. *Radiology,* **132**:693–96, 1979.

Blackshear, W.M.; Phillips, D.J.; Chikos, P.M.; Harley J.D.; Thiele, B.L.; and Strandness, D.E.: Carotid artery velocity patterns in normal and stenotic vessels. *Stroke,* **11**:67–71, 1980.

Blaisdell, F.W.: Routine operative arteriography following carotid endarterectomy. *Surgery,* **83**:114–15, 1978.

Blaisdell, F.W.; Lim, R., Jr.; and Hall, A.D.: Technical result of carotid endarterectomy. Arteriographic assessment. *Am. J. Surg.,* **114**:239–46, 1967.

Coelho, J.C.U.; Sigel, B.; Flanigan, D.P.; Schuler, J.J.; Spigos, D.G.; and Nyhus, L.M.: Detection of arterial defects by real-time ultrasound scanning during vascular surgery: an experimental study. *J. Surg. Res.,* **30**:535–43, 1981.

DeWeese, J.A.; Blaisdell, F.W.; Foster, J.H.; Garrett, H.E.; and DeWolfe, V.G.: Report of Inter-Society Commission for Heart Disease Resources. *Circulation,* **53**:A39–A50, 1976.

Dillon, M. L.; Reeves, J.W.; and Postlethwait, R.W.: Carotid artery flows and pressures in twenty-two patients with cerebral vascular insufficiency. *Surgery,* **58**:951–55, 1965.

Ekestrom, S.: Continuous flow-measurement during reconstruction of the carotid artery. *Scand. J. Thorac. Cardiovas. Surg.,* **2**:51–6, 1968.

Hobson, R.W.; Rich, N.M.; Wright, C.B.; and Fedde, C.W.: Operative assessment of carotid endarterectomy: internal carotid arterial back pressure, carotid arterial blood flow, and carotid arteriography. *Am. Surg.,* **41**:603–10, 1975.

Keitzer, W.F.; Lichti, E.L.; Brossart, F.A.; and DeWeese, M.S.: Use of the Doppler ultrasonic flowmeter during arterial vascular surgery. *Arch. Surg.,* **105**:308–12, 1972.

Kremen, J.E.; Gee, W.; Kaupp, H.A.; and McDonald, K.M.: Restenosis or occlusion after carotid endarterectomy: a survey with ocular pneumoplethysmography. *Arch. Surg.,* **114**:608–10, 1979.

Lane, R.J., and Appleberg, M.: Real-time intraoperative angiosonography after carotid endarterectomy. *Surgery,* **92**:5–10, 1982.

Mozersky, D.J.; Sumner, D.S.; Barnes, R.W.; and Strandness, D.E.: Intraoperative use of a sterile ultrasonic flow probe. *Surg. Gynecol. Obstet.,* **136**:279–80, 1973.

Rich, N.M.; and Hobson, R.W.: Carotid Endarterectomy under regional anesthesia. *Am. Surg.* **41**:253–59, 1975.

Rosenthal, J.J.; Gaspar, M.R.; and Movius, H.J.: Intraoperative anteriography in carotid thromboendarterectomy. *Arch. Surg.,* **106**:806–8, 1973.

Scott, S.M.; Sethi, G.K.; and Bridgman, A.H.: Perioperative stroke during carotid endarterectomy: the value of intraoperative angiography. *J. Cardiovasc. Surg. (Torino),* **23**:353–58, 1982.

Sigel, B.: *Operative Ultrasonography.* Lea & Febiger, Philadelphia, 1982.

Sigel, B.; Coelho, J.C.U.; Flanigan, D.P.; Schuler, J.J.; and Spigos, D.G.: Ultrasonic imaging during vascular surgery. *Arch. Surg.,* **117**:764–67, 1982.

Spencer, M.P., and Reid, J.M.: Quantitation of carotid stenosis with continuous-wave (C-W) Doppler ultrasound. *Stroke,* **10**:326–30, 1979.

Stoney, R.J., and String, S.T.: Recurrent carotid stenosis. *Surgery,* **80**:705–10, 1976.

Sundt, T.M.: The ischemic tolerance of neural tissue and the need for monitoring and selective shunting during carotid endarterectomy. *Stroke,* **14**:93–8, 1983.

Sundt, T.M; Sharbrough, F.W.; Piepgras, D.G.; Kearns, T.P.; Messick, J.M.; and O'Fallon, W.M.: Correlation of cerebral blood flow and electroencephalographic changes during carotid endarterectomy. *Mayo Clin. Proc.,* **56**:533–43, 1981.

Towne, J.B., and Bernhard, V.M.: Vascular endoscopy—an adjunct to carotid surgery. *Stroke,* **8**:569–71, 1977.

Turnipseed, W.D.; Berkoff, H.A.; and Crummy, A.: Postoperative occlusion after carotid endarterectomy. *Arch. Surg.,* **115**:573–74, 1980.

Waltz, A.G.; Sundt, T.M.; and Michenfelder, J.D.: Cerebral blood flow during carotid endarterectomy. *Circulation,* **45**:1091–96, 1972.

Zierler, R.E.; Bandyk, D.F.; Berni, G.A.; and Thiele, B.L.: Intraoperative pulsed Doppler assessment of carotid endarterectomy. *Ultrasound Med. Biol.,***9**:65–71, 1983.

Zierler, R.E.; Bandyk, D.F.; and Thiele, B.L.: Intraoperative assessment of carotid endarterectomy. *J. Vasc. Surg.,* **1**:73–83, 1984.

Zierler, R.E.; Bandyk, D.F.; Thiele, B.L.; and Strandness, D.E.: Carotid artery stenosis following endarterectomy. *Arch. Surg.,* **117**:1408–15, 1982.

19

The Routine Application of Temporary Shunting in Carotid Surgery

JOHN M. KESHISHIAN

In the field of extracranial cerebrovascular surgery, no topic has evoked more controversy or generated more discussion than the matter of how to protect the brain during carotid endarterectomy. This controversy has inspired a plethora of articles, many of which have scientific merit and all of which project the concept fostered by the specific senior author, usually firmly documented by statistically valid figures. The debate is not less lively in private discussions with our colleagues, for we surgeons occasionally generate more heat than light and are firmly convinced that our own concepts are probably the only logical ones—an attitude that reflects the strong personalities many surgeons possess. Yet, with all the difficulties these attitudes created, they have also fostered a striving for excellence and improvement of surgical results and a net benefit for patient and profession.

Protecting the brain from injury has, of course, always been a concern to the surgeon, but never more so than during restoration of blood flow through one of its damaged feeder arteries. What is, then, the optimum means of cerebral preservation in such a situation? Undoubtedly, the most effective way to protect the brain during carotid endarterectomy is to maintain uninterrupted carotid blood flow. This requires the application of a temporary indwelling shunt. If we accept the postulate that the application of indwelling shunts has advantages as well as disadvantages, then the reason for these different views is readily apparent. Evidently surgeons who never use shunts are convinced that the disadvantages of the shunt outweigh its advantages; those who always use shunts profess the opposite, whereas those who sometimes use shunts believe that the balance between the advantage and disadvantages of the shunt should be determined on an individual, patient-by-patient basis.

Because the first two positions are relatively simplistic, let us for the moment discuss the third view, that the use of the shunt should be determined according to the individual hemodynamics of the patient who is being operated upon. Such a decision naturally must be based on careful evaluation of the patient's cerebrovascular status and determination of specific parameters obtainable before or during surgery. By obtaining such information, then we may establish certain guidelines to determine when a patient will be especially at risk of cerebral ischemia during crossclamping. Unfortunately, it is the interpretation of these guidelines by the various investigators which continues to be the root of the controversy. Therefore, let us address this issue at the outset.

The initial evaluation of the patient suspected of having transient cerebral ischemia (TIA) naturally should begin with appropriate questioning and physical examination, followed by specific studies. We usually begin these studies with oculoplethysmography (OPG), which enables us to infer what pressures are present in the ophthalmic arteries and compare them with each other. If there is a difference of ±4 mm or more between them, we usually perform a study delineating the anatomical status of the arteries, e.g., arch-angiography, selective cerebral arteriograms, or some form of computer-enhanced arterial visualization. At the same time we also carry out fundoscopic examination of the retina to detect debris or refractive crystalline material that may have been dislodged from the carotid bifurcation. After establishing the diagnosis of clinically significant carotid bifurcation disease, thus the indication for surgery, we proceed with the following steps:

1. Determine the functional status of the brain by obtaining all or some of the following tests: electroencephalograms (EEG), contrast-enhanced computed tomography (CT) scans, cerebral blood flow (CBF) measurements, as well as psychometric and other tests.
2. Choose the type of anesthesia.
3. Consider the advisability of a shunt.

DETERMINATION OF THE FUNCTIONAL STATUS OF THE BRAIN

A standard EEG is necessary if there is a question of cerebral dysfunction. It is both a baseline and a graph of reference when EEG monitoring is carried out during the operation. It has been demonstrated that slow cerebral activity preoperatively may become even slower under anesthesia, depending on its concentration and depth, which in turn may affect blood pressure and blood flow rates.

A CT scan of the brain enhanced with radiopaque contrast is obtained primarily to establish a baseline and enhance understanding of the status of cerebral perfusion. Nonperfused or ischemic areas are noted. A repeat CT scan after endarterectomy may show reperfusion in some of these areas (surgery for acutely ischemic episodes is discussed elsewhere). In some centers, psychometric tests are carried out to determine the emotional status of the patient. I also have observed clearly that in some cases endarterectomy may reverse a deteriorating personality; in other instances; patients who have been diagnosed as schizophrenic have become normal after endarterectomy.

In an important publication, Rowed and Vilaghy (1981) describe a technique for measuring CBF using 16 collimated scintillation detectors mounted in probes which are positioned in predetermined areas over the cerebral hemisphere. In this manner they were able to predict which patients were at risk for internal carotid artery occlusion during endarterectomy.

THE CHOICE OF ANESTHESIA (REGIONAL VERSUS GENERAL)

Rich and associates (1980) have long pondered which form of anesthesia is optimal for endarterectomy. Rainer and associates (1968) and Basiljevac and Farha (1980) have also been concerned with this problem. Their results with local anesthesia are shown in Table 19–1.

All these investigators resorted to shunting when an alteration in the neurological level was observed, and in addition Rich and associates (1980) switched to a general anesthetic at the same time. Contrast these figures with the much later results of Thompson (1968), who used a standardized approach to all carotid endarterectomies, i.e., general anesthesia, routine shunt, and patching when indicated (see Table 19–2).

Andersen, working with Rich (Andersen *et al.*, 1980) later examined their more recent data and concluded that the use of general anesthesia with a shunt had not significantly changed the mortality rate or incidence of postoperative neurological complications when compared with results from their earlier report on surgery under local anesthesia (see Table 19–3).

Table 19–1. Results of Endarterectomy Under Local Anesthesia

SOURCE	CASES (N)	MORTALITY N (%)	PERMANENT STROKE N (%)	TEMPORARY NEUROLOGICAL DEFICIT N (%)
Rich and Hobson, 1980	232	6 (2.6)	5 (2.5)	7 (30)
Rainer *et al.*, 1968	257	2 (0.8)	2 (0.7)	7 (2.7)
Basiljevac and Farja, 1980	166	2 (1.2)	6 (3.6)	6 (3.6)

Table 19–2. Results of Endarterectomy Under General Anesthesia

SOURCE	CASES (N)	MORTALITY N (%)	PERMANENT STROKE N (%)	TEMPORARY NEUROLOGIC DEFICIT N (%)
THOMPSON (1968)	748	20 (2.7)	20 (2.7)	4 (0.5)

From: Thompson, J.E.: *Surgery for Cerebrovascular Insufficiency,* 1968. Courtesy of Charles C Thomas, publisher, Springfield, Illinois, with permission.

It is of interest to note that the current method of performing this procedure at Rich's parent institution utilizes general anesthesia and elective shunting in almost every case. It is my impression from personal interviews and site visits that most institutions use general anesthesia for this operation and that the use of local anesthesia is the exception.

CONSIDERATION OF THE ADVISABILITY OF SHUNTING

The decision is generally based on the following parameters obtained preoperatively or during the operation:

1. *Stump pressure,* also known as *back pressure,* is pressure within the internal carotid artery above a deliberately occluded portion of the vessel. It may represent the true blood pressure in the collaterals and may correlate with a simultaneous OPG measurement. It is not an indicator of cerebral perfusion, and it is probably a poor indicator for the need for shunting (Bernstein *et al.,* 1983; Brewster *et al.,* 1980; Hertzer *et al.,* 1978, etc.).

2. The EEG demonstrates cerebral energy and may reflect alterations in CBF, levels of anesthesia, and blood volume when evaluated in the proper context. It may be used with other indexes in evaluating changes in the tracing (Blondeau *et al.,* 1982; Bostoen *et al.,* 1979; Brewster *et al.,* 1980, etc.).

3. CBF measurements using Xenon 133 have suggested that flow rates at or around 20 ml/100 g of brain tissue/min are consistent with normal cerebral function when the artery is clamped. With "low" stump pressures and low hemispheric flow shunting is recommended. Our philosophy is that shunting, and shunting alone, will eliminate the necessity for the foregoing tests (Jernigan and Hamman, 1982; Owens *et al.,* 1982, etc.), especially when investigations are under way. I doubt their real value as an everyday procedure.

4. A graphic display of the affected vessels is a sine qua non. Properly obtained, it can locate the diseased area and identify any cross-cerebral collaterals that may exist and unusual conditions, such as siphon stenosis, that may represent a contraindication to surgery. When contralateral disease is present, most surgeons opt for insertion of a temporal shunt. But in the presence of unilateral disease the angiograms should not be a deciding factor for or against shunting. In the series of Rowed and Vilaghy (1981), 35 patients underwent 38 operations (see Table 19–4). After the carotid vessels were opened, the stump pressure was measured. Then, depending on cerebral blood flow levels, endarterectomy was performed with or without shunt. Shunting was employed when the mean cerebral blood pressure was less than 30 ml/100 g of brain tissue/min. The figure 20 ml was considered a critical level, but Sundt and associates (1981) reported that EEG changes did not occur until the occluded CBF was less than 18 ml/20 g of brain tissue/min. Yet the significance of the EEG change at that flow rate, which was considered a critical predictor of postoperative neurological deficit, is not agreed upon by other investigators (Rich *et al.,* 1980). Therefore, to minimize the possibility of neurological deficit, Rowed and Vilaghy (1981) selected the value of 54 torr as a mean

Table 19–3. Results of Endarterectomy Under General Anesthesia

SOURCE	CASES (N)	MORTALITY N (%)	PERMANENT STROKE N (%)	TEMPORARY NEUROLOGIC DEFICIT N (%)
Anderson *et al.,* 1980	189	1 (0.5)	5 (2.6)	5 (2.6)

From: Anderson *et al.* Carotid endarterectomy: regional versus general anesthesia. *Am. Surg.* **46**:323–27, 1980, with permission.

Table 19–4. Indications for Endarterectomy

INDICATION (PATIENTS, N=35)	ENDARTERECTOMIES N (%)	SEX		AGE (YEARS)
		MALE N (%)	FEMALE N (%)	
Cerebral insufficiency:	22 (58)	23(61)	14(39)	44-71
Transient ischemic attack	10 (26)			
Asymptomatic severe stenosis	6 (16)			

Adapted from: Rowed, D.W., and Viloghy, M.I.: Intraoperative regional blood flow during carotid endarterectomy. *Can. J. Neurol. Sci.*, **8**(3):235–241, 1981.

stump pressure of adequate cerebral perfusion. As pointed out earlier, however, there is not complete agreement on the validity of this view. Other investigators have suggested that a lower mean stump pressure is consistent with adequate intraoperative cerebral perfusion (Sublett *et al.*, 1974; Boysen, 1973).

Of importance is the finding (Rowed and Vilaghy, 1981) that the internal carotid arterial stump pressures and mean CBF agreed in only 17 of the 38 patients in whom both procedures were recorded; the internal carotid arterial stump pressures were falsely low in ten patients, and the stump pressure was below the 50 mm pressure, while the recorded CBF actually exceeded 20 ml/100 g of brain tissue/min. Additionally, the internal carotid arterial stump pressure was falsely high in six patients (18 percent). In 32 of the patients, there was no change in neurological status postoperatively, but in four patients there was a neurological deficit that cleared within two to seven days even though intraoperative shunts were used.

In my opinion, one of the worst possible indexes for determining whether a shunt is necessary is the stump pressure, as first proposed by Moore in 1969 (Moore *et al.*, 1973). There is very little agreement on what adequate stump pressure should be. Back pressure from the distal carotid artery may be obtained by a number of different methods during the operative procedure. Depending on the particular surgeon, the acceptable figures range from 25 to 75 mm Hg, without considering that there may be fluctuations of the pressure from moment to moment, depending on a number of physiological and pharmacological factors, such as anesthesia, blood loss, carbon dioxide partial pressure, and other well-known parameters. Moreover, it is now generally recognized that stump pressures do not represent flow rates; however, it is the opinion of some investigators that flow rates may be even more important than the pressures.

With these controversial data on the value of the stump pressure, it is not surprising that there is no general agreement on the value of stump pressures and the use of shunts. One investigator may demonstrate that stump pressure is important, while another points out that no two surgeons accept the same stump pressures as critical. Surgeons also disagree on the proper indication for shunts, and some surgeons even believe that shunts are not required and, indeed, may be harmful. Somewhere in this mass of data there may be a set of circumstances, a common denominator, that eventually will lead to a clearer understanding of shunting. How can we explain that one patient presents with a "good" stump pressure and even though shunted, ends with a neurological insult, while another patient operated on without a shunt does quite well? How can we explain that patients in whom the carotid artery is temporarily clamped during surgery may not necessarily have strokes or develop deficits in the central nervous system despite the fact that the stump pressures are low and angiograms show no crossover collaterals? We must assume that such pathways exist even though they are not visualized by arteriograms, supporting the concepts of String and Callahan (1983) that angiography does not predict the adequacy of collateral flow.

Baker has advocated that temporary shunts not be used during carotid endarterectomy (Baker *et al.*, 1977). A total of 940 patients operated on without shunts had very few complications except when the back pressure was less than 50 mm Hg and contralateral occlusion existed. Here the incidence of permanent deficit was 11 percent, compared with 2.8 percent when either factor was present and 0.9 percent when neither existed. It is suggested that the use of a shunt in this group might be beneficial, and in fact Baker uses a shunt when he believes that a patient who has risk potentials may be better served with intraoperative perfusion (Baker, personal communication).

In regard to the question of EEG monitoring

during carotid endarterectomy, a series of 125 patients was reviewed by Rosenthal and associates (1981). Of these patients, 89 were operated on while under continuous 16-lead EEG monitoring. Of 36 patients not monitored but shunted, 8 percent had postoperative neurological deficits. Of 48 patients monitored by EEG and stump pressures, 9 percent had postoperative deficits despite normal readings; no shunts were used in these patients. A total of 41 patients with "normal" stump and EEG pressures were nevertheless shunted and had no problems. The investigators conclude that stump pressures and EEG tracings are unreliable indicators of cerebral perfusion in patients who have had reversible ischemic neurologic deficit or stroke.

String and Callahan (1983) believe that EEG studies alone as a reflection of hemispheric flow are not helpful and must be correlated with preclamp readings, depth of anesthesia, and intraoperative blood-pressure levels. When the hemispheric flow was low shunting was used. Even then, however, clinically manifest neurological deficits still occurred, suggesting that shunting alone may not be the answer. If shunting will not restore hemispheric flow to a state where EEG changes revert to normal, despite normal carbon dioxide partial pressure, anesthesia, and blood-pressure levels, where does the problem lie? Eisengart and Towne (1980) observed that when intraoperative EEG monitoring was used as a sole determinant for cerebral function, some patients had dramatic flattening of the EEG when the artery was clamped. This was a warning to the surgeon that the neurological status of the patient was deteriorating and a shunt was required. After shunting, the EEG gradually returned to its preclamped symmetry (30 to 120 seconds) after reestablishment of flow; when the vessel was reclamped for removal of the shunt, almost all of the patients had recurrence of the same preclamp EEG changes, but again reverted to normal after restoration of flow in the repaired artery. In one patient, return to normal took ten minutes; in this instance it was felt that the EEG changes may have resulted from embolization of atheromatous debris from the carotid bifurcation.

After a thorough review of the literature, I have concluded that no one has the full answer to the problem of cerebral protection during endarterectomy. However, I agree in principle with the concept promulgated by Rowed and Vilaghy (1981) that most patients (two thirds) can tolerate complete occlusion of the carotid artery during endarterectomy without sustaining a neurological deficit but that in the remainder CBF should be maintained with an intraluminal shunt, even though we are aware that this does not always prevent intraoperative neurological deficits. As stated earlier, these deficits are probably caused by embolic phenomena.

It appears that the controversy will continue. Those who favor shunts will continue to use them and those who choose not to use them will probably not change their views. Those who use a shunt selectively will do so when in their opinion the situation demands it. Thus, despite sincere efforts to arrive at a logical consensus based on the interpretation of published reports, I am unable to do so.

Because of this and my personal bias, I continue to advocate a protocol consisting of routine use of temporary shunts, general anesthesia, controlled blood pressure, and, occasionally, EEG monitoring of my patients. I do not measure stump pressures. My results since adopting this regimen have been well within the 2 percent mortality and 2 percent complication rate. It should be pointed out that there is some danger in the insertion of a shunt into a diseased vessel despite all efforts to ensure that no debris is present when the shunt is introduced. I repeatedly emphasize the necessity for extending the arteriotomy several millimeters above the distal end of the plaque so as to assure safe passage of the upper end of the shunt through a relatively disease-free portion of the vessel, or at least an area in which there are no ulcerations or friable bits of tissue. Gentleness in manipulation of the carotid bifurcation during dissection will also prevent the dislodgement of atheromatous material. It is these two situations which may result in perioperative embolic phenomena.

For some surgeons the shunt procedure may be a nuisance because it requires practice to attain dexterity. Constant practice and familiarity with the procedure, however, will eliminate fumbling when it becomes necessary to insert a shunt, and the practiced surgeon will be able to perform this procedure in a manner that becomes almost routine. My surgical program has established a goal of being able to insert a shunt and have it functioning within three minutes. This is the arbitrary length of time that I would accept without requiring cerebral perfusion.

TECHNICAL ASPECTS OF SHUNTING

Types of Shunts

The temporary shunt applied in the course of carotid operations is a conduit which perfuses the brain for a short period of time while endarterectomy or a related procedure is being performed. The first carotid shunts were needles inserted above and below the blockage and connected with a section of tubing. This was a true external shunt. Since then many different types of shunts have evolved, all having the same basic purpose — maintaining cerebral perfusion during the operation.

Shunts differ in appearance and construction. Of the many in use today, a few are worthy of special mention. These are the Javid bypass tube (see Figure 19-1A), the Brener carotid bypass shunt (see Figure 19-1B), the Sundt shunts, both internal and external (see Figure 19-2, A and B), as well as the Hallin shunt (see Figures 19-2C and 19-3) and my modification of it. Some surgeons fashion their own shunts at the operating table by cutting a small piece of surgical tubing 3 to 4 mm in diameter and securing the center portion of the shunt with a tie so as to be able to remove it at the completion of the operation.

The Javid bypass tube is made of a polyvinyl material in one size only. It is approximately 27.7 cm in length, tapering from 17 French scale at one end to 10 French scale at the other. It has a flange at each end to accomodate specially designed clamps which secure the shunt within the artery lumen. Because of its length, the shunt can be looped to allow better positioning and to adapt to different lengths of the artery. The Brener shunt is made of similar material with a flange at either end. It can be inserted in similar fashion but does not require clamps. It is tapered in the same fashion as the Javid shunt and may be secured with umbilical tapes and tourniquets.

The Sundt shunts are constructed of a silicone elastomer reinforced with stainless-steel springs to minimize the possibility of kinking. At each end of the shunt is a cone-shaped bulb or flange to facilitate fixation of the shunt within the vessel. Tourniquets may be required distally and are always required proximally to prevent the shunt from slipping out of the artery. The shunts come in various sizes and diameters; because of their nonwettable surface, their thrombosis is unlikely. The Sundt internal shunt is a short length of straight tubing that lies wholly within the lumen of the artery. The Sundt external shunt

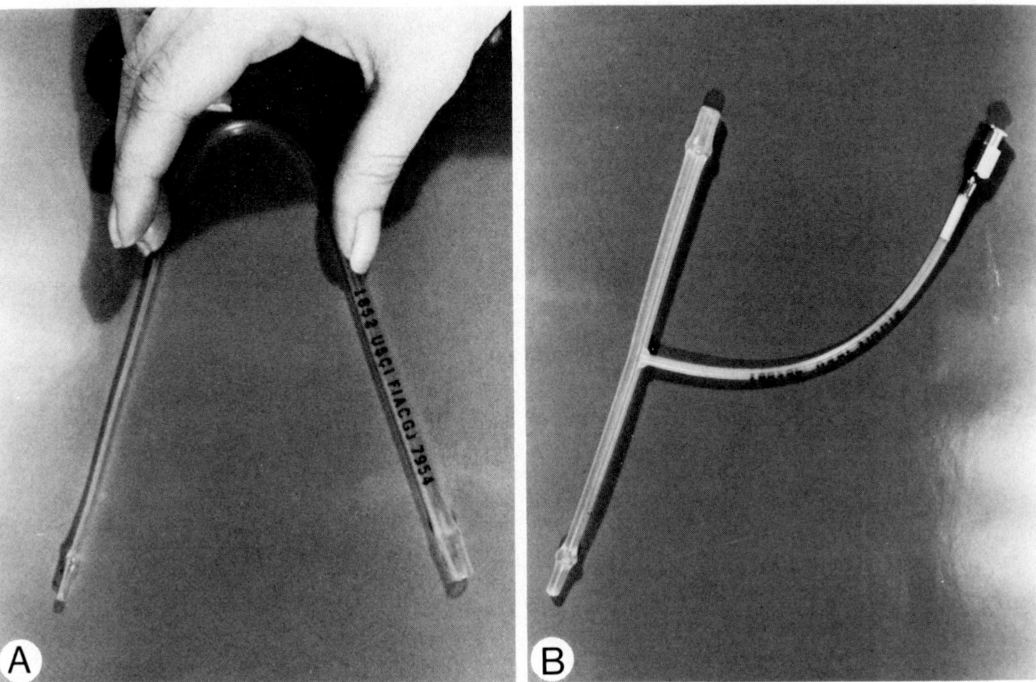

Figure 19-1. The Javid (*A*) and the Brener (*B*) shunts designed for temporary carotid bypass.

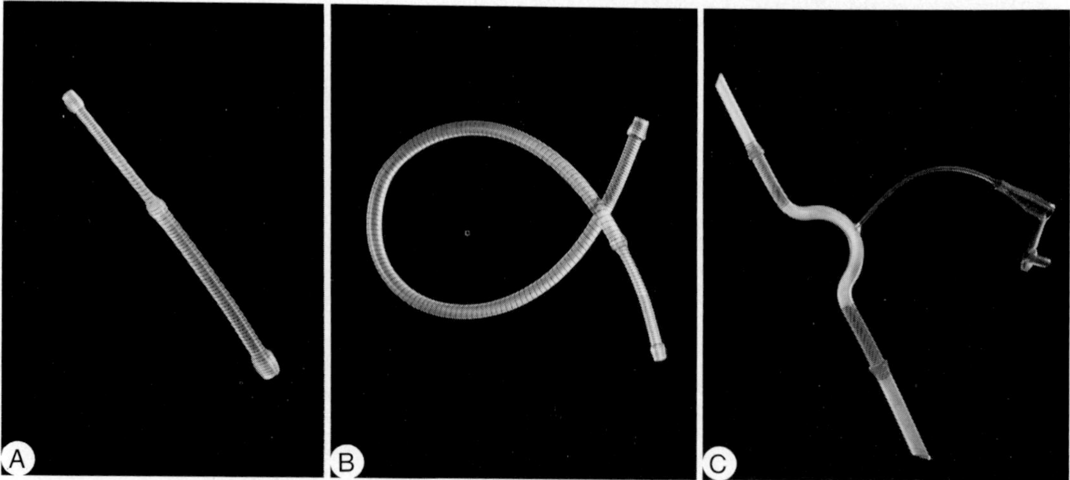

Figure 19-2. The straight (intraluminal) (*A*) and the looped (external) varieties of the Sundt shunt (*B*). The Hallin shunt (*C*).

(a misnomer) is 30 cm long to allow formation of an external loop after the ends have been placed within the artery.

The Hallin shunt is a similar elastomer with reinforced wire coils and bulbs at its ends which allow the shunt to be secured with proximal and distal tourniquets after insertion. Although it may be used without a distal tourniquet, in many instances such a tourniquet will prevent inadvertent dislodgement. The center section of the Hallin shunt has a U configuration with a sidearm extending from it that allows the introduction of heparin or the removal of blood or bubbles. If the determina-

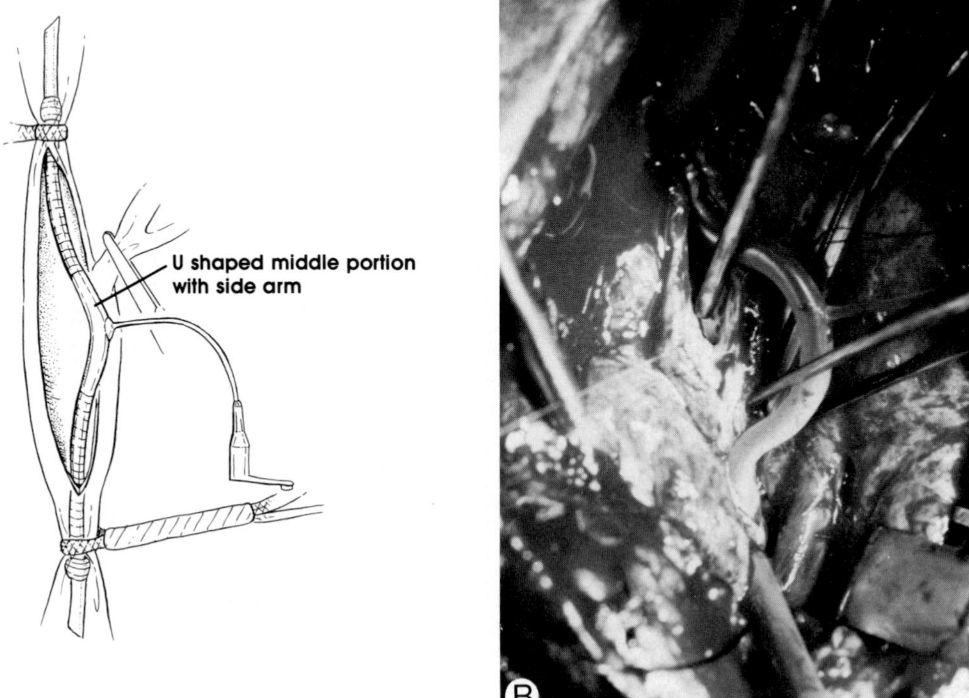

Figure 19-3. Artist's depiction (*A*) and operative photograph (*B*) of Hallin shunt in position.

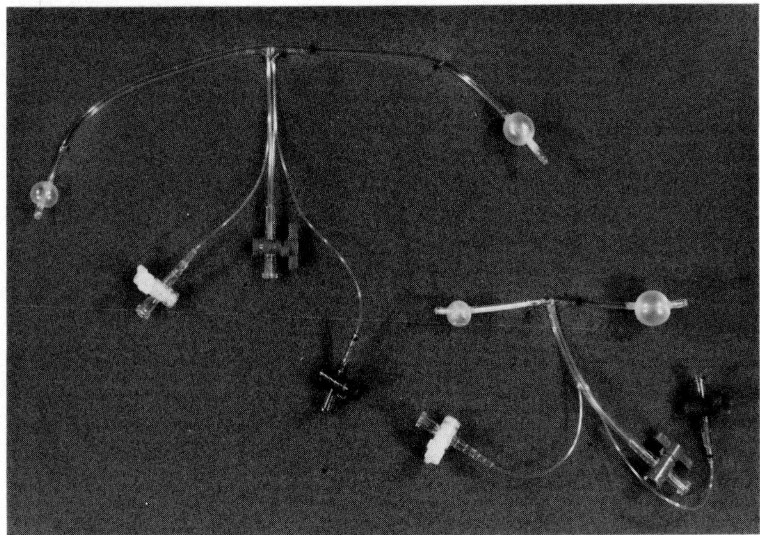

Figure 19–4. Different versions of the Pruitt-Inahara shunt.

tion of intracarotid pressures is desirable, this can be easily handled through the sidearm. By gentle manipulation of the sidearm, the assistant can move the shunt from one side to the other to facilitate the exposure. Hallin shunts come in several sizes with 1 mm differentials in the taper from top to bottom. My preferred shunt size is 4.5 to 5.5 mm.

Recently, a novel type of shunt known as the Pruitt-Inahara shunt was introduced (see Figure 19–4). It has two small balloon catheters at each end which when inflated secure the shunt within the vessel lumen. There are several attractive features to this shunt. Each balloon is inflated through a separate small line with a dedicated syringe. The length of the shunt allows it to be looped or to be placed well away from the endarterectomy site. When the procedure has been completed, the balloons are deflated and easily withdrawn from the site. Like the Hallin shunt, with a loop or U configuration, this shunt can be kept well away from the area of dissection.

Before describing my routine shunt insertion, it may be appropriate to comment on one or two simple principles that are occasionally overlooked by the busy surgeon or house officer. The printed material that accompanies the shunt suggests that it has a one-time use. In actual practice I have found that, if the shunt has been carefully handled and rinsed, it can be used again. This decision must be made by the individual surgeon and operating-room supervisor. This brings me to another point, which I cannot emphasize too strongly. It has been my observation that house officers and students often ask questions about the shunt at a point during the operation when I am unable to respond. I suggest that a wealth of information can be found in the circular enclosed in each package and in the manufacturer's catalog (there is very little printed material elsewhere, including textbooks of surgery). I liken this situation to the purchase of a new camera. The complicated dials and buttons on the camera can be easily mastered when one reads the directions. It has been my observation that most new camera owners tend to get into trouble and *then* refer to the directions. So it is with shunts. I suggest that one become thoroughly familiar with the manufacturer's directions. These directions describe in painstaking detail the diameters and composition of the shunt, note the caveats, and cite the appropriate literature.

The Management of the Shunt During Surgery

Surgeons must have a working familiarity with the type of shunt they plan to use. I generally advise the scrub nurse that I will be using a shunt and suggest that two or three sizes be available, even though I may need only one. These should be placed on the table before the procedure. It saves a great deal of frantic scurrying in the event that a shunt is inadvertently dropped. I also request the nurse to immerse

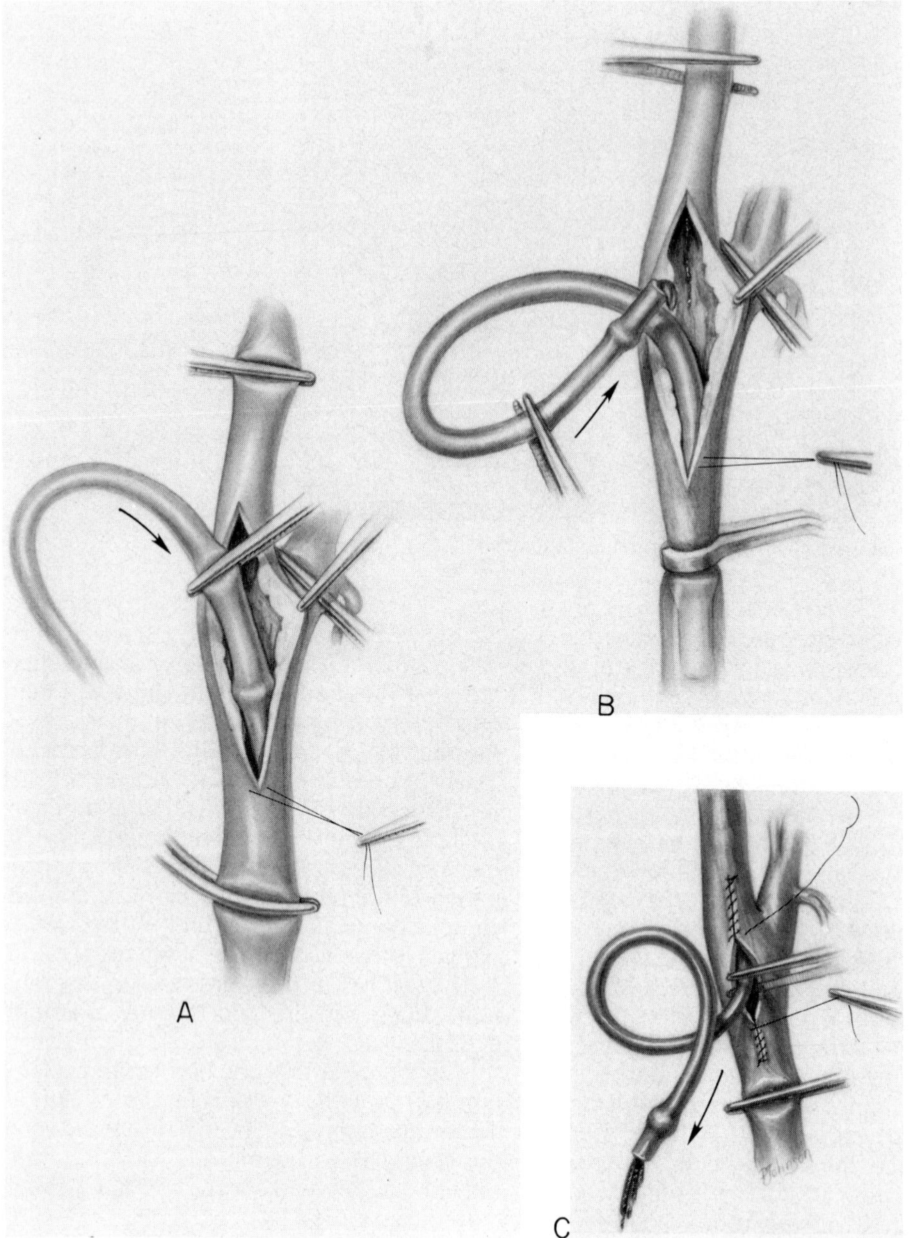

Figure 19–5. Insertion of the Javid shunt. The shunt is inserted proximally (*A*) and then allowed to seep some blood while being introduced into the internal carotid artery (*B*). The patency of the shunt is tested at the time of removal (*C*).

the shunt in a heparin-saline solution, remove any bubbles, and wet all surfaces. After the vessels have been exposed and are under control and the patient has undergone systemic heparinization, the vessels are clamped; a linear incision is made from the carotid at a point well below the plaque and extending up through the plaque and into the internal carotid several millimeters above the end of the pathology, at least to an area where there is no loose material. I back-bleed the vessels with a brief release of the clamps. The Hallin shunt is now removed from the heparin solution, and the sidearm is occluded with its own stopper. A small clamp is placed below the sidearm and the upper end of the shunt, which will be inserted first into the internal carotid. It is grasped with fine forceps and, as it is being inserted through the arteriotomy in a coordinated move, the upper clamp is released and the shunt is slipped in.

If a tourniquet is used (and I recommend it), it is snugged around the shunt at some point below the flange. Because the Hallin shunt has a reinforcing spring coil, it is virtually impossible to occlude the shunt with a tourniquet. Clamping the shunt in this location, however, would damage the coil. Therefore, if clamping is necessary, it is done in the area of the sidearm, hence no coils extend to that region. The sidearm is briefly released, and backflow is confirmed. Next the shunt is clamped *above* the sidearm, and in similar fashion the lower portion is placed in the common carotid and slipped down quickly while the tourniquet is tightened in this location. Again the sidearm is opened, and forward bleeding through the sidearm is confirmed. Finally, just before commencing full shunting, I make certain that no bubbles remain in the upper portion of the U arm. If any are present, they are quickly "tapped out" or aspirated with a small syringe. At this point all the clamps occluding the shunt have been removed, and perfusion is started. As stated earlier, this can be easily done in less than three minutes by a fumble-free team.

Close to the end of the procedure, at a point where just one or two stitches are left to close the arteriotomy, the shunt is removed. Several methods of shunt extraction can be applied. With the shunt still in place and functioning, I release the external carotid to obtain back-bleeding and eliminate small bubbles, then clamp the shunt and remove it from the internal carotid. I allow back-bleeding from this artery and then slowly occlude this vessel in such a manner that the internal and external carotids have free communication. Next the shunt is removed from the common carotid, which is flushed and clamped. At this point one has several options. A smoothly functioning team can quickly complete the suturing and slowly unclamp the common carotid, forcing out any air bubbles. Then, with the thumb and forefinger controlling the common carotid, the remaining upper clamp is removed, and circulation is restored. Another option is to remove the shunt and apply a partly occluding clamp so that the remaining few sutures can be applied and tied in a blood-free field before circulation is restored (see Figure 19–5).

In summary, it appears that some patients will maintain normal or acceptable CBF when their carotid arteries are clamped but not shunted and that others will not. Which one will behave how, unfortunately is not always predictable. Therefore, until reliable methods can be worked out and made available for easy general application, I recommend routine application of shunting in the course of carotid endarterectomy because, aside from the dangers of embolism or improper insertion of shunts, it appears that patients have excellent chances for trouble-free results. This approach also eliminates the need to perform several esoteric and costly diagnostic steps which might indicate the necessity for shunt with a dubious degree of reliability. Thus, by using the shunt we have a good common denominator; even if the shunt proves to be unnecessary, at least no harm is done. Moreover, the risks of not using the shunt far outweigh the dangers in the use of the shunt, provided it is managed by skilled hands.

REFERENCES

Andersen, C.A.; Rich, N.M.; Collins, G.J., Jr.; and McDonald, P.T.: Carotid endarterectomy: regional versus general anesthesia. *Am. Surg.*, **46**:323–27, 1980.

Baker, W.H.; Dorner, D.B.; and Barnes, R.W.: Carotid endarterectomy: is an indwelling shunt necessary? *Surgery*, **82**:321–26, 1977.

Baker, W.H.; Littooy, F.N.; Hayes, A.C.; Dorner, D.B.; and Stubbs, D.: Carotid endarterectomy without a shunt. *J. Vasc. Surg.*, **1**(1):50–6, 1984.

Basiljevac, J.E., and Farha, S.J.: Carotid endarterectomy: results using regional anesthesia. *Am. Surg.*, **46**:403–08, 1980.

Bernstein, E.F.; Humber, P.B.; Collins, G.M.; Dilley, R.B.; Devin, J.B.; and Stuart, S.H.: Life expectancy and late stroke following carotid endarterectomy. *Ann. Surg.*, **198**:80–6, 1983.

Blondeau, C.; Herbert, F.; Ducasble, G.; Watelet, J.; Testart, J.; and Samson-Dollfus, D.: Electroencephalographic surveillance during carotid endarterectomy. *Rev. Electroencephalogr. Neurophysiol. Clin.*, **12**(3):238–42, 1982.

Bostoen, H.; Allegaert, W.; and De Mol, J.: Revascularization of the extracranial carotid vertebral and subclavian arteries in a small peripheral hospital. *Acta. Chir. Belg.*, **78**:127–35, 1979.

Boysen, G.: Cerebral hemodynamics in carotid surgery. *Acta Neurol. Scand.*, **49**(Suppl. 52):3–86, 1973.

Brewster, D.C.; O'Hara, P.J.; Darling, R.C.; and Hallett, J.W., Jr.: Relationship of intraoperative EEG monitoring and stump pressure measurements during carotid endarterectomy. *Circulation*, **62**:14–17, 1980.

Eisengart, M., and Towne, J.W.: Intraoperative EEG monitoring during carotid endarterectomy. *J. Maine Med. Assoc.*, **71**:46–8, 1980.

Hertzer, N.R.; Beven, E.G.; Greenstreet, R.L.; and Humphries, A.W.: Internal carotid back pressure, intraoperative shunting, ulcerated atheromata, and the incidence of stroke during carotid endarterectomy. *Surgery,* **83**:306–12, 1978.

Jernigan, W.R., and Hamman, J.L.: The causes and prevention of stroke associated with carotid artery surgery. *Am. Surg.,* **48**:79–84, 1982.

Moore, W.S.; Yee, J.M.; and Hall, A.D.: Collateral cerebral blood pressure. *Arch. Surg.,* **106**:520–23, 1973.

Owens, M.L., and Wilson, S.E.: Prevention of neurologic complications of carotid endarterectomy. *Arch. Surg.,* **117**:551–55, 1982.

Rainer, W.G.; Guillen, C.J.; Bloomquist, C.E.; and McCrory, C.B.: Carotid artery surgery. *Am. J. Surg.,* **116**:678, 1968.

Rich, N.M., and Hobson, R.W.: Carotid endarterectomy under regional anesthesia. *Am. Surg.,* **41**:253–59, 1975.

Rosenthal, D.; Stanton, P.E., Jr.; and Lamis, P.A.: Carotid endarterectomy: unreliability of intraoperative monitoring in patients having had stroke or reversible ischemic neurologic deficit. *Arch. Surg.,* **116**:1569–75, 1981.

Rowed, D.W., and Vilaghy, M.I.: Intraoperative regional cerebral blood flow during carotid endarterectomy. *Can. J. Neurol. Sci.,* **8**(3):235–241, 1981.

String, S.T., and Callahan, A.: Critical manipulable variables of HLF during carotid surgery. *Surgery,* **93**:46–9, 1983.

Sublett, J.W.; Seidenburg, A.B.; and Hobson, R.W.: Internal carotid artery stump pressure and blood gas analysis under regional anesthesia. *Anesthesiology,* **41**:505–8, 1974.

Sundt, T.M., Jr.; Sharbrough, F.W.; Piepgras, T.F.; Kearns, T.P.; Messick, J.M., Jr.; and O'Gallon, W.M.: Correlation of cerebral blood flow and electroencephalographic changes during carotid endarterectomy. *Mayo Clin. Proc.,* **56**:533–43, 1981.

Thompson, J.E.: *Surgery for Cerebrovascular Insufficiency.* Charles C Thomas, Springfield, Illinois, 1968.

20

Carotid Endarterectomy in the Awake Patient

JOHN E. CONNOLLY

Although indications and technical aspects of carotid endarterectomy are now fairly standardized among vascular surgeons, two of the issues that remain controversial are whether the operation should be performed in the awake or anesthetized patient and whether an indwelling shunt should be used during carotid crossclamping.

DeBakey and associates (1959), reporting on their initial experience with carotid endarterectomy, stated that the operation is performed under local anesthesia to prevent cerebral depression and reduction in blood pressure and to permit close observation of any neurological changes during operation: " . . . The internal carotid artery is temporarily clamped and the patient observed for five minutes. In most cases collateral circulation is adequate to maintain normal function during operation and temporary occlusion does not produce neurologic deficits. Under these circumstances the operation is performed without employing methods designed to protect the cerebrum during operation."

On the technique of endarterectomy, Spencer and Eiseman (1962) wrote that combined local and regional anesthesia is essential to the safety of the operation. They stated that only by having the patient awake and alert can the surgeon determine the safety of temporary occlusion of the carotid artery and decide whether or not a temporary vascular shunt is needed: " . . . A simple way of expediting the operation has been to perform a posterior cervical block with 1% xylocaine before the operative field is prepared and draped. Little subsequent infiltration of the operative field itself with local anesthesia is then required."

CAROTID ENDARTERECTOMY UNDER GENERAL ANESTHESIA

Despite the initial enthusiasm for operation in the awake patient, most vascular surgeons perform carotid endarterectomy with the patient under general anesthesia because major surgery is customarily performed this way and because it is believed to be easier on both the patient and the surgeon. However, with the patient asleep it is much more difficult if not impossible to ascertain whether shunting is necessary during crossclamping of the carotid artery. Methods were devised to protect the brain during crossclamping under general anesthesia, including hypothermia, hypercarbia, hypocarbia, and systemic arterial hypertension (Peitzman *et al.*, 1982). Time and experience have disproved the alleged usefulness of all of these ancillary modalities. Those surgeons who continue to advocate operation under general anesthesia may either always or never employ a shunt, or use the device selectively based upon back pressure (stump pressure) in the internal carotid artery, observation of the backflow and color of blood from the distal internal carotid artery, jugular vein oxygen saturation, or continuous electroencephalographic (EEG) monitoring to identify those patients needing shunting. Surgeons who always use a shunt do so because of their belief that none of the foregoing indicators is completely reliable.

CAROTID ENDARTECTOMY WITH SHUNTING

We were among the first in the 1960s to perform carotid endarterectomy in patients under local anesthesia only to switch soon thereafter to general anesthesia with the use of a routine shunt. However, we ultimately concluded that the shunt itself posed potential complications, such as air or particulate embolization, the raising of a flap in the internal carotid artery, and, finally, the technical disadvantage of performing endarterectomy encumbered by a shunt. Therefore, in 1972 we again began to perform the operation in the awake patient which allowed accurate selection of the few patients (5 to 10 percent) who needed shunting (Connolly *et al.*, 1977). Not only did we find that shunting was usually unnecessary, but, even more important, we discovered that we could operate without the cardiac risks secondary to general anesthesia in a group of patients who had a high incidence of concomitant significant coronary artery disease.

Identifying the Need for Shunting

We also observed that operation in the awake patient provided an excellent opportunity to assess the reliability of the two most popular modalities used by advocates of general anesthesia to identify the need for shunting, namely, stump pressure and EEG monitoring. We measured stump pressures in 125 consecutive patients undergoing carotid endarterectomy in the awake state and found that 101 (80.8 percent of the total group) tolerated crossclamping without neurological change during the procedure (Kwaan and Connolly, 1980) and their stump pressures ranged from 20 to 90 mm Hg. It was of particular interest that 25 of the 101 patients without neurological symptons during crossclamping had stump pressures below 50 mm Hg. These 25 patients would have been unnecessarily shunted if they had been operated upon under general anesthesia and stump pressures of lower than 50 mm Hg had been used to determine the need for shunting.

On the other hand, 24 patients (19.2 percent of the 125) lost consciousness within one minute of test clamping of the carotid artery. In this second group, the internal carotid artery back pressures ranged from 15 to 85 mm Hg. Also of special interest was the fact that eight patients (33 percent) had stump pressures of 50 mm Hg or higher, yet collateral circulation was not adequate to maintain cerebral perfusion as ascertained by the development of neurological deficit during crossclamping. These eight patients therefore required shunting. If they had been operated upon while under general anesthesia, and if a stump pressure of over 50 mm Hg had been used as the criterion not to employ a shunt, they might have sustained an intraoperative neurological deficit or even died. There were no strokes or deaths in this consecutive series of 125 patients.

From these data we concluded that the levels of 25 to 50 mm Hg carotid stump pressure recommended by various investigators as indicative of adequate collateral cerebral blood flow during carotid crossclamping are unreliable and that their absolute acceptance will lead to a small but real incidence of stroke when operation is performed with patients under general anesthesia. Likewise, if stump pressure is used as the criterion for shunting under general anesthesia, some patients will be unnecessarily shunted.

The other modality used during general anesthesia to select patients for shunting is EEG monitoring. Our experience with EEG monitoring in the awake patient indicates that an abnormal tracing is a less reliable predictor of cerebral ischemia than a normal tracing is of adequate cerebral perfusion. A few of our patients had neurological changes during crossclamping without a clearly abnormal EEG. On the other hand, a number of our awake patients have had an abnormal EEG during carotid crossclamping without any clinical neurological deficit, which would have led to unnecessary shunting if the operation had been performed with the patients under general anesthesia.

Neurological Changes

As our experience with carotid endarterectomy has increased in recent years, we have noted that fewer patients have neurological changes during crossclamping in the awake state, often even when the contralateral internal carotid artery is chronically occluded. A review of our last 100 consecutive cases has shown that only 6 percent have had neurological change during carotid crossclamping, thus requiring intraoperative shunting.

TECHNIQUE

Since 1972, all of our carotid endarterectomies have been performed in the awake patient under supplemented local anesthesia (Connolly *et al.,* 1977). One to two hours before the operation 2 ml of a solution containing 0.5 mg of fentanyl citrate and 2.5 mg of droperidol per ml is given intravascularly as premedication. The skin and wound are then infiltrated with 1 percent lidocaine before incision and lidocaine infiltration is added as necessary during operation.

In addition, the anesthesiologist gives fentanyl citrate intravenously as necessary to control restlessness during the operation. Most patients require 1 to 4 ml of supplemental fentanyl during the procedure. The combined effect of these drugs is sometimes referred to as neuroleptanalgesia, characterized by general quiescence, reduced motor activity, and profund analgesia. Loss of consciousness does not occur from these drugs in the dosages employed. Some anesthesiologists prefer to use other agents such as diazepam or alphaprodine hydrochloride as a tranquilizer before and during the procedure, with equally good results.

Superficial and Deep Cervical Block

More recently we have performed a number of carotid endarterectomies in patients under superficial and deep cervical block (Bosiljevac and Farha, 1980). Regional neck block, performed by the anesthesiologist, consists of blocking C2, C3, and C4 nerves at the transverse process. A mixture of 0.75 bupivacaine (15 ml) and 3 percent chloroprocaine (15 ml) is employed using 3 to 7 ml to block each nerve. A total of 10 ml is additionally infiltrated along the anterior border of the sternocleidomastoid muscle to block the cutaneous nerves. With a satisfactory neck block, the only supplemental anesthesia necessary is lidocaine infiltration of the carotid sheath before opening it. Care must be taken by the anesthesiologist not to inject the anesthetic blocking agent into an artery.

The head is turned to the opposite side, and the chin is taped in place. A Mayo stand is placed over the head of the patient and towels are taped to the stand to keep them off the face. This detail is very important for providing patient comfort and, therefore, acceptance of the awake technique. An incision is made over the anterior border of the sternocleidomastoid muscle from the angle of the jaw extending halfway to the sternal notch. After the carotid bifurcation is exposed, the vessels are temporarily clamped, and during a two-minute test period the patient is assessed for changes in consciousness, seizures, motor function, or visual disturbances. Almost invariably if any neurological changes occur, they do so within the first minute of crossclamping. If there are any changes, an intraluminal shunt is inserted. If the patient tolerates the test period well, the operation proceeds in the usual manner without a shunt.

DISCUSSION

Carotid endarterectomy in the awake patient appears to offer a number of advantages (Bosiljevac and Farha, 1980; Connolly, *et al.,* 1977; Peitzman *et al.,* 1982; Yared *et al.,* 1979). It allows the surgeon constant knowledge of the patient's neurological status throughout the operation. Trial crossclamping of the carotid artery in the awake patient is the only absolutely accurate method of identifying patients who do not require intraoperative shunting. We believe that this is important because of the inherent dangers associated with shunting previously discussed. From our experience with selective shunting we agree with those who conclude that the operation is easier and safer when a shunt is not employed, which makes selectivity of its use important.

Operation in the awake patient also allows accurate identification of the time and, probably, origin of an intraoperative stroke, thus permitting immediate, and hopefully, successful institution of corrective measures. Hertzer and associates (1978) reported that 92 percent of their patients who had intraoperative neurological deficits had ulcerated carotid lesions that could be seen on preoperative arteriograms. From this experience they concluded that embolization during carotid dissection is the most significant factor in the etiology of intraoperative neurological deficits. Several authors (Peitzman *et al.,* 1982; Yared *et al.,* 1979) have described permanent neurological deficit occurring with crossclamping of the carotid artery along with disbandment of operation without arteriotomy, which substantiates the potential dangers of embolization during dissection or crossclamping of the carotid arteries. We cannot stress enough the need to avoid unnecessary dissection or palpation of the carotid vessels and also the potential prophylaxis against embolization afforded by early crossclamping of the internal carotid artery distal to its disease end point.

With operation in the patient under supplemented local or regional block anesthesia, we avoid the cardiac risks associated with general anesthesia. Despite the high incidence of coronary artery disease in patients with carotid artery disease, most of these patients do not have sufficiently severe cardiac disease to warrant coronary artery surgery, have unrecognized coronary artery disease, or have disease too advanced for bypass surgery. In this regard Peitzman and associates (1982) noted a nonneurological complication rate for carotid endarterectomy under general anesthesia to be 12.9 percent compared with 2.8 percent under regional block. We have been impressed with the relatively stable blood pressures observed during operations performed in awake patients and by the absence of perioperative myocardial infarctions. Operation under local or regional anesthesia has allowed us to perform carotid endarterectomy safely in patients who had been rejected for coronary artery bypass surgery because of severe triple-vessel disease and poor ventricular performance. As we have gained experience with carotid surgery in the awake patient, we have become increasingly aware of the advantages of avoiding general anesthesia in patients with concomitant cardiac disease. During the 12 years that we have used endarterectomy in the awake patient, our morbidity rate has been 1.1 percent and the mortality rate 0.85 percent. In the last group of 100 consecutive patients there was one death and no permanent neurological deficit. The death occurred in a patient who had bilateral surgery.

Operation in the awake patient is a procedure that is comfortable and safe for both patient and surgeon. We believe that the technique of carotid endarterectomy in the awake patient has not been widely employed because of lack of knowledge of its many advantages.

REFERENCES

Bosiljevac, J.E., and Farha, S.J.: Carotid endarterectomy: results using regional anesthesia. *Am. Surg.*, **46**:403–8, 1980.

Connolly, J.E.: Carotid endarterectomy in the awake patient. *Am. J. Surg.*, **150**:159–165, 1985.

Connolly, J.E.; Kwaan, J.H.; and Stemmer, E.A.: Improved results with carotid endarterectomy. *Ann. Surg.*, **186**:334–42, 1977.

DeBakey, M.E.; Crawford, E.S.; Cooley, D.A.; and Morris, G.C.: Surgical considerations of occlusive disease of innominate, carotid, subclavian and vertebral arteries. *Ann. Surg.*, **149**:690–710, 1959.

Hertzer, N.R.; Beven, E.G.; Greenstreet, R.L.; and Humphries, A.W.: Internal carotid back pressure, intraoperative shunting, ulcerated atheromata and the incidence of stroke during carotid endarterectomy. *Surgery*, **83**:306–12, 1978.

Kwaan, J.H.M.; Connolly, J.E.; and Peterson, G.J.: Stump pressure: an unreliable guide for shunting during carotid endarterectomy. *Arch. Surg.*, **115**:1083–86, 1980.

Peitzman, A.B.; Webster, M.W.; Loubeau, J.M.; Grundy, B.I.; and Bahnson, H.T.: Carotid endarterectomy under regional (conductive) anesthesia. *Ann. Surg.*, **196**:59–64, 1982.

Spencer, F.C., and Eiseman, B.: Technique of carotid endarterectomy. *Surg. Gynecol. Obstet.*, **115**:114–17, 1962.

Yared, I.; Martinis, A.J.; and Mack, R.M.: Carotid endarterectomy under local anesthesia: a retrospective study. *Am. Surg.*, **45**:709–14, 1979.

21

Perioperative Complications of Carotid Endarterectomy

FRANCIS ROBICSEK

Possible complications of carotid endarterectomy, like those of any other major vascular procedure performed in an arteriosclerotic patient, include a wide spectrum of unwanted events, ranging from pulmonary embolism to myocardial infarction. For practical purposes, this chapter is limited to complications which are particular to this procedure. Discussion of problems such as hypertension and hypovolemia, which are dealt with in Chapter 12, will not be repeated here, but complications that may have occurred during surgery but manifest during the postoperative period, such as peripheral nerve injuries, are, indeed, included.

To prevent the occurrence of postoperative complications, it is most important to have the patient adequately prepared for surgery. The indication should be impeccable, contraindications should be nonexistent, and the patient should enter the operating room in a stable, well-hydrated condition with any abnormality of the electrolytes, blood pressure, and cardiac function corrected as much as possible.

COMPLICATIONS INVOLVING THE OPERATIVE INCISION

Swelling

Some degree of swelling of the incision during the early postoperative period is common. Unless it is associated with infection, it usually subsides within a few days. In some patients in whom either the parotid gland lies low or the carotid bifurcation is abnormally high and the parotid gland must be retracted, postoperative swelling and tenderness in the upper part of the incision may continue for several days or even weeks.

Hematoma

The occurrence of a hematoma can be minimized by careful hemostasis and by neutralization of heparin, if it is used in the course of the operation. Hypertension predisposes for formation of postoperative hematomas. If the wound appears very "oozy" at the termination of the procedure, 12-hour drainage with a small cigarette drain introduced through a separate stab wound will almost certainly prevent the formation of hematomas. If a patient develops a sizable hematoma after surgery, he should be returned to the operating room without further ado; the wound should be reopened, the clot evacuated, and the bleeding brought under control.

Infection

Infection can be a very serious complication of carotid surgery. Initially, it should be treated with broad-spectrum antibiotics alone. However if there is no appropriate improvement within a reasonable time or if clinical signs of progression appear, the wound should be adequately drained, and, pending specific sensitivity studies, antibiotic therapy should be continued. If the infection extends to the operated artery and erodes the suture line itself, after the bleeding is brought under control, any foreign materials, such as synthetic patches or grafts, should be removed and replaced with autogenous vein; the wound should be adequately drained and energetic antibiotic therapy should be instituted. If bleeding recurs, ligation of the involved artery becomes a necessity and, if feasible, the carotid circulation should be restored by extraintracranial bypass. Fortunately, infection as a postoperative complication of carotid endarterectomy is rare. In our own series of more than 600 carotid endarterectomies, we had only one serious wound infection. The cause of this is probably the natural resistance of wounds of the face and neck to bacterial invasion.

PERIPHERAL NERVE INJURIES

Surgical trauma to various nerves is important from both a functional and a cosmetic viewpoint. Most of the nerve injuries are transient and at worst bothersome, but their occurrence can mar an otherwise successful operation. The prevention of cranial nerve injury in carotid surgery requires a thorough knowledge of anatomy (see Figure 21–1), precision in technique, and attention to detail.

Although superficial segmental sensory nerves are frequently divided to obtain proper exposure of the carotid artery with the minor discomfort of temporary paresthesia after surgery, every effort should be made to avoid injury to more important nerves, especially those of motor function. Injury to a single cranial nerve is usually transient and fairly well tolerated. Multiple nerve injuries, however, may create precarious, sometimes life-threatening situations, especially if they occur in connection with bilateral operations, even if staged. For reasons difficult to comprehend, progress in the technical aspects of carotid surgery does not seem to have decreased the number of associated nerve injuries. As a matter of

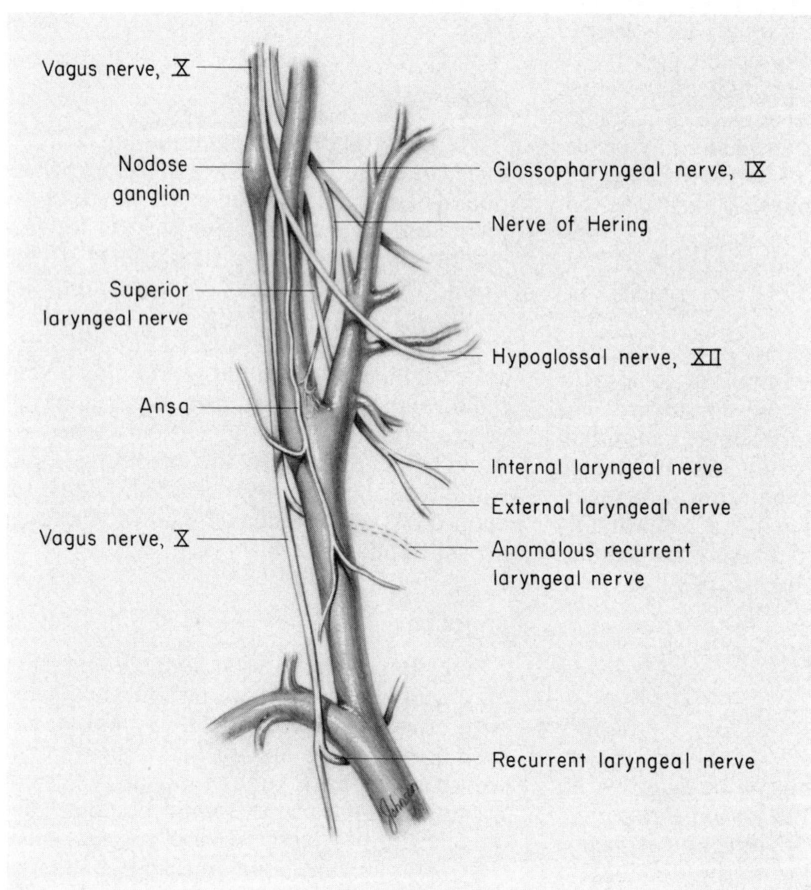

Figure 21–1. Peripheral nerves adjacent to the carotid artery.

fact, their number seems to be on the increase. The nerves most likely to be damaged are the great auricular nerve, the mandibular branch of the facial nerve, the hypoglossal, and the vagus with its cervical tributaries. Less frequently involved in surgical mishaps are the glossopharyngeal and spinal accessory nerves.

Great Auricular Nerve and Mandibular Branch of the Facial Nerve

As the surgeon cuts through the subcutanous fat and the platysma, care should be exercised to avoid damage to the great auricular nerve and to the mandibular branch of the facial nerve. The most common area in which the greater auricular nerve may be injured is the upper corner of the incision, where the nerve, after having perforated the deep fascia, ascends on the sternocleidomastoid muscle and divides into anterior and posterior branches. The former provides sensory innervation to the skin over the parietal gland, the latter to the lower part of the ear and the skin covering the mastoid process. The great auricular nerve is especially exposed to injury if the skin incision is made in the submandibular fashion and is carried too laterally. Division of the great auricular nerve causes unpleasant anesthesia around and below the ear which may last for months or even be permanent.

The mandibular branch of the facial nerve may be exposed by either of the two types of skin incisions if the dissection is carried too close to the ramus mandibule, where the nerve lies just under platysma on the deep fascia and provides motor innervation to the angle of the mouth and the lower lip. The most common cause of injury is an overextended or improperly placed self-retaining retractor. Damage to the nerve leads to partial paralysis of the corner muscles and asymmetry of the lip, both of which usually resolve in two to three months. If the nerve is injured bilaterally, the patient may have difficulty managing saliva and liquids.

Hypoglossal Nerve

Probably the most common nerve-induced complication of carotid surgery is dysphagia caused by damage to the hypoglossal nerve, either during division of the common facial vein or at a later stage of the operation. The hypoglossal nerve exits from the skull through the jugular foramen, but, unlike the vagus, it passes medially in front of the internal and external carotid arteries toward the tongue. It usually lies out of harm's way 3 to 5 cm above the carotid bifurcation; but if the bifurcation is abnormally high, this passage may occur in front of the carotid bulb itself. Sometimes the hypoglossal nerve is entangled in one or two branches of the external carotid artery which feed the sternocleidomastoid muscle. For the nerve to be retracted off the internal carotid, these small muscular branches of the external carotid need to be divided.

Damage to the hypoglossal nerve manifests itself in tongue biting and deviation of the tongue to the injured side. If the injury is unilateral, problems of deglutition are usually moderate and temporary. If the damage is caused by retraction or if only a branch is divided, the effects are transient; however, they are long-lasting if the main trunk of the hypoglossal nerve is severed. An especially dangerous situation can develop if in the course of bilateral carotid artery operations both hypoglossal nerves are injured. Such a bilateral palsy may lead to marked swallowing difficulties, inability to phonate, and acute upper-airway obstruction. The division of the descending branch, which provides motor innervation to the omohyoid muscle, is of no clinical consequence.

Vagus Nerve

Because the vagus is intimately associated with both the internal and the common carotid arteries in their entire cervical course, injury to it may occur at any stage of the operation. The vagus leaves the skull through the jugular foramen, normally lies posteriorly between the jugular vein and the carotid artery, and continues down the chest, sending the recurrent nerve back along the trachea to supply the vocal cords. In approximately 5 percent of patients, however, the vagus is anteromedial to the carotid artery, thus particularly vulnerable to injury (Callow, 1982).

The fibers that become the recurrent laryngeal nerve are especially easily injured by both retraction and pressure. Because, except for the tensor arytenoid muscle, which is innervated by the superior laryngeal nerve, the entire motor innervation of the larynx derives from the recurrent branch of the vagus, injury to these fibers leads to paralysis of the ipsilateral vocal cord with resultant hoarseness and in some cases also to breathing difficulties.

Vocal-cord weakness and impaired phonation may also be caused by damage to another motor tributary of the vagus, the superior laryngeal nerve. This nerve rises from the inferior ganglion, passes behind the internal and external carotid arteries, and then bifurcates. The internal branch traverses the thyrohyoid membrane and innervates the mucosa of the larynx above the vocal cord. The external tributary of the nerve largely follows the course of the superior thyroid artery and innervates the cricothyroid muscles. The latter nerve branch can easily be injured when the posterior surface of the external carotid artery is dissected or the superior thyroid artery is divided, with resultant weakness in vocal-cord motion. The voice of a patient whose superior laryngeal nerve is injured is monotonous, tires easily, and is of lower pitch.

The vagus may also be damaged during carotid surgery when clamps are placed on the common or the external carotid arteries. The jaws of the instrument may overextend the boundaries of the vessels and inadvertently grasp and crush the nerve, which lies just behind them. This mishap is especially likely to occur if the tape sling around the common carotid artery is misplaced and encircles the vagus as well (see Figure 21–2). The surgeon should also be aware that because the vagus may occasionally lie medially or even anteriorly to the common carotid artery it can be mistaken for the descending branch of the hypoglossal nerve and thus divided.

Another anatomical variety of the vagus is the "nonrecurrent laryngeal nerve," a nerve that anomalously rises from the midcervical portion of the vagus. Such an aberrant nerve will cross anteriorly to the carotid and can easily be injured. This type of anomaly is most likely to occur in the presence of abnormalities of the branches of the aortic arch. Injury to the recurrent nerve may also occur, though rarely, in the course of carotid surgery even if the nerve follows a normal path. Such injury produces ipsilateral vocal-cord paralysis and consequential hoarseness. This may be caused by pressure of a self-restraining retractor if the medial arm presses against the thyroid area or by compression of a postoperative hematoma. Bilateral recurrent nerve injury leads to life-threatening respiratory distress with both vocal cords blocking the entry of air to the deeper airways.

Glossopharyngeal Nerve

Injury to the glossopharyngeal nerve during carotid endarterectomy is rare but may occur if the dissection is more extensive, as may be necessary to resect a large aneurysm. If it occurs, the patient will have long-lasting diffi-

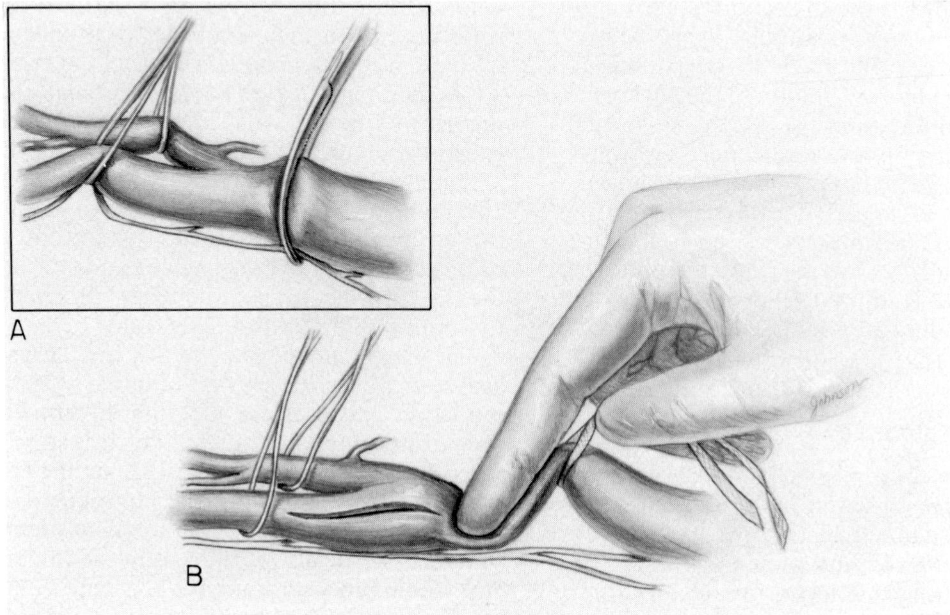

Figure 21–2. Injury to the vagus nerve by careless clamping of the common artery (*A*). Temporary occlusion of the common carotid artery by finger pressure (*B*).

culties in deglutition and occasional aspiration pneumonia.

Spinal Accessory Nerve

The spinal accessory nerve may be threatened by the surgeon's scissors if the dissection is carried close to the mastoid process. Injury to this nerve causes dysfunction of the sternocleidomastoid muscle and paralytic torticollis.

AIRWAY OBSTRUCTION

Postoperative airway obstruction is a serious complication of carotid artery surgery which may be caused by motor-nerve injury, compression by a hematoma, or laryngeal edema owing to intubation. The patient may also have acute respiratory distress if for various reasons consciousness does not return soon after anesthesia.

Tracheostomy in the management of respiratory complications should be avoided in the immediate postoperative period because of the danger of infection of the adjacent operative wound. Patients in respiratory distress therefore should be managed with endotracheal intubation; tracheostomy, if necessary, should be delayed for six to eight days, until there is healing of the operative incision.

CENTRAL NEUROLOGICAL DEFICITS

It is ironic that carotid endarterectomy, which is undoubtedly the most effective way to prevent the occurrence of stroke, has one most-dreaded complication, the most common cause of both morbidity and mortality: appearance of a new central neurological deficit or aggravation of a previously existing one. Some of these deficits are transient and well tolerated; others are permanent, could be crippling, and may result in death.

By and large, perioperative strokes of carotid artery reconstruction fall into two categories: (1) those caused by the trauma of the operation, including episodes of cerebral ischemia owing to anesthetic mishaps, carotid crossclamping, embolization of cholesterol debris, etc., and (2) those caused by acute thrombotic occlusion of the operated carotid artery. Although perioperative strokes belonging to the first group will not respond to reoperation, those of the second category may well benefit from it. In determining to which group a patient with a perioperative stroke belongs, the time of onset of the postoperative stroke is very important. Because all these complications manifest themselves in impairment of specific functions, most do not become apparent until surgery is over and the patient awakes (unless, of course, the operation is performed under local anesthesia). If the patient awakes with a stroke from anesthesia, he may belong to either category. If, however, there is a symptom-free interval between awakening and the occurrence of hemiparesis or hemiplegia, the diagnosis of acute thrombosis is most likely.

Embolization can occur at any phase of the operation or even postoperatively. Many postoperative neurological deficits are caused by upstream dislocation of atherosclerotic debris, platelet aggregate, or thrombi from necrotic atheromatous ulcers. This event may occur even before the carotid artery is opened, during dissection. For this reason rough handling, squeezing, or unnecessary manipulation of the artery should be avoided. Another stage of the operation at which cerebral embolization is likely is the moment of insertion of a temporary indwelling shunt (see Figure 21 – 3A). Because users of the shunt believe that the time between clamping of the carotid and the reestablishment of the blood flow through the shunt should be as short as possible, shunts may be introduced with haste, and debris may be pushed with the "nose" of the shunt into the internal carotid artery and from there into the cerebral circulation.

Another cause of shunt-induced embolization is inadequate clearance of the shunt conduit of air bubbles that may stubbornly cling to its wall. For this reason it is preferable to fill the shunts with heparinized saline solution which, having a lower viscosity than that of blood, is less likely to trap minute air bubbles. Shunt-induced air embolism may also occur if just before the moment of insertion of the distal end the tube is buckled and then released (see Figure 21 – 3B). This may force from the shunt a drop or two of fluid, which will then be immediately replaced with air. These mishaps can be prevented by using T-shaped shunts, which allow alternate backflow from both directions. However, this places an additional piece of tubing into the middle of the operative field, a feature that makes them less than desirable (See also Chapter 19). Other shunt-induced complications that may result in postoperative carotid thrombosis are "snow-pile" intimal damage of the common carotid (see Figure 21 – 3C) and development of a T-

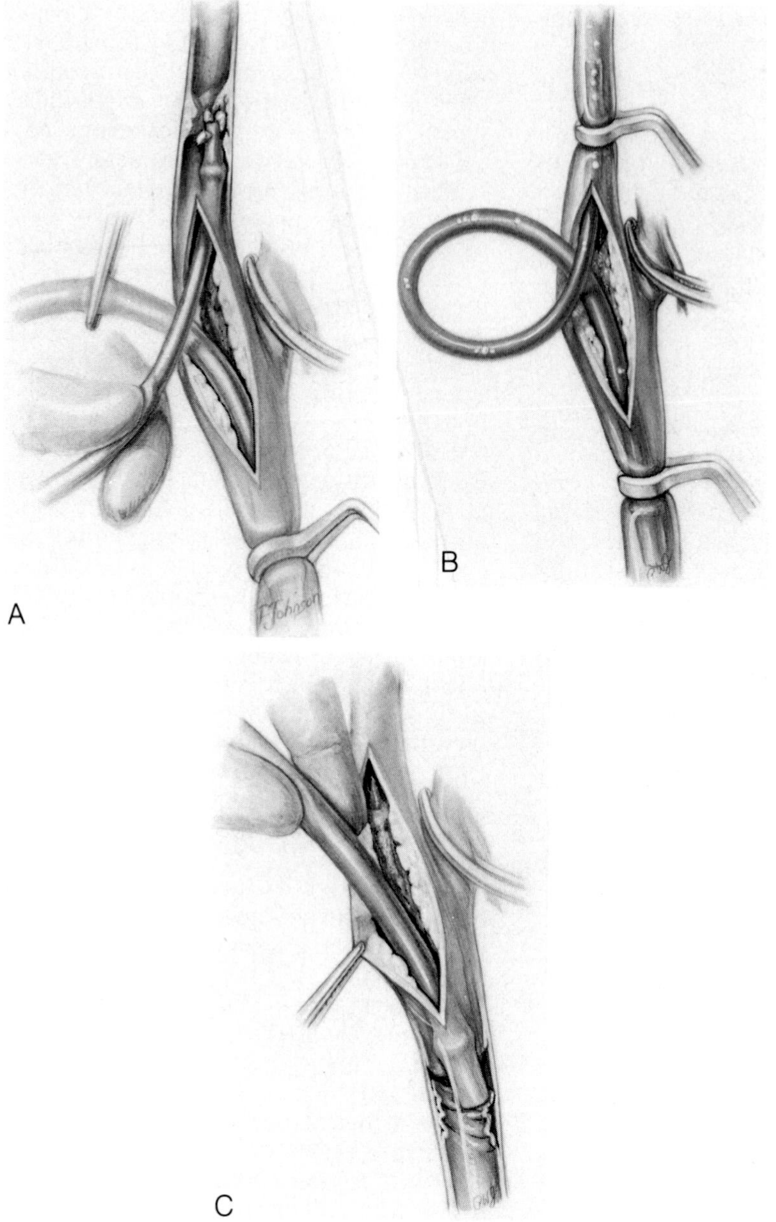

Figure 21–3. Some of the technical mishaps that may occur with the Javid shunt. Dislodgement of atherosclerotic debris (*A*). Air embolism (*B*). Proximal "snow-pile" intimal damage (*C*).

shaped tear and consequential suture-line stenosis of the distal end of the arteriotomy (see Figure 21–4).

Probably the most critical time period regarding intraoperative cerebral embolization is the moment of restoration of normal blood flow to the internal carotid artery, when flakes of debris or trapped air can readily be carried to the brain if the interior of the carotid bifurcation has not been properly cleaned out and evacuated. The exact time of embolization can be detected only if the patient is under continuous electroencephalographic monitoring or under local anesthesia (Hafner and Tew, 1981).

Intraoperative strokes may also be caused by temporary cessation of blood flow through the operated carotid artery. It appears certain that, although many patients can tolerate temporary interruption of carotid blood flow in the

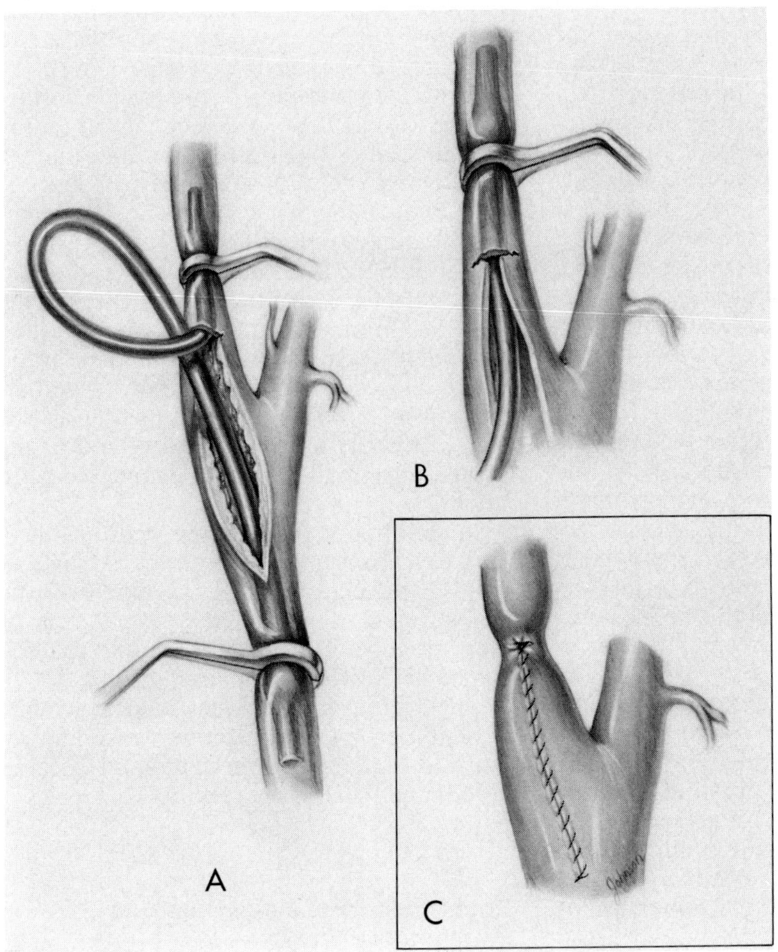

Figure 21–4. Careless raising of the distal end of the shunt may lead to a T-shaped tear (*A*) and (*B*) and suture-line stenosis (*C*).

course of carotid arterioplasty, there are also some in whom the postoperatively manifest neurological deficit can definitely be traced to intraoperative ischemia induced by the operative technique itself. Denial of the fact that hypoperfusion and ischemia of the brain occur every time a carotid artery is temporarily occluded would also imply that surgery to relieve carotid artery stenosis is unnecessary. Although the physiological importance of this hypoperfusion varies from patient to patient and is of minimal consequence in most patients, the potential danger of significant clinical damage exists every time a carotid artery is temporarily occluded by surgical instrumentation.

Because comparable results are being reported by those who use shunts routinely, selectively, or not at all, the controversy continues about whether all or most mishaps can be prevented by routine shunting, whether the persons in whom shunting is needed are identifiable by various means, or whether the shunt itself is the culprit in some of these disasters. Thompson, a long-term champion of shunting, calls special attention to patients who have previously had strokes, those whose contralateral carotid is occluded, and those who have extensive vertebral-basilar disease as being especially vulnerable to temporary internal carotid clamping (Thompson, 1983). Although we have not found appreciable differences between shunted and nonshunted patients, in the aforementioned categories of patients we continue to use temporary indwelling shunts (see also Chapters 19 and 20).

Another cause of postoperative stroke is acute thrombosis of the carotid artery. Because this can occur intraoperatively as well as postoperatively, it is mandatory that before the closure of the operative incision the operator palpate the entire length of the cervical internal carotid artery and immediately take appropriate steps if pulsation is weak or absent.

Acute thrombosis of the carotid artery during surgery may be attributable to several causes. If the carotid artery is clamped during endarterectomy without the use of a shunt, two "blind" pockets containing blood are created in the proximal common and distal internal carotid arteries. Clot may form in either cul-de-sac and cause complete or partial occlusion either in loco or by embolization. Such a thrombus may also develop in the presence of a malfunctioning shunt. Because of the danger of clot formation, most surgeons apply heparin systematically during endarterectomy. Although this practice is certainly logical, there is no direct clinical or experimental evidence of its protective effect. The most important single factor in the prevention of intra- or postoperative carotid thrombosis is the proper handling of the distal intimal edge during endarterectomy. At the end of the procedure the transitional zone between the endarterectomized segment and the intact intima must be smooth and free of bumps, flakes, or flaps. Application of metallic clamps to the internal carotid should be avoided for the same reason. Narrowing of the arterial lumen by improper suturing of the arteriotomy can also lead to complete thrombosis in the immediate postoperative period or to false "recurrent" stenosis of the carotid artery later on (see Figure 21–4).

Thrombosis of the endarterectomy site may develop, however, even if the operation is performed with a "perfect" technique, owing to the deposition of platelets and fibrins on the denuded vascular wall. If the lumen is otherwise satisfactory, this occurs very infrequently because of the high flow in the carotid artery. Other causes of postoperative carotid thrombosis are the presence of secondary pathology, such a second stricture high up in the intracranial portion of the carotid.

Early postoperative occlusion may also be caused by failure to correct abnormal elongation or kinking of the internal carotid artery. This tortuosity may be present preoperatively, or it may manifest itself clinically only after the internal carotid artery is dissected free from the connective tissue attachments that hold the artery in proper position. If such an elongation exists, the artery should be shortened and its course straightened (see Figure 17–2).

A rare case of intraoperative or early postoperative carotid artery occlusion may be caused by a dissecting aneurysm of the common carotid artery. This can occur retrograde if the proximal plaque is not divided in a "streamlined," appropriate fashion. Again, this is a rare mechanism, because the flow is directed toward the head, and the "sheer" effect on the proximal intima is much less significant than that on the intima of the distal internal carotid artery. Dissection of the common carotid artery during carotid endarterectomy can also be caused by forcing a large-caliber indwelling shunt into a small or stenotic common carotid artery.

In addition to the above, postoperative stroke can have other causes, such as hypotension, hypertension, hypovolemia, hypoxia, and cerebral ischemia occurring during or after surgery. These complications are discussed in Chapter 12 on anesthesia.

Angiography has also been implicated in the development of perioperative stroke and reperfusion damage by Bruetman and associates (1963) and by Hass and associates (1966).

Recommendations for Minimizing Perioperative Stroke

To minimize the occurrence of perioperative strokes, several recommendations have been put forward.

The following recommendations are generally accepted:

1. Manipulation of the carotid artery as little as possible until crossclamping to prevent embolization from the atheroma. The artery may be gently palpated to gain information on the extent of the disease, but it should never be squeezed.
2. Routine direct arterial blood pressure monitoring and meticulous control of arterial blood pressure during and after surgery. Prompt and energetic control of either hypotension or significant hypertension.
3. Liberal use of computed tomographic scans preoperatively to avoid surgery in patients with unrecognized acute infarcts.

Some measures are thought to be useful by some but not as valuable as the foregoing:

4. Systemic heparinization during cross-clamping.
5. Routine intraoperative angiography to discover and rectify technical errors during surgery.

Still other measures are widely debated:

6. Local rather than general anesthesia and selective shunting.
7. Stump pressure measurement and selective shunting.
8. Routine shunting.

Because internal carotid artery thrombosis may occur during either the immediate or the late postoperative period, it is highly advisable to keep the patient in the recovery room or intensive care unit under close observation at least overnight.

The management of acute stroke which manifests itself in the period after carotid endarterectomy is a special situation in which "the status of the cerebral circulation is known, the cause of stroke is suspect with a high degree of probability, and restoration of circulation may be possible before permanent brain damage" (Treiman *et al.,* 1981). If signs of stroke or impending stroke develop, the patient should be taken back to the operating room immediately and the carotid artery reexplored under local anesthesia. If satisfactory pulsation of the internal carotid artery is lacking, the arteriotomy should be reopened, the thrombus removed, and its cause investigated and, if found, corrected. This should be carried out within one to two hours, after which ischemic brain damage will likely remain irreversible (Lindberg *et al.,* 1975; Najafi *et al.,* 1971).

We regard this approach of immediate reoperation as the most effective method of handling perioperative stroke which—at the price of minimal trauma of reexploration—provides the fastest and therefore the most effective avenue to salvage brain tissue from the threat of irreversible ischemic changes. Efforts to determine carotid patency short of reexploration by use of noninvasive techniques or angiography consume valuable time, are unreliable, and—in the case of angiography—may increase the damage that has already occurred; therefore, they should not be relied upon.

In the clinical material of 26 perioperative strokes evaluated by Treiman and associates (1981), they found that (1) only patients who were taken back to the operating room from the recovery room benefited, (2) only patients who were reoperated within two hours after the onset of symptoms had improvement after reoperation, and (3) only patients who were reoperated within an hour had a full return of function. Similar findings were reported by Kwaan and Connolly (1977), who reoperated three patients with perioperative stroke within one hour after the onset of symptoms.

Postoperative Headache

Occasionally stubborn headache occurs after carotid endarterectomy; it usually follows a self-limited course and responds to standard pain relievers. Distention of a vascular bed long accustomed to reduced flow and opening of collaterals has been suggested but not proven to be the cause of the headache (Fisher, 1968). The surgeon should keep a wary eye on a patient with severe postoperative headache, which may signify a cerebral complication such as edema or hemorrhage. Neurological consultation should always be obtained in such cases, and the patient and family should never be assured that "it is nothing serious" until the headache subsides.

DEATH

The ultimate complication of any operation is, of course, death. In recent years there has been a gradual but significant improvement in the early results of carotid endarterectomy. These days the operation is performed with a surgical mortality rate of 1 to 2 percent and a rate of significant morbidity rate of less than 4 percent (DeWeese, 1983; Thompson *et al.,* 1970). The rate of operative mortality in patients operated on for fixed neurological deficits has been reported by Thompson (1983) as 5.1 percent; in patients with transient ischemia, 1.1 percent; and in patients with asymptomatic bruits, none.

REFERENCES

Bruetman, M.E.; Fields, W.S.; Crawford, E.S.; and DeBakey, M.E.: Cerebral hemorrhage in carotid artery surgery. *Arch. Neurol.,* **9**:458–67, 1963.

Callow, A.D.: Recurrent stenosis after carotid endarterectomy. *Arch. Surg.,* **117**:1082–85, 1982.

DeWeese, J.D.: Long-term result of surgery for carotid artery stenosis. In Bergan, J.J., and Yao, J.S.T. (eds.): *Cerebrovascular Insufficiency.* Grune & Stratton, New York, 1983.

Fisher, C.M.: Migraine accompaniments versus arteriosclerotic ischemia. *Trans. Am. Neurol. Assoc.,* **93**:211–13, 1968.

Hafner, C.D., and Tew, J.M.: Surgical management of the totally occluded internal carotid artery: a ten-year study. *Surgery,* **89**:710–71, 1981.

Hass, W.K.; Clauss, R.H.; Goldberg, A.F.; Johnson, A.L.; Imparato, A.M.; and Ransohoff, J.: Special problems associated with surgical and thrombolytic treatment of strokes. *Arch. Surg.,* **92**:27–31, 1966.

Kwaan, J.H.M., and Connolly, J.E.: Peripheral atheroembolism: an enigma. *Arch. Surg.,* **112**:987–90, 1977.

Lindberg, B.; Norback, B.; and Svendsen, P.: Carotid endarterectomy: a review of 104 operations. *J. Cardiovasc. Surg.,* **16**:161–70, 1975.

Najafi, H.; Javid, H.; Dye, W.S.; Hunter, J.A.; Widerman, F.E.; and Julian, O.C.: Emergency carotid thromboendarterectomy: surgical indications and results. *Arch. Surg.,* **103**:610–14, 1971.

Thompson, D.; and Patman, R.D.: Clinical endarterectomy for cerebrovascular insufficiency: long-term results in 592 patients followed up to thirteen years. *Ann. Surg.,* **172**:663–79, 1970.

Thompson, J.E.: Operative mortality following carotid endarterectomy. *Stroke,* **14**:115–17, 1983.

Treiman, R.L.; Cossman, D.V.; Cohen, J.L.; Foran, R.F.; and Levin, P.M.: Management of postoperative stroke after carotid endarterectomy. *Am. J. Surg.,* **142**:236–38, 1981.

22

Long-Term Results of Carotid Endarterectomy

VINCENZO GALLUCCI and GIORGIO M. ARU

The long-term results of surgery for carotid artery stenosis are not well known, and what is known is disturbing. The late results need to be evaluated regarding the following: (1) residual or new symptoms, (2) morphological changes in the operated carotid artery, (3) progression of the disease in the rest of the cerebrovascular system, and (4) late mortality.

LONG-TERM FUNCTIONAL RESULTS

In viewing the postoperative relief of symptoms, the approach must be careful because a significant number of patients operated upon for severe carotid stenosis were asymptomatic before surgery; in these, of course, symptomatic improvement is not at issue. Also, in an unknown number of patients the symptoms which were attributed to a lesion that was finally corrected may actually have been caused by other pathology, such as medication, emotional problems, diffuse intracranial vascular disease, or inoperable lesion of the contralateral carotid artery. Even a technically highly successful operation will not relieve such symptoms. Also, whereas symptomatic improvement resulting from the operation can indeed be graded, symptomatic worsening which may have been surgically prevented cannot. For example, it is possible that a person operated upon for tight carotid stenosis who was dizzy preoperatively and who remained dizzy postoperatively may have been spared from a stroke by the surgery. These factors should be taken into consideration in evaluating symptoms after carotid endarterectomy.

The exhaustive studies of DeWeese and Rob (DeWeese, 1983) included 103 patients who were operated on for carotid artery stenosis, 88 of whom had "classic" transient ischemic attacks (TIAs) and who were followed for more than ten years postoperatively. Twenty-four percent of these patients continued to have or developed clearly identifiable neurological symptoms after surgery, including seven deaths from stroke. From close analysis of this clinical material, DeWeese concluded that, while 11 percent of the 103 patients had late symptoms or death probably related to the operated carotid artery, in the additional 13 percent who continued to have atypical nonhemispheric symptoms, such as dizziness, syncope, headache, seizures, and confusion, the persisting symptoms were due to vertebral-basilar intracranial vascular disease or other physical or emotional problems.

View and results similar to DeWeese's were reported by Thompson and associates (1970) and by Lees and Hertzer (1981). Thompson's study encompasses 293 patients who clinical status was monitored for a time period varying from six months to 13 years. Of these patients, 40 (19 percent) continued to have neurological symptoms referable to the operated carotid artery. Of the 335 patients followed by Lees and Hertzer (1981) for an average of 8.6 years, 38 (11 percent) developed TIAs appropriate to the carotid artery operated upon.

The percentage of late strokes after carotid endarterectomy also varies widely in published series. In the series of Wylie and Ehrenfeld (1970) and Lees and Hertzer (1981), late stroke related to endartectomy was found to be 3 and 7 percent, respectively. These reports and others strongly indicate that about 10 percent of patients have recurrence of symptoms of cerebral ischemia owing to related changes in the operated carotid artery.

In patients who have already had frank strokes, any long-term amelioration in the neurological status obtainable from cerebral revascularization is difficult to assess in terms of how much of the improvement can be attributed to surgery and how much to the natural history and spontaneous improvement of the disease. Therefore, in the analysis of the results of surgery, attention must be dedicated primarily to its effectiveness in preventing TIAs and primary or recurrent strokes.

The primary goal of surgery is the long-term relief of "classic" carotid symptoms, such as contralateral motor and sensory loss, ipsilateral amaurosis, and dysphasia, which disappear after the operation in 80 to 90 percent of cases (Thompson *et al.,* 1982; Rob, 1978). Ten to 20 percent of the operated patients, however, will continue to have symptoms similar to those they had preoperatively that were seemingly appropriate to the affected artery. It must also be noted that these symptoms, as well as other nonhemispheric disturbances such as dizziness, syncope, headache, seizures, and confusion, may also occur from concomitant vertebral-basilar or intracranial carotid arterial involvement (DeWeese *et al.,* 1973; Lees and Hertzer, 1981; Thompson *et al.,* 1982). Therefore, it is difficult if not impossible to determine the real incidence of TIA or even stroke related to the endarterectomized segment of the carotid artery because of the differences in reporting methods and the varying lengths of follow-up time reported in the literature.

RECURRENT STENOSIS

The true incidence of restenosis of an endarterectomized internal carotid artery is uncertain, and no one investigator's experience is conclusive. The presence of bruits on the operative side is neither a reliable sign of restenosis nor of persistence of the presurgical lesion. Scarring, edema, and deformity of the arterial lumen can cause turbulence and thus audible bruits even in the absence of hemodynamically significant stenosis. Sudden change in the auscultatory findings, such as disappearance of murmurs previously present, however, carries a definite clinical significance.

Most studies documenting the low percentage of restenosed carotid arteries suffer from the same drawback; i.e., arteriographic controls have been performed in only a small minority of patients, and in those patients usually only because of the recurrence of neurological symptoms. Thus, most asymptomatic patients, even those presenting with loud carotid bruits, have not been restudied. With the recent development of sophisticated noninvasive detection techniques as well as digital angiography there appears to be a trend toward more careful investigation and follow up. Another important conclusion emerging from all published series is that a great number of patients are lost to vascular follow up because of intervening major cardiac diseases that often cause death (Bernstein *et al.,* 1983; DeWeese *et al.,* 1973). Thus, the incidence of carotid restenosis reported in older series as varying from 0.5 to 4.5 percent (Callow, 1980; Kartchner and McRae, 1978; Thompson *et al.,* 1982) probably fails to reflect the real significance of the problem. Finally, we must realize that the incidence of late postoperative occlusion is much greater than the incidence of recurrent symptoms and that there is no strict correlation in the literature between good clinical results and continuing patency of the operated carotid artery (Baker *et al.,* 1983; Zierler *et al.,* 1982).

If we consider more recent reported series in which noninvasive control techniques were routinely used, the percentage of recurrent stenoses is significantly higher—3.5 to 9 percent (Baker *et al.,* 1983; Hertzer *et al.,* 1979; Kremen *et al.,* 1979; and our own series). Identification of the asymptomatic recurrent stenosis is obviously very important because even if asymptomatic, the patient is still at risk for stroke, and the extent of this hazard is not yet clearly defined (Callow, 1980). Therefore, it seems advisable to follow closely and periodically carefully evaluate all patients after carotid surgery.

PATHOLOGY OF RECURRENT LESIONS

Speculations on the possible causes of late restenosis or occlusion of the endarterectomized carotid artery are generally based on the observations of Stoney and String (1976), which were confirmed by others (Callow, 1980; Hertzer *et al.*, 1979; Zierler *et al.*, 1982) with histological and electron microscopic examination of removed fragments of the restenosed arterial wall.

The typical early (within 24 months) recurrent stenotic plaque is white, smooth, and glistening; has no cleavage plane; and shows the histological features of myointimal cell proliferation, which could be the consequence of an abnormal exuberance of the arterial reparative process that would normally follow the surgical trauma to the arterial wall (Callow, 1980; Stoney and String, 1976). The cause of this process, which occurs in only a minority of patients, is not known. On the other hand, late restenoses, generally developing two years or more after surgery, usually have the well-known gross and microscopic features of atherosclerosis. These two apparently distinct processes may in fact be different phases of the same arteriosclerotic disease which in different human hosts modifies the plaque by hemorrhagic, calcific, and lipidic infiltrations. It is likely, however, that a sizable number of restenoses are due to iatrogenic technical factors, probably caused by trauma owing to application of vascular clamps, incomplete endarterectomies leaving residual intimal or medial flaps or tags, failure to remove the distal shelf of the atherosclerotic lesion, or improper suture of the arteriotomy.

FOLLOW-UP EVALUATION OF THE CAROTID ARTERIES BY NONINVASIVE AND INVASIVE METHODS

Before noninvasive carotid studies became available, the postoperative status of extracranial carotid arteries could be evaluated only by direct angiography, the use of which was obviously limited to sympomatic patients and to those willing to undergo such tests. The recent introduction and wide acceptance of digital subtraction angiography has made contrast studies both more common and acceptable, but it, too, is an invasive investigation requiring transvenous introduction of contrast media, a procedure that is probably not suitable to routine control studies. It appears, therefore, more appropriate for the routine follow up of both operated and nonoperated patients to use the more recent noninvasive techniques of varied sophistication. The most popular of these are oculoplethysmography (Kremen *et al.*, 1979), carotid phonoangiography, and ultrasonic duplex scanner with spectral analysis (which combines real-time B-mode imaging of the artery and pulsed Doppler flow detection in the same system). A high degree of accuracy (more than 90 percent), however, is obtainable only by performing all three tests and combining the results. The duplex scanning technique seems to be particularly useful for identifying high-grade stenoses and differentiating between stenosis and occlusion (Zierler *et al.*, 1982). For lesser-grade lesions it is much less accurate. With perfection of these techniques it is possible to assess both anatomical and functional hemodynamic components of carotid lesions responsible for bruits, thus making postoperative follow up, as well as screening in general, much easier and more precise. If the results are suggestive of restenosis, the indication for reoperation should naturally be confirmed by arteriography.

An important limitation of the noninvasive techniques is the low yield in the diagnosis of ulcerated nonstenosing plaques, well-known causes of repeated cerebral embolization that are identifiable only by conventional arteriography.

LATE STROKE AFTER CAROTID ENDARTERECTOMY

To understand the cause of postoperative TIAs and strokes, one must consider the overall patency rate of the operated cervical carotid, the recurrence of stenosis at the bifurcation, and the possible existence and severity of atherosclerotic disease in the intracranial vessels.

According to expectations expressed in the literature, once the immediate postoperative period with its morbidity and mortality risk of 1 to 7 percent for perioperative strokes or myocardial infarctions (Bernstein *et al.*, 1983; Callow, 1980), is past, patients should be fairly well protected against subsequent strokes. In reality, however, classic neurological symptoms, such as amaurosis fugax, speech disturbances, and contralateral motor and sensory deficits, recur in an average of 10 to 24 percent of patients within five years (DeWeese *et al.*, 1973; Lees and Hertzer, 1981; Thompson *et al.*, 1982). These symptoms may be caused by recurrence of stenosis at the endarterectomy site, but more frequently (in about 21 percent of patients) they are due to lesions in the carotid artery contralateral to the endarterectomized vessel (DeWeese *et al.*, 1973; Lees and Hertzer, 1981; Thompson *et al.*, 1982). The likelihood of occurrence of such late strokes is lowest after surgery for asymptomatic carotid bruits and just slightly higher after surgery for TIAs (8 to 10 percent at five years; Bernstein *et al.*, 1983). The patients of the highest risk are those who were operated on the side "not matching" their hemispheric symptoms—a 36 percent incidence of stroke at five years, a much higher percentage than that for patients with asymptomatic bruits, TIAs, or even prior stroke with full recovery (Bernstein *et al.*, 1983). It should be added that there is a difference in favor of the patient with asymptomatic bruit whereas the TIA group has a continuing higher incidence of stroke.

The data concerning patients with asymptomatic carotid stenosis show that this causes stroke in 12 to 20 percent of the cases in a two-to-six year interval after discovery unless they have undergone contralateral carotid endarterectomy previously. In the latter case the stroke incidence is much lower, usually preceded by ischemic attacks, and in the 0 to 7 percent range after five to six years (Bernstein *et al.*, 1983). In Lees and Hertzer's experience, the patients who had bilateral carotid stenosis but underwent surgery on only one side had stroke in the late postoperative period with an incidence of 29 percent, 16 percent of which involved the contralateral cerebral cortex. Of patients who had bilateral surgery, however, only 18 percent had late strokes (Lees and Hertzer, 1981). Moreover, those who had complete occlusion on one side and stenosis on the other and who were successfully operated upon, presented a surprisingly low incidence of subsequent strokes. The reason for this may be that there was an adequate collateral flow and no danger of embolization from a stenotic and/or ulcerated contralateral vessel.

The foregoing data seem to indicate that the incidence of late strokes among patients operated upon for extracranial carotid lesions is much higher than that for the general population and that only a limited number of such incidents can be blamed for recurrent stenosis. Several factors seem to influence such trends, which seem to especially endanger patients who have already had frank strokes (Bardin *et al.*, 1982; Lees and Hertzer, 1981). Among these factors are stenosis or occlusion of the contralateral carotid, occlusive disease in the remainder of the brachiocephalic vessels, and the progression of preexisting atherosclerotic lesions or the development of new ones in other arteries that are responsible for late strokes in the contralateral cerebral cortex or the midbrain, especially if the collateral circulation is inadequate. Finally, especially in hypertensive patients, late neurological disasters and deaths can be due to cerebral hemorrhage.

"EXTRAVASCULAR" FACTORS INFLUENCING LONG-TERM PROGNOSIS

In carotid surgery, as in other major vascular surgery fields, much influence on long-term results and survival can be exerted by extravascular factors, some of which are known as true "risk" factors. Among these are age, sex, race, smoking, diabetes, hypertension, and hyperlipidemia. Some but not all of these factors can be modified by medical treatment.

Older patients understandably carry a higher risk: the late mortality rate (five years) is 18 percent for patients in the sixth decade, 38 percent for those in the seventh decade, and 52 percent for those in the eighth decade (DeWeese *et al.*, 1973).

Smoking, diabetes, and hyperlipidemia exert a definite influence not only on the evolution of all cardiovascular diseases but also on the patients' tolerance of operation and on the late prognosis, although no statistical data are available with regard to carotid lesions. Of hypertensive patients operated upon for carotid stenosis, 20 percent had late strokes, compared with 10 percent of those without hypertension, the cause probably being related to hemorrhage into the atheroma (Lees and Hertzer, 1981).

Presence of associated conditions, especially coronary artery disease, can also profoundly affect the late results of carotid surgery by radically altering the patient's life expectancy. Coronary lesions coexist in as many as 49 percent of the cases treated for carotid stenosis (Ennix *et al.*, 1979). This condition needs to be treated concomitantly because fatal myocardial infarction can occur soon after surgery as well as in the late follow-up period (Lees and Hertzer, 1981; Thompson *et al.*, 1970).

Progression of atherosclerosis can often be slowed if not arrested by radical modification of some of the aforementioned risk factors (diabetes, hyperlipidemia, and hypertension). Cessation of smoking can also make a great contribution to this difficult task. Early detection and treatment (medical and surgical) of associated diseases, both cardiac (mostly coronary) and vascular (especially aortic aneurysm) can substantially improve the late prognosis of carotid patients.

The use of antiplatelet drugs (aspirin, dipyridamole) in the postoperative period of these patients with the purpose of decreasing the incidence of recurrent TIAs and strokes has so far failed to yield conclusive results.

LATE MORTALITY

The percentage of late mortality after carotid endarterectomy has been reported as being high by most investigators: DeWeese (1983) reports 32 percent at two months to seven years; Riles and associates (1982) report 22 percent at five years; Hertzer and associates (1979) and Lees and Hertzer (1981) report 27 percent at five years and 48 percent at 11 years, respectively. Our own series was 27 percent at 10 years. Late mortality appears to be directly related to the patient's age at the time of surgery (mentioned previously among the risk factors) as well as to a history of coronary heart disease (56 percent compared with 27 percent of patients without such histories; DeWeese, 1983). The neurological symptoms on which the operative indication was based also greatly affect the long-term results. In asymptomatic patients, the incidence of late mortality at seven years was found to be 22 percent, becoming 27 percent of those with TIAs and 35 percent of those with progressive or frank stroke (DeWeese, 1983). A favorable survival rate has been recently reported by Lord in Australia (1984). He followed 236 patients who underwent 310 carotid endarterectomies for TIAs for a period varying from 30 months to 12 years, and found a survival rate of 65 percent after 12 years. This is a statistic comparable to that of the general population of the same age.

We found late death owing to myocardial infarction or its complications in more than 50 percent of the cases, to stroke or brain hemorrhage in 15 percent, to cancer in 8 to 10 percent, to ruptured aortic aneurysm in 2 to 3 percent, and to other causes in the remaining 22 to 25 percent. Similar results were reported by most other investigators. There is also agreement that aortocoronary bypass surgery can produce a significant improvement in the otherwise worrisome late survival rate of most of these patients (see also Chapter 27 on combined carotid-coronary surgery).

In our practice, before aortocoronary bypass surgery, we presently require that every patient with a previous history of TIAs, stroke, and/or carotid bruits, even if asymptomatic, be studied by both coronary arteriography and four-vessel arteriogram. This practice has led to the discovery of many unsuspected severe stenotic or ulcerated lesions of the carotid arteries and to a sizable increase in the number of simultaneous interventions. This procedure was found to be valid also for patients referred primarily for carotid surgery but who had a history of angina and/or positive electrocardiograms under stress.

REFERENCES

Baker, W.H.; Hayes, A.C.; Mahler, D.; and Littooy, F.N.: Durability of carotid endarterectomy. *Surgery,* **94:**112–15, 1983.

Bardin, J.A.; Bernstein, E.F.; Humber, P.B.; Collins, G.M.; Dilley, R.B.; Devin, J.B.; and Stuart, S.H.: Is carotid endarterectomy beneficial in prevention of recurrent stroke? *Arch. Surg.,* **117:**1401–7, 1982.

Bernstein, E.F.; Humber, P.B.; Collins, G.M.; Dilley, R.B.; Devin, J.B.; and Steward, S.H.: Life expectancy and late stroke following carotid endarterectomy. *Ann. Surg.,* **198:**80–6, 1983.

Callow, A.D.: An overview of the stroke problem in the carotid territory. *Am. J. Surg.,* **140:**181–91, 1980.

DeWeese, J.A.: Long term results of surgery for carotid artery stenosis in cerebrovascular insufficiency. In Bergen, J.J., and Yao, J.S.T. (eds.): *Cerebrovascular Insufficiency.* Grune & Stratton, New York, 1983.

DeWeese, J.A.; Rob, C.G.; Satran, R.; Marsh, D.O.; Joynt, R.J.; Summers, D.; and Nichols, C.: Results of carotid endarterectomies for transient ischemic attacks: five years later. *Ann. Surg.,* **178:**258–64, 1973.

Ennix, C.L., Jr.; Lawrie, G.M.; Morris, G.C., Jr.; Crawford, E.S.; Howell, J.F.; Reardon, M.J.; and Weatherford, S.C.: Improved results of carotid endarterectomy in patients with symptomatic coronary disease: an analysis of 1,545 consecutive carotid operations. *Stroke,* **10:**122–25, 1979.

Hertzer, N.R.; Martinez, B.D.; Benjamin, S.P.; and Beven, E.G.: Recurrent stenosis after carotid endarterectomy. *Surg. Gynecol. Obstet.,* **149:**360–64, 1979.

Kartchner, M.M., and McRae, L.R.: Non-invasive assessment of the progression of extracranial carotid disease. In Diethrich, E.B. (ed.): *Non-Invasive Cardiovascular Diagnosis: Current Concepts.* University Park Press, Baltimore, Maryland, 1978.

Kremen, J.E.; Gee, W.; Kaupp, H.A.; and McDonald, K.M.: Restenosis or occlusion after carotid endarterectomy: surgery with ocular pneumoplethysmography. *Arch. Surg.,* **114:**608–10, 1979.

Lees, C.D., and Hertzer, N.R.: Postoperative stroke and late neurologic complications after carotid endarterectomy. *Arch. Surg.,* **116:**1561–68, 1981.

Riles, T.S.; Imparato, A.M.; Kopelman, I.; Wintzer, R.; *et al.:* Comparison of results of bilateral and unilateral carotid endarterectomy five years after surgery. *Surgery,* **91**:258–62, 1982.

Rob, C.: Occlusive disease of the extracranial cerebral arteries: a review of the past 25 years. *J. Cardiovasc. Surg.,* **19**:487–98, 1978.

Stoney, R.T., and String, S.T.: Recurrent carotid stenosis. *Surgery,* **80**:705–10, 1976.

Thompson, J.E.; Austin, D.J.; and Patman, R.D.: Carotid endarterectomy for cerebrovascular insufficiency: long-term results in 592 patients followed up to thirteen years. *Ann. Surg.,* **172**:633–79, 1970.

Thompson, J.E.; Patman, R.D.; Talkington, C.M.; and Garrett, W.V.: Restenosis following carotid endarterectomy. In Keith, F.J. (ed.): *Critical Problems in Vascular Surgery.* Appleton-Century-Crofts, New York, 1982.

Wylie, E.J., and Ehrenfeld, W.K.: *Extracranial Occlusive Cerebrovascular Disease: Diagnosis and Management.* W.B. Saunders, Philadelphia, Pennsylvania, 1970.

Zierler, R.A.; Bandyk, D.F.; Thiele, B.L.; and Strandness, D.E.: Carotid artery stenosis following endarterectomy. *Arch. Surg.,* **117**:1408–15, 1982.

23

The Neuropsychological Effects of Carotid Endarterectomy

SAMUEL E. WILSON and PHILLIP POLIDO

The clinical spectrum of cerebral vascular disease (including extracranial vascular disease) ranges from no symptoms (in which case detection of the stenosis is usually prompted by a bruit) to transient ischemic attacks (TIAs), unilateral paresis and paralysis, profound coma, and death.

In the early 1950s, Fisher (1951a,b; 1954) suggested the potential neuropsychiatric importance of arteriosclerotic disease of the carotid arteries. After observation of several patients with dementia associated with both unilateral and bilateral carotid artery occlusion, Fisher proposed that "carotid occlusion may well explain some cases of senile dementia which previously were not attributed to a cerebrovascular lesion" (Fisher, 1954). Hurwitz and associates (1959), in a summary of their findings from the Cornell-Bellevue Stroke Study, reinforced Fisher's thesis when they too described impaired mentation as a manifestation of carotid arterial occlusive disease and added that it was one of several syndromes providing a warning of impending stroke. A year before, Williams and Bruetsch (1958) had stated that internal carotid arterial occlusion "should be borne in mind particularly in instances of rapidly developing dementia."

Severe bilateral carotid artery disease was recognized to have particular significance in relation to neuropsychological alterations. Of ten such patients described by Fisher, five were associated with "senile dementia." He noted that "in the long history of the study of senile dementia the state of the carotid vessels carrying the major blood supply to the brain has never before been investigated" (Fisher, 1954). Eisenbrey and associates (1955), in their study of bilateral thrombosis of the internal carotid artery, suggested that dementia may be a prominent feature of bilateral carotid artery occlusive disease and emphasized the role of collateral circulation in the degree of symptomatology. Groch and associates (1960) and Sours (1960), however, presented several cases in which patients did not manifest dementia; both studies concluded that "bilateral carotid artery disease is not always necessarily associated with dementia" (Groch *et al.*, 1960). These observations confirm the varied spectrum of symptoms and signs caused by carotid artery disease.

NEUROPSYCHOLOGICAL DEFECT IN EXTRACRANIAL DISEASE

Since the 1950s, dementia has been shown to be associated with a decrease in total hemispheric blood flow (Freyhan *et al.*, 1951; Fazekas *et al.*, 1953; Lassen *et al.*, 1957). The diminished oxygen content of cerebral venous blood suggests that relative anoxia of brain in some cases could be held responsible for the patient's mental aberrations. Beginning in 1970, alterations in regional blood flow to the brain have been investigated, particularly the diminished blood flow to the fronto-temporal regions in demented patients. O'Brien and

Mallet (1970) studied the cerebral perfusion rate in patients with primary dementia as well as those with dementia secondary to vascular disease. Their results showed that decreased perfusion of the cerebral cortex occurred in direct relation to loss of tissue bulk and metabolic demand. In those patients who had dementia owing to vascular disease, the cerebral cortex perfusion rates were diminished early in the disease, and this reduction was out of proportion to the degree of cortical atrophy (O'Brien and Mallet, 1970).

Other investigators have also collected evidence supporting the relationship of decreased cerebral blood flow and dementia. Ingvar and associates (1965) noted a reduction in cerebral blood flow and in "gray weight" in senile and presenile dementia, with the severity of dementia being roughly proportionate to the degree of reduction of cerebral blood flow. Reduced flow in both presenile and senile dementia was also confirmed by Simard and associates (1971). O'Brien and Mallett (1970) suggested that cortical perfusion rates were lower in patients with cerebrovascular dementia as compared with primary neuronal degeneration. These studies, however, have included various pathological types of dementia; historically, recognition of these diagnostic categories has been beset by difficulties in clinical classification and in correlation of the clinical and pathological findings. The possibility of misclassification of certain patients under study could alter the findings of the investigators. Clear separation of various types of dementia would seem to be an important and essential prerequisite to accurate study and treatment of the disease.

Patients with significant arteriosclerotic disease of the cerebral vessels also have an elevated cerebral vascular resistance and a constantly decreased cerebral blood flow (Freyhan *et al.*, 1951; Scheinberg, 1950; Fazekas *et al.*, 1953). Freyhan and associates (1951) studied ten such patients with "psychotic changes in personality." Freyhan's group found significant reductions in cerebral blood flow, cerebral oxygen consumption, and the oxygen content of cerebral venous blood, along with an increase in cerebrovascular resistance. This increase in cerebrovascular resistance and consequent decrease in flow may be a physiological reflection of the vascular changes caused by arteriosclerosis. It appears that the reduction of blood flow was partly compensated for by an increase in mean arterial blood pressure.

An alternative theory first advanced by Simard and associates (1971) holds that cerebrovascular dementia is not caused by longstanding diminished blood supply owing to arteriosclerosis but by acute stroke or primary degeneration. In 1968, Fisher proposed that dementia may be the result of large strokes or multiple small strokes (lacunar state). Simard and associates (1971) studied regional blood flow in demented patients by carotid angiography, pneumoencephalography, electroencephalography, and cortical biopsy as a means of classifying their patients. Three of their 24 patients were considered to have dementia caused by vascular lesions. The researchers reasoned that dementia in the arteriosclerotic patient is not due to gradual narrowing of the cerebral arteries, because these arteries can still dilate and constrict normally, but probably results from stroke or a primary degenerative disease of the brain (Simard *et al.*, 1971). More recently, Owens and associates (1980) determined that "small infarcts detectable only by scan cause a deterioration in intellectual function which can readily be assessed by psychometric testing."

PSYCHOLOGICAL TESTING

Discussion of the neuropsychological effects of carotid artery surgery requires objective measurements applicable to clinical investigation. Psychological tests are viewed as constituting a refinement and extension of the neurological examination. By certain test methods, one can evaluate intellectual capacities such as orientation, retention, memory, and language function in an objective and precise manner. These tests can also assess perceptual changes such as reaction time, problem-solving ability, visuoperceptive ability, and constructional praxis. Thus, the psychological examination can provide an inventory or profile of behavioral (both intellectual and perceptual) capacities (Benton, 1977).

Four cogent arguments can be made for psychological testing of patients with cerebrovascular disease. First, it provides an accurate and unbiased determination of various aspects of a patient's behavioral capacity. This determination can be used as a guide to patient management, as well as a basis for modifying treatment plans and as a baseline to which future changes may be compared. Second, the psychological examination is an aid in determining the presence of neurological disease that is not readily apparent on physical examination. Third, the psychological examination is helpful in determining focal cerebral disease manifested behaviorally, such as minor aphasic disturbance, visuoperceptive and visuoconstructive disability, impairment of planning activity, and other special characteristics of a patient's performance profile. Fourth, neuropsychological test results may be used as objective data in neurological research.

After administration of the battery of tests, the performance of the patient is evaluated. The number of defective performances contributes to an "impairment index." Studies by Chapman and Wolf (1959) revealed that the Halstead Battery did significantly discriminate between intact subjects and patients with cerebral lesions. Another study by Reitan (1959) also determined that the Halstead Battery may be somewhat more effective than the Wechsler Adult Intelligence Scale (WAIS) in identifying patients with cerebral disease. However, like the Wechsler tests, the various Halstead subtests are of unequal value in differentiating the brain-damaged patients from the control subjects. The categories "Speech Discrimination" and "Form Board" appear the most objective in discrimination, whereas the Flicker and "Time Estimation" tests appear not to be as discriminating. The "Categories" and "Tactual Form Board" tests have also proved to be valuable in the study of brain-damaged patients and are more widely used than the other tests. Depending on the exact nature of the particular neuropsychological condition, a series of flexible tests can also be constructed to identify a subject's level of functional performance. The categories of functional impairment include the evaluation of: (1) retention, memory, and orientation, (2) reasoning and problem solving, (3) visuoperception, (4) constructional praxis, (5) psychomotor performance, (6) language abilities, and (7) personality.

THE NEUROPSYCHIATRIC EFFECTS OF CAROTID ENDARTERECTOMY

That carotid artery reconstruction prevents the recurrence of focal neurological defects has been convincingly demonstrated. Carotid endarterectomy in such patients is thus "prophylactic," that is, an attempt to prevent future deterioration. The positive impact of carotid endarterectomy on neurophsychological function, however, is, to say the least, controversial. Arteriosclerotic cerebrovascular disease is associated with alterations in intellect, cognition, and personality, including memory loss, dementia, and emotional instability (Fisher, 1951a,b; Fisher and Adams, 1951; Fisher, 1954, Hurwitz *et al.,* 1959), but whether these can be reversed by the vascular surgeon is uncertain.

In the early history of carotid endarterectomy the initial observations of improved postoperative function were anecdotal. The reports appeared to show an associated benefit from carotid endarterectomy, but the data were subjective, consisting primarily of comments by patients, their families, and their physicians about improved psychological functioning. As such they did not permit valid conclusions.

Williams and McGee (1964) provided one of the first studies using neuropsychological tests to assess pre- and postoperative intellectual functioning. They studied 11 men aged 48 to 71, nine of whom had evidence of partial carotid stenosis and two of whom had total occlusion of one carotid artery. The patients were evaluated pre- and postoperatively with a battery of neuropsychological tests, including the Wechsler-Bellevue Intelligence Scale, Form I; the Wechsler Memory Scale; the Trail Making Test; and the Rorschach Test. The authors did not use matched controls but compared their results with average scores reported for normal persons in approximately the same age groups. The preoperative results revealed that the 11 patients had psychological function at the low-normal levels and tended to be moderately deficient in psychomotor functions and realistic perception of the environment. The greatest deficits appeared to be in the four patients with bilateral carotid disease.

Postoperative follow up was difficult but was attained in six of nine who underwent endarterectomy. At one month postoperatively, the investigators found some measure of improvement in 50 percent of the patients, but they were unable to demonstrate any significant improvement in memory function, psychomotor functions, productive energy, and Rorschach's "constructive fantasy activity." (Constructive fantasy activity is regarded as the experience of movement associated with Rorschach's inkblot interpretation, which suggests that the more complex a fantasy developed around an inkblot and the greater the quantity of fantasy the deeper is one's withdrawal and the more autistic the solution to a problem; Becker, 1952.) The examiners did, however, describe the patients as clinically somewhat less depressed and anxious, less somatically preoccupied, and more hopeful. Caution should be used in interpreting these subjective findings because they may be due in part to the feeling of well-being after surgery, possibly thought to be a "placebo effect" produced simply by undergoing a surgical procedure.

Duke and associates (1968) published another of the earlier reports of changes in neuropsychological functions as studied by psychological tests after carotid endarterectomy in 47 patients. They concluded that "vascular surgery has a differential effect for different skills." They felt that the failure of the Trail Making and Finger Tapping tests to demonstrate improvement reflected their insensitivity in detecting subtle deficits. The superior performance of the group with small-vessel disease compared with that of the group with large-vessel disease was thought to be related to the greater severity of the disease in the group with large-vessel disease. The patients with small-vessel disease had clinical signs of organic pathology, but their arteriograms did not show any large-vessel pathology. The deficits on the arteriograms and the clinical manifestations of the patients with large-vessel disease were significantly worse, suggesting more advanced disease. The important conclusion of this study was that the operation did not restore lost skills but halted the deterioration associated with vascular disease.

Goldstein and Scheerer (1941) studied the neuropsychological changes associated with carotid endarterectomy in six patients aged 57 to 72 years. The Halstead-Reitan Battery of Neuropsychologic Tests, the Trail Making Test, the Wechsler-Bellevue Intelligence Scale, and the Aphasia Screening Test were administered three to four days preoperatively and approximately three months postoperatively. The six patients had presented with TIAs, and all had bilateral carotid artery stenosis; one patient had greater than 90 percent stenosis of both carotid arteries. The results (see Figures 23–1 and 23–2) in general indicated that performance after surgery was somewhat better than before; however, the higher level attained was still consistent with the subnormal level of persons with cerebrovascular disease. The comparative scores were the normative data from normal control subjects developed by Reitan (1959).

Perry and associates (1974) studied 20 patients preoperatively and three months post-

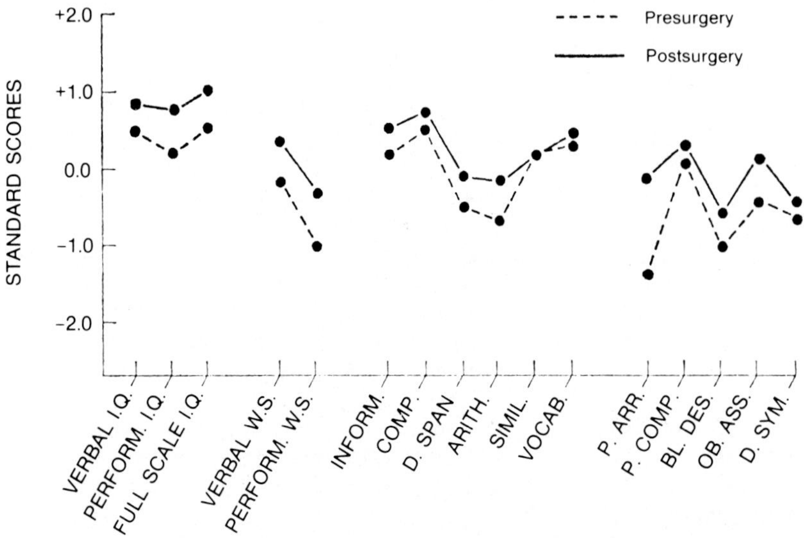

Figure 23–1. Mean performance levels of patients on Wechsler-Bellevue Intelligence Scale, Form I, pre- and postoperatively. From Goldstein, K., and Scheerer, M.: Abstract and concrete behavior: an experimental study with special tests. *Psychol. Monogr.*, **3**:2, 1941.

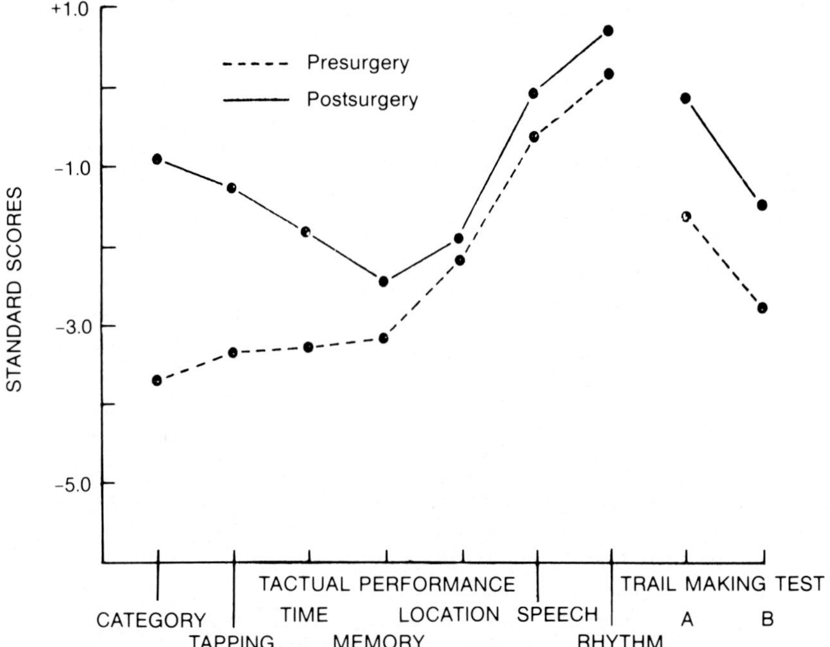

Figure 23–2. Mean performance levels on Halstead's tests and Trial Making Test pre- and postoperatively (as standard scores). From Goldstein, K., and Scheerer, M.: Abstract and concrete behavior: an experimental study with special tests. *Psychol. Monogr.*, **3**:2, 1941.

operatively using eight of the standard psychological tests of Halstead. A composite score labeled "impairment index" was used to evaluate these patients: the greater the index, the more impaired the patient. Blood flow through the carotids was also measured using an electromagnetic flowmeter, before and after repair. The results indicated that preoperatively the patients were impaired mentally as compared with the normal population. After operation, there was significantly improved cerebral function; however, there was no correlation between internal carotid blood flow preoperatively and the impairment index.

Haynes and associates (1976) examined 17 symptomatic patients with at least 50 percent carotid artery stenosis. The control subjects were nine hospitalized patients, matched for age, sex, and education, without carotid artery disease admitted for nonneurosurgical operative procedures. All patients were tested 24 hours before surgery and four to eight weeks after surgery with the following neuropsychological tests: verbal comprehension and perceptual organization-Cohen factors (Cohen, 1957), subtests of the WAIS, the Trail Making Test, and the Minnesota Multiphasic Personality Inventory. The patients undergoing carotid endarterectomy had significant improvement in verbal intelligence, perceptual-organization intelligence, and Trail Making Test scores, suggesting improvement in cognitive function and perceptual motor ability. The group also achieved improved scores on the Minnesota Multiphasic Personality Inventory, suggesting reduction in levels of anxiety, suspicion, distrust, and nervousness, characteristics common to senility.

King and associates (1977) repeated the study by Haynes *et al.*, (1976), again showing that the study and control groups were comparable. The endarterectomy group had no significant change in verbal intelligence; however, the perceptual-organization intelligence scores increased significantly, indicating an average increase in intelligence quotient (IQ) of 12.5 points. The Trail Making Test was accomplished in shorter time, and the Minnesota Multiphasic Personality Inventory results revealed that postendarterectomy patients had significant improvement in symptoms of confusion, suspicion, disorientation, and communication difficulties.

The six foregoing studies form the basis of the concept that carotid endarterectomy provides patients with an improved quality of living through better intellectual functioning and also possibly reduces the anxiety associated with senility.

On the other hand, Matarazzo and associates (1979), in evaluating the effects of carotid endarterectomy on IQ and neuropsychological change, produced results contrary to these studies. They compared four populations: (1) 35 patients with the diagnosis of chronic schizophrenia, (2) 16 nonsurgical patients with diffuse cerebrovascular disease, (3) 29 healthy young patrolmen, who were control subjects, and (4) 17 patients (15 males, two females) who underwent carotid endarterectomy for symptoms of cerebral ischemia. The Halstead-Reitan battery and the WAIS were administered to these patient groups. The patrolmen scored in the normal range both at the initial test and at the retest 20 weeks later. The 16 nonsurgical patients with diffuse cerebrovascular disease had no improvement, remaining in the abnormal range initially and on retest 12 weeks later. The group of schizophrenic patients had abnormal *mean* scores on initial testing and on reexamination 52 weeks later. Examination of the *individual* scores, however, demonstrated significant variability; in fact, several patients actually improved spontaneously and significantly, which apparently is not unusual in the natural history of schizophrenia. The pre- and postoperative results of the 17 patients who underwent carotid endarterectomy remained in the abnormal range. The slight improvement demonstrated early was attributed to the "practice effect," which is the improvement achieved by repetition or by "practice." The Matarazzo study concluded that carotid endarterectomy did not produce any improvement in intellectual and cognitive functioning, though they conceded that surgery may be helpful for certain subgroups—an explanation for the improvement seen in other studies.

Kelly and associates (1980) studied 35 patients who had carotid endarterectomy for either 70 percent or greater stenosis or ulcerated carotid artery plaque. The neuropsychiatric and personality tests were administered within 72 hours before surgery, and postoperative testing was performed four to eight weeks later. The battery of neuropsychological and personality tests (see Table 23-1) showed that (1) the carotid endarterectomy group did not differ preoperatively from the other group in any tests, (2) only the carotid endarterectomy group showed postoperative improvement on the Wechsler Memory Scale ($p < 0.01$) and the Benton Controlled Word Association Test, and (3) both the carotid endarterectomy group and the control group had postoperative improvement on the Educational Testing Service Hidden Patterns Test and the Spreen Benton Right-Left Discrimination Test.

Table 23-1. Neuropsychological and Personality Batteries

TEST	GENERAL FUNCTIONS
Neuropsychologic Battery	
Wechsler Memory Scale	Recent and remote memory, attention
Wells-Ruesch Memory for Objects Test	Recent memory
Minnesota Test for Differential Diagnosis of Aphasia, Sentence Production Subtest	Expressive language
Benton Controlled Word Association Test	Expressive language (fluency)
Peabody Picture Vocabulary Test	Receptive language, verbal IQ
Rush-Presbyterian-St. Luke's Tests of Stereognosis and Praxis	Stereognosis, ideational, and ideomotor praxis
Spreen-Benton Right-Left Discrimination Test	Right-left discrimination
Stanford-Binet Intelligence Test, Picture Absurdities Subtest	Social judgment
Educational Testing Service Hidden Patterns Test	Perceptual analysis
Wells-Ruesch Arithmetical Reasoning Test	Numerical problem solving
Gotham Proverbs Test (partial)	Verbal problem solving
Personality Battery	
State-Trait Anxiety Scale	State and trait anxiety
Mini-Mult	General psychopathology

Source: Kelly, M.P., Garron, D.C., Javid, H.: Carotid artery disease, carotid endarterectomy and behavior. *Arch. Neurol.*, **37**:743, 1980.

Analysis of the variance in the results led the investigators to conclude that the endarterectomy group did not differ preoperatively from the control group on any tests (see Table 23-2). One important observation was that "age and education have been shown to be related to recovery of cognitive abilities following non-progressive brain insults; the present data provide additional evidence that recovery of function is more likely to occur in younger and better educated individuals (Kelly *et al.*, 1980)." The relationship between altered mental function as a consequence of carotid endarterectomy and the many demographic and medical variables suggested that "evalua-

Table 23–2. Characteristics of Patients Improved and Not Improved Behaviorally After Carotid Endarterectomy

	PATIENTS*		SIGNIFICANCE	
PROGNOSTIC CHARACTERISTICS	IMPROVED ($N = 16$)	NOT IMPROVED ($N = 19$)	t	χ^2
Demographic Factors				
Age, year (mean)	59.19	64.95	2.14†	
Education, year (mean)	14.11	11.29	2.43†	
Associated Diseases				
Hypertension	8.00	13.00		1.10
Diabetes	0	4.00		2.00
Other atherosclerotic disease	7.00	15.00		3.22‡
Chronicity of Symptoms				
Symptom duration > 3 months	9.00	9.00		0.23
Admission Data				
Abnormal electrocardiogram	6.00	14.00		2.01
Chest roentgenogram cardiomegaly	3.00	7.00		0.64
Systolic blood pressure, mm Hg (mean)	143.19	161.37	2.04†	
Diastolic blood pressure, mm Hg (mean)	85.00	82.79	0.71	
Angiogram				
Presence of ulceration	6.00	10.00		0.80

Source: Kelly, M.P., Garron, D.C., Javid, H.: Carotid artery disease, carotid endarterectomy and behavior. *Arch. Neurol.*, **37**:748, 1980.

* Unless otherwise noted.

† $p < 0.05$.

‡ $p < 0.10$.

tion of simple preoperative and postoperative group changes in behavior alone may not be the most enlightening method of analysis."

Three contemporary studies performed by two surgical groups hold some promise for reversibility of the neuropsychological symptoms of cerebral ischemia. Owens *et al.* (1980) studied 28 males, average age 63 years, who had unilateral elective carotid endarterectomy. Eleven of the 28 patients had evidence of previous stroke. The report is important: earlier studies had not related intellectual changes to anatomical and physiological variables such as blood flow and degree of arteriosclerotic vascular disease but this study attempted to consider those variables. The investigators noted that patients undergoing carotid artery surgery do so because there is no adequate medical therapeutic approach; thus, a comparable nonoperable group may not exist, and an adequate equivalent control group may not be possible. The 28 males were examined preoperatively, three to ten days postoperatively, and again at three months. Seven psychological tests and several physiological and anatomical measurements were used, including (1) computed axial tomography (CT) of the brain, (2) computed radionuclide angiogram with static-delayed imaging, (3) four-vessel cerebral angiogram, (4) intraoperative electromagnetic flow measurements of the internal carotid artery, and (5) oculoplethysmography, phonoangiography, and supraorbital Doppler examinations preoperatively and postoperatively.

The neuropsychological tests used were a test of general intelligence—the Ravens Standard Progressive Matrices; tests of spatial orientation, vocabulary, arithmetic, and short-term memory; and Finger Tapping tests. At three months, the reexaminations revealed that the patients with flow-restrictive stenosis did not score as well as they had immediately postoperatively. They concluded that carotid endarterectomy improves certain aspects of intellect and related this to an increase in blood flow, because the greatest improvements were in patients who underwent correction of flow-restrictive lesions (see Figure 23–3). They also found that small infarcts detectable only by scanning may have caused deterioration in intellectual functioning: "while acknowledging the role of marginal perfusion in deterioration of intellectual function, we must conclude that small cerebral infarcts due to clinically occult emboli may be a more important cause" (Owens *et al.*, 1980).

Jacobs and associates (1982) studied "cognitive improvement after extracranial reconstruction for the flow-endangered brain."

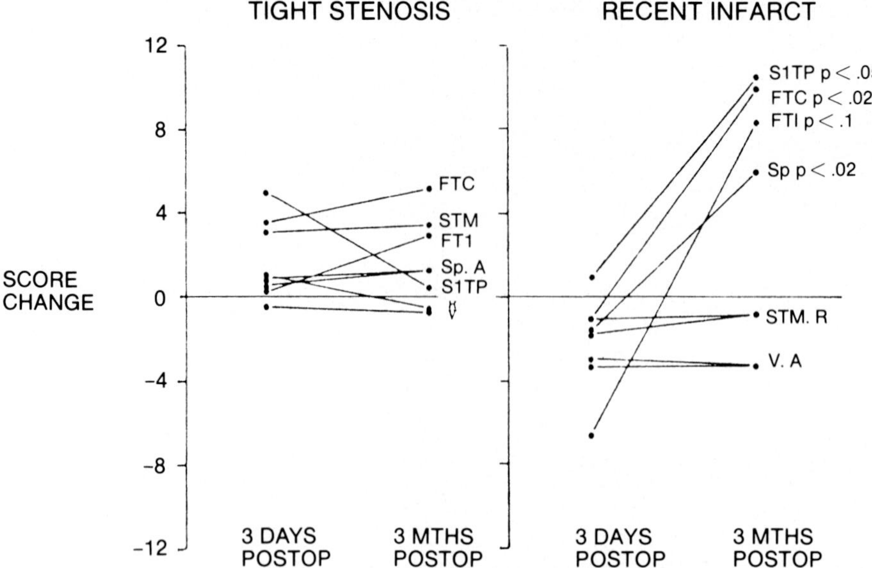

Figure 23–3. Postoperative scores on psychological tests of patients with small cerebral infarcts. Such patients show improvement on psychometric tests when repeated at three months. Other patients' scores are improved preoperatively and then remain unchanged. The differences may be due to recovery from the effects of small infarcts. From Owens, M.; Pressman, M.; Edwards, A.; *et al.*: The effects of small infarcts and carotid endarterectomy on postoperative psychologic test performance. *J. Surg. Res.*, **28**:209, 1980.

Their study involved 12 patients who were classified as having "low flow–endangered brain" defined by Whitten and associates (1981) on the basis of angiographically demonstrable 75 percent or greater reduction in total cross-sectional area of both internal carotid arteries. The indication for operation was a clear history of transient ischemic attacks or a small, stable stroke. No patient had a fixed neurological deficit more recently than six weeks preoperatively.

All the patients underwent four-vessel angiography before entry into the study. Nine patients had complete occlusion of one internal carotid artery and stenosis of the other. Two patients had severe bilateral internal carotid stenosis, and one patient had occlusion of the left common carotid artery and stenosis of the right internal carotid artery. Five of the 12 patients had, in addition, disease of the subclavian-vertebral system. A control group of 12 patients (matched in age, education, total carotid occlusive time, duration of follow up, number of fixed strokes, and time of the neurological event) was included in the study.

The patients were given neuropsychological tests preoperatively and at one week, one month, three months, and six months postoperatively. The two groups, study and control, were well matched. All measured parameters of memory improved significantly after reconstruction. Jacobs and associates concluded that the low flow–endangered brain has a reduction of memory and cognitive ability and that carotid endarterectomy appears to improve intellectual functioning significantly, markedly improving the quality of life for patients.

The recent investigation by Bennion and associates (1985) is a prospective study of 53 patients who underwent unilateral carotid endarterectomy for progressive TIAs. The purpose of this study, too, was to assess the impact of carotid endarterectomy on intellectual functioning. The study involved right-handed males with an average age of 63 years. Eighteen patients had either history or physical examination suggestive of at least one remote cerebral infarct. These patients were studied with (1) brain CT scans, (2) computed radionuclide angiogram with static delayed imaging, (3) four-vessel angiogram with selective biplane carotid and cerebral views, and (4) oculoplethysmography, phonoangiography, and supraorbital Doppler examinations. The neurophyschological tests used were the Ravens Standard Progressive Matrices, spatial orientation, vocabulary, arithmetic, short-term memory, finger-tapping. The tests were administered preoperatively, three to seven days postoperatively, and finally three months postoperatively.

Angiographically, 43 of the 53 patients (81 percent) had greater than 50 percent reduction in cross-sectional diameter of the carotid artery to be operated upon. Of the 43 patients, 33 (77 percent) had critical stenosis greater than 75 percent, 24 had 50 percent stenosis of the contralateral carotid artery, and six had complete occlusion of the contralateral carotid artery.

Composite test scores showed significant improvement in the first postoperative week. This improvement appeared most pronounced in the subjects with high-grade stenosis and correlated with an intraoperative increase in carotid artery blood flow. However, this statistically significant improvement disappeared three months postoperatively. The subjects with carotid artery stenosis of less than 50 percent did not show improvement. Two mechanisms for the return of the early postoperative improvement to baseline scores by the third month were postulated: by way of an autoregulatory process such as intracerebral shunting or by further progression of atherosclerotic changes in ipsilateral distal sites and the contralateral circulation. The investigators concluded that early postoperative improvement indeed occurs in intellectual function but emphasized that in future studies precise tests of intellectual function should be correlated with changes in perfusion.

In conclusion, neuropsychological deficits have been observed by many investigators in patients with intracranial and extracranial cerebral disease. These deficits range from emotional instability and personality aberrations to dementia with its associated loss of memory and diminished intellectual and cognitive abilities. The intellectual deficits of cerebrovascular disease are associated with a decrease in cerebral blood inflow due to stenosis or occlusion compounded by inadequate collateral blood supply and increased cerebrovascular resistance. The increase in systemic blood pressure commonly observed in the elderly is a means of compensating for this deficit in inflow. Bilateral carotid artery disease may be associated with an increased incidence in dementia, but this finding has not been consistent. Deficits in the intellect associated with cerebrovascular disease may also be due to multiple cerebral infarcts so small as to be undetectable, recognizable only by CT scanning of the brain.

For the past 20 years, there has been an effort to assess the impact of carotid endarterectomy on the neuropsychological effects of internal carotid artery occlusive disease. Although numerous neuropsychological tests are available, no test is totally suitable for study of this aspect of vascular surgery. Demographic factors such as age, education, cultural background, and the "practice effect" have an important and difficult-to-measure influence on the test results. Measurement of the postendarterectomy intellect has shown improvement or no change or, conversely, deterioration, depending on the investigator. A recent major study has demonstrated that the postoperative improvement may be only temporary (Bennion *et al.*, 1985).

We must also conclude that the data presently available are insufficient to support a definite role for endarterectomy in permanently reversing the neuropsychological deficits produced by cerebrovascular disease. Future investigation must reduce the uncontrolled variables associated with the present studies. So far, the patient groups have been mixed with regard to the presence or absence of infarcts, the laterality of the disease, and the extent of stenosis or occlusion as well as collateral flow. The selection of control groups has been a most difficult problem; finding an ideal control group completely matched with respect to demographic factors, extent of cerebrovascular disease, and extent of preoperative neuropsychological deficits appears to be an almost overwhelming obstacle.

Study of the neuropsychological effects of carotid endarterectomy has been hampered by both the variability and small number of patients, the inadequate neuropsychological tests, an inability to obtain adequate control subjects, and the lack of correlation with blood flow. What has emerged so far is the certain knowledge that operations on the extracranial vascular system can affect the patient's neuropsychological status; what remains elusive is the ability to quantify the change.

REFERENCES

Becker, S.: *Rorschach's Test: Advances in Interpretation.* Grune & Stratton, San Francisco, 1952.

Bennion, R.S.; Owens, M.L.; and Wilson, S.E.: The effect of unilateral carotid endarterectomy on neuropsychologic test performance in 53 patients. *J. Cardiovasc. Surg.*, **26**:21–26, 1985.

Benton, A.L.: Psychologic testing. In Baker, A. (ed.): *Clinical Neurology.* Harper & Row, San Francisco, 1977.

Chapman, L.F., and Wolff, H.G.: The cerebral hemisphere and the highest integrative functions of man. *A.M.A. Arch. Neurol.*, **1**:357–62, 1959.

Cohen, J.: A factor-analytically based rationale for the Wechsler Adult Intelligence Scale. *J. Consult. Clin. Psychol.*, **21**:451–57, 1957.

Duke, R.B.; Bloor, B.M.; Nugent, G.R.; and Majzoub, H.S.: Changes in performance on WAIS, Trail Making Test and Finger Tapping Test associated with carotid artery surgery. *Percept. Mot. Skills*, **26**:399–404, 1968.

Eisenbrey, A.B.; Urrutia, A.T.; and Karnosh, L.J.: Bilateral thrombosis of the internal carotid artery. *Cleve. Clin. Q.*, **22**:174–83, 1955.

Fazekas, J.F.; Bessman, A.N.; Cotsonas, N.J., Jr.; and Alman, R.W.: Cerebral hemodynamics in cerebral arteriosclerosis. *J. Gerontol.*, **8**:137–45, 1953.

Fisher, C.: Dementia in cerebrovascular disease. In Seikert, R.J. (ed.): *Cerebrovascular Diseases: Sixth Conference,* Grune & Stratton, New York, 1968.

Fisher, M.: Occlusion of the carotid arteries. *AMA Arch. Neurol. Psychiatry,* **72**:187–204, 1954.

Fisher, M.: Occlusion of the internal carotid artery. *AMA Arch. Neurol. Psychiatry,* **65**:346–77, 1951a.

Fisher, M.: Senile dementia: a new explanation of its causation. *Can. Med. Assoc. J.*, **65**:1–7, 1951b.

Fisher, M., and Adams, R.D.: Observations on brain embolism. *J. Neuropathol. Exp. Neurol.*, **10**:92–8, 1951.

Freyhan, F.A.; Woodford, R.B.; and Kety, S.S.: Cerebral blood flow and metabolism in psychosis of senility. *J. Nerv. Ment. Dis.*, **113**:334–41, 1951.

Goldstein, K., and Scheerer, M.: Abstract and concrete behavior: an experimental study with special tests. *Psychol. Monogr.*, **3**(2), 1941.

Groch, S.N.; Hurwitz, L.J.; and McDowell, F.: Bilateral carotid artery occlusive disease. *AMA Arch. Neurol.*, **2**:130–37, 1960.

Haynes, C.D.; Gideon, D.A.; King, G.D.; and Dempsey, R.L.: The improvement of cognition and personality after carotid endarterectomy. *Surgery,* **80**:699–704, 1976.

Hurwitz, L.J.; Groch, S.N.; Wright, I.S.; and McDowell, F.H.: Carotid artery occlusive syndrome. *AMA Arch. Neurol.*, **1**:491–98, 1959.

Ingvar, D.H.; Gustafson, N.L.: Normal values of regional cerebral blood flow in man, including flow and weight estimates of gray and white matter. *Acta Neurol. Scand. (Suppl.),* **43**:42–73, 1970.

Jacobs, L.A.; Ganji, S.; Shirley, J.G.; Morrell, R.M.; and Brinkman, S.D.: Cognitive improvement after extracranial reconstruction for the low flow-endangered brain. *Surgery,* **93**:683–87, 1982.

Kelly, M.P.; Garron, D.C., Javid, H.; *et al.*: Carotid artery disease, carotid endarterectomy and behavior. *Arch. Neurol.*, **37**:743–48, 1980.

King, G.D.; Gideon, D.A.; Haynes, C.D.; Dempsey, R.L.; and Jenkins, C.W.: Intellectual and personality changes associated with carotid endarterectomy. *J. Clin. Psychol.*, **33**:215–20, 1977.

Lassen, N.A.; Munck, O.; and Tottey, E.R.: Mental function and cerebral oxygen consumption in organic dementia. *Arch. Neurol. Psychiatry,* **77**:126–33, 1957.

Matarazzo, R.G., *et al.*: IQ and neuropsychological changes following carotid endarterectomy. *J. Clin. Neuropsychol.*, **1**:97, 1979.

O'Brien, M.D., and Mallet, B.L.: Cerebral cortex perfusion rates in dementia. *J. Neurosurg. Psychiatry,* **33**:497–500, 1970.

Owens, M.; Pressman, M.; Edwards, A.; Tourtellotee, W.; Rose, J.; Stern, D.; Peters, G.; Stabile, B.; and Wilson, S.E.: The effects of small infarcts and carotid endarterectomy on postoperative psychologic test performance. *J. Surg. Res.*, **28**:209–16, 1980.

Perry, P.M., *et al.*: Neuropsychologic tests and carotid arterial disease. *Surg. Res. Soc.*, **61**:922, 1974.

Reitan, R.N.: The comparative effects of brain damage on the Halstead Impairment Index and the Wechsler-Bellevue Scale. *J. Clin. Psychol.*, **15**:281–87, 1959.

Scheinberg, P.: Cerebral blood flow in vascular disease of the brain. *Am. J. Med.*, **8**:139–47, 1950.

Simard, D.; Olesen, J.; Paulson, O.B.; Lassen, N.A.; and Skinhøj, E.: Regional cerebral blood flow and its regulation in dementia. *Brain,* **94**:273–88, 1971.

Sours, J.A.: Some neurologic and psychiatric aspects of bilateral internal carotid occlusion. *J. Ment. Sci.*, **106**:1062–67, 1960.

Whitten, R.H.; Gee, W.; Kraupp, H.A.; and McDonald, K.M.: Extracranial surgery for low flow-endangered brain. *Arch. Surg.*, **116**:1165–69, 1981.

Williams, C., and Bruetsch, W.: Mental deterioration and occlusion of the internal carotid arteries in the neck. *Am. J. Psychiatry,* **115**:256, 1958.

Williams, M., and McGee, T.F.: Psychological study of carotid occlusion and endarterectomy. *Arch. Neurol.*, **10**:293–97, 1964.

24

The Management of Trauma to The Carotid-Vertebral System

NORMAN M. RICH

Trauma to the carotid and vertebral arteries presents challenging and specific management problems. Because of the hazard of irreversible neurological damage, particularly with carotid injuries, patients with these injuries are unique among cases involving trauma to major peripheral arteries. The resultant neurological deficits can develop either from the primary injury or from temporary interruption of the circulation during arterial reconstruction. There has also been considerable controversy during the past 15 years regarding the optimal methods of managing carotid and vertebral arterial injuries and the evaluation of the extent of neurological deficits. Technical problems may also be associated with attempted repair of either carotid or vertebral arterial injuries. The hemodynamic stability of the patient is also an important consideration.

Associated injuries are also frequently present and can indeed complicate the management of trauma to the carotid-vertebral system. In a relatively small and confined space in the neck there are many important structures, including many crucial nerves and the spinal cord. Bacterial contamination can be associated with these wounds, especially if there is damage to the trachea, pharynx, and esophagus. Postoperative healing may be jeopardized if drainage occurs from any of these wounds.

INCIDENCE OF CAROTID-VERTEBRAL ARTERIAL INJURIES

In contrast to the vast majority of acute and chronic arterial injuries in both civilian and military experience in which approximately 90 percent of the injuries involve extremity arteries, carotid arterial injuries represent only about 5 percent of overall arterial injuries. Vertebral arterial injuries are even less frequent. According to the monumental review by DeBakey and Simeone in 1946 of 2,471 acute arterial injuries among American soldiers serving in the European theater in World War II, less than 1 percent of the patients had carotid arterial injuries (ten cases). The review from the Korean conflict revealed an incidence of about 4 percent (11) carotid arterial injuries of a total of 304 arterial injuries (Hughes, 1958). From the early reports of civilian arterial injuries, Morris and associates (1960) reported 18 carotid arterial injuries among 220 total arterial injuries in Houston, an incidence of 8 percent. In a comparable series from Atlanta, Ferguson and Colleagues (1961) documented a frequency of only approximately 3 percent. In 1971, Perry and coworkers described 32 carotid arterial injuries (approximately 6 percent) among 508 arterial injuries in Dallas.

In the past ten years there have been more

reports of experience in managing carotid arterial injuries in specific medical centers.

Injury to the internal carotid artery represents approximately 20 to 30 percent of total carotid arterial trauma. From the retrospective analysis of 722 patients with carotid injury, Unger and colleagues (1980), found 149 internal carotid injuries (26 percent) and 415 common carotid arterial injuries. Ledgerwood and co-workers (1980) identified ten patients with internal carotid arterial injuries among the 36 patients with carotid trauma in their series. Injuries to the external carotid artery are seldom reported because of the negligible disability associated with external arterial ligation. In an interim review from the Vietnam Vascular Registry (Rich *et al.,* 1976), there were 25 external carotid arterial injuries (9 percent) in a total of 276 carotid arterial injuries in 252 patients. Also included were 179 common carotid arterial injuries (71.4 percent) and 54 internal carotid arterial injuries (19.6 percent).

Vertebral arterial injuries are rare and usually are clinically less significant. Three such injuries were reported in World War I and none in World War II, the Korean conflict, or the Vietnam War interim reports. In eight different civilian series only six such cases were identified.

ETIOLOGY OF CAROTID AND VERTEBRAL ARTERIAL INJURIES

In military experience, injury to the carotid and vertebral arteries is most frequently of the penetrating variety resulting from fragments from exploding devices such as grenades, mortars, rockets, and mines. Fragment wounds accounted for 88 percent of the carotid arterial injuries in the Vietnam War (Rich *et al.,* 1970a,b). In the interim report from the Vietnam Vascular Registry of 1,000 acute major vascular injuries, 50 carotid injuries or 5 percent were noted (Rich *et al.,* 1970a,b). Characteristically, most carotid injuries from high-velocity gunshot wounds are fatal because of exsanguination within minutes after wounding. The early civilian experience with carotid and vertebral arterial injuries showed that about one half were due to stab wounds, and the other half were due to gunshot wounds, as reported from Houston by Beall *et al.* (1963) and Monson *et al.* (1969). Now this proportion seems to change in favor of gunshot wounds, reflecting the recent increase in the use of guns rather than knives in the civilian community.

Carotid arterial injuries after percutaneous puncture of the carotid artery for cerebral angiography have been reported in the past, but this approach now has largely been abandoned. Three such cases were documented at Walter Reed General Hospital (Rich and Spencer, 1978). Of the 11 cases of major vascular injury occurring during the course of elective operative procedures, one carotid artery injury occurred during an emergency tracheostomy and the other during a radical neck dissection (Rich and Spencer, 1978). Similar injuries can occasionally be found in major reports of vascular injuries during the past 30 years.

Although still relatively rare compared with penetrating injuries of the carotid and vertebral arteries, increasing numbers of carotid and vertebral injuries from blunt trauma to the neck have been reported. In 1967, Yamada and co-authors described one case and found 52 cases published by others of carotid arterial occlusion after nonpenetrating trauma.

The exact mechanism of injury to the carotid arteries by nonpenetrating trauma is not completely understood. The etiology of 52 cases reviewed in the literature is outlined in Table 24–1. Fleming and Petrie (1968) suggested four possible mechanisms: (1) a direct blow, (2) stretching of the carotid artery by hyperextension and lateral flexion of the neck, (3) trauma to the peritonsillar area by a foreign object in the mouth, (4) injury to the intrapetrous portion of the carotid artery in association with a basal skull fracture. Injuries with intraoral foreign bodies occur frequently in children as when a child falls with a foreign object in his mouth, such as a pencil, stick, or toothbrush.

Extrinsic compression of the internal carotid artery is an unusual mechanism of trauma. Mandelbaum and Kalsbeck (1970) reported the case of a 20-year-old nurse injured in an automobile accident; there was hemorrhagic infarction of a group of lymph nodes which subsequently compressed the left internal carotid artery at the level of the first cervical vertebra.

The first known report of traumatic carotid arterial thrombosis was that by Hirshfeld in 1858; a similar case was reported by Verneuil in 1872 in which thrombosis followed forced rotation of the head (Javid, 1963). Hockaday (1959) noted that in most patients with trau-

Table 24–1. English Literature Review of Carotid Arterial Trauma, 1952–1979, and University of Virginia Experience, 1958–1977

SERIES	PATIENTS (N)	MEAN AGE (YEARS)	MALE/ FEMALE	LEFT/RIGHT	COMMON INTERNAL CAROTID	STAB WOUNDS	GUNSHOT WOUNDS	OTHER PENETRATING WOUNDS	BLUNT INJURIES
Current Literature	19	36	17/2	8/11	7/12	1	9	2	7
15 cases	171	33	71/13	69/25	69/52	23	32	29	52
15 cases	532	27	288/34	158/78	339/85	66	203	102	14
Total	722	28	376/49	235/107	415/149	90	244	133	73

Source: Unger, S.W.; Tucker, W.S.; Medeza, M.A.; Wellons, H.A., and Chandler, J.G.; Carotid arterial trauma. *Surgery* **87**:477–87, 1980.

matic thrombosis of the internal carotid artery, the site of obstruction was about 2 cm above the birfucation of the common carotid artery. In his review, nine of ten cases with autopsy findings showed injury to the intima and media with localized thrombus formation. Delayed onset of hemiplegia and aphasia in some patients was thought to be caused by distal embolism from the intraluminal thrombus.

Penetrating injuries of the vertebral artery are fortunately rare; because they are usually of minimal clinical significance, the majority are treated by ligation. Trauma to the vertebral artery has also occurred in the course of percutaneous angiography. Thrombosis of the vertebral artery has been associated with nonpenetrating injuries (Murray, 1957; Ford and Clark, 1956). Gurdjian and associates (1963) reported thrombosis of the vertebral artery which also caused thrombosis of the carotid arteries in two of five patients with cervical trauma.

CLINICAL PATHOLOGY

In those patients who survive, most of the carotid arterial injuries are lacerations. In 50 carotid arterial injuries reported from Vietnam, the great majority were lacerations and perforations (Rich *et al.*, 1970a). Two patients had transsection with thrombosis of the severed ends, three had contusion of the carotid artery, and two had acute arteriovenous fistulas. Among 18 civilian injuries reported by Beall and associates (1963), approximately two-thirds were lacerations, and five resulted in arteriovenous fistulas. Transsection occurred only twice, and one patient had thrombosis of false aneurysm. As noted by Yamada and colleagues (1967), intimal tear and thrombosis occurred most frequently due to nonpenetrating injury.

Early recognition of an acute arteriovenous fistula involving the carotid or vertebral vessels could easily be missed because the classical continuous murmur may not be audible for several days, probably evolving as surrounding clot is resorbed. A continuous thrill is readily felt with the classical arteriovenous fistula, and dilated regional veins may pulsate visibly. The diagnosis can be further substantiated by obliterating the continuous bruit with digital pressure and noting a concomitant slowing of the heart rate, the Branham-Nicoladoni sign (Rich and Spencer, 1978). False aneurysms may also result from trauma, representative reviews of which include those by Cooper (1859), Hunt and Snyder (1979), Lai and colleagues (1966), Matas (1893), and Rich and colleagues (1975b).

CLINICAL FEATURES

Injury to the carotid artery should be suspected in a patient who either has bright red bleeding from a neck wound, particularly if it is pulsating, or presents with a rapidly expanding hematoma. However, even the mere presence of a penetrating neck wound in proximity to the carotid vessels should suggest the diagnosis, because tangential injuries may be temporarily sealed by a thrombus. Absence of distal pulsations with penetrating wounds is not very useful clinically because hematomas often make accurate palpation difficult. When head injuries are also present, a neurological deficit may be due either to the head trauma itself or to the ischemia from injury to the carotid artery. If the patient is fully conscious despite the presence of a severe neurological deficit, the likelihood of the cause being an ischemic injury is prevalent. The absence of neurological injury, however, is not a particularly helpful sign in excluding carotid arterial injury, because neurological deficits are present in only approximately one third of all carotid arterial injuries (Thal *et al.*, 1974).

An unusual feature of nonpenetrating injuries is the delayed appearance of symptoms, as outlined by Yamada and colleagues (1967). Only three of 52 patients were admitted to the hospital with an established diagnosis of carotid arterial injury. Of the 52 patients, 23 percent had significant head injures which may have obscured the correct diagnosis. Similarly, signs of injury to the neck, bruises or skin abrasions, existed in only one half of the patients. Only 10 percent of the patients had serious symptoms within one hour of the injury, and approximately 50 percent were asymptomatic even after ten hours. When the symptoms appeared, they were typical of carotid insufficiency with loss of consciousness, aphasia, hemiparesis, and paresthesias. Monoparesis or hemiparesis was present in all but one of the 52 patients. The reason for the frequent delay in appearance of symptoms is uncertain. The delay may be due to the gradual development of a thrombus at the site of intimal injury, or possibly be caused by subintimal dissection of the hematoma. Awareness of the late appearance of lethal carotid arterial thrombosis is one of the best aids in establishing the correct diagnosis. Jernigan and Gardner (1971), in documenting two cases and reviewing the literature, stated that Horner's syndrome was reported on the initial examination in many patients before any other neurological deficit. They concluded that trauma to the superior sympathetic chain and first ganglion sufficient to cause Horner's syndrome was also likely to injure the internal carotid artery because of the close anatomical proximity.

Roentgenograms of the neck and skull should be obtained in any patient with injuries of the head and neck. With penetrating injuries foreign bodies can be recognized, and the path of the missile can be projected. Two Vietnam patients with hemiplegia underwent successful carotid reconstruction with subsequent removal of metallic emboli from the middle cerebral artery and eventual neurological recovery (Rich and Spencer, 1978). Angiograms are not indicated in most patients with penetrating injuries, especially when overt hemorrhage makes the diagnosis obvious. In obscure cases, however, usually those in which a small laceration has become sealed by thrombus, elective angiography may be of value (see Figures 9–28 and 9–29).

MANAGEMENT OF CAROTID AND VERTEBRAL ARTERIAL INJURIES

An important concept in the treatment of penetrating injuries of the neck is that the vast majority of such injuries should be explored surgically, whether or not symptoms are present. This concept has been gradually recognized in the last several years in both civilian and military injuries. With such an approach clinically undetectable lacerations of the carotid artery that are temporarily sealed by thrombus can be identified and repaired with the avoidance of subsequent development of secondary hemorrhage, false aneurysm, or arteriovenous fistula. Penetrating neck injuries with hemorrhage must be treated with great urgency. Control of hemorrhage may be particularly difficult because tourniquets or pressure dressings cannot be applied without obstructing the trachea; direct pressure with a finger while the patient is being taken to the operating room may be the only effective method. Intubation of the trachea should be performed rapidly because airway obstruction often evolves rapidly, either from expanding hematoma or from edema of the vocal cords.

At operation the best incision is a diagonal one along the medial border of the sternocleidomastoid muscle. Once the incision has been made, the hematoma should be quickly evacuated, the nature and the extent of the injury identified, and hemorrhage controlled by proximal and distal control of the artery. Appropriate debridement of injured soft tissues should be performed, combined with liberal irrigation with saline solution (Rich and Spencer, 1978).

Lateral suture repair may be performed in many patients, especially when the defect has been produced by a sharp instrument or a small fragment (see Figure 24–1A). A patch of autogenous vein may be used to avoid constriction of the lumen. With a more extensive injury, excision of the traumatized segment followed by an end-to-end anastomosis should be performed (see Figure 24–1B). The latter method was utilized in 22 percent of the Vietnam injuries included in the interim report from the Vietnam Vascular Registry (Rich *et al.*, 1970a). Otherwise, a vascular graft, preferably the greater autogenous saphenous vein, should be used. Prosthetic material should generally be avoided in contaminated wounds.

Whether a shunt, either internal or external, should be utilized in managing carotid arterial injuries is a major unresolved question. Some advocate utilizing a shunt because this method will maintain blood flow to the brain through the carotid artery at the time of repair (see Figure 24–1C). Abundant data, however, are available from operations performed for arteriosclerotic stenosis of the carotid artery under local anesthesia which indicate that many patients tolerate temporary occlusion of the carotid artery very well because of adequate collateral circulation. In the Vietnam experience, most patients were treated without shunts (Rich *et al.*, 1975a and 1976; Cohen, 1970; Buchman *et al.*, 1972). In 1970, Cohen and associates emphasized that they were unable to relate morbidity or mortality to interruption of cerebral flow and did not believe that shunts were necessary.

It is well established, however, that a small percentage of patients will not tolerate temporary occlusion or permanent occlusion of the carotid artery. It is uncertain how this group can be identified. In all likelihood, however, those patients who have no neurological ab-

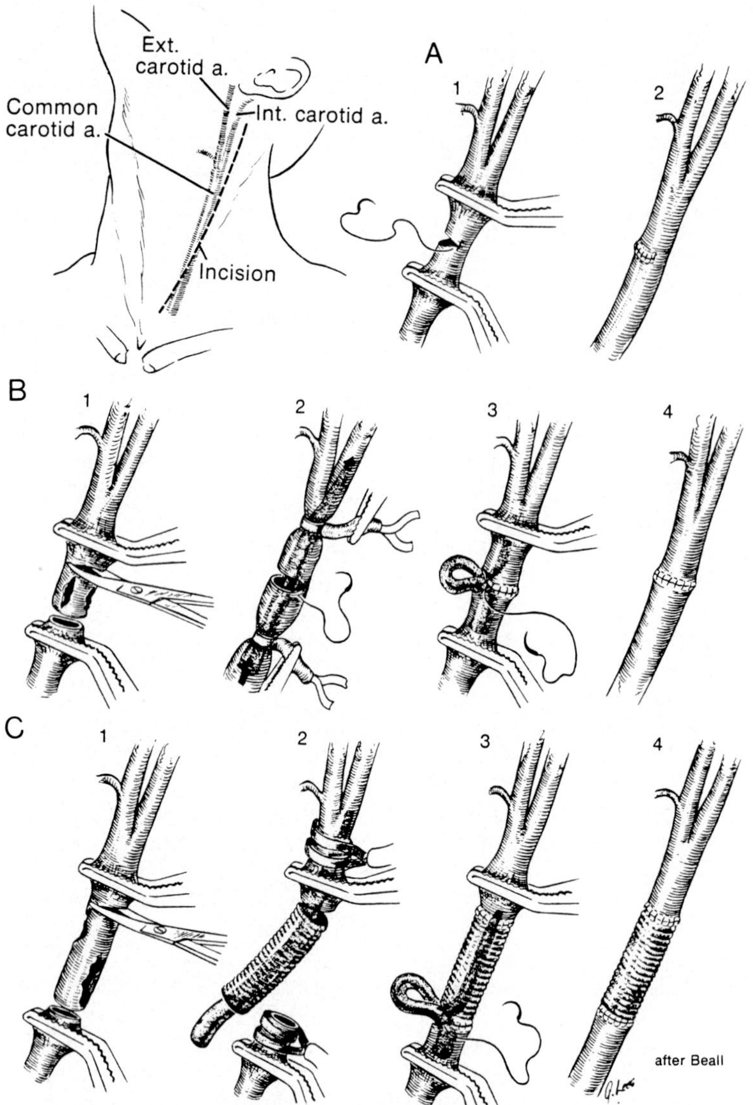

Figure 24–1. Different techniques used in the repair of common carotid artery injuries. Suture closure of a laceration (*A*). Resection of injured segment and end-to-end anastomosis using a temporary indwelling shunt (*B*). Resection of the damaged segment and graft replacement using a temporary indwelling shunt (*C*). From Rich, N.M., and Spencer, F.C.: *Vascular Trauma.* W.B. Saunders, Philadelphia, Pennsylvania, 1978.

normalities associated with complete interruption of the carotid arterial flow after injury can be operated upon safely without a shunt. If a neurological injury is present beforehand, it is particularly difficult to evaluate the situation and the final clinical results.

There is a second unsettled question involving possible adverse effect of restoration of carotid arterial flow in patients with abnormal neurological findings after carotid artery trauma. In a report on patients injured in the Vietnam War, Cohen and co-workers (1970) emphasized that arterial repair resulted in a significant morbidity and mortality rate. They noted the clinical similarity between such patients and those undergoing immediate or early operation for acute stroke, with probable conversion of an infarction to a hemorrhagic infarction after increase in carotid arterial blood flow. Although this question also remains unresolved, ligation of the carotid artery in such a situation may be the safest procedure, particularly if the patient presents with a dense neurological deficit associated with the appropriate hemisphere of the brain.

Adjacent soft tissues should be closed over the repair site after carotid arterial reconstruction. Most cervical incisions can be closed primarily. If, however, there is extensive contamination of the wound, the skin and subcutaneous tissues may be left open for delayed primary suture in three to six days. Concomitant venous injuries, usually to the internal jugular vein, can be safely treated by ligation. Small lacerations of the jugular vein can be closed by lateral suture to control hemorrhage before arterial repair. If there are any questions regarding the adequacy of the arterial repair, an intraoperative arteriogram is useful in identifying technical errors, distal thrombi, or additional sites of injury.

If carotid arterial injury is suspected in a patient with blunt trauma to the neck, angiography will confirm the diagnosis. If occlusion is fund, surgical exploration with thrombectomy should be performed promptly, unless there is already a complete hemiplegia. A Fogarty balloon catheter can be helpful for removal of distal propagating thrombus. Towne and associates (1972) have emphasized that nonoperative treatment is the best choice for the patient with thrombosis in the internal carotid artery after blunt cervical trauma when there has been a resultant hemiplegia. They established that this clinical situation was similar to an acute stroke and that restoration of blood flow to a softened ischemic brain would often result in hemorrhagic infarction. They also concluded that efforts should be directed toward aiding the collateral blood flow and in preventing propagation and embolization of thrombus. Heparin, dextran, and steroids have been utilized in efforts to prevent these complications. Zelenock and associates (1982) reviewed their experience with extracranial internal carotid artery dissections (noniatrogenic traumatic lesions) and suggested that direct cerebral revascularization, staged internal carotid artery constriction and ligation, as well as intensive nonoperative therapy were valid therapeutic options to consider in such lesions.

Most vertebral arterial injuries can be treated by ligation without sequelae. Near the origin of the vertebral artery, however, it may be possible to perform a resection and end-to-end anastomosis (see Figure 24–2).

POSTOPERATIVE CARE

It is extremely important to provide careful neurological monitoring of the patient in the immediate postoperative period. A complete neurological examination should be performed and documented as soon as the patient is reactive. Development of any new neurological deficits could herald an impending catastrophe. Reoperation, with or without a postoperative arteriogram, may be mandatory in the early postoperative period.

Although postoperative arteriograms are not generally performed, valuable information can be obtained from them. The unexpected finding of a false aneurysm at a repair site in one Vietnam casualty is an example. It was possible to successfully repair this false aneurysm.

COMPLICATIONS

Beall and coworkers (1963) emphasized that in their series of 26 patients there were two deaths and that all major complications were related to neurological ischemic injury. This problem remains a principal one with carotid arterial reconstruction, but it is difficult to correlate it with technical results of the repair. Because of the rich blood supply of the neck, infection is seldom seen.

Although thrombosis of the carotid artery repair could lead to late cerebral infarction, four patients seen at Walter Reed General Hospital with occlusion of the reconstructed artery had no neurological defects. An arch arteriogram is the best means of determining whether an arterial repair has failed if pulses cannot be felt.

A separate question is the importance of residual stenosis after an arterial repair, which is probably not significant unless more than 80 percent of the lumen is occluded. Two patients seen at Walter Reed General Hospital after carotid repair had audible high-pitched carotid artery bruits but remained asymptomatic. In a patient who after a gunshot wound had an end-to-end anastomosis of the common carotid to the internal carotid artery with the use of an internal shunt, vague dizziness developed. An arch arteriogram showed marked-stenoses. Elective reconstruction with a vein graft was performed with success.

After lateral repair of the common carotid artery complications are frequent. Buchman and associates (1972) reported a patient at Valley Forge General Hospital with an arteriovenous false aneurysm which had developed after a lateral repair. A patient who returned to Walter Reed General Hospital was found to have thrombosis of the right common carotid artery after a lateral repair had been performed with an autogenous venous patch graft.

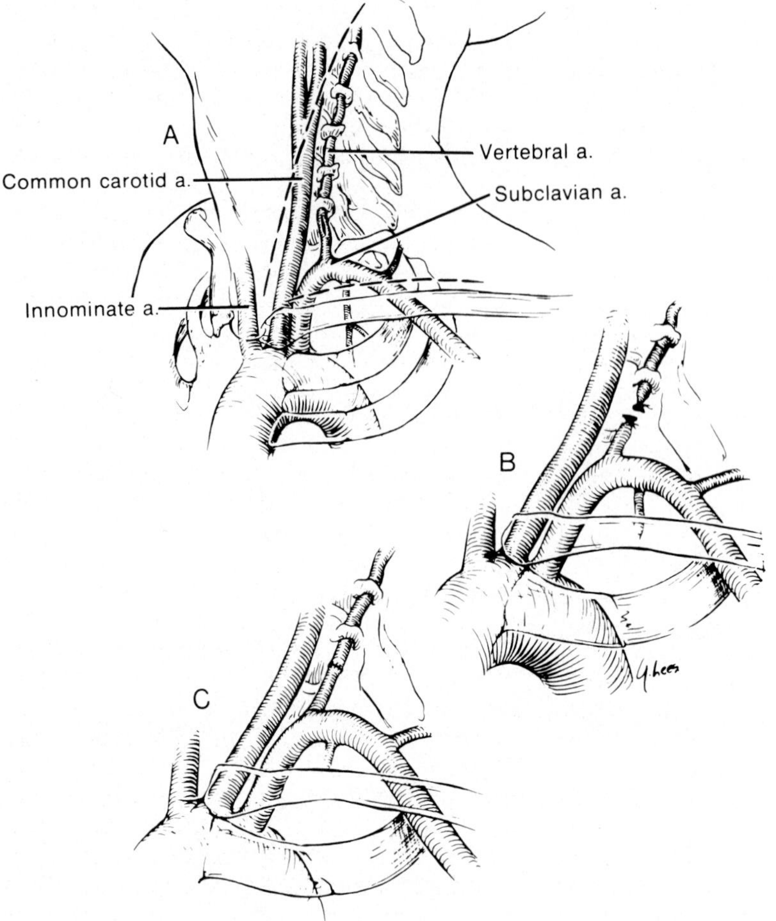

Figure 24–2. Laceration of the proximal left vertebral artery and its management either by end-to-end anastomosis or ligation. From Rich, N.M., and Spencer, F.C.: *Vascular Trauma.* W.B. Saunders, Philadelphia, Pennsylvania, 1978.

RESULTS

Makins (1919) reported a neurological deficit rate of 30 percent involving 128 carotid arterial injuries among British troops. Lawrence and co-workers (1948) reported a 47 percent mortality rate among 17 Americans wounded in World War II, including one case in whom lateral suture was successfully used and another case with an unsuccessful anastomosis and thrombosis of a Blakemore tube. DeBakey and Simeone (1946) recorded a 30 percent morbidity rate (three of ten patients who had cerebral complications) in their review of 2,471 American casualties in World War II who had acute arterial injuries. Summarizing the entire experience from the Korean conflict, Hughes (1958) recorded only four carotid arterial repairs among 11 injuries. The repairs included two by lateral suture, one end-to-end anastomosis, and one with an autogenous vein graft. Five patients with pulsating hematomas or arteriovenous fistulas did not require emergency surgery and were evacuated to be operated upon at a later time. Two patients were treated by ligation with resulting hemiplegia.

In the early Vietnam experience, lateral suture was used in 19 repairs, and was the method most often employed (Rich *et al.*, 1970a). End-to-end anastomosis and autogenous vein grafts were used with almost equal frequency. Only three patients were treated by arterial ligation. Four of the vein grafts were known to have thrombosed. In a series of 85 carotid arterial injuries, including both Vietnamese and American casualties, Cohen and associates (1970) reported a mortality rate of 15 percent among 82 patients. This mortality was only 6 percent if death from associated injuries was excluded. Eight of the 82 patients had neurological deficits on admission. In two it later cleared completely, in two it became worse, one remained unchanged, and three died after arterial repair.

I have reported the cases of seven patients seen at Walter Reed General Hospital with complications after carotid arterial repair in Vietnam, including one infection, four thromboses, and two stenoses. In most of these patients there were no significant neurological sequelae which could be related to inadequate arterial reconstruction (see Table 24-2).

Beall and coauthors (1963), reporting a relatively large civilian series, performed definitive operations in 22 of 25 patients with carotid arterial trauma. Three died before definitive surgery could be performed. The overall mortality was 20 percent, but only two of the 22 patients died after repair of the carotid artery, a mortality rate of 9 percent. Both deaths were related to cerebral damage already evident at the time of admission. Among the 20 long-term survivors, 16 remained asymptomatic. Neurological deficits were seen after operation in four patients; hemiplegia in one patient was already present before operation and remained unchanged. Hemiparesis followed operation in the other three patients. In the three patients who had neurological injury during reconstruction, thrombosis of the anastomosis occurred in one. In another, the common carotid artery was occluded for 70 minutes during reconstruction.

In the combined review of 722 cases by Unger and colleagues (1980), the overall mortality rate was 21 percent. Of these patients, 186 presented with severe neurological deficits. Arterial repair in that group resulted in 34 percent improvement in contrast to 14 percent improvement after ligation of the carotid artery or total absence of surgical treatment. Shock or coma, independently, were significantly ominous. The investigators determined, however, that there was no evidence to show that coma is a contraindication to restoring arterial continuity. They also determined that in patients with preoperative neurological deficits, no data could be found to substantiate the contention that prompt arterial repair would yield better results than delayed repair.

Table 24-2. Management of Carotid Arterial Injuries (Vietnam Vascular Registry)

METHOD	NUMBER	(%)
Lateral Suture	19	38
Autogenous Vein Graft	14	28
End-to-end Anastomosis	11	22
Miscellaneous	6	10
Totals	50	(100)

Source: Rich, N.M.; Baugh, J.H.; and Hughes, C.W.: Acute arterial injuries in Vietnam: 1,000 cases. *J. Trauma,* **10**:359, 1970*a*.

In general, the results of treatment of carotid arterial occlusions secondary to nonpenetrating trauma are poor. In the review by Yamada and associates in 1967, 21 patients were operated upon; three died, 12 remained with a serious neurological deficit, three had moderate residual deficits, and only four were asymptomatic. Of 31 patients not operated upon, 17 died, and 14 remained with severe deficits. The overall mortality was approximately 40 percent and a severe neurological residual damage occurred in 52 percent of patients. In the report by Towne *et al.* (1972) two of three patients operated upon died, and the third did not improve. The fourth patient, who was treated nonoperatively, recovered without neurological residuals.

Again, it should be emphasized that the sequelae of managing vertebral arterial injuries is usually minimal. Most of the reported cases provide only anecdotal information.

FOLLOW UP

Buchman and colleagues (1972) reported 15 patients seen at Valley Forge General Hospital over a six-year period after carotid arterial injuries in Vietnam. Thirteen patients had carotid arterial reconstruction; there were good immediate results in nine. Two who were hemiparetic before arterial reconstruction continued with similar neurological deficits afterward. Additional operations were required in five of the 15 patients, including two aorto-carotid bypasses, one thrombectomy, one closure of an arteriovenous fistula, and one ligation of the internal carotid artery. Both patients treated with bypass had complained of dizziness, and one had had recurrent syncope. Both became asymptomatic after reconstruction. Twelve of the 13 patients eventually had a good result, excluding the two patients who were hemiparetic immediately after injury.

Among the early follow-up reviews, Haller (1962) obtained a retrograde aortic arch study which revealed patent common carotid arteries one month after bilateral carotid arterial repair by end-to-end anastomoses approximately 1 in proximal to each carotid bifurcation. The patient was able to return to work as a heavy laborer approximately six weeks after injury and had had no subsequent difficulty up to the time of the report. An unusual complication of carotid arterial reconstruction was reported by Carrasquilla and Weaver (1972), who found aneurysmal dilation of a saphenous vein graft which had been used to repair the common carotid artery in a Vietnam casualty. Another unusual case also involved a Vietnam casualty in whom multiple repairs had been attempted by lateral suture of the innominate artery. Thrombosis ensued, and there was reversal of flow in both the right common carotid artery and the right vertebral artery. The patient was dizzy and could not work. Restoration of anterograde arterial flow through both the common carotid and vertebral arteries on the patient's right side was possible with an aorto-innominate bypass.

Unger and associates (1980) in their review of 703 patients with carotid arterial trauma emphasized that follow-up status at one year was available for only 40 cases from the entire literature. They added 19 cases from their own experience with a mean of 4.6 years' follow up after injury which uncovered multiple, persistent neurological defects, one stenotic arterial repair, two aneurysms, and an arteriovenous fistula. It is obvious that further efforts must be made to provide long-term follow up along with efforts to solve the problems of managing these difficult injuries.

REFERENCES

Beall, A.C.; Shirkey, A.L.; and DeBakey, M.E.: Penetrating wounds of the carotid arteries. *J. Trauma,* **3**:276–87, 1963.

Buchman, R.J.; Thomas, P.A., Jr.; and Park, B.: Carotid artery injuries—follow-up of 15 patients treated in Vietnam. *Angiology,* **23**:97–102, 1972.

Carrasquilla, C., and Weaver, A.W.: Aneurysm of the saphenous graft to the common carotid artery. *Vasc. Surg.,* **6**:66–68, 1972.

Cohen, A.; Brief, D.; and Mathewson, C., Jr.: Carotid artery injuries: an analysis of 85 cases. *Am. J. Surg.,* **120**:210–214, 1970.

Cooper, E.S.: Aneurysm of the right carotid and subclavian arteries. *Am. J. Med. Sci.,* **38**:398, 1859.

DeBakey, M.E., and Simeone, F.A.: Battle injuries of arteries in World War II: an analysis of 2,471 cases. *Ann. Surg.,* **123**:534–79, 1946.

Ferguson, I.A., Sr.; Byrd, W.M.; and McAfee, D.K.: Experiences in the management of arterial injuries. *Ann. Surg.,* **153**:980–86, 1961.

Fleming, J.F.R., and Petrie, D.: Traumatic thrombosis of the internal carotid artery with delayed hemiplegia. *Can. J. Surg.,* **11**:166–72, 1968.

Ford, F.R., and Clark, D.: Thrombosis of the basilar artery with softenings in the cerebellum and brain stem due to manipulation of the neck—a report of two cases with one post-mortem examination. Reasons are given to prove that damage to the vertebral arteries is responsible. *Bull. Johns Hopkins Hosp.,* **98**:37–42, 1956.

Gurdjian, E.S.; Hardy, W.; Lindner, D.W.; and Thomas, L.M.: Closed cervical cranial trauma associated with involvement of carotid and vertebral arteries. *J. Neurosurg.,* **20**:418–27, 1963.

Haller, J.A.: Bullet transection of both carotid arteries with immediate repair and survival.. *Am. J. Surg.,* **103**:532–35, 1962.

Hockaday, T.D.R.: Traumatic thrombosis of the internal carotid artery. *J. Neurol. Neurosurg. Psychiatry,* **22**:229–31, 1959.

Hughes, C.W.: Arterial repair during the Korean War. *Ann. Surg.,* **147**:555, 1958.

Hunt, J.L., and Snyder, W.H.: Late false aneurysms of the carotid artery: repair with extraintracranial arterial bypass. *J. Trauma,* **19**:198–200, 1979.

Javid, H.: Vascular injuries of the neck. *Clin. Orthop.,* **28**:70–78, 1963.

Jernigan, W.R., and Gardner, W.C.: Carotid artery injuries due to closed cervical trauma. *J. Trauma,* **11**:429–35, 1971.

Lai, M.D.; Hoffman, H.B.; and Adamkiewicz, J.J.: Dissecting aneurysms of internal carotid artery after nonpenetrating neck injury. *Acta Radiol. Diag. (Stockh.),* **5**:290–95, 1966.

Lawrence, K.B.; Shefts, L.M.; and McDaniel, J.R.: Wounds of common carotid arteries: report of 17 cases from World War II. *Am. J. Surg.,* **76**:29–37, 1948.

Ledgerwood, A.M.; Mullins, R.J.; and Lucas, C.E.: Primary repair vs. ligation for carotid artery injuries. *Arch. Surg.,* **115**:488–93, 1980.

Makins, G.H.: *Gunshot Injuries to the Blood Vessels.* John Wright and Sons, Bristol, England, 1919.

Mandelbaum, I., and Kalsbeck, J.E.: Extrinsic compression of internal carotid artery. *Ann. Surg.,* **171**:434–37, 1970.

Matas, R.: Traumatisms and traumatic aneurysms of the vertebral artery and their surgical treatment with report of a cured case. *Ann. Surg.,* **18**:477, 1893.

Monson, D.P.; Saletta, J.D.; and Freeark, R.J.: Carotid-vertebral trauma. *J. Trauma,* **9**:987–99, 1969.

Morris G.C., Jr.; Beall, A.C., Jr.; Roof, W.R.; and DeBakey, M.E.: Surgical experience with 220 acute arterial injuries in civilian practice. *Am. J. Surg.,* **99**:775–81, 1960.

Murray, D.S.: Post-traumatic thrombosis of the internal carotid and vertebral arteries after non-penetrating injuries of the neck. *Br. J. Surg.,* **44**:556–61, 1957.

Perry, M.D.; Thal, E.R.; and Shires, G.T.: Management of arterial injuries. *Ann. Surg.,* **173**:403–408, 1971.

Rich, N.M., and Spencer, F.C.: *Vascular Trauma.* W.B. Saunders, Philadelphia, Pennsylvania, 1978.

Rich, N.M.; Baugh, J.H.; and Hughes, C.W.: Acute arterial injuries in Vietnam: 1,000 cases. *J. Trauma,* **10**:350–69, 1970a.

Rich, N.M.; Baugh, J.H.; and Hughes, C.W.: The significance of complications associated with vascular repairs performed in Vietnam. *Arch. Surg.,* **100**:646–51, 1970b.

Rich, N.M.; Collins, G.J., Jr.; and Anderson, C.A.: Carotid arterial trauma, unpublished data. Presented at the 24th Scientific Meeting of the International Cardiovascular Society (North American Chapter), June 19, 1976, Albuquerque, N. M.

Rich, N.M.; Hobson, R.W. II; and Collins, C.J., Jr.: Elective vascular reconstruction following trauma. *Am. J. Surg.*, **130**:712–19, 1975a.

Rich, N.M.; Hobson, R.W. II; and Collins, C.J., Jr.: Traumatic arteriovenous fistulas and false aneurysms: a review of 558 lesions. *Surgery,* **78:** 817–28, 1975b.

Thal, E.R.; Snyder, M.H., III; Hayes, R.J.; and Perry, M.O.: Management of carotid artery injuries. *Surgery,* **76**:955–62, 1974.

Towne, J.B.; Delbert, D.N.; and Smith, J.W.: Thrombosis of the internal carotid artery following blunt cervical trauma. *Arch. Surg.*, **104**:565–68, 1972.

Unger, S.E.; Tucker, W.S.; Medeza, A.N.; Wellons, H.A.; and Chandler, J.G.: Carotid arterial trauma. *Surgery,* **87**:477–87, 1980.

Yamada, S.; Kindt, G.W.; and Youmans, J.R.: Carotid artery occlusion due to nonpenetrating trauma. *J. Trauma,* **7**:333–42, 1967.

Zelenock, G.B.; Kazmers, A.; Whitehouse, W.M.; Graham, L.M.; Erlandson, E.E.; Cronenwett, J.L.; Lindenauer, S.M.; and Stanley, J.C.: Extracranial internal carotid artery dissections: noniatrogenic traumatic lesions. *Arch. Surg.*, **117**:425–32, 1982.

25

Aneurysms and Dissecting Aneurysms of the Cervical Carotid Artery

FRANCIS ROBICSEK

ANEURYSMS OF THE CERVICAL CAROTID ARTERIES

Aneurysms of the extracranial carotid arteries are infrequent in comparison to the occurrence of occlusive or ulcerative carotid lesions or to the total number of aneurysms of other parts of the arterial system. Houser and Baker (1968) found the incidence of aneurysms of the extracranial carotid artery to be about eight in every 5,000 angiograms. Despite this relative rarity of cervical carotid aneurysms, most vascular surgeons have the opportunity to operate on a few during their professional careers, and when they do, they may be faced with some particular problems.

Etiology

The etiology of cervical carotid aneurysms is similar to that of aneurysms of other vessels, with arteriosclerosis the primary cause in up to 75 percent of all cases. The second most common cause is trauma, either closed or penetrating. Winslow (1926), reviewing 106 carotid aneurysms, found 26 to be of traumatic origin. Less frequent causes are congenital defects, Marfan's syndrome, and fibromuscular dysplasia. Carotid aneurysms have also been reported after radiation, angiography, and carotid reconstruction. Before the era of antibiotics many resulted from local cervical or pharyngeal infections. Severe hypertension occurs in approximately 62 percent of the patients and may be a contributing factor (Rhodes *et al.,* 1976).

Types of Cervical Carotid Aneurysms

The most common sites for extracranial carotid aneurysm are the common carotid artery and its bifurcation. Aneurysms of the common carotid artery are twice as frequent as those of the cervical internal or external carotid arteries (Coleman and Kittle, 1973).

The review of the cases reported show three anatomical types of cervical carotid aneurysms. The most common type is fusiform, usually arteriosclerotic in origin, which occurs with about equal frequency on the internal and common carotid arteries. Saccular aneurysms are less frequent and are usually caused either by infection or by trauma, about half of them being mycotic. Others are associated with fibroelastic dysplasia or are congenital. The third type is diffuse enlargement of the carotid sinus, which occurs mainly in hypertensive patients. Despite many similarities, there are also features that may distinguish cervical carotid aneurysms from other peripheral artery aneurysms, primarily those of the femoropopliteal region. The male-to-female ratio of carotid artery aneurysms is 2.5 to 1 in Zwolak's series (Zwolak *et al.,* 1984), which is distinctly lower than the 30 to 1 male-to-female ratio associated with femoral and popliteal arteries (Graham *et al.,* 1980). Another difference between cervical carotid aneurysms and other peripheral artery aneurysms is that only 15 percent of bilateral lesions occur in the neck (Bole *et al.*, 1978), whereas 60 to 90 percent of the aneurysms in the femoral and popliteal arteries occur bilaterally (Graham *et al.*, 1980).

False aneurysm of the carotid artery is sometimes caused by nonsurgical trauma (See also Chapter 24 on carotid trauma), but it also occurs as a complication of carotid endarterectomy (Ehrenfeld and Hays, 1972). In an overwhelming number of cases the development of postoperative aneurysms can be traced to the technique of the suturing and to the suture material itself rather than to the weakness of the residual arterial wall, which, even though paper-thin, if properly treated will be able to contain the pressure of circulating blood. Patch grafts, particularly patch grafts sewed in with silk, are especially thought to predispose to postoperative false aneurysm formation. Since the introduction of nonabsorbable suture materials, postendarterectomy carotid aneurysms have been seen only rarely, and if they do occur, they usually develop from communicating postoperative hematomas or are caused by infection.

Diagnosis

Because of the relatively superficial course of the cervical carotid arteries, the presence of a carotid aneurysm usually becomes apparent early, diagnosed simply by observing or feeling an expansively pulsating tumor on the neck. Aneurysms of the internal carotid artery can sometimes be palpated best from inside the pharynx. Despite easy recognition, aneurysms of the carotid artery are occasionally misdiagnosed and have been incised as peritonsillar abscesses with fatal outcome; others have been biopsied as inflammatory or neoplastic masses, causing alarming hemorrhage.

In the differential diagnosis of pulsating cervical masses, elongated and buckled carotid arteries, carotid body tumors, and lymph nodes closely attached to the carotid arteries need to be considered and sometimes can be differentiated only by angiography (see Fig. 9–26). Angiography is recommended even if the diagnosis of aneurysm is equivocal because it may not only detect unsuspected associated pathology of the involved carotid artery, such as atherosclerotic stricture, occlusion, or multiple aneurysm formation involving the intracranial portion, but also supply valuable data on the status of the contralateral carotid artery and the interhemispheric collateral circulation, information important to the operative planning.

Symptoms

Although some carotid aneurysms remain asymptomatic except for the presence of a palpable mass and/or a bruit, others produce symptoms early in their course. Compression upon neighboring structures may cause hoarseness, atrophy of the sternocleidomastoid muscle, hemiatrophy of the tongue with deviation on protrusion, and Horner's syndrome. About half of the patients present with cerebral or eye symptoms owing to embolization of fibrinoplatelet clots or red thrombus commonly lining the interior of the dilated segment (McEntyre *et al.*, 1967). Cerebral ischemia may also develop because of thrombotic occlusion of the aneurysm itself. In Zwolak's series (Zwolak *et al.*, 1984), amaurosis fugax was present in 33 percent of patients, hemispheric transient attacks in 21 percent, and stroke in 8 percent. Nonspecific symptoms, such as headache and dizziness, were associated with 17 percent of the cases, and only 33 percent presented with asymptomatic cervical masses. Although rupture and hemorrhage are infrequent, aneurysms of both the internal and the external carotid arteries have been reported to burst and cause contained hematoma in the neck (Kaupp *et al.*, 1972), bleeding into the pharynx, or to hemorrhage into either the external auditory canal or through the eustachian tube into the nose (Busby *et al.*, 1968).

Treatment

The fate of most cases of nonoperated carotid aneurysm is dismal. About 50 percent of the patients with untreated aneurysm end with strokes (Zwolak *et al.*, 1984). In the series of 35 nonoperated patients collected by Winslow (1926), there were only three "cures," probably owing to spontaneous thrombosis, and 25 died from the effects of the aneurysms.

The various operations recommended for the treatment of cervical internal or common carotid aneurysms can be grouped as follows:

Procedures that do not restore carotid blood flow:

1. Proximal ligation
2. Proximal and distal ligation (with or without excision)

3. Staged occlusion using gradually occluding clamps or partial ligatures

Operations that promote collateral blood flow to the ipsilateral hemisphere after occlusion of the carotid artery:

1. Cervical sympathectomy after occlusion or excision of the carotid aneurysm
2. End-to-end anastomosis between the distal stumps of the external and internal carotid arteries—Conley procedure (Conley, 1965)

Operations that either preserve or restore carotid flow:

1. Endoaneurysmorrhaphy
2. Wall reinforcement with or without partial resection
3. Excision with primary anastomosis
4. Anastomosis of the ipsilateral proximal external to the distal internal carotid after excision of the aneurysm
5. Proximal and distal ligation with bypass graft
6. Excision and graft replacement

Until the early 1950s, ligation with or without concomitant cervical sympathectomy or ganglionectomy remained the preferred treatment. Because this approach resulted in hemiplegia in 15 to 25 percent of patients, procedures with permanent interruption of the carotid flow are now performed only under the most unusual circumstances, and the generally accepted method of extracranial carotid aneurysm has become resection with arterial reconstruction (Bole *et al.*, 1978). Exceptions to this rule may be patients with asymptomatic chronically occluded aneurysms or those in whom the aneurysmal dilatation, and thus the ligation, involves only the external carotid artery, and whose ipsilateral internal carotid is normal. Surgical treatment of carotid aneurysms once also included aneurysmorrhaphy, a procedure rarely applied today, though it may be considered for a smooth-walled fusiform aneurysm.

The exposure of the carotid aneurysm is by and large identical to the surgical approach described for carotid endarterectomy. Depending on the size of the aneurysm, however, it may need to be more extensive than exposure for endarterectomy. Occasionally a very proximal common carotid aneurysm may necessitate resection of the clavicle or exposure of either the innominate artery or the aortic arch. Because many aneurysms contain clot that may not show on angiograms, careless handling before crossclamping can easily cause distal embolization.

The operative procedure for saccular aneurysm with a narrow neck is resection with primary closure (see Figure 25–1A). If the neck of

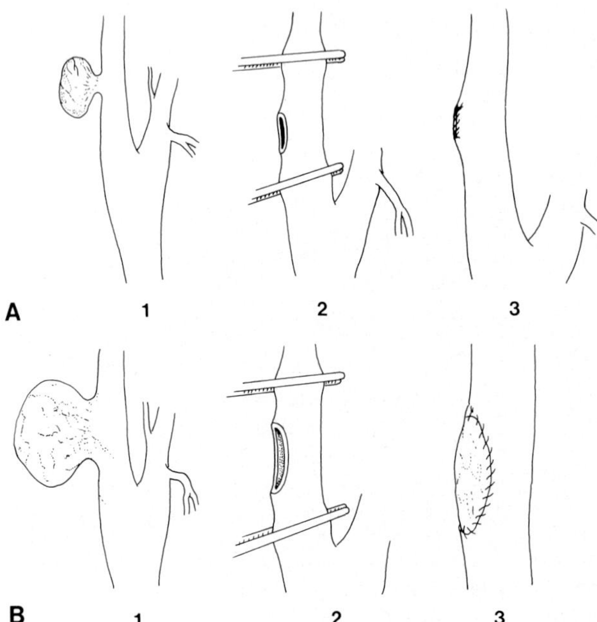

Figure 25–1. Surgical management of relatively small saccular aneurysms of the internal carotid artery by resection (*A*), and by lateral suture and patch angioplasty (*B*).

the aneurysm is wide, it is preferable to close the site of the resection with a patch to provide a more reliable suture line and at the same time to prevent narrowing (see Figure 25-1B). The surgical treatment of large saccular or fusiform aneurysms necessarily includes resection of the involved carotid segment. If this segment is relatively short, end-to-end anastomosis can usually be achieved as a means of restoring carotid blood flow, especially if the course of the carotid artery is tortuous. An additional length may be obtained by extensive mobilization and by division of the external carotid artery (see Figures 25-2, 25-3, and 25-4A).

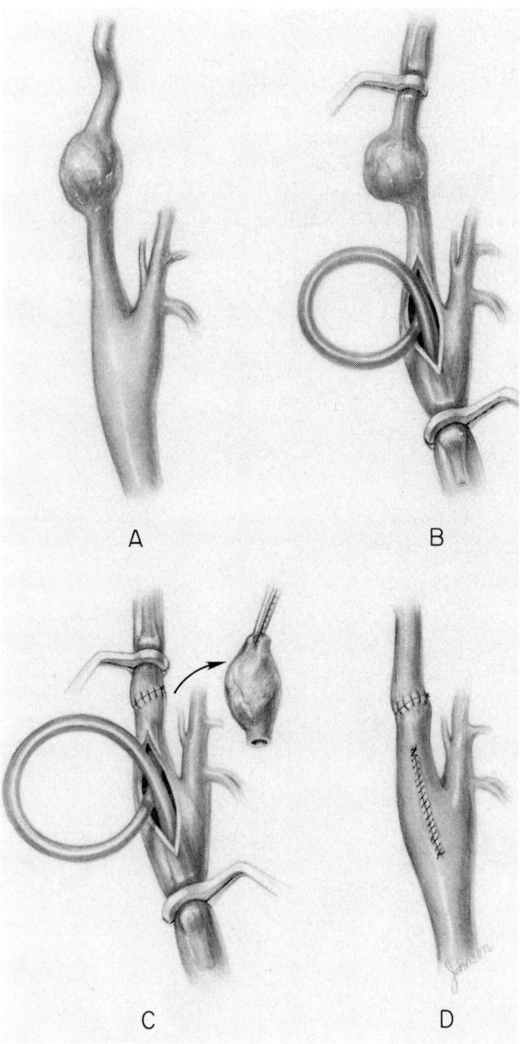

Figure 25-2. Surgical management of internal carotid aneurysm by resection and end-to-end anastomosis under the protection of an indwelling shunt. The exposed aneurysm (*A*), insertion of the shunt (*B*), resection and end-to-end anastomosis (*C*), and the completed procedure (*D*).

If direct anastomosis is not feasible, the resected segment of the internal carotid artery should be replaced with a graft, preferably a segment of autogenous saphenous vein. If, for some reason, vein graft is not available or there is a significant discrepancy between the vein and the artery, synthetic vascular prostheses are acceptable alternatives. Because of its physical properties, which allow easier handling and the use of finer suture material, my preference is the Gore-Tex vascular prosthesis if the internal carotid artery needs to be replaced (see Figure 25-4B). In grafting of the common carotid artery, the choice of the prosthetic material matters very little.

Exposure of a very large or a very high carotid artery aneurysm may be difficult and may require the dismantling of the vertical ramus of the mandible. This can best be accomplished with a vertical osteotomy extending from the angle to the incision. The outward rotation of the posterior fragment combined with the anterior retraction of the mandible provides exposure of the internal carotid artery up to the bony foramen (Wylie, 1983). If this is not feasible, Krupski and associates (1983) recommend that if the stump pressure exceeds 65 mm Hg the carotid artery should simply be ligated. If the stump pressure is low, extraintracranial saphenous vein bypass should be considered, under the protection of which the cervical carotid aneurysm can be excised (Hunt and Snyder, 1979).

The "to-shunt or not-to-shunt" controversy discussed in previous chapters also emerges in the management of carotid artery aneurysms. Although the "shunters" recommend that all cervical carotid artery aneurysms be resected under the protection of temporary indwelling shunts, the results of other surgeons indicate that this not only is unnecessary but could even be harmful. In the series of Zwolak and associates (1984), all four strokes occurred in patients whose aneurysms were resected under the "protection" of indwelling shunts.

INFECTION

The management of mycotic aneurysms of the extracranial carotid arteries presents a particular problem. The damage may be inflicted by direct spread of the infection, septic emboli, or extraneous destructive processes such as tumorous invasion or radiation, the latter being the most common offender. In such cases

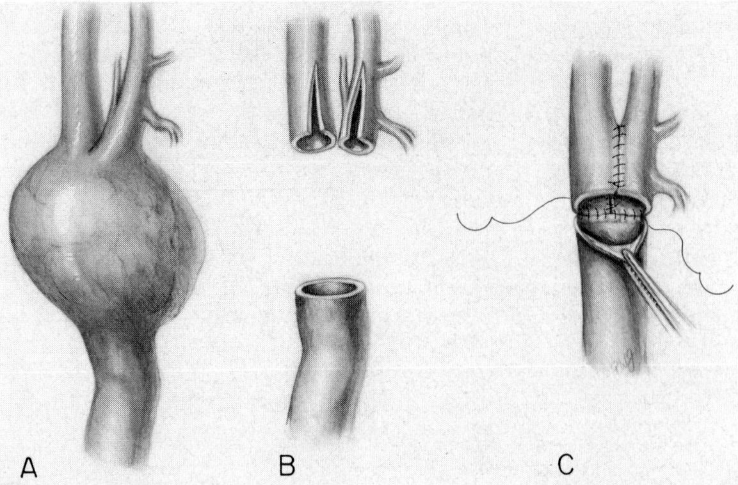

Figure 25–3. Treatment of fusiform aneurysm (*A*) of the carotid sinus by resection (*B*) and by reconstruction of the bifurcation by arterioplasty (*C*).

every effort should be made to restore carotid blood flow without insertion of a graft, preferably by direct anastomosis. This, however, should be performed only if the surgeon is satisfied that after all of the necrotic wall has been resected the arterial ends can be brought together without any tension on the suture line; otherwise, disruption of the anastomosis is virtually guaranteed. If grafting appears to be an absolute necessity, arterial (Stoney and Wylie,

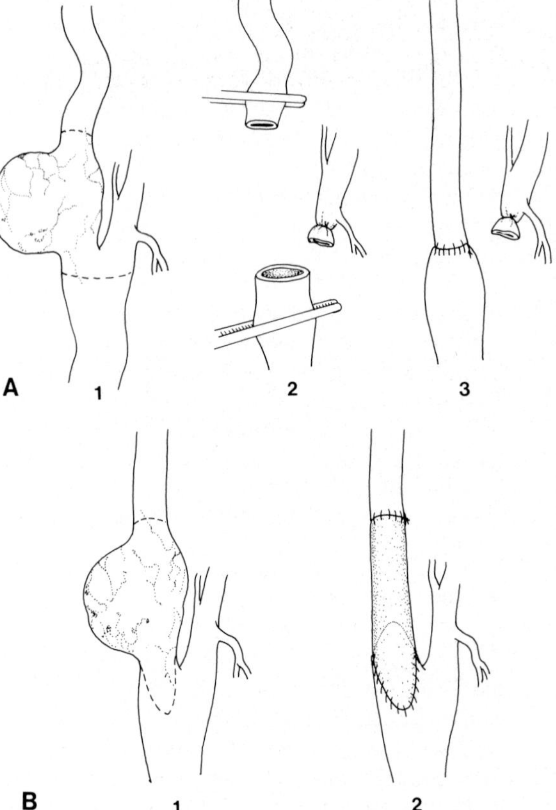

Figure 25–4. Aneurysm of the proximal internal carotid artery. Treatment with resection and end-to-end anastomosis between the internal and common carotid arteries (*A*) and by graft replacement (*B*).

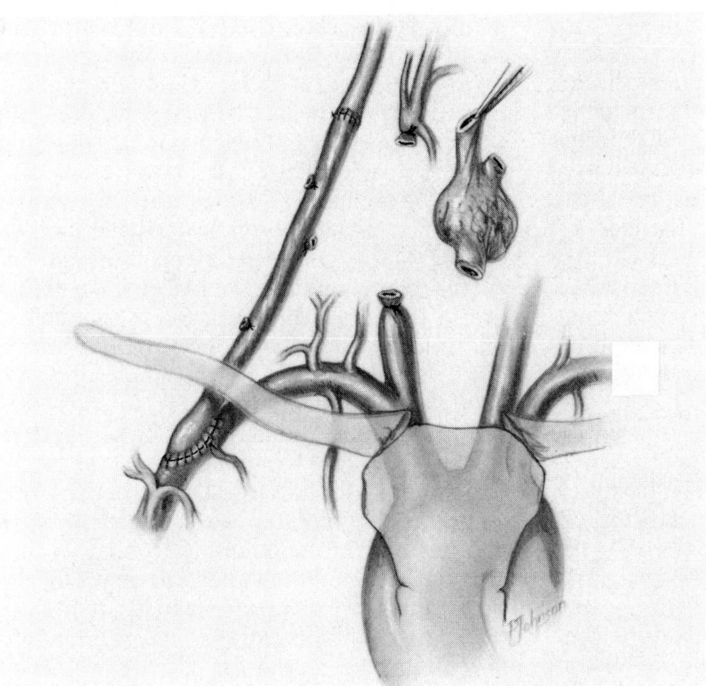

Figure 25–5. Restoration of blood flow after resection of a mycotic aneurysm of the carotid bifurcation using autogenous saphenous vein bypass graft between the axillary and internal carotid arteries.

1970) or saphenous vein (Conley, 1965) autografts should be utilized. If the infection appears to be especially virulent, or if skin necrosis or fistula is present, the stage is set for arterial disruption and hemorrhage (Wylie, 1983). In such patients any vascular procedure other than simple ligation should be avoided in the infected area because the infection may attack even autogenous saphenous veins as well as the suture lines. A preferred method is simply to excise the aneurysm, ligate the artery, carry the vein graft through an uninfected area, and perform extraanatomical bypass either between the two carotid bifurcations or between the cervical and intracerebral carotid arteries (see Figure 25–5). The same strategy should be used in cases of impending carotid artery rupture after radiation or in the course of radical neck dissection when neighboring tissues are infected and/or necrotic.

The results of operations performed for carotid aneurysm indicate that the risk is appreciably higher than in surgery for aneurysms of other peripheral vessels. This evidently reflects the special problems associated with carotid surgery (Kaupp, 1972). Nevertheless, despite the high rate of morbidity and mortality, because an aneurysm of the cervical carotid artery is such a significant threat to both life and health and the risk of nonoperative management is so forbiddingly high, surgery is almost invariably indicated.

DISSECTING ANEURYSMS OF THE CAROTID ARTERY

A dissecting aneurysm occurs when the bloodstream penetrates the arterial wall through an intimal tear and separates its layers. Because in most cases the widening of the artery is only moderate and may even be absent, the term dissecting aneurysm, is not entirely correct. The cleavage within the arterial wall may occur between the media and the intima or within the media itself. The process is usually self-perpetuating and may extend in either or both directions, usually downstream. The fate of the patient, if not operated upon, depends on the further course of the dissection; the false channel of the "double-barrel" vessel may cease expanding and reenter the true lumen, with the situation more or less stabilizing. In the unfavorable situation, however, the patient may develop acute distress either because of aneurysmal dilatation and rupture or, more frequently, because of interruption of the carotid blood flow caused by compression of the true lumen by expanding false channel (Robicsek and Guarino, 1985).

From an anatomical point of view, dissecting aneurysms of the extracranial carotid arteries may be divided into two principal groups: (1) dissections limited to the carotids and (2) those originating in the aortic arch.

A localized dissection of the carotid artery may be either spontaneous or induced by trauma. A patient with spontaneous dissection of the cervical carotid artery was first described by Anderson and Schechter (1959). Since then, such cases have been reported with increasing frequency, a number of them associated with fibromuscular dysplasia.

Traumatic dissections may be caused by blunt injury to the neck, surgical instrumentation, or invasive diagnostic studies (Robicsek *et al.*, 1967). Localized dissections of the carotid artery and intramural hematomas were especially common in the 1960s and early 1970s, when most carotid angiograms were performed by the direct needle-puncture technique and were frequently complicated by intramural injection of contrast material. In dissection of the carotid associated with aortic arch dissecting aneurysm, the primary site is invariably the aorta.

The management of carotid dissection depends on its location, extent, and symptoms. Acute localized asymptomatic dissections, especially those caused by invasive diagnostic procedures, can be handled conservatively unless they severely encroach upon the carotid lumen. Most localized cases, however, present as acute vascular occlusions, and they should be treated as such with immediate surgery, preferably by complete excision of the involved segment and graft replacement (see Figure 25–6). Similarly, because of the possibility of sudden thrombotic occlusion, chronic cases, symptomatic or not, should be operated upon. A dissenting opinion to this was sounded by Krupski and associates (1983), in whose series of 14 patients there were eight documented failures of surgical repair; this compared unfavorably with 14 patients who had not undergone attempted arterial reconstruction, none of whom had neurological symptoms. They recommended, therefore, that surgical intervention on carotid artery dissection be reserved for patients who continue to have recurrent transient ischemic attacks. In contrast to the foregoing, we believe that surgery is indicated for every localized carotid artery dissection unless it appears to be

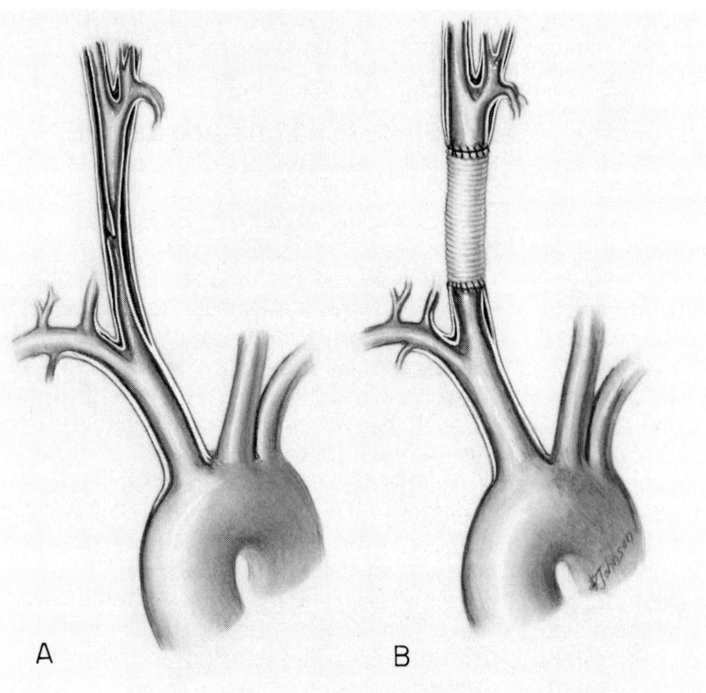

Figure 25–6. Dissecting aneurysm of the right carotid artery (*A*). Treatment with segmental resection and graft replacement (*B*).

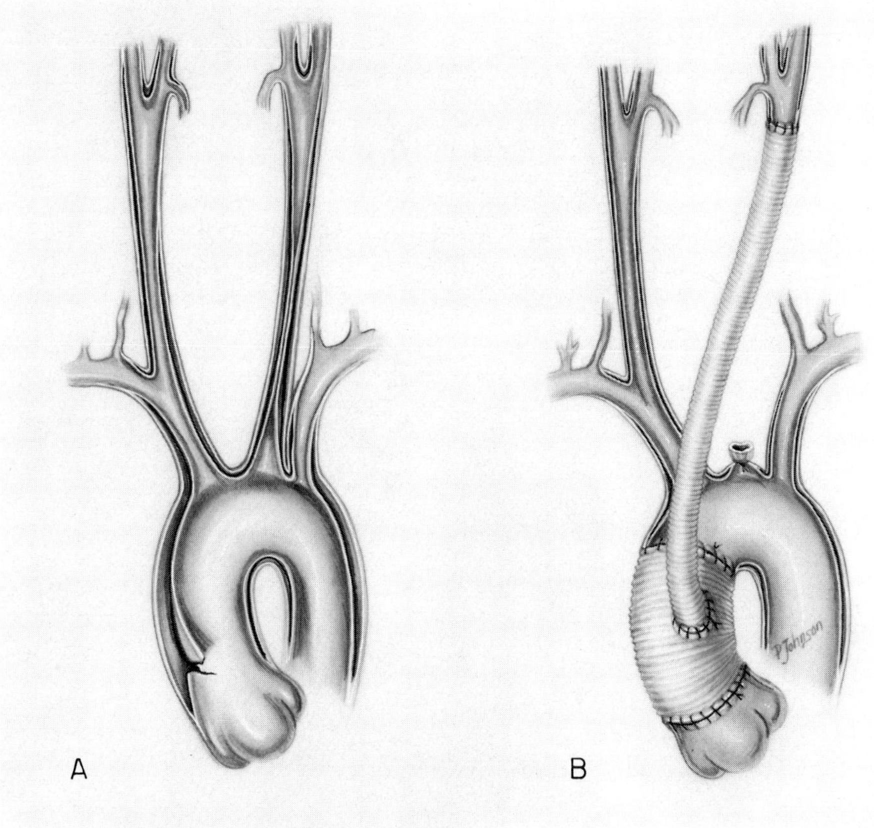

Figure 25–7. Dissecting aneurysm of the aortic arch causing occlusion of the left common carotid artery (*A*). Treatment with graft replacement of the ascending aorta and grafting of the left common carotid artery (*B*).

trivial, especially if it has been caused by instrumentation and the patient has no ischemic symptoms.

The situation is different if the dissection of the carotid artery is due to extension of a dissecting aneurysm of the aortic arch. In such cases, the dissection should be attacked at its source, i.e., the aorta, rather than by surgery on the carotid artery itself. Redirection of the flow from the false to the true lumen in the aorta will usually restore free circulation through its tributaries, including the carotid arteries.

There are, however, certain exceptions to this practice. One such exception occurs when an otherwise seemingly successful repair of aortic dissection fails to correct the obstruction of the blood flow in one or both carotid arteries. If this condition is recognized while the chest is still open, a sidearm should be brought out of the aortic graft and anastomosed end-to-end to the bifurcation of the involved carotid artery (see Figure 25–7). If, however, carotid occlusion develops or is recognized only after the aortic operation is over, the involved carotid artery should be explored in the neck and the situation remedied by a local "reentry" procedure. In the course of such an operation, the intimal tube is divided, a portion of the proximal intima is resected, and the distal intima is circumferentially tacked to the remainder of the arterial wall (see Figure 25–8). If the circulation through the other branches of the aortic arch appears to be normal, one can also consider the insertion of a subclavian carotid bypass graft, the distal end of which should be anastomosed to the divided peripheral stump of the carotid artery.

Another situation in which direct correction of a carotid artery occlusion owing to aortic dissection is considered arises when the primary presenting signs are those of severe brain ischemia that needs to be resolved before the aorta itself can be repaired. A bold approach to correcting such a situation was applied by

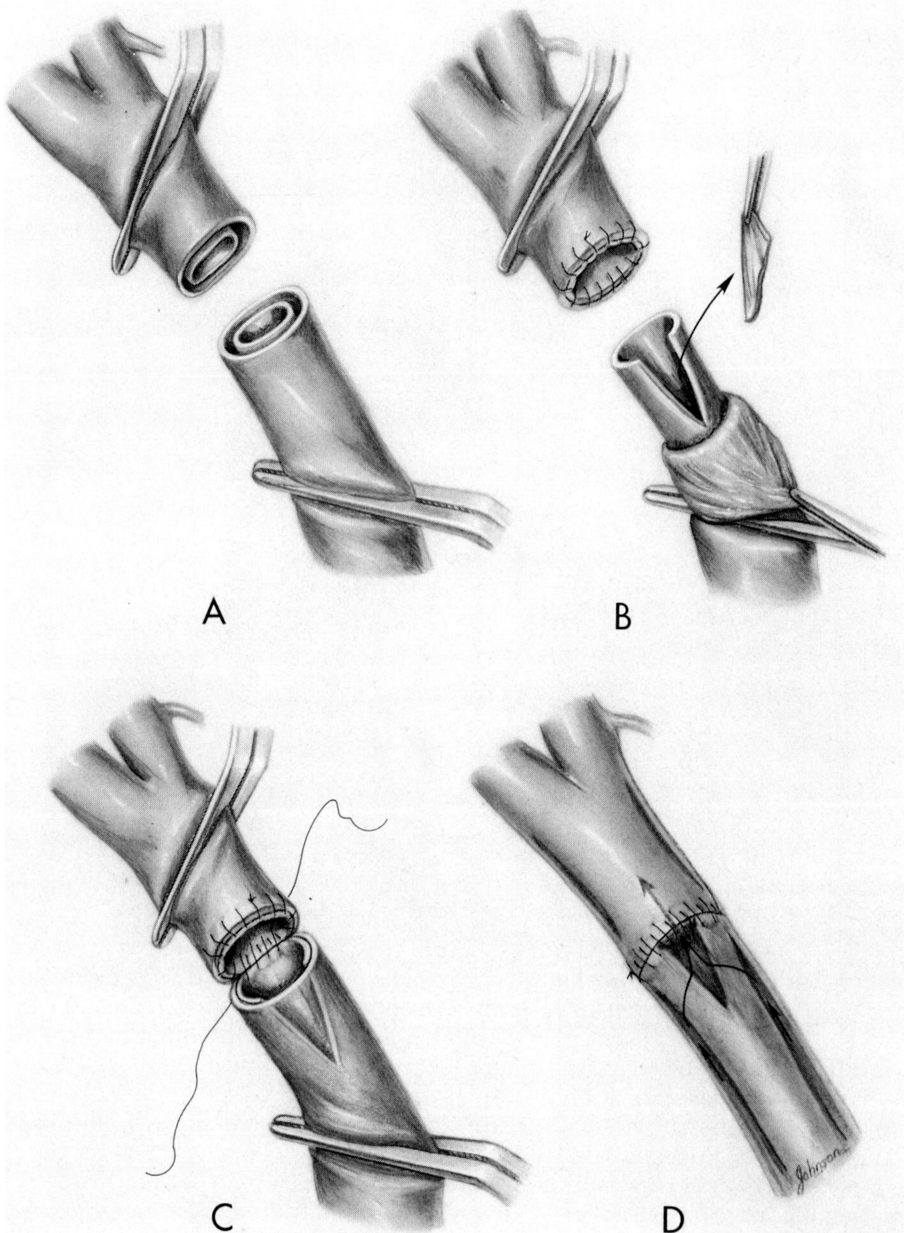

Figure 25–8. Carotid reentry procedure. Division of the dissected artery (*A*), closure of the distal portion of the false channel and removal of a wedge-shaped portion of the proximal intima (*B*), end-to-end anastomosis (*C*), and the completed procedure (*D*).

Borst (personal communication, 1984). He successfully brought a graft in a comatose young man from the uninvolved ipsilateral femoral artery to his common carotid, which was occluded by dissection, before repair of the aortic dissection itself was undertaken.

In conclusion, all patients with symptomatic dissecting aneurysms of the carotid artery require immediate surgical attention. If the dissection is confined to the carotid artery, it should be treated by resection of the involved segment and graft replacement. In cases in which the dissection originates in the aorta, attention should first be given to the source of the dissection, and if that does not restore carotid flow, a concomitant procedure should be performed on the carotid artery itself. At the present stage of vascular surgery it also appears advisable to consider resection and replacement in all dissecting aneurysms of the carotid artery even if the patient is asymptomatic. Exceptions to this are acute intramural hematomas caused by needle puncture in the course of direct angiography, if they do not significantly encroach upon the carotid lumen, and small asymptomatic intramural hematomas that do not occlude the lumen by more than 50 percent. These cases may be well handled by anticoagulant treatment.

REFERENCES

Anderson, R.M., and Schechter, M.M.: A case of spontaneous dissecting aneurysms of the internal carotid artery. *J. Neurosurg. Psychiatry,* **22:**195–201, 1959.

Bole, P.V.; Babu, S.; and Clauss, R.H.: Planned extra-anatomic cerebral revascularization for carotid artery ligation. *Surgery,* **83:**440–44, 1978.

Busby, D.R.; Slemmons, D.H.; and Miller, T.F., Jr.: Fatal epistaxis via carotid aneurysm and eustachian tube. *Arch. Otolaryngol.,* **87:**295–98, 1968.

Coleman, P.G., and Kittle, C.F.: Aneurysms of the common carotid artery. *Surg. Clin. North Am.,* **53:**231–40, 1973.

Conley, J.J.: The carotid body tumor: a review of 29 cases. *Arch. Otolaryngol.,* **81:**187–93, 1965.

Ehrenfeld, W.K., and Hays, R.J.: False aneurysm after carotid endarterectomy. *Arch. Surg.,* **104:**288–91, 1972.

Graham, L.M.; Zelenock, G.B.; Whitehouse, W., Jr.; Erlandson, E.E.; Dent, T.L.; Lindenauer, S.M.; and Stanley, J.C.: Clinical significance of arteriosclerotic femoral artery aneurysms. *Arch. Surg.,* **115:**502–7, 1980.

Houser, O.W., and Baker, H.L.: Fibrovascular dysplasia and other uncommon diseases of the cervical carotid artery: angiographic aspects. *A.J.R.,* **104:**201–12, 1968.

Hunt, J.L., and Snyder, W.H.: Late false aneurysm of the carotid artery: repair with extra-intracranial arterial bypass. *J. Trauma,* **19:**198–200, 1979.

Kaupp, H.A.; Haid, S.P.; Jurayj, M.N.; Bergan, J.J.; and Trippel, O.H.: Aneurysms of the extracranial carotid artery. *Surgery,* **72:**946–51, 1972.

Krupski, W.C.; Effeney, D.J.; and Ehrenfeld, W.K.: Fibromuscular dysplasia, aneurysms and spontaneous dissection of the carotid artery. In Bergan, J.J., and Yao, J.S.T. (eds.): *Cerebrovascular Insufficiency.* Grune & Stratton, New York, 1983.

McEntyre, J.M.; Keates, E.; and Whitley, W.: Retinal embolus from extracranial carotid artery aneurysm. *Arch. Ophthalmol.,* **77:**317–19, 1967.

Rhodes, E.L.; Stanley, J.C.; Hoffman, G.L.; Croenwett, J.L.; and Fry, W.J.: *Arch. Surg.,* **111:**339–43, 1976.

Robicsek, F., and Guarino, R.L.: Compression of the true lumen by retrograde perfusion during repair of aortic dissection. *J. Cardiovasc. Surg. (Torino),* **26:**36–40, 1985.

Robicsek, F.; Daughtery, H.K.; Sanger, P.W.; and Gallucci, V.: Intermittent cerebrovascular insufficiency: a frequent and curable cause of stroke. *Coll. Works Cardiopulm. Dis.,* **13:**72–74, 1967.

Stoney, R.S., and Wylie, E.J.: Arterial autografts. *Surgery,* **67:**18–25, 1970.

Winslow, N.: Extracranial aneurysm of the internal carotid artery. *Arch. Surg.,* **13:**689–729, 1926.

Wylie, E.J.: Overview: minisymposium: unusual problems in carotid surgery. *Surgery,* **93:**297–98, 1983.

Zwolak, R.W.; Whitehouse, W.M.; Knake, J.E.; Bernfeld, B.D.; Zelenock, G.E.; *et al.:* Atherosclerotic extracranial carotid artery aneurysms. *J. Vasc. Surg.,* **1:**415–22, 1984.

26

Carotid Body Tumors and Hypersensitive Carotid Sinus Syndrome

FRANCIS ROBICSEK

The carotid body develops from the third branchial branch of the mesenchyma in close proximity to the third aortic arch, from which the carotid artery later evolves. Is is already recognizable in the six- to seven-week-old embryo. The fully developed carotid body lies between the medial and adventitial layer of the carotid bifurcation and is composed of chemoreceptor cells that are reactive to the oxygen and to carbon dioxide tension of the blood. When these receptor cells are stimulated by either hypoxia or hypercarbia, they evoke an increase in the rate and depth of ventilation via the efferent fibers of the glossopharyngeal nerve and the respiratory center of the medulla.

Tumors of the carotid body are relatively uncommon. Until 1973, only about 500 cases had been reported in the literature (Singhabhandhu *et al.*, 1973). The rate of occurrence of such tumors is about equal in both sexes, which contrasts with the preponderance of glomus jugulare tumors in women. Although the average patient with a carotid body tumor is in the fourth decade of life, it also has been found in the very young as well as in the very old. Familial occurrence of carotid body tumors has also been reported, almost a third of them being bilateral compared with only 5 percent bilateral occurrence of nonfamilial tumors (Singhabhandhu *et al.*, 1973).

On microscopic examination, the cells in the carotid body tumor are of epitheloid nature and are separated by a vascular stroma (see Figures 26 – 1 and 26 – 2). The three histologic types include (1) those apparently composed of normal carotid body cells, (2) the adenoid type, and (3) the angiomal-like pattern (LeCompte, 1948). Most carotid body tumors grow slowly; however, some expand rapidly and in some cases malignancy with metastasis does occur. The reported rate of malignancy varies from 5 to 50 percent (Pettet *et al.*, 1953). This wide range of difference reported by various investigators undoubtedly reflects their definition of malignancy, which for some is based only on the histologic appearance. Although all carotid body tumors can be considered potentially malignant, the degree of this potential cannot always be determined on the basis of histology. Metastases may occur by hemotologic spread as well as through the lymphatics. Even recurrence is not an absolute proof of malignancy because it can simply be the consequence of inadequate primary excision. In a series of 62 patients, only three tumors proved malignant by the presence of lymph node metastases (Rob, 1976). Currently, only a few pathologists would go so far as to state that the carotid tumor is malignant unless metastases are already evident.

Symptoms, if present, are usually caused by compression on adjacent structures and may consist of pain, difficulty in swallowing, hoarseness, stridor, Horner's syndrome, deviation of the tongue, headache, and carotid sinus hypersensitivity syndrome.

Diagnosis of the carotid body tumor is usually made by its location. A hard mass palpable at the level of the carotid bifurcation,

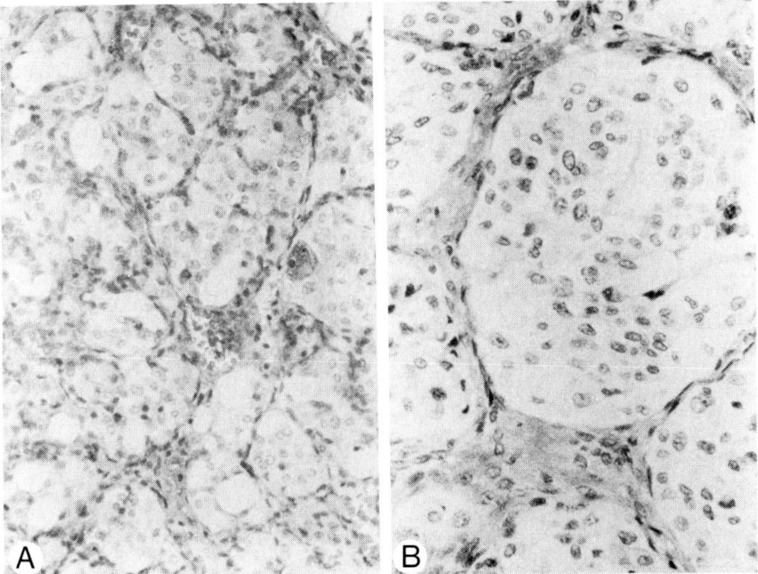

Figure 26–1. Histologic picture of a carotid body tumors shows a paraganglioma with prominent sinusoids and the well-circumscribed cell-nests (*A*). Note the granular and clear cytoplasm of the tumor cells (*B*).

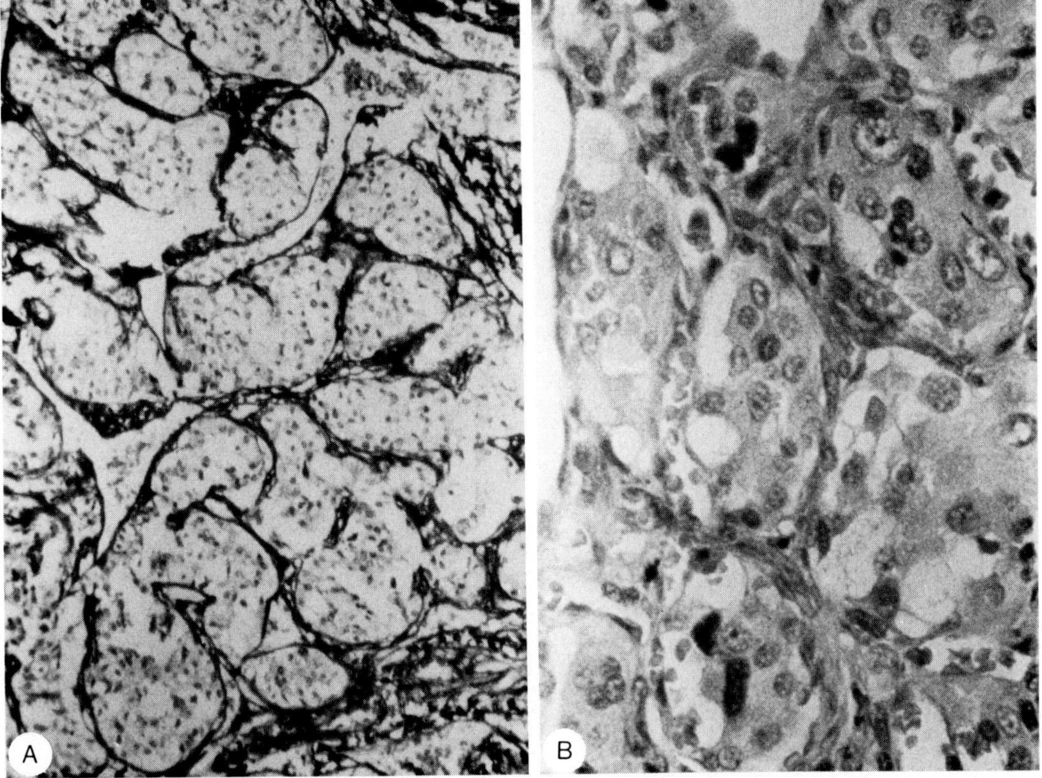

Figure 26–2. Microphotograph of a carotid body tumor shows the variable size of the cell nests (*A*) and cellular pleomorphism (*B*) which in this endocrine tumor does not indicate malignancy per se.

which may be moved horizontally but not vertically, should suggest a carotid body tumor. Such a neoplasm usually extends either upward or downward, but medial extension with the tumor protruding into the oral pharynx (Westbury, 1967) has also been reported. The diagnosis can be confirmed by needle biopsy or, more properly, by angiography (see Figure 9–27). The typical angiographic picture shows widening of the carotid bifurcation owing to the presence of the tumor and a typical "tumor filling" of a network of small vessels at the carotid bifurcation. Conditions simulating the presence of a carotid body tumor include enlarged lymph nodes, lymphoma, metastatic carcinoma, carotid aneurysm, brachial cyst, or salivary gland tumors.

Surgical excision is the only effective cure for carotid body tumor. The possibility of damage to the carotid artery during removal of the tumor is considerable. Shamblin *et al.* (1971) reviewed 90 cases and found 16 surgical postoperative deaths among 72 operative procedures. This and the generally slow growth of the tumor have been used in the past as an argument against such surgery. This reasoning, which may have been valid in the 1950s, is no longer acceptable at the present stage of modern vascular surgery. Carotid body tumors present special technical problems because of their vascularity and close proximity to the carotid arteries. Therefore, whenever surgery is contemplated, the groin should be prepared for removal of the saphenous vein, should grafting become necessary.

The exposure of the carotid body tumor is by and large identical to that of carotid endarterectomy. If, however, the growth is very large or adheres to the adjoining tissues, extension of the exposure either upward or downward may be necessary. Occasionally, the styloid process needs to be resected to allow complete removal. After dividing the superficial fascia, the internal jugular vein is retracted laterally, and the common carotid artery is encircled with tapes. Before beginning dissection, it is advisable to identify and ensnare the hypoglossal nerve, which is usually in close association with the tumor. It is seldom difficult to dissect the distal external carotid artery free and pass a silastic rubber tape around it, but it may not be so easy to gain control over the distal internal carotid artery. If such a difficulty arises, distal dissection of the internal carotid should be abandoned, and any retrograde bleeding owing to vascular injury should be controlled with an internal balloon occluder.

The modern technique of excising a carotid body tumor is based upon recognition that the carotid body develops embryologically within the adventitia of the carotid vessels without involving the medial layer (Boyd, 1937). The cleavage plane of removal between the tumor and the media has been identified by various investigators as either subadventitial or adventitial. The safest plane for the dissection is undoubtedly the subadventitial loose areolar tissue. The tumor should preferably be first dissected off the external carotid artery to assure optimal mobilization and then separated from the internal carotid. Several small arteries supplying the tumor, usually originating from the external carotid artery, must be ligated as well as the small vessel that as a rule rises from the "crotch" of the bifurcation (see Figures 26–3 and 26–4).

Although most carotid body tumors can be removed without injury to the carotid artery, vascular damage is certainly not uncommon, especially if the tumor has infiltrated the medial layer. For this reason, removal of a carotid body tumor should be undertaken only by a surgeon who is versatile in vascular surgery. The repair of vascular injuries can be difficult because the carotid stripped of its adventitia is fragile and holds sutures poorly. If the cleavage plane is properly followed, injury to the carotid artery usually can be avoided. If injury occurs, the carotid should be clamped, and the arterial repair should be carried out with 7-0 polypropylene sutures or a vein patch (see Figure 26–5).

More extensive involvement of the vessel may require either insertion of a vein patch or block resection and replacement of the damaged segment with autogenous saphenous vein or with a synthetic graft.

If the integrity of the internal carotid artery is maintained, injury to the external carotid need not be repaired, but the vessel may be ligated with impunity (see Figure 26–6). Because of the space left after removal of the tumor, it is advisable to drain the operative area with a small cigarette drain inserted through a separate stab wound.

A somewhat different method of removing carotid body tumors is used by Rob (1976). After initial dissection, he divides the external carotid artery, temporarily clamps both the common and the internal carotid arteries, and performs the removal of the tumor in an avas-

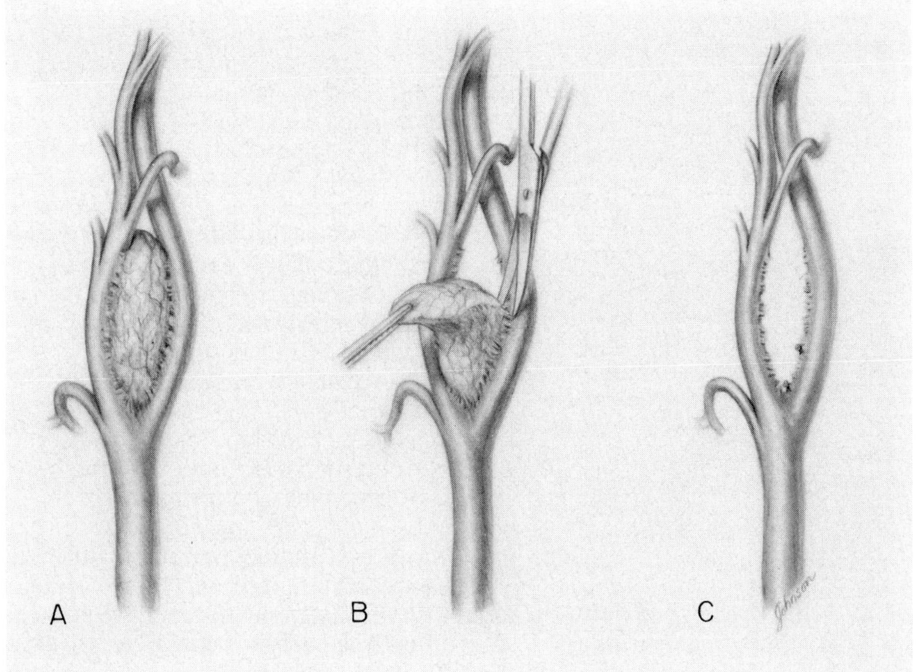

Figure 26–3. The treatment of carotid body tumor (*A*) by surgical removal (*B* and *C*).

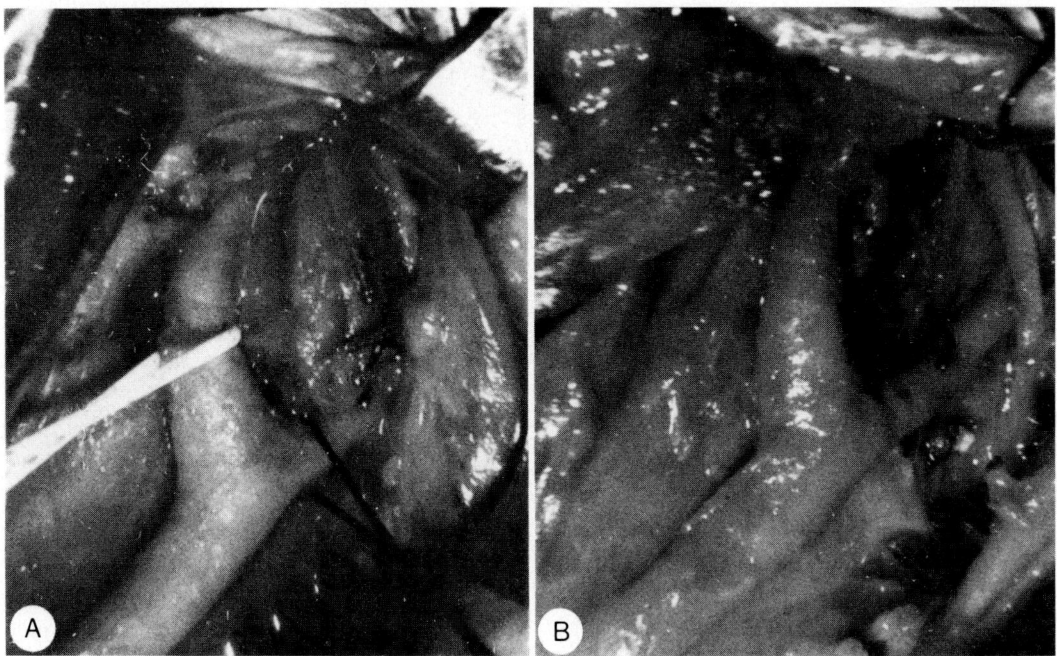

Figure 26–4. Large carotid body tumor (*A*). Carotid bifurcation after removal of the tumor (*B*).

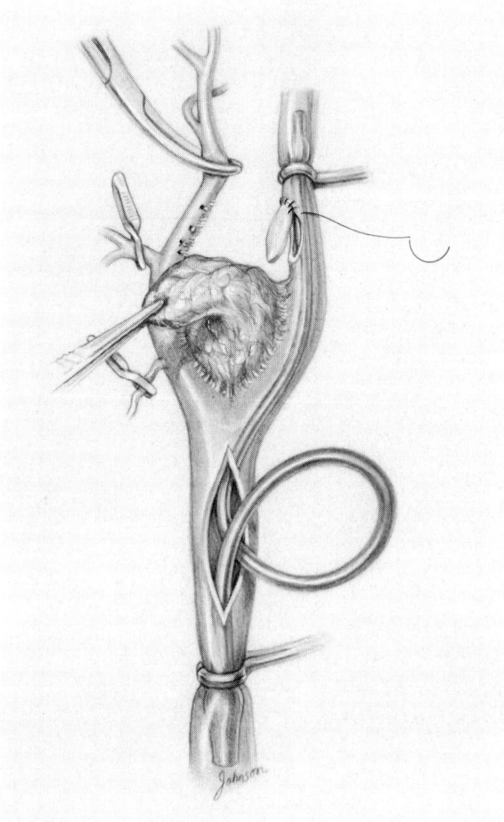

Figure 26-5. Repair of injury to the common carotid artery during resection of carotid body tumor with patch graft angioplasty.

cular field. I find this method to be seldom necessary and believe that, because the collapsed vessels cannot be easily differentiated from the tumor tissue, the technique predisposes to vascular injury.

HYPERSENSITIVE CAROTID SINUS SYNDROME

The carotid sinus is a group of specialized nerve endings situated in the wall of the slightly bulbously enlarged proximal portion of the internal carotid artery and perhaps a short contiguous portion of the common and external carotid arteries. Four nerves contribute to the innervation of receptors in the carotid sinus and the adjacent carotid body: the glossopharyngeal, vagus, cervical sympathetic, and hypoglossal. These nerves show considerable variation in their anatomical arrangements.

Reflexes originating from the carotid sinus can produce changes in both blood pressure and heart rate. Decrease in blood pressure in the carotid sinus evokes diffuse vasoconstriction in the body. This reflex was described by Herring (1927) and studied in depth by Heymans *et al.* (1933). Similar groups of receptors have also been described in the wall of large veins and in the atria (Hamby, 1952), with their nerve fibers mainly carried by the vagus. Interestingly enough, the receptors of the carotid sinus are stimulated not by the low arterial pressure itself but by the reflex changes invoked by cessation of stimulation by the normal arterial pressure waves. Even in the normal person, pressure upon the carotid sinus baroreceptors may both slow the heart rate and decrease blood pressure to some degree (Abel and McCutcheon, 1979), but usually will not produce symptoms. If these changes are pronounced and cardiovascular instability results from minimal mechanical stimulation, the patient is considered to have carotid sinus hypersensitivity syndrome (Brown and Watson, 1982; Weiss and Baker, 1933).

Besides cardioinhibitory, bradycardiac, and vasomotor hypotensive responses, Peretz *et al.* (1973) also describe a third type of "cerebral" reflex with loss of consciousness but no change in general hemodynamics. The existence of this reflex is in doubt, and the loss of consciousness is attributed by some (Thomas, 1969) to occlusion of carotid flow by pressure rather than to any reflex activity.

Two distinct types of hypersensitive carotid sinus syndrome have been recognized: (1) the bradycardia-asystole type, with response mediated through the efferent vagal fibers, and (2) the vasodilator-hypotensive form, which is mediated through the sympathetic system. When abnormal sensitivity of the carotid sinus reflex exists, increased efferent impulses may also result in a variety of symptoms of autonomic overreactivity, depending on which of these two principal pathways is implicated.

Clinically, events of carotid sinus hypersensitivity consist of sudden, usually unexpected episodes of lightheadedness or fainting. These spells occur frequently and may be reproducible under special circumstances, such as by exerting pressure on the neck or turning the head sharply sideways or upward. The episodes are sometimes preceded by visual, vertiginous, auditory, or hallucinatory phenomena and usually last but a few seconds. Recovery is

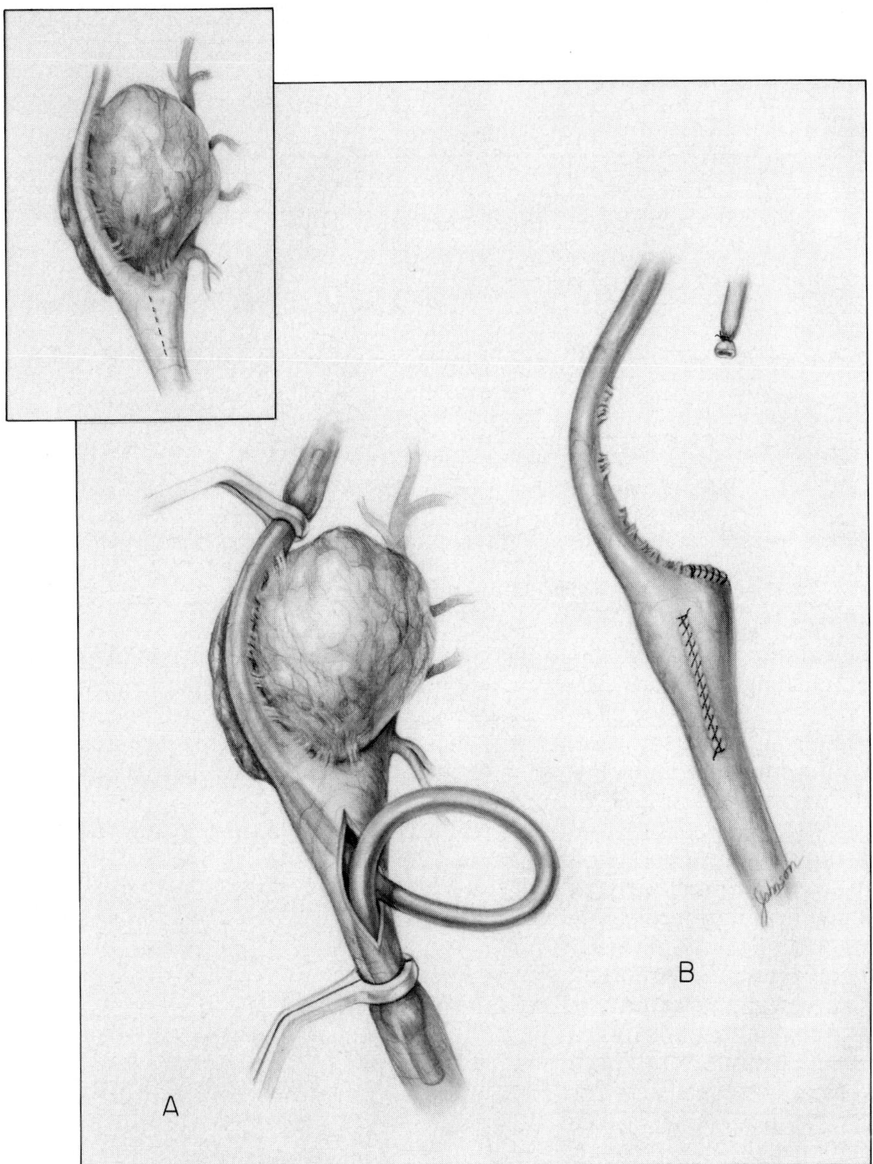

Figure 26-6. Injury to external carotid artery occurring during removal of carotid body tumor (*A*) handled by ligation of the distal and suture closure of the proximal external carotid artery (*B*).

usually prompt and complete. The simplest means of invoking the carotid sinus hypersensitivity response is by massage of the carotid bifurcation area (see Figure 26-7). The test is considered to have a positive result if asystole lasts longer than three seconds or a drop in blood pressure greater than 50 mm Hg occurs within 20 seconds of the provocation (Franke, 1963). Patients with such positive responses are considered candidates for surgery. Besides presenting itself as a disease per se, carotid sinus hypersensitivity syndrome may also develop owing to tumors of the neck or occlusive atherosclerosis or may manifest itself in the course of operations on the carotid bifurcation.

The incidence of carotid sinus hypersensitivity increases with age, and some drugs, such as digitalis, predispose for the disease (Nichol and Strauss, 1943). In the differential diagnosis of carotid sinus hypersensitivity syndrome, Stokes-Adams attacks, the so-called sick-sinus syndrome and epilepsy should be considered. Sick-sinus syndrome may especially closely

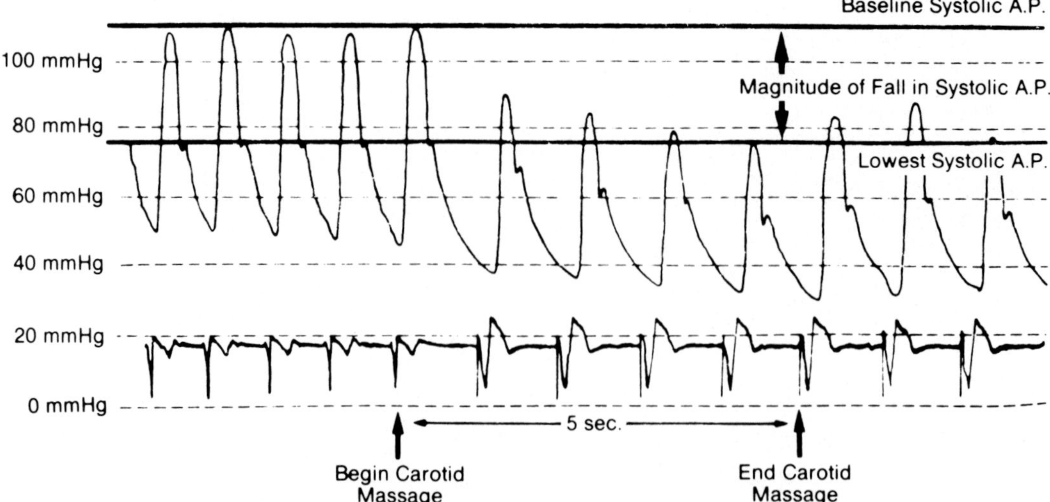

Figure 26–7. Vasodepressor response during carotid sinus massage in a patient with carotid sinus hypersensitivity syndrome. From Madigan, N.P.; Flaker, G.C.; Curtis, J.J.; Reid, J.; Mueller, K.J.; and Murphy, T.J.: Carotid sinus hypersensitivity: Beneficial effects of dual-chamber pacing. *Am. J. Cardiol.*, **53**:1034–40, 1984.

mimic hypersensitive carotid sinus activity but can easily be differentiated by the typical electrocardiographic finding of a wandering pacemaker indicated by changing configuration of P waves, as well as by the difference in the P-R interval, by episodes of sinus arrest, and by junctional escape beats.

The treatment of carotid sinus hypersensitivity syndrome that is uncomplicated by other conditions may be pharmacological, electrophysiological, or surgical. In the selection of the proper therapy it is most important not only to establish the degree of severity of the condition but also to distinguish between the two principal types of the disease; pacing or anticholinergic drugs may be effective in the cardioinhibitory type but not in the vasodepressive type. Association of the two types may create a combined form (Brown and Watson, 1982) which can be diagnosed by pacing during carotid sinus massage.

The most common operation to relieve carotid sinus syndrome is removal of the nerve plexus of the wall of the carotid sinus. During the operation the carotid bifurcation is dissected free, and the adventitia is stripped from the carotid bulb along with the first 1.5 cm of the internal and 1 cm of the external carotid arteries (see Figure 26–8). The small artery and the nerve rising from the carotid body are divided, and the carotid body is removed. After the surgical denervation, the same area may be painted lightly with phenol solution. Because the operation is often complicated by dysrhythmias and hypotension, it requires extraordinary attention and special measures by the anesthesiologist, including the insertion of a temporary transvenous pacemaker electrode.

As an alternative to carotid sinus denerva-

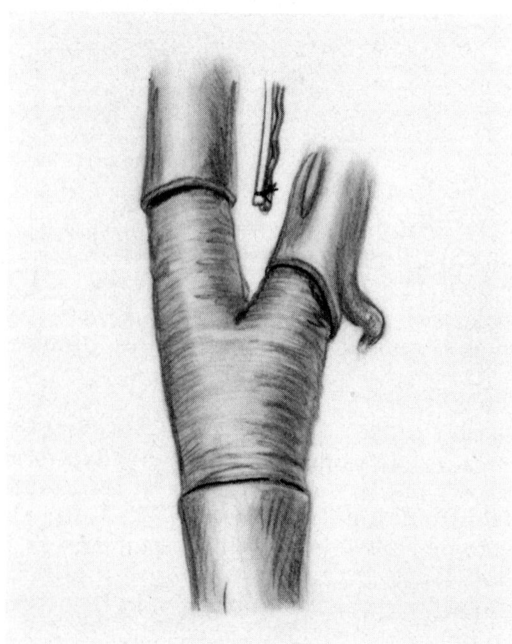

Figure 26–8. The appearance of the carotid bifurcation after adventitial stripping and carotid body resection for carotid sinus hypersensitivity.

tion, intracranial resection of the glossopharyngeal nerve was recommended for the treatment of the syndrome by Ray and Stewart (1948).

Among other modalities of treatment, irradiation for carotid sinus (Greeley *et al.*, 1955) and the administration of sympathomimetic and parasympathomimetic agents (Thomas, 1969) were also recommended. With the ease, effectiveness, and low risk of pacemaker insertion first used in the therapy for carotid sinus syncope by Voss and Magnin (1970), drug therapy is seldom utilized today.

Initially, ventricular demand pacing was the generally applied treatment of choice (Braunwald, 1980; Maur *et al.*, 1972). Because of the possibility of His-Purkinje block (Borst *et al.*, 1982; Fisher, 1981) or sinus arrest, atrial synchronous pacing is not recommended (Madigan *et al.*, 1984). If atrial preloading is desirable, unless the patient has atrial fibrillation, most cardiologists now prefer a dual-chamber ventricular-inhibited system to ventricular demand pacing. Recent reports (Madigan *et al.*, 1984; Morley *et al.*, 1983) also indicate that pacing may be ineffective in some cases because of a continuing significant vasodepressor component (Madigan *et al.*, 1984). Even in this age of highly sophisticated electrophysiological measures, the need for surgical intervention in carotid sinus hypersensitivity syndrome has not been eliminated, especially in patients in whom the vasodepressive component is significant. Madigan recommends that before a definite decision is made for the type of therapy, i.e., pacemaker, denervation, or both, the patient should be evaluated for blood pressure changes due to carotid sinus massage while paced temporarily (Madigan *et al.*, 1984). If there is a significant decrease in pressure, pacing alone is unlikely to relieve the patient's symptoms. Another way to evaluate vasodepressor response is by repeating carotid sinus massage after administering 1 mg of atropine. If a significant decrease in blood pressure occurs despite normalized heart rate, vasodepressor response is present and significant; and surgical denervation of the carotid sinus should receive due consideration.

REFERENCES

Abel, F.L., and McCutcheon, E.P.: *Cardiovascular Function: Principles and Applications.* Little, Brown, Boston, pages 319–20, 1979.

Borst, C.; Karemaker, J.; and Dunning, A.: Prolongation of atrioventricular conduction time by electrical stimulation of the carotid sinus nerves in man. *Circulation,* **65**:432–34, 1982.

Boyd, J.: The development of the human carotid body. *Contrib. Embryol. Carnegie Inst.,* **26**:1, 1937.

Baunwald, E.: *Heart Disease: A Textbook of Cardiovascular Medicine.* Vol. 1. W.B. Saunders, Philadelphia, Pennsylvania, pages 957–8, 1980.

Brown, C.W., and Watson, C.B.: Carotid sinus syndrome intraoperative management facilitated by temporary transvenous demand pacing. *Anesthesiology,* **56**:151–53, 1982.

Fisher, J.A.: Role of electrophysiological testing in the diagnosis and treatment of patients with known and suspected bradyarrhythmias and tachyarrhythmias. *Prog. Cardiovasc. Dis.,* **1**:24–30, 1981.

Franke, H.: *Uber das Karotissinus-Syndrome and den sogennante hyperactiven Karotissinus-Reflex.* Friedrich Karl Schottayer Verlag, Stuttgart, page 149, 1963.

Greeley, H.P.; Smedal, M.I.; and Most, W.: The treatment of the carotid sinus syndrome by irradiation. *N. Engl. J. Med.,* **152**:91–4, 1955.

Hamby, W.B.: *Intracranial Aneurysms.* Charles C Thomas, Springfield, Illinois, 1952.

Herring, H.E.: *Die Karotissinus Refexe auf Herz and Gefässe von normal physiologischen pathologischphysiologischen und klinischen Standpunkt (Gleichzeitig über die bedeutung der Blutdruck augler fur den Normalen and abnormalen Kreislauf).* Steinkopff, Leipzing, 1927.

Heymans, C.; Bouckaert, J.J.; and Reginiers, P.: *Le sinus carotidien et la zone homologue cardio-aortique.* In Doin, G. (ed.): Paris, pages 281–303, 1933.

Jonas, E.; Kosowsky, B.; and Ramaswamy, K.: Complete His-Purkinje block produced by carotid sinus massage. *Circulation,* **50**:192–96, 1974.

LeCompte, P.M.: Tumors of the carotid body. *Am. J. Pathol.,* **24**:305–21, 1948.

Madigan, N.P.; Flaker, G.C.; Curtis, J.J.; Reid, J.; Mueller, K.J.; and Murphy, T.J.: Carotid sinus hypersensitivity: beneficial effects of dual-chamber pacing. *Am. J. Cardiol.,* **53**:1034–40, 1984.

Maur, K.V.; Nelson, E.W.; Holsinger, J.W.; and Eliott, R.S.: Hypersensitive carotid sinus syncope treated by implantable demand cardiac pacemaker. *Am. J. Cardiol.,* **39**:209–10, 1972.

Morley, C.A.; Perrins, E.J.; Chan, S.L.; and Sutton, R.: The role of rate hysteresis pacing in the hypersensitive carotid sinus syndrome. *PACE,* **6**:1224–28, 1983.

Nichol, A.D., and Strauss, H.: The effect of digitalis, arginin, congestive cardiac failure, and atropine on the hyperactive carotid sinus. *Am. Heart. J.,* **25**:746–59, 1943.

Peretz, D.; Gerein, A.; and Miyagishima, R.: Permanent demand pacing for hypersensitive carotid sinus syndrome. *Can. Med. Assoc. J.,* **108**:1131–34, 1973.

Pettet, J.R.; Woolner, L.B.; and Judd, E.S., Jr.: Carotid body tumors (chemodectomas). *Ann. Surg.,* **137**:465–77, 1953.

Ray, B.S., and Stewart, H.J.: Role of the glossopharyngeal nerve in the carotid sinus reflex in man: relief of carotid sinus syndrome by intracranial section of the glossopharyngeal nerve. *Surgery,* **23**:411–24, 1948.

Rob, C.: Excision of carotid body tumors. In Rob, C., and Smith, R. (eds.): *Operative Surgery.* Butterworths, London, pages, 327–31, 1976.

Shamblin, W.R.; Remine, W.H.; and Sheps, S.G.: Carotid body tumor (chemodectoma): clinicopathologic analysis of ninety cases. *Am. J. Surg.,* **122:**722–29, 1971.

Singhabhandhu, B.; Gray, S.W.; Bryant, M.F.; and Skandalakis, J.E.: Carotid body tumors. *Am. Surg.,* **39:**501–8, 1973.

Thomas, J.E.: Hyperactive carotid sinus reflex and carotid sinus syncope. *Mayo Clin. Proc.,* **44:**127–39, 1969.

Voss, D.M., and Magnin, G.E.: Demand pacing and carotid sinus syncope. *Am. Heart. J.,* **79:**544–7, 1970.

Weiss, S., and Baker, J.P.: The carotid sinus reflex in health and disease: its role in the causation of fainting and convulsions. *Medicine (Baltimore),* **12:**297–354, 1933.

Westbury, G.: Carotid body tumors. *J. R. Coll. Surg. Edinb.,* **12:**107–20, 1967.

27

Surgical Management of Carotid Obstruction and Coronary and/or Peripheral Vascular Disease in the Same Patient

ELLIS L. JONES, RICHARD A. MICHALIK, JOSEPH M. CRAVER, and CHARLES R. HATCHER, JR.

The coexistence of extracranial carotid obstruction with peripheral vascular and/or coronary disease has been of interest to clinicians for many years. The important relationship of these entities is best expressed by the known but highly variable incidence of myocardial infarction after carotid endarterectomy and by the devastating effects of neurological injury that occasionally occurs after routine coronary bypass or peripheral vascular reconstructive surgery. The actual incidence of atherosclerotic carotid vascular obstruction in patients with ischemic cardiac or peripheral vascular disease is unknown. However, the occurrence of significant internal or carotid bifurcation stenosis in candidates for myocardial revascularization has been reported to be from 6 to 16 percent (Barnes *et al.*, 1981; Mehigan *et al.*, 1977). The incidence of carotid artery disease in patients undergoing peripheral vascular reconstruction is probably higher, with asymptomatic cervical bruits said to occur in 5 percent of the stroke-age population and 16 to 32 percent in patients undergoing peripheral vascular reconstruction (Hart and Easton, 1983). Such reported incidence varies with the intensity of the search for the condition. Conversely, coronary artery disease (manifest by angina pectoris or prior myocardial infarction) may coexist with carotid obstructive disease in as many as 49 percent of patients (Ennix *et al.*, 1979).

MANAGEMENT OF PATIENTS WITH COEXISTING DISEASES

Because of the frequent association of carotid and coronary disease, the fear of infarction after isolated carotid endarterectomy and concern for neurological injury after coronary bypass or peripheral vascular reconstructive procedures, there has been a recent trend to standardize surgical care for all patients found to have such coexisting conditions. Combined or simultaneous operations using carotid endarterectomy with coronary bypass grafting and carotid endarterectomy with peripheral vascular surgery have been recommended for these patients with the anticipation that risk and mortality will be similar to those of coronary, peripheral, vascular, or carotid surgery alone (Craver *et al.*, 1982; Mehigan *et al.*, 1977; Okies *et al.*, 1977; Urschel *et al.*, 1976). Other investigators, however, have recommended staging certain categories of patients with coronary and carotid disease and combining the operations only when definite clinical indications exist (Craver *et al.*, 1982; Hertzer *et al.*, 1978). Still others advise that the carotid component of the combined disease be ignored entirely under certain circumstances (Hart and Easton, 1983).

Selection of a particular approach is further influenced by the fact that many strokes occurring at the time of elective coronary bypass are embolic in origin and are not due to a low-flow state secondary to carotid vascular obstruction. In addition, several recent studies have demonstrated that patients with extracranial carotid obstruction can safely undergo noncardiac surgical procedures with a very low incidence of perioperative stroke (Carney *et al.*, 1977; Hart and Easton, 1983).

The Combined Approach

A combined approach for the treatment of carotid and coronary disease was first described by Bernard and colleagues (1972) and later by Urschel and associates (1976). Both groups noted frequent complications often necessitating emergency intervention when patients undergoing carotid endarterectomy suddenly had unstable angina or acute myocardial infarction in the postoperative period or, in reverse, when patients undergoing myocardial revascularization had perioperative or late strokes. It was believed that by combining the two procedures the number of both immediate and delayed complications could be significantly reduced. Since these early reports, it has remained unclear which patients really need the combined form of therapy.

Fatal myocardial infarction after carotid endarterectomy has been reported to occur with a frequency of from 3 to 5 percent (Hertzer *et al.*, 1978; Thompson *et al.*, 1970), but its true frequency depends on the clinical state of the patient. This incidence is 1 percent in persons with no history of coronary disease but increases to 7 percent in patients with a history of coronary disease and even to 17 percent in cases of unstable angina pectoris (Sundt *et al.*, 1975; Thompson *et al.*, 1970).

Risk Factors

Perioperative stroke constitutes a major potential risk of both carotid endarterectomy and myocardial revascularization. In experienced hands, this risk should not exceed 2 to 3 percent after isolated endarterectomy (Ennix *et al.*, 1979; Thompson *et al.*, 1970). The incidence of neurological injury after carotid endarterectomy for asymptomatic bruit is, of course, less than that for transient ischemic attacks or stroke (Schwartz *et al.*, 1982). Any attempt to extrapolate such data to patients undergoing combined carotid surgery or coronary bypass alone becomes difficult because the cause of stroke as a complication of isolated carotid endarterectomy may be quite different from that of stroke after coronary artery bypass. The reported incidence of neurological injury after coronary bypass is approximately 2 percent (Barnes and Marzalek, 1981; Breuer *et al.*, 1980; Hertzer *et al.*, 1978; Reul *et al.*, 1972) and has occurred at a rate of just under 1 percent in our own series of patients having coronary bypass surgery alone.

The etiology of stroke after routine elective coronary bypass has been difficult to elucidate. At present, stroke remains a major source of morbidity after this procedure. Possible causes include reduced flow through stenotic extra- or intracranial vessels, dislodgement of ulcerated plaques from the carotid artery, embolization of atherosclerotic material or platelet debris from the ascending aorta, and embolization of postinfarction left ventricular mural thrombus. Because of confusion regarding the origin of stroke, patients with a positive neurological history or asymptomatic cervical bruit scheduled for elective coronary bypass surgery have generated justifiable concern in creating a protocol for preoperative evaluation and treatment.

Several recent studies, mostly involving patients having peripheral vascular reconstruction, have failed to demonstrate a direct relationship between cervical bruit, severity of carotid disease, and the incidence of perioperative stroke (Hart and Easton, 1983). Some of this confusion arises because only about half of the patients found to have asymptomatic cervical bruits preoperatively had significant carotid stenosis, and many patients without clinical signs or symptoms indeed had severe carotid occlusive disease. For many years the presence of a carotid bruit in association with peripheral vascular and ischemic heart disease has complicated the surgical management of patients. Fear of perioperative strokes secondary to low-flow states through stenosed carotid arteries has been responsible for the development of numerous noninvasive tests to detect significant carotid disease. However, once such obstructions have been found, there has continued to be controversy regarding the optimal method of management.

Noninvasive tests now in use for evaluation of carotid bruits are pulsed and continuous-wave Doppler scans, real-time B-mode scans, carotid phonoangiography, ophthalmosonometry, and oculopneumoplethysmography (OPG). A routine battery of such tests applied to patients with asymptomatic cervical bruits can be quite expensive, often confusing, and cost-ineffective. In experienced hands, however, noninvasive evaluation of cervical bruits is capable of detecting 75 percent or greater cross-sectional reduction in lumen with a sensitivity of 90 percent (Hart and Easton, 1983).

Asymptomatic cervical bruits are present in approximately 10 percent of patients scheduled to undergo coronary artery bypass, but only approximately one half turn out to have carotid stenosis detected by noninvasive studies. It is interesting that the incidence of both cervical bruits and carotid stenosis documented by these tests is consistently less in coronary bypass patients than in patients having peripheral vascular reconstruction (Hart and Easton, 1983).

The occurrence of perioperative stroke is slightly higher in patients undergoing peripheral vascular procedures who have had prior cerebral ischemic symptoms; this is true whether or not cervical bruits are present. There does not appear to be an increase in perioperative stroke in patients with carotid stenosis (whether asymptomatic or symptomatic) as defined by Doppler studies (Barnes *et al.*, 1981). However, Kartchner and McRae (1981), using OPG, found that the perioperative stroke rate was 1 percent in patients with normal OPG findings and 17 percent in those with moderate flow reduction. One possible explanation for this difference in findings may be the variation in specificity for higher degrees of stenosis in the latter test (Hart and Easton, 1983).

Unfortunately, the events relating perioperative stroke to cervical bruits and carotid stenosis in patients undergoing coronary bypass have been less intensively studied than those for patients undergoing peripheral vascular operations. However, all data available and our own experience support the contention that cervical bruits do not effectively identify subgroups of cardiac patients at increased risk for perioperative stroke. One study, however, has demonstrated that if Doppler study shows obstructions greater than 50 percent in lumen diameter the stroke rate is slightly increased (Hart and Easton, 1983).

The literature supports the postulate that, for patients undergoing peripheral vascular reconstruction, cervical bruits do not identify a subset of those at risk for perioperative stroke. There are no data to support the necessity for perioperative carotid arteriography and endarterectomy in the patient with asymptomatic cervical bruit before undergoing a major vascular procedure. Although less well studied, these same conclusions are valid for patients undergoing cardiac surgical procedures. In approximately 1,500 consecutive patients screened for carotid bruits before cardiac surgical procedures by Ivey and associates (1981), asymptomatic patients with and without hemodynamically significant stenoses safely underwent cardiopulmonary bypass without carotid endarterectomy. Therefore, in most such patients the carotid bruit can be ignored and a battery of expensive noninvasive tests is unjustified.

Balderman and associates (1983), using OPG, screened 500 patients underoing coronary bypass surgery for asymptomatic carotid disease. Patients with abnormal OPG results had cerebral angiography. The incidence of carotid bruit in the 500 patients was 6 percent. Abnormal OPG findings in addition to the carotid bruit were found in 2 percent. Of those with abnormal OPG results, two thirds had significant carotid artery stenosis and had endarterectomy two weeks to two months before cardiac surgery. Significant carotid stenosis was found in one third of patients without cervical bruits but with positive OPG findings. With this approach to the management of patients undergoing coronary revascularization, the incidence of perioperative stroke was 0.4 percent. They concluded that patients without hemodynamically significant carotid disease verified by OPG can be spared from cerebral angiography. Two patients had perioperative stroke after coronary revascularization; one had normal OPG results, and the other had severe bilateral carotid disease.

Hertzer and associates (1983) reported 331 patients who had simultaneous carotid and coronary surgery from 1973 to 1981. The hospital mortality rate was 5.7 percent. These 331 patients represented 1.7 percent of all patients who had coronary artery revascularization during the eight-year period. Permanent neurological deficit occurred perioperatively in 4.5 percent. Although postoperative stroke increased with advancing age of the patient (zero in those less than 50 years of age, 9 percent in those 60 to 69 years, and 14 percent in those over 70 years), these differences did not attain statistical significance. The incidence of stroke in patients with asymptomatic carotid bruit was 8 percent and increased to 21 percent if the patient had a prior stroke. One of the most important factors in predicting the likelihood of stroke after coronary revascularization and carotid endarterectomy is the presence and extent of disease in the contralateral carotid artery. If the latter has less than 50 percent stenosis, the stroke rate is 7 percent; if the degree of stenosis is greater than 90 percent, it increases the stroke rate to 20 percent (Hertzer *et al.*, 1983).

Etiology of Perioperative Stroke. The suggestion of an embolic cause for most perioperative strokes was initially made by Franco at the Cleveland Clinic Foundation (unpublished data). He noted that the incidence of stroke after coronary bypass was 9 percent in patients who had preoperative angiographic evidence of left ventricular thrombus and only 2 percent for those without this angiographic finding (Franco *et al.*, personal communication). Mural thrombus is frequently found in patients with a large previous infarction, and dislodgement may occur at the time of intraoperative cardiac manipulation. Intraoperative factors such as left ventricular venting may also contribute to an increased incidence of perioperative neurological injury either by the introduction of air into the cardiac chambers or by dislodgment of mural thrombus.

Except for patients with extensive bilateral carotid disease, it is probable that, contrary to what was once thought, the cause of most cerebral vascular injuries after routine coronary bypass is totally unrelated to known or occult extra- or intracranial cerebral vascular obstructions. The superb autoregulatory mechanisms of the cerebral circulation, use of systemic hypothermia, and the salutary effects of hemodilution appear to be sufficient to protect the brain from low-flow states which might theoretically occur when the extracranial circulation is obstructed or even occluded.

In our own experience with patients undergoing isolated coronary bypass and having asymptomatic cervical bruit, a prior history of stroke or transient ischemic attack, (TIA), or a prior history of carotid endarterectomy, the incidence of perioperative stroke was 3 percent in patients with bruit, 8.6 percent in patients with prior neurological symptoms, and 5.1 percent in those with a prior carotid endarterectomy (Jones *et al.*, 1984). The almost 9 percent incidence of perioperative stroke in patients with a prior history of stroke or TIA who had coronary bypass only would suggest that these patients should be treated differently and should have a most careful and thorough evaluation (including angiography) before elective bypass surgery. When significant carotid vascular disease is found in these patients with a prior neurological history, a combined carotid-coronary operation should be performed.

In our initial investigation of the problem of simultaneous occurrence of carotid and coronary disease, we felt that all patients having extracranial carotid vascular obstruction should be treated with carotid endarterectomy at the time coronary bypass was performed. Therefore, early in our series there was no selectivity of patients for the staged versus the combined procedure, and all patients found to have significant carotid obstruction were subjected to the combined procedure. We found that simultaneous procedures could be performed safely and with low morbidity and hospital mortality rates (Craver *et al.*, 1982; Jones *et al.*, 1984). During this time, perioperative complications were not significantly more frequent in patients having the combined procedure when compared with patients without carotid disease having coronary bypass only. Hospital mortality for the combined procedure was 2 percent and less than 1 percent for those having isolated coronary bypass. The incidence of stroke after each procedure was 1.6 and 0.6 percent, respectively. These differences were not statistically significant.

In a review of our own experience of patients having stroke after isolated coronary bypass, the only contributory factors appear to be advanced age and the presence of extensive atherosclerosis in the ascending aorta. The latter finding implies an embolic origin for the stroke event.

A number of reports have indicated a high incidence of left main coronary disease in candidates for carotid endarterectomy and coronary bypass. The incidence varies from 16 to 40 percent (Mehigan *et al.*, 1977; Schwartz *et al.*, 1982), and some have noted the occurrence to be three times that in patients with coronary disease but without carotid obstruction (Ennix *et al.*, 1979; Hertzer *et al.*, 1978). Schwartz reported a 37 percent incidence of left main coronary disease in patients having the combined carotid-coronary operation and a hospital mortality rate of 11 percent compared with a less than 1 percent mortality in all other patients having coronary bypass surgery for left main disease. The reason for the difference could not be explained, but they recommend that in these patients the more time-honored method of performing the coronary bypass operation first followed at a later date by carotid endarterectomy should be pursued. The high incidence of left main coronary disease in their study cannot be explained in light of our own series incidence of 15 percent, which was not statistically different from the percentage in patients having coronary bypass alone.

In our own experience and that of others, the difference in hospital mortality rate of patients having the combined procedure may relate to the operative technique. The carotid portion of the combined operation is performed first to avoid producing potential deleterious pressure and flow gradients through the carotid circulation during cardiopulmonary bypass. Factors felt to be important in performance of the carotid portion of the procedure are systemic heparinization; internal carotid shunt, leaving a smooth adherent intimal margin at the distal end of the artery; and use of patch grafting if necessary, especially for patients with restenosis. In most cases the carotid endarterectomy is performed while veins are removed from the leg. However, in extremely unstable patients or patients with high-grade left main coronary obstruction, the chest may be opened before the carotid portion of the operation and the heart prepared for rapid cannulation should hemodynamic instability occur.

Based on experience at our own institution and that of others, the following recommendations can be made for the treatment of patients with both carotid and coronary atherosclerotic disease. Simultaneous carotid-coronary operation should be performed when there is symptomatic neurological disease (TIA or prior stroke), and when carotid artery obstruction is associated with unstable angina pectoris, significant left main obstruction, or diffuse multivessel disease. Although the evidence is not substantial, we also recommend the combined approach in elderly patients (more than 70 years old) and in patients under 50 who have asymptomatic carotid artery disease. In the former group, extracranial vascular obstruction has an increased likelihood of being associated with intracerebral arterial disease; the combined effect of the two could potentially cause reduced cerebral blood flow during cardiopulmonary bypass. However, this supposition is totally unproven at this time. In patients less than 50 years old the combined approach is justified by the extended longevity of most of these patients with an increased likelihood of later symptoms secondary to extracranial carotid artery obstruction.

Simultaneous carotid-coronary surgery in patients having recent or prior neurological symptoms is justified by the low incidence of perioperative stroke in patients having the combined procedure for TIAs or prior stroke history (see Figure 27-1). This is particularly true in light of the almost 9 percent incidence of perioperative stroke in patients with a prior history of stroke or TIA having coronary artery bypass alone.

A simultaneous approach to carotid coronary disease is also recommended whenever bilateral carotid and severe or unstable coronary artery disease coexist. However, the treatment of bilateral extracranial carotid vascular obstruction presents several difficult problems. Previous studies have demonstrated that bilateral obstruction can be effectively managed as an isolated staged procedure in patients free of coronary disease even when there is ipsilateral total occlusion of one carotid and significant contralateral stenosis of the other (Thompson *et al.*, 1970). However, for patients with unstable angina and bilateral carotid disease the situation is different, and the operative risk is high; death, cerebral accident, or transient deficit are reported in as many as 20 percent of patients (Mehigan *et al.*, 1977). Patients with unstable angina and severe bilateral carotid disease should be treated by first performing endarterectomy on the carotid (which contributes most of the cerebral blood flow) and then performing coronary bypass as

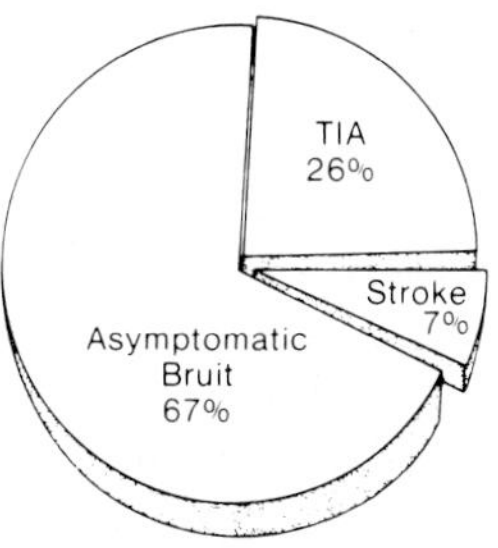

Figure 27-1. Indications for cerebral angiography in 104 patients having simultaneous carotid-coronary surgery. Combined carotid/coronary surgery indications for cerebral angiography ($n = 104$). (From Jones, E.L.; Craver, J.M.; Michalik, R.A.; Murphy, D.A.; Guyton, R.A.; Bone, D.K.; Hatcher, C.R.; and Reichwald, N.A.: Combined carotid and coronary operations: when are they necessary? *J. Thorac. Cardiovasc. Surg.*,**87**:7-16, 1984.

part of the combined procedure. The second carotid obstruction is treated surgically as an isolated procedure at a later date.

Justification of the combined approach is certainly easier when the clinical setting is ideal for complex operations. In many centers such optimal conditions are present, and both procedures can be performed together safely. If this is not the case, it may be more desirable to separate the two procedures, first performing the operation that satisfies the patient's most immediate needs.

All of the aforementioned guidelines for myocardial revascularization in patients with carotid obstruction are equally applicable to those patients having carotid disease who require peripheral vascular procedures. Staged operations should be performed except in the situation in which both cerebral and peripheral vascular circulations are in immediate jeopardy. Except in patients with prior or active neurological symptoms, reconstruction of the peripheral vascular circulation can be accomplished as an isolated procedure with satisfactory results.

Preference for the staged approach, i.e., carotid endarterectomy first followed at some later date by myocardial revascularization, should be exercised only when the patient has clinically stable angina pectoris. In this setting, patients having TIAs associated with significant carotid disease, complicated carotid revascularization procedures, or significant bilateral carotid disease should have the carotid portion of the operation performed first as a separate procedure. Advocates of such a policy have noted the low mortality rate associated with the staged approach and have accepted a fatal infarction and overall hospital mortality rate after isolated carotid endarterectomy of no greater than 1 and 2 percent, respectively (Hertzer and Lees, 1981). In one large series (Hertzer *et al.,* 1978), the hospital mortality rate after the carotid portion of the staged procedure was 1.5 percent and approximately the same after subsequent myocardial revascularization. The mortality rate was 4 percent when the combined approach was used. Anginal pattern or extent of anatomical coronary disease should dictate whether the combined or the staged approach is used.

Complicated carotid revascularization procedures may frequently be necessary in cases where there is restenosis at a prior endarterectomy site. In such a situation, operating time and the extent of the grafting procedures are less predictable, and it is probably best to perform the operation staged whenever possible. A staged procedure (carotid first) is also indicated for a neurologically unstable patient with severe carotid disease associated with asymptomatic coronary disease and in most patients requiring peripheral vascular operations.

Coronary artery bypass may be performed as the only procedure in most situations in which there is discovery of an asymptomatic cervical bruit associated with unilateral carotid artery obstruction. Recently our approach to the patient with very unstable angina and asymptomatic cervical bruit has been to treat the situation with coronary bypass alone; this has produced no significant increase in stroke rate. In many of these patients with cervical bruit coronary bypass was performed without the benefit of prior cerebral or carotid angiography. Patients with prior stroke and very unstable angina may be similarly treated, although the stroke rate will probably be increased. In the latter situation the risk of extensive diagnostic cerebral arteriographic studies during a time of cardiac instability is probably higher than the risk of stroke after myocardial revascularization alone. An algorithm for the workup of patients with carotid and coronary disease that has been useful at our institution is presented in Figure 27–2.

Because of the suspected embolic nature of most perioperative strokes after coronary bypass surgery, we have concentrated on certain principles that might reduce the likelihood of these events. This has consisted of careful placement of the aortic cannulation site away from diseased areas of the ascending aorta, careful placement of side-biting and crossclamps on the aorta, and nontraumatic introduction of the Swan-Gantz catheter about the area of the carotid artery. Extraction of left ventricular thrombus should be performed when demonstrated angiographically.

The introduction of digital vascular imaging and noninvasive tests has done much to simplify and make safe the diagnostic workup of patients with carotid and coronary disease (Wood *et al.,* 1983). It is possible that in the future our approach will be to study larger numbers of patients with these techniques; this may modify the guidelines slightly. However, the incidence of false-negative and false-positive results from both of these procedures must be established with great certainty before we abandon the traditional definitive diagnostic techniques.

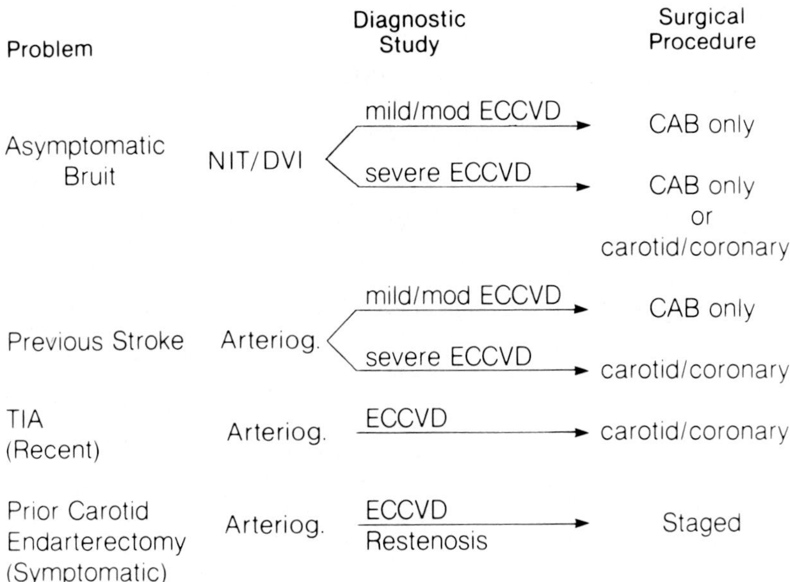

Figure 27–2. Algorithm of preoperative evaluation of patients with evidence of carotid-coronary disease. DVI = digital vascular imaging; ECCVD = extracranial carotid vascular disease; CAB = coronary artery bypass; arteriog. = cerebral and extracerebral arteriogram; NIT = noninvasive testing procedures. (From Jones, E.L.; Craver, J.M.; Michalik, R.A.; Murphy, D.A.; Guyton, R.A.; Bone, D.K.; Hatcher, C.R.; and Reichwald, N.A.: Combined carotid and coronary operations: when are they necessary? *J. Thorac. Cardiovascular. Surg.*, **87**:7–16, 1984.)

Finally, it is difficult to design a diagnostic and treatment protocol that is suitable for all clinical situations. It is hoped that the experience cited will be helpful in most instances in the management of these often difficult cases. Morbidity and mortality rates from carotid endarterectomy and coronary bypass vary considerably from hospital to hospital. Guidelines have been described in an effort to minimize operative complications for the many types of patients with carotid, coronary, and peripheral vascular disease.

REFERENCES

Balderman, S.C.; Gutierrez, I.Z.; Maukla, P.; Bhayana, J.N.; and Gage, A.A.: Noninvasive screening for asymptomatic carotid artery disease prior to cardiac operation. *J. Thorac. Cardiovasc. Surg.*, **85**:427–33, 1983.

Barnes, R.W., and Marszalek, P.B.: Asymptomatic carotid disease in the cardiovascular surgical patient: is prophylactic endarterectomy necessary? *Stroke*, **12**:497–500, 1981.

Barnes, R.W.; Liebman, P.R.; Marzalek, P.B.; *et al.*: The natural history of asymptomatic carotid disease in patients undergoing cardiovascular surgery. *Surgery*, **90**:1075–83, 1981.

Bernard, J.M.; Johnson, W.D.; and Peterson, J.J.: Carotid artery stenosis: association with surgery for coronary artery disease. *Arch. Surg.*, **105**:837–40, 1972.

Breuer, A.C.; Hanson, M.R.; Furlan, A.J.; *et al.*: Central nervous system complication of mycoardial revascularization: a prospective analysis of 400 patients. *Stroke*, **11**:136, 1980.

Carney, W.I.; Stewart, W.B.; DePinto, D.J.; Murcha, S.J.; and Roberts, B.: Carotid bruit as a risk factor in aortoiliac reconstruction. *Surgery*, **81**:567–70, 1977.

Craver, J.M.; Murphy, D.A.; Jones, E.L.; Curling, P.E.; Bone, D.K.; Smith, R.B., III; Purdue, G.D.; Hatcher, C.R.; and Kandrach, M.: Concomitant carotid and coronary artery reconstruction. *Ann. Surg.*, **195**:712–20, 1982.

Ennix, E.L.; Lawrie, G.M.; Morris, G.C.; *et al.*: Improved results of carotid endarterectomy in patients with symptomatic coronary disease: an analysis of 1,546 consecutive carotid operations. *Stroke*, **10**:122–25, 1979.

Hart, R., and Easton, J.D.: Management of cervical bruits and carotid stenosis in preoperative patients. *Stroke*, **14**:290–97, 1983.

Hertzer, N.R., and Lees, D.C.: Fatal myocardial infarction following carotid endarterectomy. *Ann. Surg.*, **194**:212–18, 1981.

Hertzer, N.R.; Loop, F.D.; Taylor, P.C.; and Beven, E.G.: Staged and combined surgical approach to simultaneous carotid and coronary vascular disease. *Surgery*, **84**:803–11, 1978.

Hertzer, N.R.; Loop, F.D.; Taylor, P.C.; and Beven, E.G.: Combined myocardial revascularization and carotid endarterectomy. *J. Thorac. Cardiovasc. Surg.*, **85**:577–89, 1983.

Ivey, T.D.; Strandness, D.E.; Williams, D.B.; Langlois, Y.; Misbach, G.A.; and Kruse, A.P.: Management of patients with carotid bruit undergoing cardiopulmonary bypass. *J. Thorac. Cardiovasc. Surg.*, **87**:183–89, 1984.

Jones, E.L.; Craver, J.M.; Michalik, R.A.; Murphy, D.A.; Guyton, R.A.; Bone, D.K.; Hatcher, C.R.; and Reichwald, N.A.: Combined carotid and coronary operations: when are they necessary? *J. Thorac. Cardiovasc. Surg.*, **87**:7–16, 1984.

Kartchner, M.M., and McCrae, L.P.: Guidelines for non-invasive evaluation of asymptomatic carotid bruits. *Clin. Neurosurg.*, **28**:412–28, 1981.

Mehigan, J.T.; Buch, W.S.; Pipkin, R.D.; and Fogarty, T.J.: A planned approach to coexistent cerebrovascular disease in coronary artery bypass candidates. *Arch. Surg.*, **112**:1403–09, 1977.

Okies, J.E.; MacManus, Q.; and Starr, A.: Myocardial revascularization and carotid endarterectomy: a combined approach. *Ann. Thorac. Surg.*, **23**:560–2, 1977.

Reul, G.J.; Morris, C.G.; Howell, J.R.; *et al.*: Current concepts in coronary artery surgery. *Ann. Thorac. Surg.*, **14**:243–59, 1972.

Schwartz, R.L.; Garrett, J.R.; Karp, R.B.; and Kouchoukos, N.T.: Simultaneous myocardial revascularization and carotid endarterectomy. *Circulation*, **66**(Suppl. 1):97–101, 1982.

Sundt, T.M.; Sandok, B.A.; and Whisnant, J.P.: Carotid endarterectomy complications and preoperative assessment of risk. *Mayo Clin. Proc.*, **50**:301, 1975.

Thompson, J.E.; Austin, D.J.; and Patman, R.D.: Carotid endarterectomy for cerebrovascular insufficiency: long-term results in 592 patients followed up to thirteen years. *Ann. Surg.*, **172**:663–79, 1970.

Urschel, H.C.; Razzuk, M.A.; and Gardner, M.A.: Management of concomitant occlusive disease of the carotid and coronary arteries. *J. Thorac. Cardiovasc. Surg.*, **72**:829–34, 1976.

Wood, G.W.; Lukin, R.R.; Tomsick, T.A.; and Chambers, A.A.: Digital subtraction angiography with intravenous injection: assessment of carotid bifurcations. *A. J. R.*, **140**:855–59, 1983.

UNIT IV

Management of Diseases of the Brachiocephalic and Vertebral Vessels

28

Atherosclerotic Occlusive Disease of the Innominate and Subclavian Arteries

FRANCIS ROBICSEK

THE AORTIC ARCH SYNDROME

Occlusive disease of the extracranial cerebral vessels may impede blood flow to the brain in two regions: (1) the carotid system, which supplies the anterior and middle cerebral segments (hemisphere, peduncles, midbrain, basal ganglia, and the eyes) and (2) the subclavian-vertebral system, which supplies the hindbrain (brainstem, medulla oblongata, cerebellum, and the occipital lobes.

Occlusive disease of the brachiocephalic vessels has been known under various names: anisosphygmia, pulsus incongruens, pulseless disease, aortic arch syndrome, and pulsus differens. A special form of the syndrome, arteritis, occurring primarily in young women, was named Takayasu's disease for a Japanese ophthalmologist (See also Chapter 29 on Takayasu's Disease).

In the joint study of extracranial arterial occlusion (Fields and Lemak, 1972), 6,534 case reports were submitted. Of these 1,111 (17 percent) showed evidence of subclavian or innominate arterial occlusion or stenosis of 30 percent or more. Among these patients, more than 80 percent had associated lesions in more than a single extracranial cerebral artery.

The most common underlying pathology of stenotic lesions of the branches of the aortic arch is arteriosclerosis, which, though a generalized disease, makes its most prominent appearance at the origin of bifurcation of major arteries (Najafi *et al.*, 1979). (see Figure 28 – 1). Syphilitic aortitis with or without aneurysm has also been mentioned as a major etiological factor in aortic arch syndrome; its significance, however, has decreased steadily as the treatment and prophylaxis of the disease have progressed. Other conditions, such as congenital atresia, injuries from surgical intervention, trauma, and nonspecific arteritis may occasionally also lead to occlusion. Much less common lesions are thrombosed aneurysms or emboli of distant origin. Impediment of the innominate, carotid, or subclavian blood flow may also occur from dissection extending from the aortic arch. The surgical treatment of the latter, however, primarily involves management of the underlying process in the aorta itself and rarely necessitates brachiocephalic reconstruction (Najafi *et al.*, 1979).

Asymptomatic brachiocephalic lesions are usually limited to a single vessel and are nonulcerated, whereas symptomatic brachiocephalic occlusive disease usually involves more than one artery and is often ulcerated. The symptoms of impaired blood flow through the brachiocephalic vessels is variable and depends primarily on the following factors: (1) the degree of obstruction, (2) the location of the occlusion or stenosis, (3) the status of the collateral circulation, and (4) the length of duration. Cerebral symptoms of innominate or common carotid stenosis resemble those of carotid bifurcation occlusion, whereas those of subclavian disease may indicate vertebral-basilar insufficiency; thus, the clinical manifestations include brief attacks of blurring of vision or blindness, vertigo, paresthesia, and discoor-

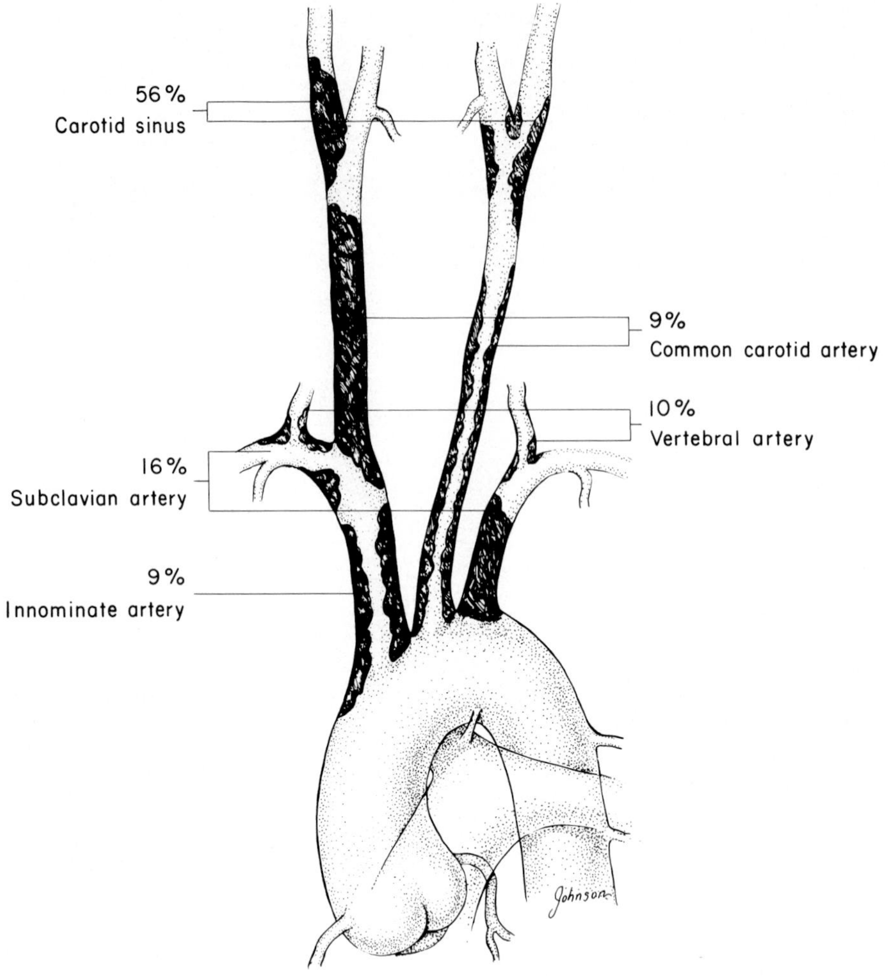

Figure 28–1. The relative frequency of occlusive lesions in the brachiocephalic vascular system.

dination, which may progress into frank blindness or stroke. These are caused either by the decrease in forward flow through the vessel involved or by the reversal of flow away from that particular area of the brain. Sometimes in aortic arch syndromes there are also pronounced mental changes, such as loss of motivation, apathy, and drowsiness, resulting in inability to work and sexual difficulties over a long period. Characteristically, all of these symptoms will be joined by those of upper-extremity underperfusion, such as pain and discomfort of varying degree, which usually worsen with exercise ("claudication of the arms"). When vertebral steal syndrome is present, the cerebral symptoms are usually those of basilar insufficiency and tend to occur when the involved arm is used.

In about two thirds of the cases the diagnosis of aortic arch syndrome can be established by physical examination alone, primarily by absence or weakness of the pulse over the involved extremity which is confirmed by measurement of blood pressure.

Beside absence or diminution of the pulses over the involved extremity, bruits are one of the most common signs of brachiocephalic disease. These bruits are usually stystolic but sometimes continuous, resembling those of arteriovenous fistulas (Ross and McKusick, 1953). To establish the final diagnosis and elucidate the pathological anatomy, appropriate angiographic studies are required. The optimal technique of angiography is percutaneous transfemoral entry into the aortic arch with a catheter. Among the various noninvasive screening tests, ultrasound, especially Doppler ultrasound, has achieved particular popularity (Mozersky *et al.*, 1973; Widder, 1977). Other studies, such as the carotid compression test, brachio-oscillometry, ophthalmodynamometry, dye dilution curves, and digital subtraction studies, contribute little if anything to the angiographic findings.

In contrast to carotid bifurcation stenosis, in arteriosclerotic disease of the brachiocephalic vessels disabling symptoms frequently occur, but irreversible neurological damage is rare (Edwards and Mulheim, 1983). Surgical intervention, therefore, is less frequently pressing and seldom urgent.

The operative indication in brachiocephalic disease is a matter of some controversy; in general, however, it can be stated that (1) symptomatic lesions require surgery, (2) significant lesions threatening cerebral flow should be operated on even if asymptomatic, and (3) surgical indication in asymptomatic subclavian steal is debatable.

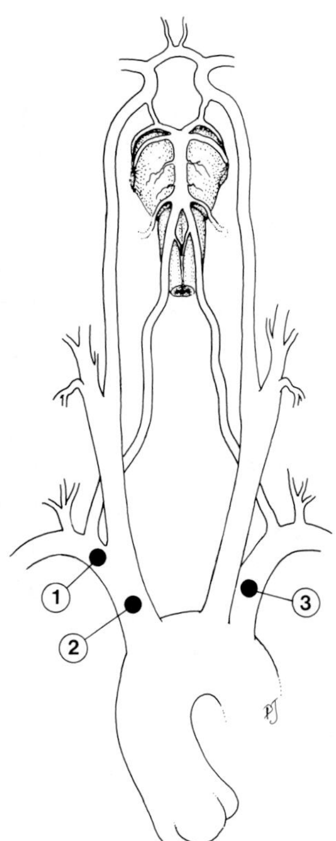

Figure 28–2. The areas of brachiocephalic occlusion that may result in steal syndromes: right subclavian artery (*1*), innominate artery (*2*), and left subclavian artery (*3*).

THE SUBCLAVIAN STEAL SYNDROME

The term "subclavian steal" was coined by Fisher (1961) in an editorial appearing in the *New England Journal of Medicine* as a substitute for such expressions as "brain drain," "subclavian snitch," "grand larceny of the vertebral," and "centrifugal cerebral ischemia." The pathological and anatomical basis for the subclavian steal syndrome is that occlusion of the innominate, or of the subclavian artery proximal to the rise of the vertebral artery creates a low-resistance vascular pool into which a portion of the cerebral arterial blood flow can readily drain (see Figure 28–2). This drainage may occur via the circle of Willis, depending on the site of occlusion, through either of the two vertebral arteries or through the right carotid artery (see Figures 9–14, 9–15 and 28–3). If the diversion of blood flow reaches a significant degree, or if the brain is already deprived of part of its blood flow because of associated cerebrovascular disease, symptoms of cerebral ischemia may develop. Simultaneous subclavian steals on both sides do occur, but very rarely.

The subclavian steal phenomenon may result from any condition that interferes with blood flow from the proximal subclavian into the vertebral artery but leaves the subclavian outflow intact. The most common cause of subclavian or innominate artery occlusion, and hence subclavian steal, is arteriosclerosis. Congenital anomalies, embolization, as well as surgical or traumatic occlusions may also produce reversal of vertebral blood flow. Classic subclavian steal syndrome has been seen after Blalock-Taussig anastomosis or secondary to occlusion of a left carotid-to-subclavian bypass graft. A particular form of the subclavian steal syndrome may develop in patients with arteriovenous shunts of the arm created for the purpose of renal dialysis.

Symptoms of vertebral-basilar insufficiency caused by the subclavian steal, e.g., dizziness, visual disturbances, ataxia, lightheadedness, syncope, and headaches, may be difficult to differentiate from those caused by "simple" vertebral or basilar artery occlusion. One clue

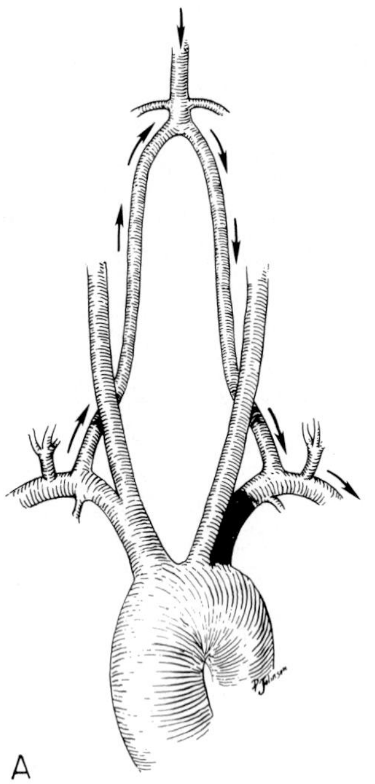

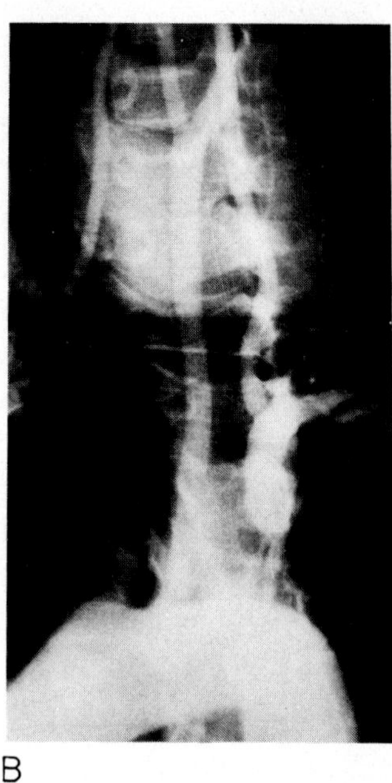

Figure 28–3. Subclavian syndrome owing to proximal occlusion of the left subclavian artery. **A:** Schematic presentation. **B:** Radiographic picture.

is that occasionally subclavian steal-induced symptoms of vertebral-basilar ischemia can be triggered by exercising the arm of the same side. In vertebral or basilar artery occlusion not associated with "steal," this will not occur. In the differentiation between symptoms of cerebral ischemia caused by carotid or subclavian artery disease it is helpful to remember that the latter usually coexist with those of impaired circulation to the arm. (Robicsek *et al.*, 1967).

About 20 percent of patients with subclavian steal remain asymptomatic providing the steal is not excessive and the blood supply to the brain is otherwise not impaired. In such cases the presence of subclavian steal may be suspected only because of the difference in the quality of the pulses and a difference in blood pressure between the two arms.

With regard to the indication for surgical repair of subclavian steal syndrome, some questions are settled whereas others are still the subject of debate:

1. It is generally agreed that repair of the subclavian steal syndrome is indicated when symptoms of cerebral perfusion deficit are present. Subclavian occlusive disease should also be corrected in the presence of clinically manifest upper-extremity ischemia consisting of arm "claudication" or, in more advanced cases, pain at rest or threatened gangrene of the hand.

2. The indication for operation in subclavian steal is uncertain in patients who have fixed neurological deficits as a result of previous stroke.

3. Because the subclavian steal syndrome is often associated with occlusive lesions in the carotid arteries, an increased surgical cure rate in this group of patients can be achieved by identification and correction of other significant extracranial stenoses.

4. Surgical indication in an asymptomatic subclavian steal syndrome is debatable. Although some believe that surgical therapy is warranted only for relief of disabling symptoms, vertebral vascular insufficiency, or arm ischemia, others, including myself, recommend that whenever subclavian steal is documented by angiography it should be corrected even if asymptomatic, especially if there is angiographic evidence of associated carotid or contralateral vertebral disease. The reason for this is that restoration of forward vertebral flow opens up and preserves an important collateral pathway to the brain, which could make

the difference between stroke and no stroke and even between life and death if carotid disease develops later.

SURGICAL TREATMENT

The type of operative procedure designed to treat cerebral perfusion deficits caused by occlusive disease of the brachiocephalic vessels in general and by subclavian steal syndrome in particular depends on both the anatomical distribution and extent of the lesion. Generally, it involves one of the following three basic techniques:

1. Operations that do not restore blood flow.
2. Operations that restore blood flow by an "anatomical approach," that is, by either cleaning out the involved artery with endarterectomy or replacing it with a graft in the normal anatomical position (in a variation of the latter, the artery is not resected but simply bypassed in its anatomical course). Most of these operations are carried out through the transthoracic approach.
3. Procedures that restore blood flow using extraanatomical bypasses, which usually do not involve the opening of the chest.

Vertebral Artery Ligation

Because the vertebral artery may be ligated without producing harmful effects in most patients, it appears logical that in the subclavian steal syndrome, where this vessel not only fails to deliver cerebral flow but siphons it away from the brain, it could be ligated with beneficial effects. At first glance, ligation of the vertebral artery seems to be the simplest method of eliminating the steal phenomenon. In the past, simple ligation of the involved vertebral artery has been used in a number of cases for the treatment of subclavian steal syndrome. It eliminated the steal and provided symptomatic relief (Cameron and Wright, 1964; Rob, 1965).

The problem with this approach is that in the subclavian steal syndrome, blood flow in the involved vertebral artery is not necessarily unidirectional, i.e., away from the brain, but may be reversible in a way that in some situations, it flows in the cerebrifugal and, in others, in the cerebripetal direction. In these instances, the steal of blood through the vertebral artery is only intermittent, and because its ligation eliminates the possibility of forward cerebral flow, cerebral insufficiency may occur. The latter is especially likely if the contralateral vertebral artery is unable to deliver the necessary amount of blood to the basilar circulation. Severe, sometimes deadly, brain ischemia has been reported after unilateral occlusion of the vertebral artery either occurring spontaneously or caused by surgical ligation (Carpenter, 1961).

To eliminate this problem, a unique method of correcting subclavian steal was recommended by Clark and Perry (1966), i.e., to dissect the vertebral artery at its origin, divide it, ligate proximally, and anastomose the distal stump end-to-side to the carotid artery. Despite the ingenious principle behind it, the procedure never gained wide acceptance because of the difficulty associated with handling this small fragile vessel (See also Chapter 30 on vertebral artery surgery).

Beside the possibility of producing basilar ischemia, ligation of the vertebral artery (as well as carotid-vertebral anastomosis) may have another undesirable effect: because the vertebral artery is the principal collateral to the arm when the subclavian artery is occluded, its interruption may induce or aggravate already existing symptoms of arm ischemia (Cameron and Wright, 1964).

For the aforementioned reasons, I believe that vertebral artery ligation for the treatment of subclavian steal syndrome no longer has a place in modern cerebrovascular surgery. Furthermore, I agree with those who believe that simple vertebral artery ligation for other reasons should also be avoided if possible (Hafner and Tew, 1981).

"Direct" Operations Restoring Blood Flow

The Innominate Artery. It has been estimated that only about 1.5 percent of atherosclerotic extracranial lesions occur in the innominate artery (Wylie and Ehrenfeld, 1970). Atherosclerotic occlusion of the innominate artery is virtually unknown in nonsmokers (Brewster *et al.*, 1985). Localized occlusion of the innominate artery may impair cerebral flow and cause hemispheric, global, or ocular symptoms by three different mechanisms: (1) obstruction to the innominate flow per se, (2) reversal of the flow through the carotid or vertebral arteries depending on whether the innominate bifurcation is occluded, and (3) embolization. If peripheral vessels are patent, obstruction of the innominate artery may often cause substantial disability but seldom results in irreversible cerebral insult.

The innominate artery may be exposed through several different approaches. During the 1960s and early 1970s, most investigators advocated exposure through the base of the neck with resection of the head of the right clavicle or through a so-called trapdoor incision. The latter involved the axial division of the manubrium of the sternum, then extension of the incision into the right fourth intercostal space (Shumacker, 1973).

Although some investigators recommend splitting only the upper third of the sternum, in my view an incision that completely divides the sternum gives better exposure and is easier to close. Such an incision can be made swiftly and easily, affords good exposure with simple retraction or division of the left innominate vein, and provides an excellent approach not only to the innominate artery but also to the proximal segments of the left common carotid and left subclavian arteries (see Figure 3–2). In addition, it is relatively painless postoperatively and causes essentially no chest-wall instability. The incision may also be extended to the neck along the anterior border of either the right or left sternocleidomastoid muscle to gain access to the innominate bifurcation, the right subclavian, the common carotid, or the contralateral carotid and subclavian vessels (see Figure 28–4) (Wylie and Effeney, 1979).

In the course of such an exposure, both the neck and the anterior chest are draped and made available for the procedure. The skin incision follows the median axis of the sternal bone from the suprasternal notch to the xyphoid process. After dividing the subcutaneous layers, the midline of the sternum is marked with electrocautery, split with an oscillating electric saw, and spread with an appropriate self-restraining retractor. The innominate vein as well as the confluence of the superior cava are dissected free and snared to be elevated for dissection at deeper levels. The innominate artery is usually easily located and is dissected free from its origin to its bifurcation. Silastic rubber tapes are passed around the right common and subclavian arteries.

Endarterectomy. The innominate artery is usually amenable to endarterectomy because in most cases the disease is localized to its origin from the aortic arch or to its proximal third (Brewster *et al.*, 1985) and the distal runoff is good. The advantage of the endarterectomy is, naturally, that it allows the restoration of blood flow without the introduction of prosthetic graft material. To perform an endarterectomy safely on the innominate artery, the consistency of the aortic wall should be such that the application of a partially occluding vascular clamp will exclude the aortic portion of the lesion without significantly encroaching upon the aortic lumen (see Figure 28–5). Clamping of the innominate artery is usually well tolerated unless bilateral carotid disease is also present. "Blind" endarterectomy without clear view of the proximal end of the atheroma of the proximal innominate artery is possible, but it is with obvious hazards and therefore not recommended.

Grafting of the Innominate Artery. Occlusive lesions of the innominate artery that appear unsuitable for endarterectomy are treated by grafting. Because the distal portion of the innominate artery is usually spared by the occlusive process, the grafting can be easily carried out from the aorta to the bifurcation of the innominate artery. The ascending aorta is carefully palpated for the presence of calcification and/or plaques, and a suitable site—preferably on the anterolateral surface—is selected for the insertion of the proximal end of the graft. An appropriate segment of the ascending aorta is excluded with a partially occluding clamp, and a vertical aortotomy about 1 cm long is made using a No. 11 blade. The edges of the incision are held open with 6-0 polypropylene sutures. A 10 mm crimped Dacron prosthesis is then anastomosed end-to-side to the ascending aorta with a 4-0 polypropylene running suture buttressed over a circular strip of thin Teflon felt. After the anastomosis is tested for leaks, the vascular prosthesis is clamped with a hemostat at its origin to prevent the formation of a "blind" pocket that may promote thrombosis within the graft while the distal anastomosis is performed.

Distal occlusion of the innominate artery may be accomplished by placing a curved nontraumatic vascular clamp at its distal portion (see Figure 28–6); or, if the occlusive process involves the bifurcation, the two principal branches are individually occluded. The innominate artery is cross-sected with Potts scissors distally from the occlusive lesion and is anastomosed end-to-side with the peripheral

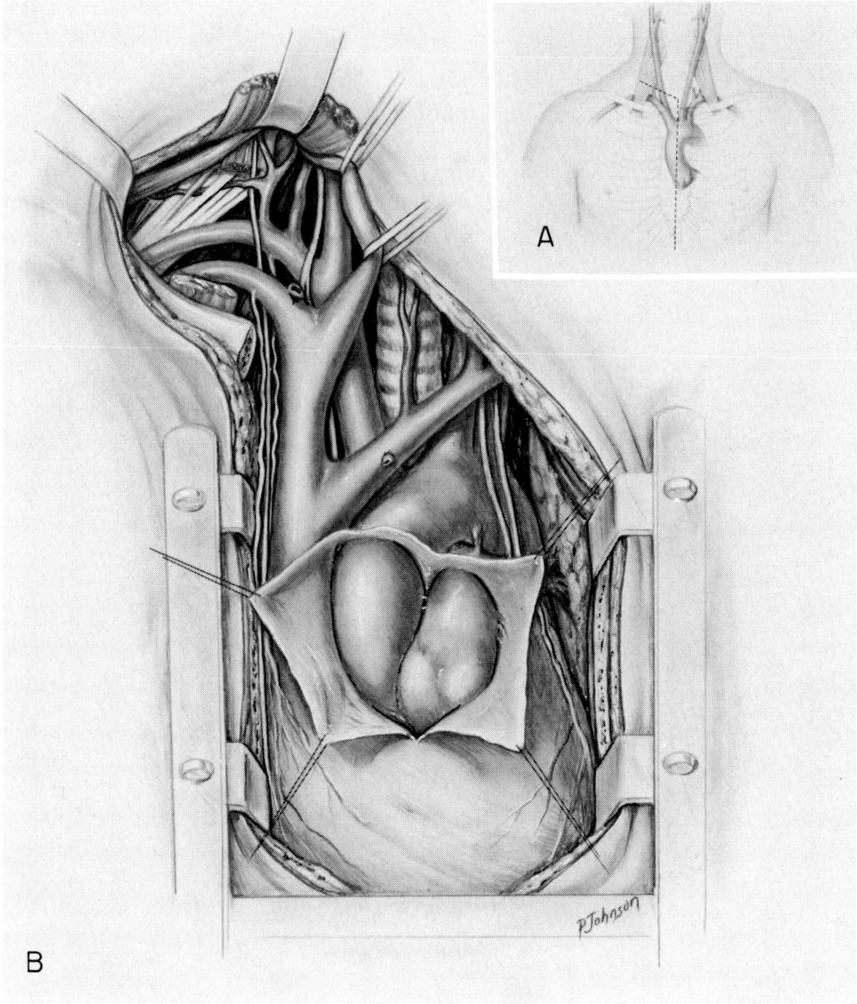

Figure 28–4. Exposure of the aortic arch and the innominate artery and its branches through a sternum-splitting anterior mediastinotomy that is extended along the anterior border of the right sternocleidomastoid muscle.

portion of the vascular prosthesis using a 4-0 polypropylene running suture.

Before the last stitches to the prosthesis are placed, air and possible debris are removed by backward and forward flush. After completing the procedure, patency of the peripheral arteries is tested by palpating the right carotid pulse on the neck as well as the radial pulse in the right arm. The pericardium is preferably left open, the mediastinum is drained through a single substernal silastic catheter, and the sternum is closed with wire sutures (see Figure 28–7A).

If the occlusive process extends into the bifurcation of the innominate artery, several other technical options are available for the surgeon (see Figure 28–7) (1) Anastomosing of a No. 17 bifurcated vascular prosthesis to the aorta and use of the two "legs" of the prosthesis to perform individual end-to-end or end-to-side anastomoses to the right common carotid and right subclavian arteries (see Figure 28–7B,C). I prefer this option. (2) Distal endarterectomy can be combined with grafting if the occlusive process involves the bifurcation but does not extend into either the carotid or the subclavian artery. (3) The operation may be modified using a straight graft coming from the aorta and anastomosing it end-to-side to the right subclavian or (preferable) to the right common carotid artery if the occlusion is close to the bifurcation of the innominate artery but enough lumen remains to provide adequate "crossover" flow between

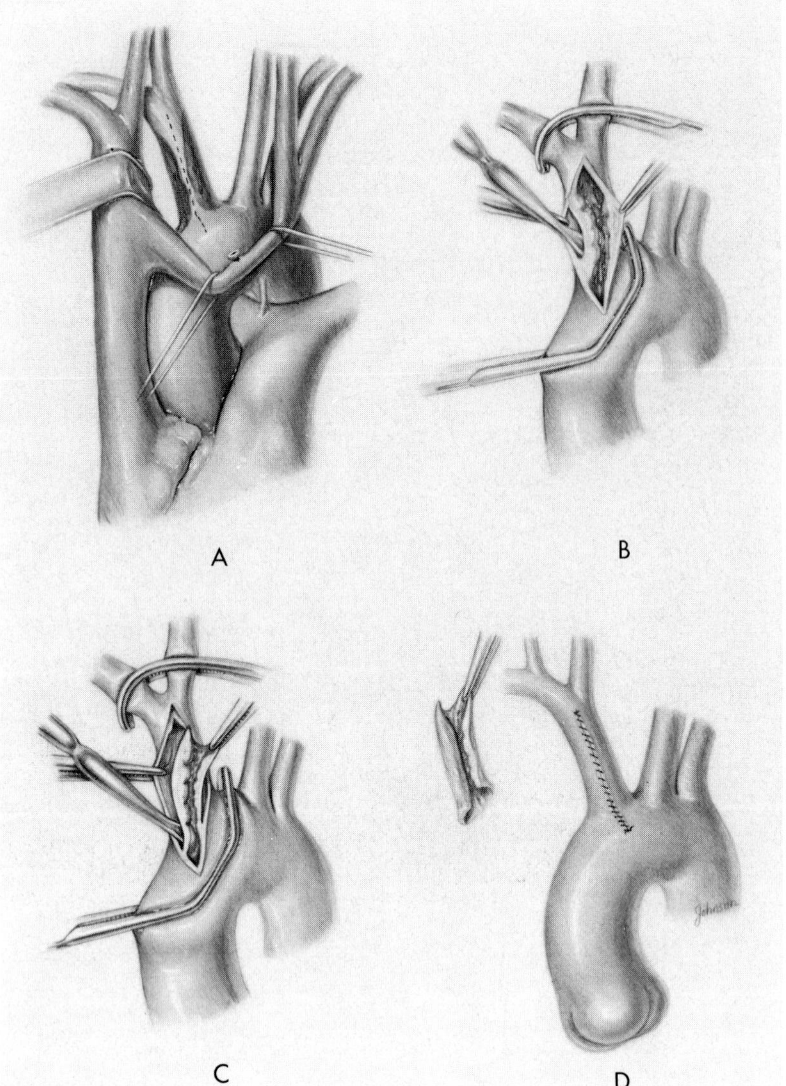

Figure 28–5. Endarterectomy of the innominate artery.

the subclavian and carotid arteries. This procedure provides forward carotid flow as well as retrograde subclavian flow through the proximal segments of the carotid artery (see Figure 28–7D,E). (4) If occlusions of the innominate artery are associated with similar lesions of other brachiocephalic vessels, a number of other anatomical or extraanatomical procedures may be applied using the intra- as well and the extrathoracic routes.

Transthoracic Operations for Proximal Left Subclavian Artery Disease. Different techniques are employed to expose the proximal portion of the subclavian arteries on the two sides of the body. Whereas the right subclavian artery can be freed its entire length through a supraclavicular cervical incision, the first portion of the left subclavian artery can be reached only through a left thoracotomy or through an anterior mediastinotomy.

To avoid the trauma associated with a thoracotomy, most surgeons prefer to use the supraclavicular approach and different types of extraanatomical bypass procedures on occlusive lesions of the left subclavian artery and its tributaries and apply the direct approach through a posterolateral thoracotomy incision only if carotid crossclamping must be avoided at all

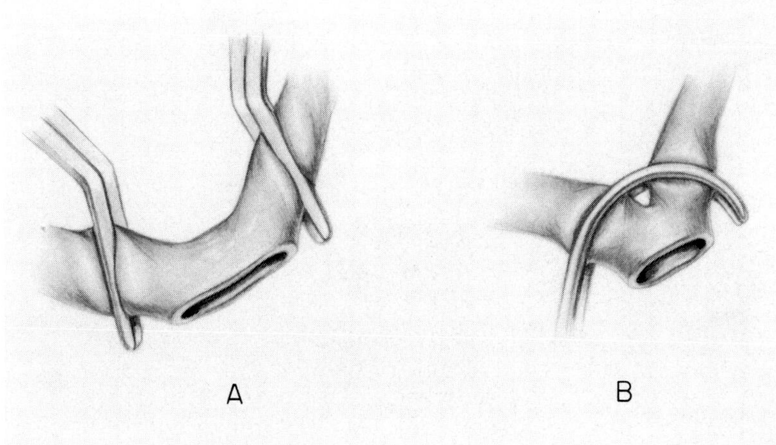

Figure 28–6. The lumen of the vessel gaps open if clamps are placed separately on the branches of the innominate artery when the vessels are divided close to its bifurcation (*A*). Such gaping does not occur if the right subclavian and carotid arteries are occluded with a single instrument, such as a curved nontraumatic clamp placed distally.

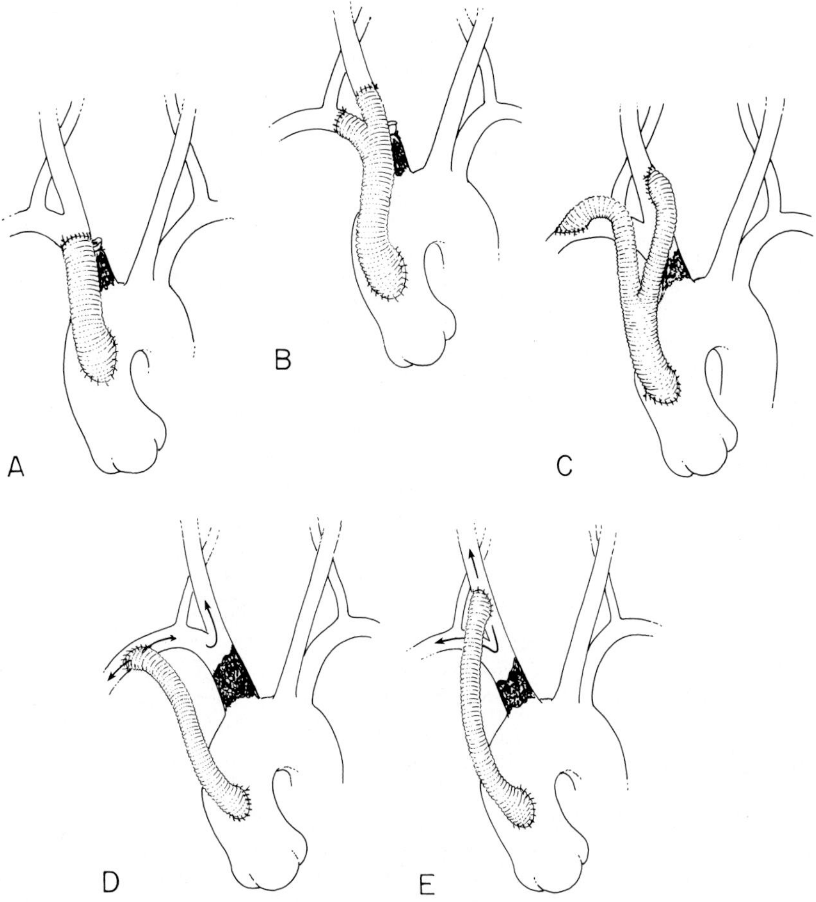

Figure 28–7. Various transthoracic anatomic grafting procedures applicable to patients with isolated occlusion of the innominate artery. Aorta-to-innominate artery bifurcation graft (*A*), aorta-to-carotid and -subclavian artery graft with distal anastomoses end-to-end (*B*), the same as (*B*) but distal anastomoses end-to-side (*C*), aorta-to-right subclavian artery graft (*D*), aorta-to-right carotid artery graft (*E*).

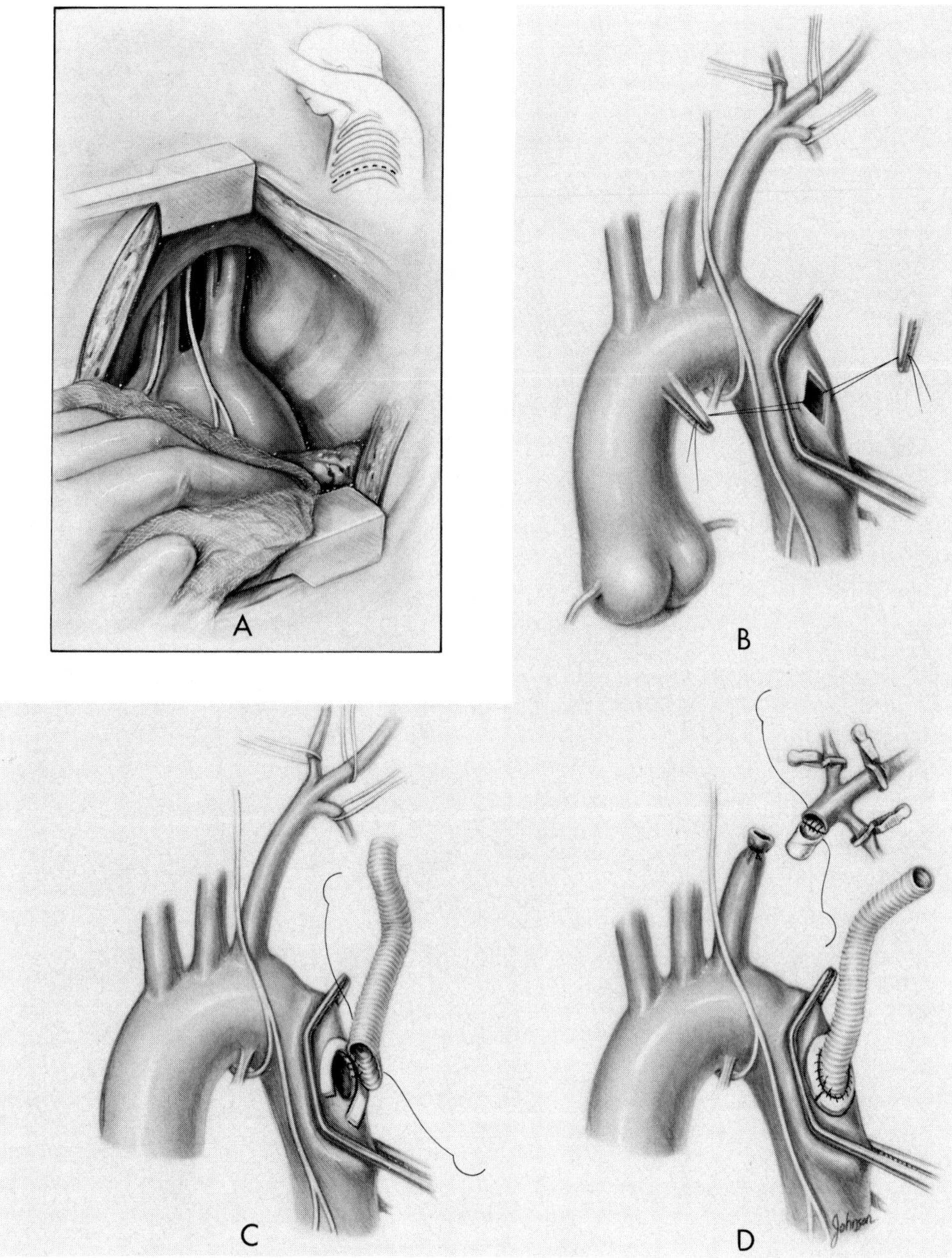

Figure 28–8. Aorta-to-left subclavian artery grafting. **A:** Transthoracic exposure of the left subclavian artery. **B:** Placement of partially occluding clamp upon the aorta. **C:** Graft-to-aorta anastomosis. **D:** Anastomosis of a short Gore-Tex graft to the distal subclavian artery.

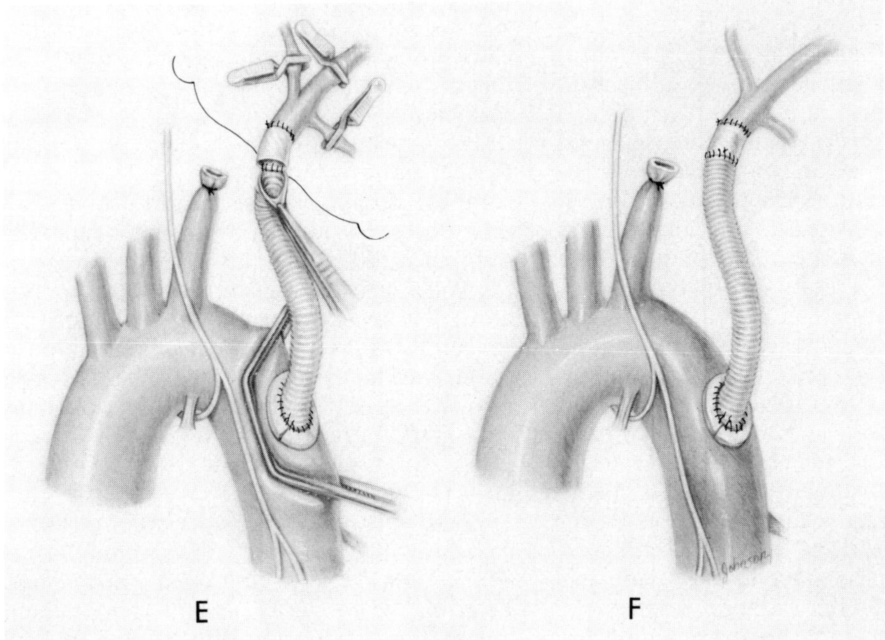

Figure 28–8. *(continued)* E and F: Completion of the procedure by anastomosing the Dacron graft to the Gore-Tex prosthesis.

costs or if an unobstructed inflow vessel is not available for extracranial bypass. Others, including myself, prefer the anatomical transthoracic approach in most cases (Sanger *et al.*, 1964).

Endarterectomy of the Proximal Left Subclavian Artery. Although transthoracic endarterectomy of the most proximal portion of the left subclavian artery with or without arterioplasty has been performed successfully in the treatment of occlusion of the left subclavian artery, because the aortic wall is frequently involved around the origin of the subclavian artery this procedure is rarely—if ever—used today.

Aorto-to-Left Subclavian Artery Graft. A high left thoracotomy incision made anteriorly, laterally, or posteriorly gives excellent exposure to the origin of the left subclavian artery and, to a lesser degree, to the left common carotid artery. I prefer a short posterolateral thoracotomy incision, entering the pleural cavity through the bed of the resected fifth rib. The lung is retracted downward, and the distal half of the intrathoracic portion of the left subclavian artery is dissected free. A double lumen endotracheal tube allows selective ventilation of the lung and greatly facilitates the exposure. More proximal dissection of the subclavian artery is not recommended because it may damage the small esophageal branch, which usually arises posteriorly from the artery near its origin, and may tear and create cumbersome bleeding. Individual branches of the subclavian trifurcation in the thoracic outlet are freed and looped with bands of silastic rubber.

The distal aortic arch is carefully examined to find an appropriate "soft spot" (preferably one on the anterolateral surface) for the proximal anastomosis (see Figure 28–8A and B). On a suitable site of the aorta, the parietal pleura, but not the adventitia, is stripped and a portion of the aorta is excluded from the circulation with a partially occluding clamp. Circular dissection, placement of tapes around the aorta, or ligation of intercostal vessels is unnecessary. The proper position of the partially occluding clamp is confirmed by checking the distal aortic pulse.

An 8 to 10 mm incision is now made on the excluded portion of the aorta with a No. 11 blade, and the edges of the aortotomy are retracted with 6-0 polypropylene sutures (see Figure 28–8B). A side-to-end anastomosis is performed between the aorta and an 8 mm crimped Dacron prosthesis with a 4-0 running polypropylene suture is buttressed over a narrow circular strip of Teflon felt (see Figure 28–8C). After completion of the anastomosis, the partially occluding clamp is removed to flush the site. Then the graft is clamped at its base so as not to create a blind pocket in which clots could form. The interior aspect of the graft is cleansed of blood with heparinized saline solution.

If the wall of the subclavian artery is of good quality, the surgeon can simply tie off the artery proximally, clamp it distally, and divide in between to allow an end-to-end anastomosis between the distal stump of the artery and the Dacron prosthesis, using a 4-0 continuous polypropylene suture. Because the distal subclavian artery more often than not is quite brittle, we prefer to perform the anastomosis by occluding the distal subclavian artery and its first two tributaries with small atraumatic bulldog clamps (instead of using a single vascular clamp) and dividing it with Potts scissors about 1 cm proximal to the trifurcation. If necessary, the distal subclavian artery is endarterectomized. The proximal end of the artery is ligated and a Gore-Tex vascular prosthesis of about 2 cm length and 8 mm diameter is anastomosed end-to-end to the distal stump of the artery with a 6-0 polypropylene suture (see Figure 28–8D). Performing the anastomosis with this short a segment of Gore-Tex graft instead of with the Dacron prothesis already anastomosed to the aorta has several advantages: (1) the anastomosis can be performed without any tension on the suture line and with fine suture material; (2) after completion of the anastomosis the interior of the vessel can be conveniently inspected; (3) additional stitches, if necessary, can be placed with ease.

The operation is completed by end-to-end anastomosis of the proximal Dacron prosthesis to the distal Gore-Tex graft (see Figure 28–8E and F). This part of the operation can be performed in a few minutes. Before the last stitches are placed, debris and air are evacuated from the grafts with both backward and forward flush of blood. A drainage tube is inserted through the seventh interspace in the midaxillary line, and the thoracotomy incision is closed layer by layer. Unless there is a special preoperatively known reason, such as associated axillary or brachial arterial disease, the patient should have clearly palpable brachial and radial pulses on completion of the procedure. Because arterial spasm commonly occurs during surgery, the quality of these pulses usually improves further during the first postoperative day.

Aorto-to-left subclavian artery anastomosis can also be made by attaching the distal end of the graft to the subclavian artery in an end-to-side fashion. Because this procedure is technically more complicated and offers no physiological advantage, I see no reason for its application.

Theoretically, the saphenous vein appears to be the most suitable arterial substitute and some may argue for its use in aorto-subclavian anastomosis. However, because it is generally of smaller caliber than the subclavian artery, it is less suitable than a synthetic substitute for aorto-subclavian grafts. Also, the claim that saphenous veins in the aorto-subclavian position have a better patency record has not been proven. In the 13 aorto-subclavian saphenous vein grafts implanted by Wylie and Effeney (1979), five occluded during the late postoperative period.

Treatment of Left Subclavian Artery and Vertebral Artery Stenosis with Simultaneous Transthoracic Aorto-Subclavian Graft and Vertebral Arterioplasty. In our view a lateral thoracotomy is the most satisfactory exposure to proximal left subclavian lesions. Contrary to the objection by Edwards and Mulheim (1980) that the origin of the vertebral artery is difficult to deal with by this exposure, we found it to be a convenient approach to perform simultaneous left aorto-subclavian grafting combined with transthoracic vertebral arterioplasty (see Figure 28–9) (Robicsek and Selle, 1985). This is done the following way: After the aorta-to-graft side-to-end anastomosis is completed, the intrathoracic portion of the subclavian artery is freed and a tape is passed around it. The dissection is now carried farther into the thoracic outlet. By exerting traction on the tape, the trifurcation of the subclavian artery is visualized, with the mammary artery heading anteriorly and inferiorly, the distal subclavian in the center, and the vertebral artery heading upward and posteriorly. These vessels can be readily exposed, encircled with silastic tapes, and closed off with small bulldog clamps. The subclavian artery is now divided distal to the plaque and its proximal end ligated. After cross-secting the subclavian artery, any thrombi can be readily extracted from the orifice of the vertebral artery. We were especially impressed by the ease with which a Fogarty catheter can be passed into the vertebral artery through this approach.

When narrowing of the vertebral artery is caused by an arteriosclerotic plaque, the distal subclavian stump is incised anteriorly, and the arteriotomy extended into and beyond the

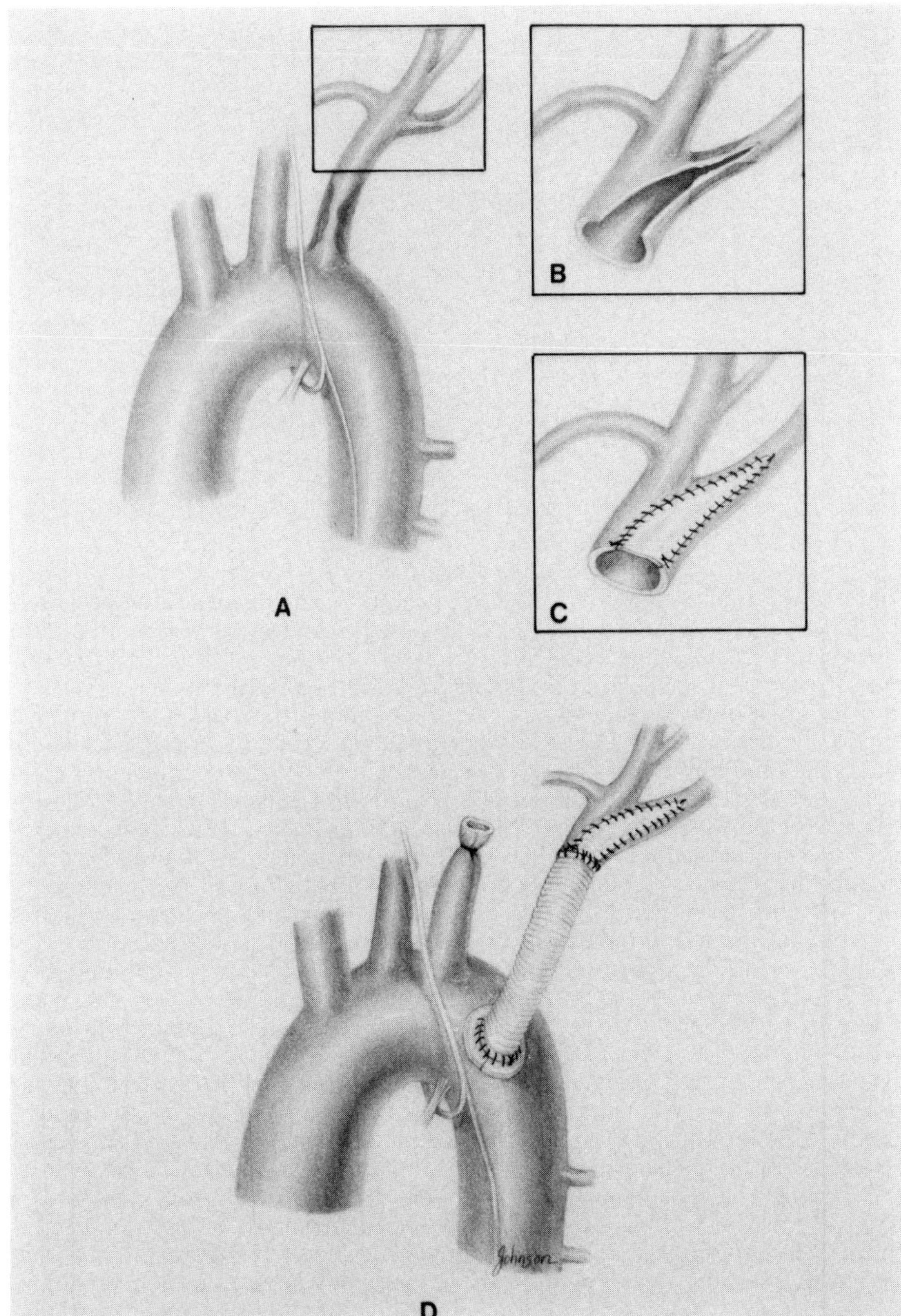

Figure 28–9. Combination aorta-to-left subclavian artery graft and transthoracic vertebral arterioplasty. **A:** Anatomic site. **B** and **C:** Subclaviovertebral patch arterioplasty. **D:** Completed operation. (From Robicsek, F., and Selle, J.G.: Transthoracic approach to the left subclavian and vertebral arteries. *J. Thorac. Cardiovasc. Surg.*, **89**:144–46, 1985, with permission.)

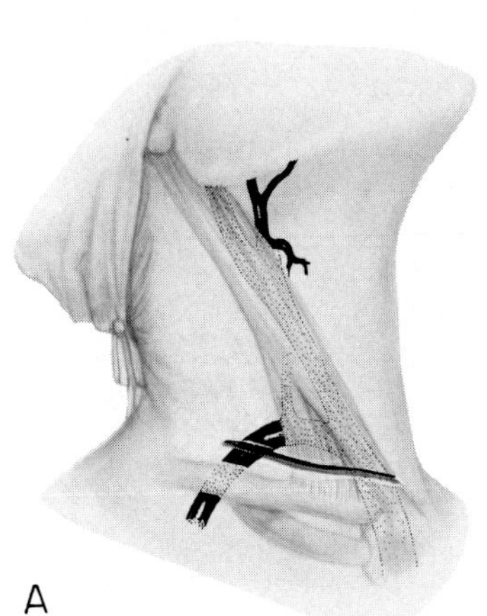

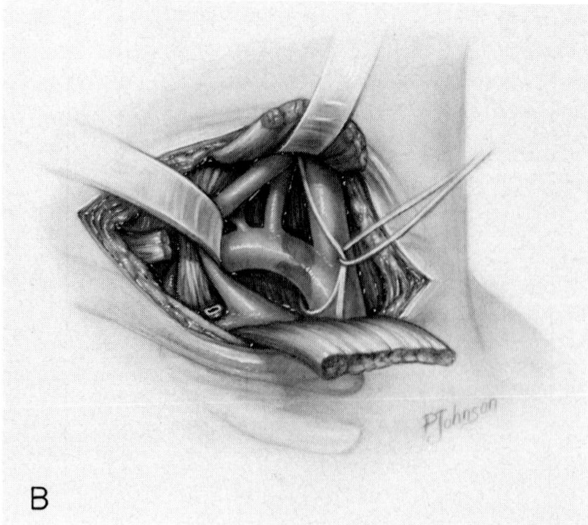

Figure 28–10. Supraclavicular exposure of the right subclavian artery **A:** Skin incision. **B:** Exposed subclavian artery.

stenosed portion of the vertebral artery (see Figure 28–9B). A satisfactory lumen is restored to the latter by performing an arterioplasty with the aid of a wedge-shaped patch of synthetic material or autogenous saphenous vein (see Figure 28–9C). The operation is completed with an end-to-end anastomosis between the vascular prosthesis and the distal subclavian artery (see Figure 28–9D).

Supraclavicular Exposure of the Right Subclavian Artery, Subclavian Endarterectomy, and Arterioplasty. Because the entire subclavian artery can be easily exposed through a cervical incision on the right side of the neck, endarterectomy is commonly used to treat occlusions of the proximal right subclavian artery. With this procedure the right side of the neck and the right upper chest are draped, the latter in case it becomes necessary to extend the operative exposure. An 8 mm incision is made just above and parallel to the right clavicle (see Figure 28–10A). The subcutaneous tissue, the platysma and the clavicular attachment of the sternocleidomastoid muscle are divided. The fat-pad on the scalene muscle is retracted superiorly. Special attention is given to major lymphatic vessels, which are carefully ligated to prevent continued drainage of lymph through the operative incision. The phrenic nerve, which runs on the anterior surface of the scalene muscle, and the vagus nerve, which crosses in front of the subclavian artery, are identified and protected throughout the procedure (see Figure 3–10B,D). The anterior scalene muscle is now lifted with a curved hemostat and divided with electrocautery, exposing the second portion of the subclavian artery (see Figure 28–10B). From this point the dissection is carried medially.

As the operation progresses, the proximal branches of the subclavian artery are carefully identified. The vertebral artery is easily recognizable as the first proximal branch. One must protect it and proceed carefully because occasionally an aberrant intercostal artery arises proximal to the origin of the vertebral artery (Mehigan *et al.*, 1978). If necessary, the mammary artery and the trunk of the anterior cervical artery may be ligated with impunity; however, it seems advisable to preserve the internal mammary artery in patients with arteriosclerotic disease because they are potential candidates for future coronary artery revascularization. Exposure of the proximal portion of the right subclavian artery may be facilitated by dividing the external jugular vein. Medial retraction of the internal jugular vein exposes the proximal portion of the common carotid artery, which is also ensnared with a silastic rubber tape. Gentle traction on the silastic tapes passed around the common carotid and the subclavian arteries will now bring the bifurcation of the innominate artery into view. This maneuver is usually not difficult, especially if the artery is elongated and tortuous because of arteriosclerosis in the patient. Care should be taken not to injure the vagus and the sympathetic chain as it arches over the subclavian artery, to leave the stellate ganglion intact, and not damage the recurrent laryngeal nerve as it courses up the neck beneath the subclavian artery.

Occasionally, in cases where the bifurcation of the innominate artery is situated more deeply, it may be difficult to properly expose and control the innominate bifurcation with the supraclavicular approach. In such patients, the proximal portion of the clavicle may be resected. Rarely, it may even become necessary to extend the exposure into a vertical sternotomy or into a trapdoor incision to gain adequate vascular control.

After exposing the innominate bifurcation, a nontraumatic curved vascular clamp is placed on the innominate artery to allow access to the bifurcation itself. The subclavian artery is occluded distally with a Bainbridge vascular clamp, and its tributaries are either controlled with small bulldog clamps or ensnared with silastic loops. An axial incision is now made into the subclavian artery with a No. 11 knife (see Figure 28 – 11A). The arteriotomy should begin distal to the plaque and extend 2 to 3 mm into the innominate bifurcation to assure adequate visualization. After the proximal portion of the atheroma has been removed, the clamp can be moved distally to restore blood flow from the innominate to the common carotid artery. During this maneuver, care should be taken to prevent air or arteriosclerotic debris from embolizing into the carotid artery. The distal portion of the plaque is now removed with a fine periosteal elevator (see Figure 28 – 11B).

As with carotid endarterectomy, one of the dangers of right subclavian endarterectomy is that a distal intimal flap may be created during dissection. Such a flap could lie across the vertebral ostium and close off the blood flow to the vertebral artery (Piccone and LaVeen, 1970). When the intima does not break "clean" distally, it may be necessary to tack it down with a few stitches of 6-0 polypropylene. After careful inspection of the interior of the subclavian artery and removal of all fragile intimal remnants, the arteriotomy is closed with either a simple continuous 6-0 polypropylene suture or, preferably, with a diamond-shaped patch of autogenous vein or prosthetic material (see Figure 28 – 11C,D). Closure of the arteriotomy should begin proximally and, after the boundaries of the innominate bifurcations

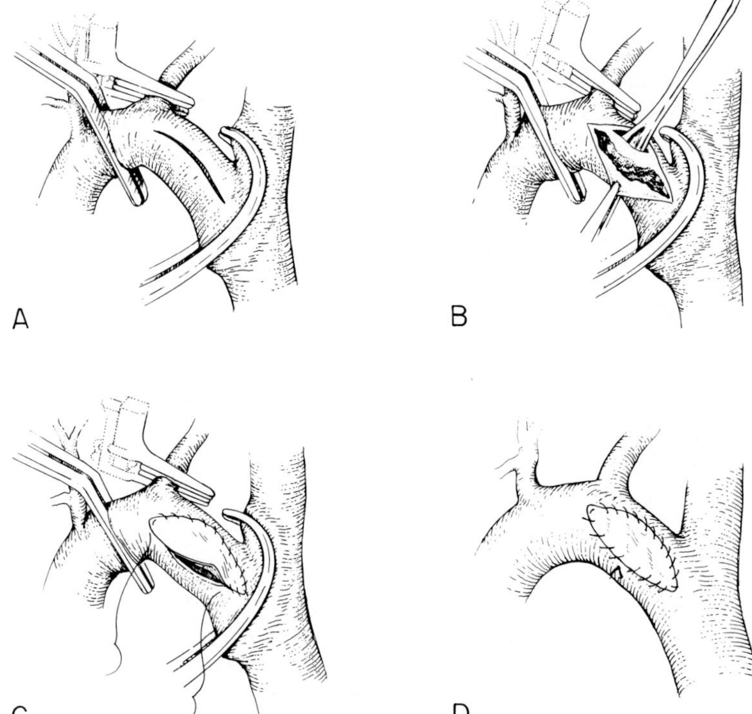

Figure 28 – 11. Right subclavian endarterectomy and patch arterioplasty. **A:** Exclusion of the subclavian artery from the circulation. **B:** Subclavian endarterectomy. **C:** Patch arterioplasty. **D:** Completed operation.

are passed, the vessel should be flushed backward from the subclavian and forward from the innominate artery to assure patency and remove air and debris. The vascular clamps are then removed. The peripheral patency of the vessels should also be confirmed by palpating vigorous distal pulses on both the neck and the right arm. The incision is then closed layer by layer. Should accidental pneumothorax occur during dissection of the innominate bifurcation, the pleural cavity is drained anteriorly with an intercostal water-sealed catheter.

Grafts from the Aorta to Multiple Branches of the Aortic Arch. A single graft with multiple distal anastomoses ("snake graft") can be used to correct multiple narrowing of brachiocephalic arteries (see Figure 28–12A). In a theoretical case of combined proximal stenosis of the innominate, left carotid, and left subclavian arteries, the procedure can be performed by exposing the ascending aorta and anastomosing a 10 mm Dacron prosthesis end-to-side to the ascending aorta as described previously. Instead of aiming the graft upward at a 45 degree angle and to the right, it is directed only slightly toward the right to meet the innominate artery in a gentle curve. At the appropriate length, an ophthalmologic burner is used to make a hole of approximately 8 mm diameter on the posterior surface of the graft. This opening is anastomosed to a similar hole made on the anterior surface of the innominate artery distal to the occlusion. The graft is now carried toward the left to meet the left

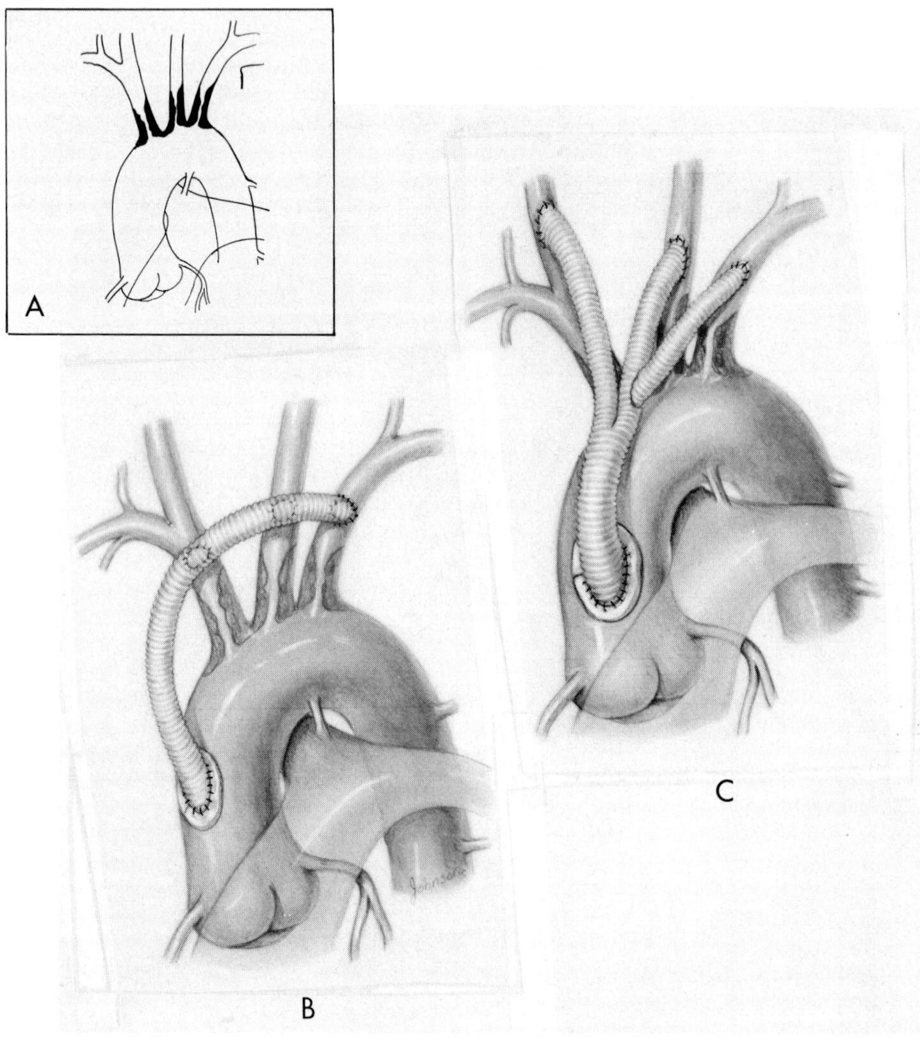

Figure 28–12. Revascularization of the three branches of the aortic arch (*A*) with a snake graft (*B*) and a "three-legged" prosthesis (*C*).

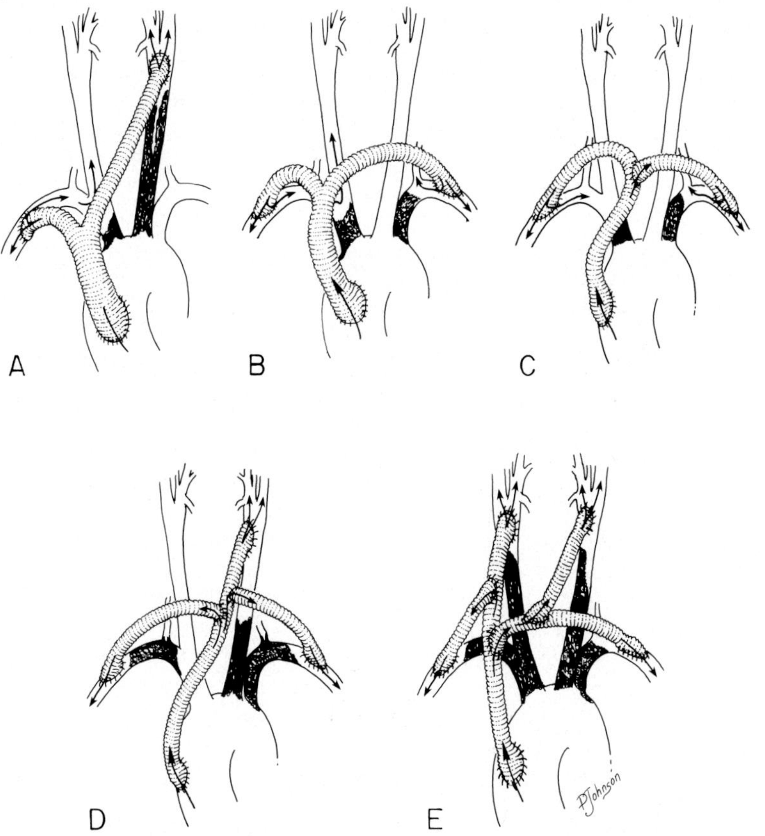

Figure 28–13. Additional transthoracic procedures applicable to patients with occlusive arterial disease involving more than one brachiocephalic vessel.

carotid artery in a similar fashion. After completing the second anastomosis, the graft is terminated by anastomosing it end-to-side (or end-to-end) to the left subclavian artery (see Figure 28–12B).

Although this method of revascularizing the brachiocephalic arteries appears attractive, it has no advantage over a simple prosthesis bearing multiple branches (see Figure 28–12C). It also has the shortcoming that if the graft fails at any specific anastomotic site, the distal portion of the graft may be jeoparized; moreover, the side-to-side technique is more cumbersome to perform than an end-to-side or end-to-end anastomosis.

If prefabricated bifurcation grafts (see Figures 28–13A,B) are used in the mediastinum, special care should be taken not to use large caliber prostheses because they may lead to tracheal or venous compression. The prosthetic graft should be isolated from the sternum by interposing thymic remnants. If, beside the innominate artery, other brachiocephalic branches are occluded as well, they can be handled with appropriate sidearms from the aorto-innominate graft (see Figures 28–13C–E).

Percutaneous Balloon Angioplasty in the Treatment of Occlusive Proximal Brachiocephalic Disease. With increasing use of percutaneous balloon angioplasty in the treatment of occlusive lesions of the coronary, renal, and iliac arteries, it was expected that this method should undergo clinical trials in the management of brachiocephalic and carotid artery disease.

Favorable experiences with this technique have been reported in both atherosclerotic (Motarjeme *et al.*, 1981) and fibrodysplastic (Belain *et al.*, 1982; Dublin *et al.*, 1983; Hasso *et al.*, 1981) occlusive disease of the carotid, vertebral, and brachiocephalic arteries. (Balloon dilatation in carotid fibrodysplastic disease is also discussed in Chapter 17).

The indications for percutaneous transluminal balloon angioplasty in extracranial cerebrovascular disease are generally ill defined and often controversial. The main advantage of percutaneous angioplasty over surgical correction of the stenosis is that, unless complications occur, it eliminates operative trauma and makes general anesthesia unnecessary. The principal shortcoming of the method is that possible complications, including acute occlusion of the vessel being dilated as well as dislodgement of thrombi, are rather formidable. Thus, dilatation of cerebral vessels may lead to disastrous and irreversible consequences, contrary to results from similar accidents in other arteries, such as the renal or even the coronary arteries, where timely surgical intervention can more likely correct such mishaps. Also one must consider the mechanism of balloon dilatation of arteriosclerotic lesions, i.e., flattening of the plaque, rupturing of the intima, and exposure of the inside of the atheroma, in other words, the creation of a situation virtually identical to that of a spontaneously ulcerated atheroma—a hotbed for formation and discharge of cerebral emboli.

For the aforementioned reasons I do not recommend percutaneous balloon angioplasty for the treatment of arteriosclerotic cerebrovascular disease. An exception to this may be a symptomatic vertebral steal syndrome resulting from short and noncalcified narrowing of the most proximal subclavian artery. Even if an acute occlusion or embolization occurs, in such a situation it is not likely to produce irreversible brain damage. Similarly, balloon dilatation may be considered in symptomatic stenosis of the innominate or intrathoracic carotid artery if direct vascular surgery is highly inadvisable because of the extremely debilitated condition of the patient, severe associated disease of other organ systems, or history of previous cardiac or mediastinal surgery.

Extraanatomical Bypass Procedures

Extraanatomical bypasses (which are usually also extrathoracic bypasses) to the different branches of the aortic arch are relatively new procedures in the armamentarium of the vascular surgeon. They are designed to deliver blood to the distal portion of a proximally occluded vessel using another peripheral artery as the source of blood supply. Such bypasses became accepted only after several investigators proved that flow through any branch of the aortic arch may substantially increase in response to a drop in peripheral resistance; thus it can serve as a donor vessel for one or more vascular beds without decreasing the supply of blood to the original area.

The term *extraanatomical bypass* is in itself controversial because etymologically it implies a "bypass outside the body" (Barker, 1983); however, it has been retained because its use is so well established. The first report of extraanatomical bypass seems to be that of Freeman and associates (1954), who performed a femoro-femoral bypass using the endarterectomized superficial femoral artery as a graft material. While operating on a ruptured abdominal aneurysm, Lewis (1961) demonstrated that the subclavian artery could be used to provide circulation to the lower parts of the body. He used a crimped nylon graft which was then anastomosed to an aortic homograft. Blaisdell and associates (1961) used a prosthesis to connect the thoracic aorta extraperitoneally to the femoral artery. A year later, the same investigator (Blaisdell *et al.*, 1962) developed the axillofemoral graft and then the axillobifemoral graft (Blaisdell and Hall, 1963). Today, the pattern and number of extraanatomical bypasses seem to be limited only by the patient's need and the surgeon's ingenuity (Barker, 1983) (see Figure 28–14).

Because the exposure of a proximal obstruction of the brachiocephalic vessels (except for that of the right subclavian artery) requires the performance of a thoracotomy, and because many patients are elderly and many have diffuse arteriosclerosis, it became a practice to apply different extraanatomical bypass techniques instead of exposing these patients to the operative risk of opening the chest.

The view that mortality and morbidity rates after surgery for brachiocephalic disease increase significantly when the thorax is opened (Fields and Lemak, 1972) derived from data by Crawford and associates (1969), who showed that the mortality rate declined from 20.2 to 5.6 percent if extrathoracic-extraanatomical bypass techniques were used to treat brachiocephalic lesions.

The validity of this postulate, however, faded during the decade of the 1980s when the risk of thoracotomy, especially that of midline anterior thoracotomy, decreased considerably primarily because of advances in anesthesia and surgical aftercare.

A recent article by Crawford and associates (1983) now reports a near-identical mortality rate, i.e., less than 2 percent in both intra- and

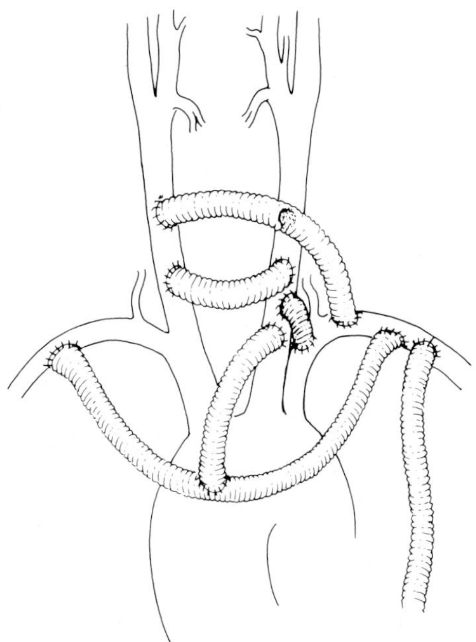

Figure 28–14. Various extrathoracic extraanatomic bypass procedures applied in the management of occlusive brachiocephalic disease.

extrathoracic procedures, with a slightly increased late-death rate for the cervical as compared with intrathoracic operations. It has always been our policy to perform direct anatomical bypass procedures on nearly all patients requiring repair of proximal brachiocephalic occlusive disease resulting in reversal of vertebral flow. During the past two decades, we have completed 52 such consecutive operations; nine patients underwent aorto-innominate grafting and/or endarterectomy, four had endarterectomy of the right subclavian artery, three had aorto-carotid grafting, four had aorto-carotid and subclavian grafting, and 24 had aorto-to-left subclavian grafting. There was no mortality in this series, and there were only two major complications; one patient had hemiplegia after endarterectomy of the innominate artery which completely cleared during her hospitalization, and another had an occlusion in the aorto-subclavian graft 12 hours after surgery. The patient was immediately and successfully reoperated. During the same period, ten patients underwent carotid-to-subclavian artery bypass by other members of our department with no mortality and one major complication (graft thrombosis). There was no difference in long-range patency between the two groups. These data certainly seem to indicate that both direct and extraanatomical procedures can be performed to treat brachiocephalic occlusions with equally low surgical risk.

Beside this significant change in the pattern of morbidity and mortality of the "direct" operations, it should also be noted that extraanatomical bypasses performed for occlusive brachiocephalic disease, especially carotid-to-subclavian grafts, also have disadvantages. Some of these have been proven and others are still under debate, including the following:

1. Because blood flow in the operated common carotid must be temporarily interrupted during surgery, this maneuver may be especially hazardous if cerebral arteries other than the ipsilateral vertebral artery are involved. It may create a situation in which the ipsilateral vertebral flow is reversed, the ipsilateral common carotid is temporarily occluded, and the contralateral cerebral vessels are diseased. The latter possibility may be as high as 80 percent (Ehrenfeld *et al.*, 1969).

2. Short-necked persons in particular have a risk of stenosis of the graft and/or of the common carotid artery through kinking by neck movements. Blaisdell and associates (1969) report a 4 percent incidence of central nervous system damage after carotid-subclavian bypass that is probably associated with such problems.

3. Subclavian-to-subclavian or axillary-to-axillary anastomoses may change the direction of blood flow 180 degrees at both ends of the anastomosis and create zones of turbulence that may invoke thrombosis. Because grafts pass anterior to the trachea or sternum, they are not only unsightly but also highly susceptible to thrombosis from external compression (Wylie and Effeney, 1979).

4. Extraanatomical bypass operations do not remove lesions from the circulation that have been or may become sources of cerebral embolization (Wylie and Effeney, 1979).

5. Carotid-subclavian grafting may jeopardize carotid flow by diverting blood into the subclavian artery especially if proximal carotid stenosis develops (Beebe *et al.*, 1980). The creation of such a bypass duplicates the hemodynamic situation which exists in the subclavian steal syndrome, i.e., it connects a high cerebral pressure to a lower brachial artery pressure.

The practical conclusions to be drawn from the foregoing considerations are as follows:

1. It is preferable to correct syndromes caused by occlusion of brachiocephalic vessels

by direct surgery (endarterectomy-arterioplasty or graft replacement) rather than by extraanatomical bypasses. In general, I prefer direct grafting procedures for the management of occlusion of the branches of the aortic arch, and utilize endarterectomy as the principal technique for short occlusions at the origin of the right subclavian artery.

2. Extraanatomical bypass should be reserved for the patient who constitutes a forbidding surgical risk for a thoracotomy or has specific anatomical or clinical justifications, such as previous operations on the aortic arch, coronary bypass, or history of mediastinal infections.

3. All extra- and intracranial cerebral and brachiocephalic vessels of the patient in whom extraanatomical bypass is contemplated should be thoroughly scrutinized for occlusive changes.

4. The carotid artery should be used as a feeding vessel for an extrananatomical bypass only if it is free of both proximal and distal occlusive disease. If extraanatomical bypass is for some reason unavoidable and carotid stenosis exists, the stenosis should be corrected before or concomitantly with the bypass operation.

5. Carotid-to-subclavian bypass should be avoided whenever possible in the presence of contralateral carotid occlusive disease.

Carotid-to-Subclavian Bypass Graft. Common carotid-to-subclavian bypass (see Figure 28–15) is one of the most common extraanatomical operations applied for treatment of occlusive brachiocephalic disease. It may be used to treat occlusions of the proximal common carotid artery by diverting blood from the intact ipsilateral subclavian artery to the carotid circulation or vice versa in patients with proximal subclavian disease or it may be used to treat subclavian steal syndrome by diverting blood from the common carotid into the subclavio-vertebral bed.

The operation may be performed through a single incision especially if the distal carotid is not involved in the occlusive process. The approach to the subclavian artery is similar to that described previously. A short supraclavicular exposure is used, but the incision is carried more medially to allow better retraction of the sternocleidomastoid muscle, thus freeing the common carotid posterior to the internal jugular vein.

If two incisions are used because of planned simultaneous carotid endarterectomy, then the distal common carotid is exposed through the route conventionally taken to free the carotid bifurcation, that is, with an approach parallel to the anterior edge of the sternocleidomastoid muscle (see Figure 28–16).

After both the common carotid and the subclavian arteries are exposed, the unoccluded donor artery which is to supply the other vessel is approached first. If it is the common carotid artery, the appropriate segment is excluded from the circulation by a Satinsky clamp, and a longitudinal arteriotomy is made on its lateral aspect. The Satinsky clamp is used as "fully occlusive" because partial occlusion of the carotid, as recommended by some, is technically impossible unless it is extremely ectatic. A crimped Dacron prosthesis or other type of graft is properly beveled and anastomosed end-to-side to the common carotid artery. A saphenous vein graft in the carotid-subclavian position performs relatively poorly (Moore, 1984). After the anastomosis is completed, the clamp is removed and the carotid artery is flushed through the graft. The prosthesis is now clamped just distal to the anastomosis. The graft may be brought either behind or in front of the jugular vein (the posterior position is preferable) for anastomosis to the subclavian artery performed in a similar fashion.

Direct Carotid-to-Subclavian Anastomosis. Anastomosis of the common carotid artery to the subclavian artery has been recommended as an alternative to graft interposition between the two vessels in the treatment of vertebral steal syndrome caused by occlusion of the proximal subclavian artery and for lesions in the orifice of the common carotid artery. The technique appears to be somewhat more complicated because of the need for extended exposure, but has the advantage of a single rather than a double anastomosis and the avoidance of prosthetic material.

The operation has three varieties: (1) With lesions of the common carotid orifice, the carotid artery is detached from its origin and implanted end-to-side into the subclavian artery, thus restoring carotid flow. (2) If the most proximal subclavian artery is obstructed, the subclavian artery is divided just after the occlusion, and the distal stump is anastomosed end-to-side to the common carotid artery to eliminate subclavian steal. (3) The third modality of direct anastomosis between the carotid and subclavian arteries is the side-to-side method, which can be used in either proximal carotid or proximal subclavian occlusion (Ed-

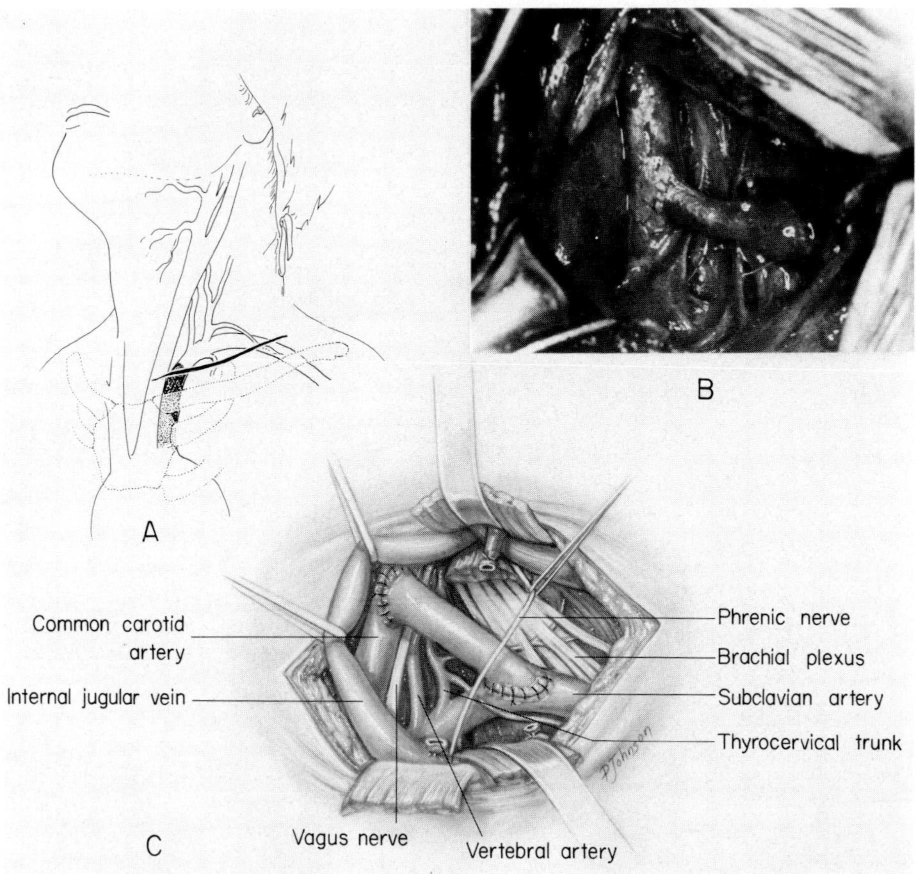

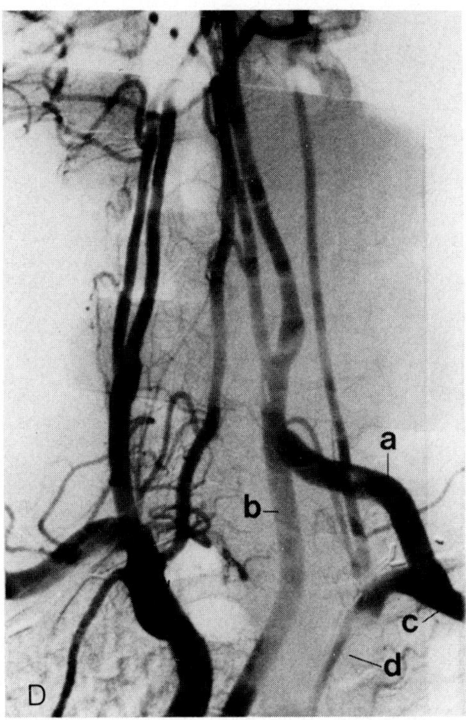

Figure 28–15. Left Carotid-to-subclavian artery bypass. **A:** Supraclavicular exposure. **B:** Operative photograph. **C:** Schematic drawing of the completed procedure. **D:** Postoperative angiogram: (*a*) Gore-Tex common carotid-to-left subclavian artery bypass graft; (*b*) left common carotid artery; (*c*) distal left subclavian artery; (*d*) occluded proximal left subclavian artery.

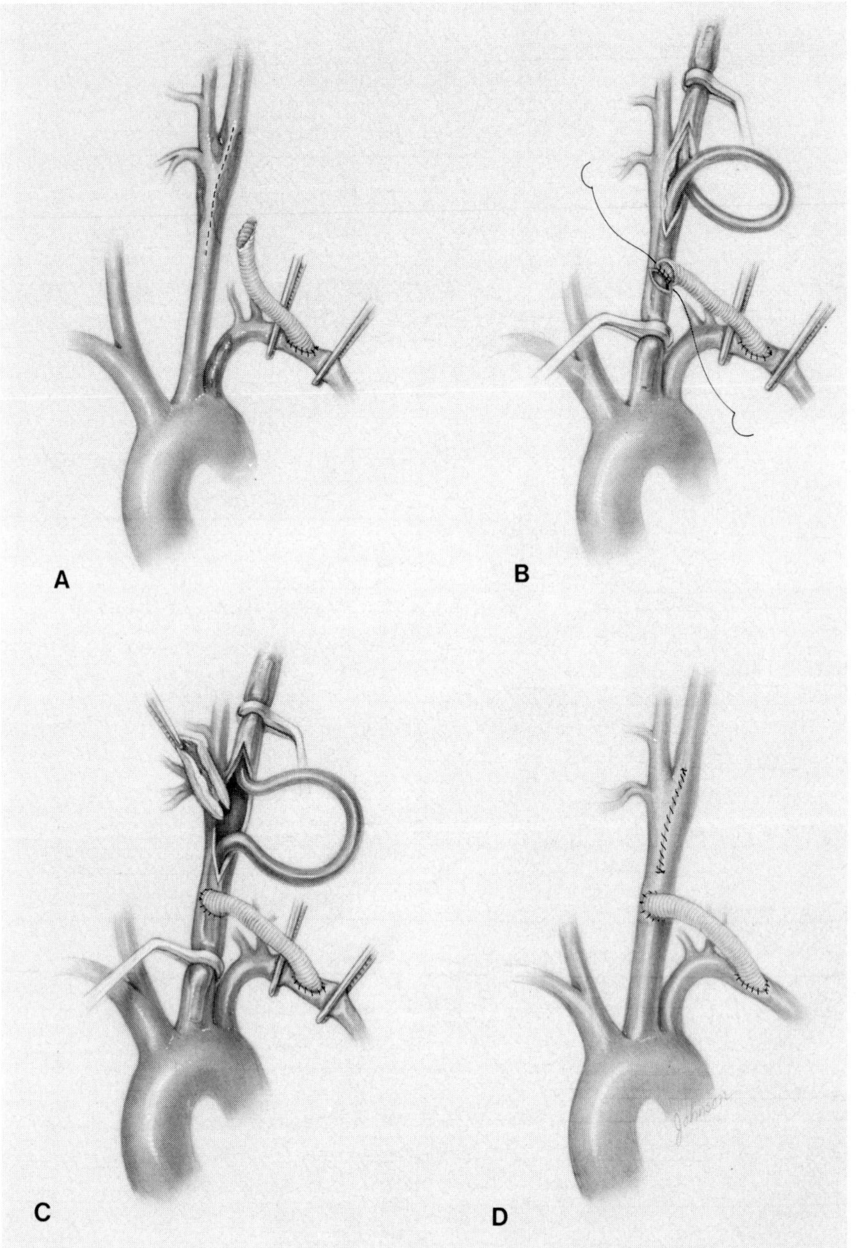

Figure 28-16. Technique of combined left carotid endarterectomy and carotid-to-subclavian artery bypass graft using the Javid shunt. **A:** Graft-to-subclavian anastomosis. **B:** Graft-to-carotid anastomosis under the protection of a Jarvis shunt. **C:** Carotid endarterectomy. **D:** Completed operation.

wards and Mulheim, 1980). The exposure, mobilization, etc., are identical for all three types of direct carotid-to-subclavian anastomoses.

The exposure of the subclavian and common carotid arteries is carried out as described previously. If the patient has proximal subclavian artery occlusion and *side-to-end carotid-subclavian anastomosis* is planned, the branches of the clavicular portion of the subclavian artery are identified. To facilitate exposure, the mammary artery is double-ligated and divided. Injury to the vertebral artery is to be avoided at all cost. The subclavian artery is snared with an umbilical tape and gently pulled upward and laterally to expose its proximal segment. Proximal dissection is carried to the level of the occlusive plaque, just above which the subclavian artery is clamped and divided.

The proximal stump of the subclavian artery is ligated, and the distal end is held by a padded bulldog clamp. Following the plane of periarterial dissection, the distal subclavian artery is entirely freed from the surrounding loose connective tissue.

The location of the anastomotic site on the carotid artery is determined by placing the stump of the mobilized subclavian artery next to the carotid while it is confirmed that the vertebral artery is neither buckled nor kinked. The appropriate segment of the carotid artery is now excluded with a Satinsky clamp and a linear arteriotomy is made on its anterolateral aspect facing the approximated subclavian artery (see Figure 28–17A). The two vessels are joined side-to-end with a 4-0 running polypropylene suture (see Figure 28–17B). Before the insertion of the last stitch, both arteries are flushed to remove air and debris. It should be confirmed that there is no tension on the anastomosis. If any exists, the procedure should be converted to grafting and a segment of saphenous vein or Gore-Tex vascular graft should be used for interposition.

If the patient has proximal common carotid artery occlusion, the situation may be remedied by *implantation of the common carotid into the ipsilateral subclavian artery.* The exposure is similar to the previously described operation; however, the dissection of the subclavian artery need not be as extensive and fewer, if any, side branches need to be sacrificed. *Side-to-side anastomosis between the common carotid and the subclavian artery* has also been recommended to bypass proximal occlusions of either the left common carotid or the left subclavian artery (Edwards, 1975). This approach uses the third portion of the subclavian artery lateral to the scalenus anticus muscle. The midportion of the clavicle may have to be resected to provide adequate exposure. It is seldom utilized because technically it is cumbersome and hemodynamically it offers little if any advantage over other carotid-to-subclavian shunts.

Carotid-to-Axillary Bypass Graft. In 1973, Shumacker extended the concept of carotid-subclavian bypass by demonstrating the feasibility of carrying the distal anastomosis down to the axillary artery. Such a bypass may be performed even if occlusive changes involve most or even all of the subclavian artery.

To perform carotid-to-axillary bypass, the common carotid artery is exposed through either a supraclavicular short transverse incision

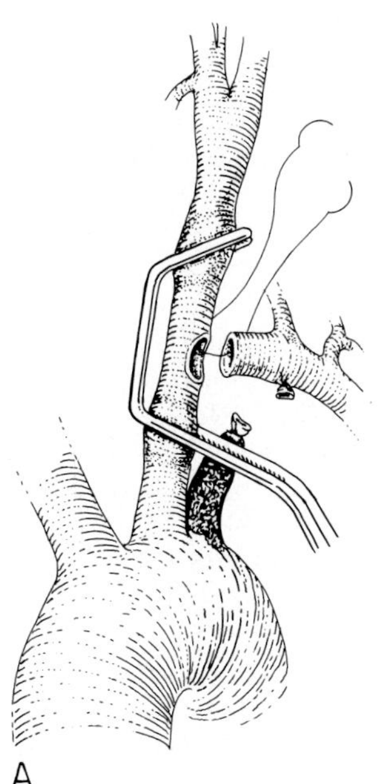

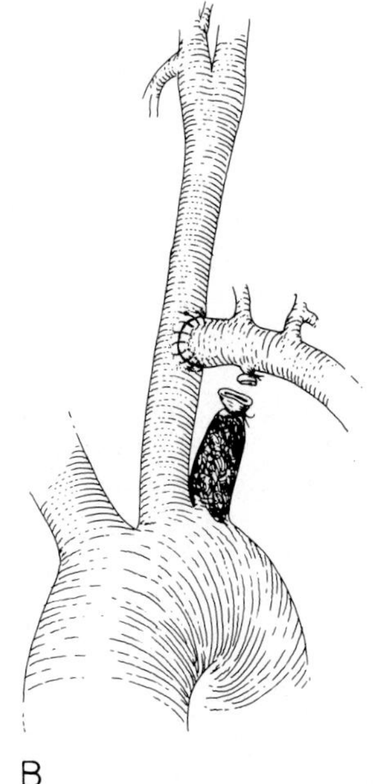

Figure 28–17. Implantation of the subclavian artery into the carotid artery. **A:** Side-to-end carotid-subclavian anastomosis. **B:** Completed procedure.

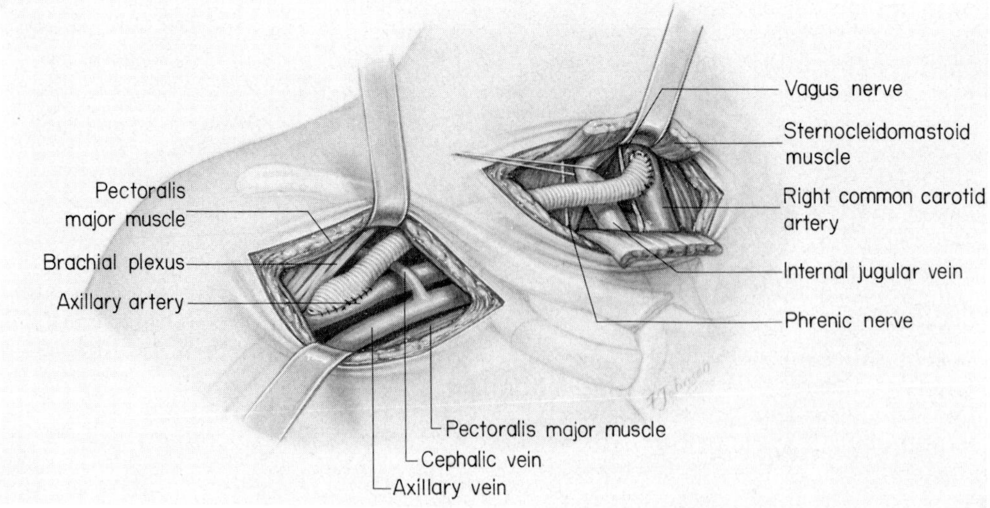

Figure 28–18. Carotid-to-axillary artery bypass graft.

or an incision made parallel to the anterior edge of the sternocleidomastoid muscle. The axillary artery is then visualized through a second incision made infraclavicularly and carried inferiorly toward the axilla. (See the section on "Axillary-Axillary Bypass Graft" in this chapter for a detailed description of the method for exposure of the axillary artery). The proximal anastomosis between the carotid artery and the graft is completed first side-to-end, and the graft is carried through either a subcutaneous or a retroclavicular tunnel to the axillary artery to be anastomosed in a similar fashion (see Figure 28–18).

Subclavian-to-Subclavian Bypass Graft. Depending on the situation, subclavian-to-subclavian or axillary-to-axillary bypass grafts can be used for the treatment of cerebrovascular insufficiency as well as to alleviate ischemic symptoms of the arm. The advantage of the subclavian-to-subclavian bypass compared with the carotid-to-subclavian or carotid-to-axillary bypass is that the carotid arterial system is not tampered with during the procedure, so that potential neurological complications associated with carotid artery surgery are obviated. Moreover, the procedure can be used in the presence of carotid artery disease. Disadvantages, however, are that a longer graft is needed, two separate incisions and bilateral exposure must be made, and it requires a good deal of dissection. Also, in isolating the subclavian arteries, which involves the division of the scalenus anticus muscles, occasionally traction or pressure is exerted on both phrenic nerves, which could cause paresis of the diaphragm, a disastrous event if it occurs bilaterally (Jacobson *et al.*, 1973).

To perform subclavian-to-subclavian artery bypass, both subclavian arteries are exposed through short transverse incisions carried about 1 cm above the medial one third of the clavicles. The clavicular heads of the sternocleidomastoid muscles and the anterior scalene muscle is divided. During the first maneuver, the phrenic nerve is identified and carefully protected. The subclavian artery is dissected free just distal to the origin of the vertebral arteries, snared with silastic bands, clamped, and longitudinally opened to be anastomosed to the beveled ends of a crimped Dacron prosthesis or an autogenous saphenous vein graft. The graft is then carried through a subcutaneous tunnel anterior to the trachea and anastomosed to the similarly exposed contralateral subclavian artery (see Figure 28–19).

If, besides unilateral subclavian artery occlusion, the patient also has impediment of the flow in one or both carotid arteries, the situation can be handled by means of one or two sidearms brought from the graft and anastomosed to the involved carotid artery or arteries distal to the level of the stenosis. Good results have been obtained with this method by Finkelstein *et al.* (1972).

Axillary-to-Axillary Bypass Graft. Depending on the situation, axillary-to-axillary bypass grafts can be used for cerebrovascular insufficiency as well as arm ischemia. The des-

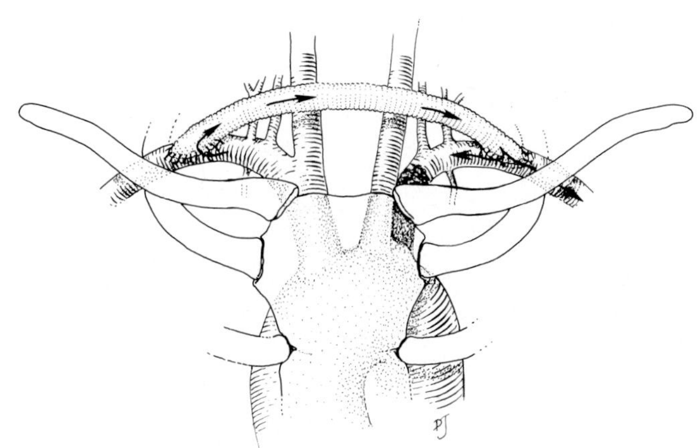

Figure 28-19. Subclavian-to-subclavian artery bypass.

ignation of the axillary-to-axillary bypass graft as opposed to the subclavian-to-subclavian bypass graft is that the anastomosis is performed distal to the outer margin of the first rib as the subclavian becomes the axillary artery (see Figure 28-20). The axillary-to-axillary bypass may have some advantages over the subclavian-to-subclavian bypass procedure because the dissection is carried out through a less "sensitive" area. It also provides an easier approach to the supplying artery and can be used even where there are diffuse but not occlusive arteriosclerotic changes in the subclavian artery of the donor side. The potential disadvantages of the method are that it requires a longer graft and that the graft may be overstretched if the anastomosis is made to the distal axillary artery and the arms are abducted (Sheiner, 1978). Also, because it places the graft in a more superficial location, the patient should be advised of the danger of compression and cautioned against lying in a prone position.

An axillary-to-axillary bypass is commonly performed with the patient under general endotracheal anesthesia but can be carried out satisfactorily under local anesthesia. The axillary arteries on each side are exposed through a bilateral transverse incision made beneath the clavicles. The incision begins 2 to 3 cm lateral to and beneath the sternoclavicular joint and arches inferiorly toward the axilla in a length of 6 to 8 cm (Mozersky *et al.*, 1973). The next step is to incise the clavipectoral fascia and split the pectoralis major muscle along its fibers in the natural cleavage plane between its sternal and clavicular origins. This will expose the first and third portions of the axillary vessels while their midportion remains covered by the pectoralis minor muscle (see Figure 28-21A). To expose the second portion of the axillary artery and vein, the pectoralis minor mus-

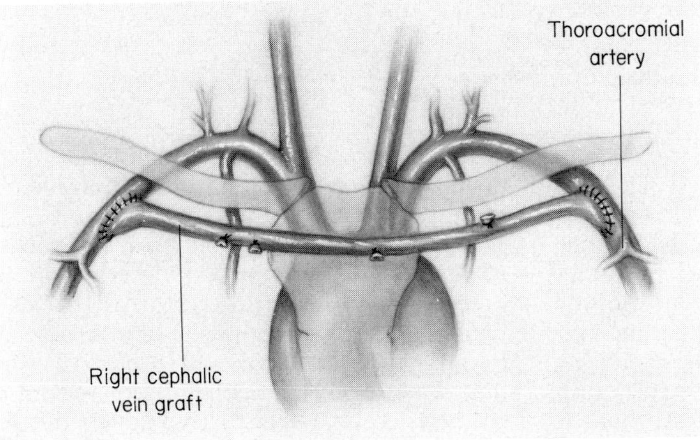

Figure 28-20. Axillary-axillary bypass.

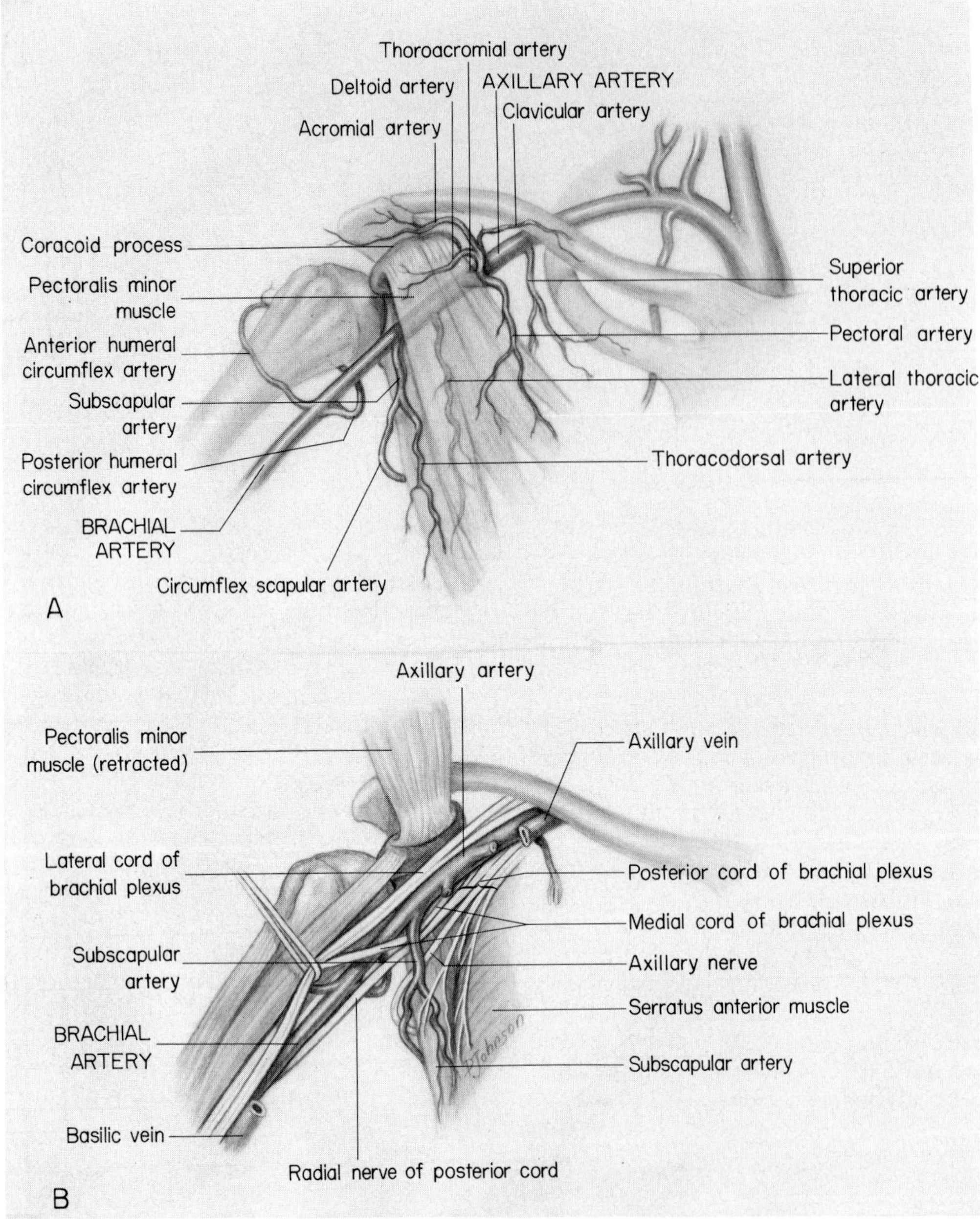

Figure 28–21. The anatomic relationship of the axillary artery to neighboring structures.

cle is retracted laterally and either divided or detached from the coracoid process. The axillary vein is mobilized and retracted to provide a better approach to the axillary artery, which lies posteriorly to the vein.

The only major tributary of the first portion of the axillary artery is the supreme thoracic artery which may not need to be sacrificed. The second portion of the axillary artery gives rise the thoracoacromial and lateral thoracic arteries, which sometimes must be ligated to obtain adequate mobilization and to facilitate the anastomosis.

The axillary vein runs anteriorly and somewhat inferiorly to the axillary artery and it is necessary to mobilize and retract it. This may require severing some smaller branches, or, if the anastomosis is performed in the lower portion, division of the cephalic vein may also become necessary. The first segment of the axillary artery is not surrounded by nerve cords, but the second and third portions are in close proximity to the tributaries of the brachial plexus. Careful dissection and judicious separation of the artery from the nerve cords in that region are required. The lateral cord lies immediately cephalad to the artery, while the medial cord runs caudal. The nerves of these cords join anterior to the artery to form the median nerve. This junction marks the limit of space available for access to the axillary artery (see Figure 28–21B). Forceful retraction or anastomosis performed too close to these cords may cause postoperative palsy of the median nerve. This can be prevented by choosing the anterior aspect of the first or second portion of the axillary artery for the anastomosis.

Similar dissection is carried out below the middle third of the contralateral clavicle, and then a subcutaneous tunnel is fashioned under the subcutaneous fascia in front of the pectoralis muscle and across the manubrium. The unoccluded axillary artery is then clamped both proximally and distally and incised on the anteromedial surface; a side-to-side anastomosis is fashioned between it and the graft. After the anastomosis is completed, the graft is occluded with a clamp just distal to the anastomosis, and the flow through the artery is restored. The graft is now carried through the tunnel over to the contralateral side, where end-to-side anastomosis is again carried out between the graft and the axillary artery.

Femoroaxillary Bypass Graft. In the past, the sine qua non for extrathoracic brachiocephalic bypass surgery was that at least one of the three brachiocephalic branches must be free of significant stenosis. This postulate, however, was disproved by the application of femoral-to-subclavian bypass for occlusive subclavian disease. The procedure was originally developed for just the opposite reason, i.e., to deliver blood from the subclavian axillary vessels to the femoral artery (Blaisdell *et al.*, 1962). If subclavian obstruction exists, however, the same operation may enhance blood flow to the subclavian and vertebral arteries. Sproul (1971) first applied this technique "in reverse" in a patient with severe stricture of the innominate artery and also with occlusions of the left common carotid and the left subclavian arteries. Because of his condition the patient was considered to be an extremely poor risk for intrathoracic procedures, and therefore blood flow in the patent portion of the innominate artery was restored by "bringing up a femoral-axillary bypass graft" and using the right femoral artery as a source of blood flow (Sproul, 1971). Femoral-to-carotid bypass was used by Borst *et al.* (1983) to treat acute cerebral ischemia caused by aortic arch dissection. Yamamoto and associates (1984) applied femoral-internal carotid artery bypass in two patients with Takayasu's disease who had symptoms of severe cerebral ischemia.

REFERENCES

Barker, W.F.: Historical comments on vascular surgery. In Moore, W.A. (ed.): *Vascular Surgery: A Comprehensive Review.* Grune & Stratton, New York, pages 1–19, 1983.

Beebe, H.G.; Stark, R.; Johnson, M.S.; Jolly, P.S.; and Hill, L.D.: Choices of operation for subclavian vertebral arterial disease. *Am. J. Surg.*, **139**:616–623, 1980.

Belain, A.; Vesela, M.; Vanek, I.; and Peregrin, T.H.: Percutaneous transluminal angioplasty of fibromuscular dysplasia of the internal carotid artery. *Cardiovasc. Intervent. Radiol.*, **5**:79–81, 1982.

Blaisdell, F.W.; DeMattei, G.A.; and Gauder, P.J.: Extraperitoneal thoracic aorta to femoral bypass graft as replacement for an infected aortic bifurcation graft. *Am. J. Surg.*, **102**:583–85, 1961.

Blaisdell, F.W.; Gauder, P.J.; and Hall, A.D.: Panarteriography in cerebrovascular insufficiency. *Arch. Surg.*, **85**:41–8, 1962.

Blaisdell, F.W., and Hall, A.D.: Axillary-femoral artery bypass for lower extremity ischemia. *Surgery*, **54**:563–68, 1963.

Blaisdell, F.W.; Clauss, R.H.; Galbraith, J.G.; Imparato, A.M.; and Wylie, E.J.: Joint study of extracranial arterial occlusion: 4. Review of surgical considerations. *J.A.M.A.*, **209**:1889–95, 1969.

Borst, H.: Personal communication, 1983.

Brewster, D.C.; Moncure, A.C.; Darling, R.C.; Ambrosion, J.J.; and Abbott, W.M.: Innominate artery lesions: problems encountered and lessons learned. *J. Vasc. Surg.*, **2**:99–112, 1985.

Cameron, D.J., and Wright, E.S.: Subclavian steal syndrome with olfactory hallucinations. *Ann. Intern. Med.*, **61**:128–33, 1964.

Carpenter, S.: Injury of the neck as cause of vertebral artery thrombosis. *J. Neurosurg.*, **18**:849–53, 1961.

Clark, K., and Perry, M.O.: Carotid vertebral anastomosis: an alternate technique for repair of the subclavian steal syndrome. *Ann. Surg.*, **163**:414–16, 1966.

Crawford, E.S., and Fields, W.S.: Roentgenographic diagnosis and surgical treatment of basilar artery insufficiency. *J.A.M.A.*, **168**:509–514, 1958.

Crawford, E.S.; Stowe, C.L.; and Powers, R.W.: Occlusion of the innominate, common carotid and subclavian arteries: long-term results of surgical treatment. *Surgery*, **94**:781–91, 1983.

Crawford, E.S.; DeBakey, M.E.; Morris, G.C., Jr.; and Howell, J.F.: Surgical treatment of occlusion of the innominate, common carotid, and subclavian arteries: a 10-year experience. *Surgery*, **65**:17–31, 1969.

Dublin, A.B.; Baltaxe, H.H.; and Cully, A.C.: Percutaneous transluminal carotid angioplasty in fibromuscular dysplasia. *J. Neurosurg.*, **59**:162–65, 1983.

Edwards, W.H., and Mulherin, J.L.: The management of brachiocephalic occlusive disease. *Am. Surg.*, **49**:465–71, 1983.

Edwards, W.H., and Mulherin, J.L.: The surgical approach to significant stenosis of vertebral and subclavian arteries. *Surgery*, **87**:20–8, 1980.

Ehrenfeld, W.K.; Chapman, R.D.; and Wylie, E.J.: Management of occlusive lesions of the branches of the aortic arch. *Am. J. Surg.*, **118**:236–43, 1969.

Fields, W.S., and Lemak, N.A.: Joint study of extracranial arterial occlusion. Subclavian steal: a review of 168 cases. *J.A.M.A.*, **222**:1139–43, 1972.

Finkelstein, M.N.; Byer, A.; and Rush, B.F., Jr.: Subclavian-subclavian bypass for the subclavian steal syndrome. *Surgery*, **71**:142–45, 1972.

Fisher, C.M.: A new vascular syndrome "the subclavian steal." Editorial. *N. Engl. J. Med.*, **265**:912–13, 1961.

Freeman, N.E.; Leads, F.H.; Elliott, W.G., and Roland, S.I.: Thromboendarterectomy for hypertension due to renal artery occlusion. *J.A.M.A.*, **156**:1077, 1954.

Hafner, C.O., and Tew, J.M.: Surgical management of the totally occluded internal carotid artery: a ten-year study. *Surgery*, **89**:710–71, 1981.

Hasso, A.N.; Bird, C.R.; Zinke, D.E.; and Thompson, J.R.: Fibromuscular dysplasia of the internal carotid artery: percutaneous transluminal angioplasty. *A.J.R.*, **136**:955–60, 1981.

Jacobson, J.H., II; Mozersky, D.J.; Mitty, H.A.; and Brothers, M.S.: Axillary-axillary bypass for the "subclavian steal" syndrome. *Arch. Surg.*, **106**:24–7, 1973.

Lewis, C.D.: A subclavian artery as the means of blood supply to the lower half of the body. *Br. J. Surg.*, **48**:574–75, 1961.

Mehigan, J.T.; Buch, W.S.; Pipkin, R.D.; and Fogarty, T.J.: Subclavian-carotid transposition for the subclavian steal syndrome. *Am. J. Surg.*, **136**:15–20, 1978.

Moore, W.S.: The management of extracranial cerebrovascular disease. In Rutherford, R.B. (ed.): *Vascular Surgery*. W.B. Saunders, Philadelphia, pages 1191–1328, 1984.

Motarjeme, A.; Keifer, J.W.; and Zuska, A.J.: Percutaneous transluminal angioplasty of the vertebral arteries. *Radiology*, **139**:715–17, 1981.

Mozersky, D.J.; Sumner, D.S.; Barnes, R.W.; and Strandness, D.E., Jr.: Subclavian revascularization by means of a subcutaneous axillary-axillary graft. *Arch. Surg.*, **106**:20–3, 1973.

Najafi, H.; Javid, H.; Hunter, J.A.; Dye, W.S.; and Julian, O.C.: Occlusive disease of the branches of the aortic arch. In Bergan, J.J., and Yao, J.S.T. (eds.): *Surgery of the Aorta and Its Body Branches*. Grune & Stratton, New York, pages 191–204, 1979.

Piccone, V.A., Jr., and LeVeen, H.H.: The subclavian steal syndrome. *Ann. Thorac. Surg.*, **9**:51–75, 1970.

Rob, C.: Subclavian occlusive disease and reversal of flow in the ipsilateral vertebral artery: treatment. In Millikan, C.H.; Sickert, R.G.; and Whisnant, J.P. (eds.): *Cerebral Vascular Diseases*. Grune & Stratton, New York, 1965, pp. 122–27.

Robicsek, F., and Selle, J.G.: Transthoracic approach to the left subclavian and vertebral arteries. *J. Thorac. Cardiovasc. Surg.*, **89**:144–46, 1985.

Robicsek, F.; Daugherty, H.K.; Sanger, P.W.; and Gallucci, V.: Intermittent cerebrovascular insufficiency: a frequent and curable cause of stroke. *Geriatrics*, **22**:96–108, 1967.

Ross, R.W., and McKusick, V.A.: Aortic arch syndromes: diminished or absent pulses in arteries arising from arch of aorta. *Arch. Intern. Med.*, **92**:701–40, 1953.

Sanger, P.W.; Taylor, F.H.; Robicsek, F.; and Tavana, M.: The subclavian steal syndrome. *South. Med. J.*, **57**:1385–90, 1964.

Sheiner, N.M.: Peripheral vascular surgery: alternate anatomical pathways and the use of allograft veins as arterial substitute. *Curr. Probl. Surg.*, **15**:1–76, 1978.

Shumacker, H.B.: Carotid axillary bypass grafts for occlusion of the proximal portion of the subclavian artery. *Surg. Gynecol. Obstet.*, **1326**:447–48, 1973.

Sproul, G.: Femoral-axillary bypass for cerebral vascular insufficiency. *Arch. Surg.*, **103**:746–47, 1971.

Widder, B.: *Entwicklung und Vergleich verschiedener Methoden zur unblutigen Vorsorgeuntersuchung auf operable Stenosen der Arteria carotid.* Dissertation, University of Ulm, 1977.

Wylie, E.J., and Effeney, D.J.: Surgery of the aortic arch branches and vertebral arteries. *Surg. Clin. North Am.*, **54**:669–80, 1979.

Wylie, E.J., and Ehrenfeld, W.K.: *Extracranial Occlusive Cerebrovascular Disease: Diagnosis and Management.* W.B. Saunders, Philadelphia, 1970, p. 27.

Yamamoto, S.; Nozawa, T.; and Aki, H.: Femoro-internal carotid artery bypass for cerebral ischemia in Takayasu's arteritis. *Arch. Surg.*, **119**:1426–33, 1984.

29

Takayasu's Disease

KAICHIRO ISHIKAWA

The history of the discovery and treatment of the disease generally known today as "Takayasu's disease" or "Takayasu's arteritis" falls into three periods, mainly according to descriptions of the locations of lesions of the aorta and its branches.

HISTORICAL PERSPECTIVE

The first period (1908–1947) may be called the "eye" period. In Japan, Takayasu (1908), an ophthalmologist, called attention to arteriovenous anastomoses of the central retinal vessels of unknown etiology that he had observed in a 21-year-old woman. In the discussion of Takayasu's presentation, Onishi and Kagoshima (Judge *et al.*, 1962) described two patients without radial pulses who had fundoscopic changes similar to those of Takayasu's patient. As similar cases were reported by ophthalmologists during this period, a profile of a distinct syndrome gradually developed, but with no eponym for the disease. Niimi (1941), also an ophthalmologist, who emphasized that the disease represents a special syndrome owing to occlusive changes caused by arteritis of the aortic arch vessels of unknown cause, was the first to call it "Takayasu's disease." He treated a 17-year-old girl with the disease and noted that almost all the 20 reported patients in Japan were young females.

Oota (1940) was the first to describe autopsy findings in a 25-year-old woman with the disease. Not only the aortic arch, its main branches, and the abdominal aorta, but also the pulmonary artery showed evidence of the disease. He designated the histological changes as panarteritis of unknown etiology. Savory (1856), an English physician, described in detail a necropsy case report entitled "Case of a young woman in whom the main arteries of both upper extremities and of the left side of the neck were throughout completely obliterated." Historically, this may be the earliest case compatible with Takayasu's disease.

The second period (1948–1960) may be called the "aortic arch" or "confused" period. Shimizu and Sano (1948, 1951) reviewed 33 cases of Takayasu's disease, including their own eight cases, and gave it the name "pulseless disease." The clinical features were characterized by loss of pulsations in the radial arteries, peculiar retinal arteriovenous anastomoses, and hypersensitivity of the carotid body and sinus. These findings were said to be due to thrombosis of the aortic arch vessels secondary to panarteritis of unknown cause.

The eponym "Takayasu's disease" first appeared outside Japan when Caccamise and Whitman (1952) collected 58 cases of "pulseless or Takayasu's disease" from Japanese literature and added one of their own from the United States. "Takayasu's or pulseless disease" was renamed by Ross and McKusick (1953) as "young female arteritis," a variety of the aortic arch syndrome, the latter caused by obliteration of the vessels branching off from the aortic arch irrespective of the etiology of the underlying diseases, as first suggested by

Frövig (1946). From then on the term "pulseless disease" was sometimes used synonymously with "aortic arch syndrome."

The third period (1961 to date) may be called the "entire aorta" period. Inada and associates (1961, 1962) differentiated three forms of arteritis: (1) pure form of "pulseless disease," in which there are no arterial lesions except in the aortic arch branches, (2) acquired form of atypical coarctation of the descending aorta without any lesions of the aortic arch branches, and (3) combination of the first two varieties. They suggested that the etiology of the three forms may be the same. Nasu (1963) described autopsy findings in 21 patients with "pulseless disease." He found pathological changes in the aortic arch vessels, in the ascending and descending aorta, in the main branches, and in the pulmonary arteries.

Strachan (1964) presented a study on the natural history of the disease and found two distinct phases: an early prepulseless phase and a late or fatal pulseless phase. Occurrence of aortic aneurysm caused by the disease was also noted in some cases. Thus, attention was directed to the entire aorta and its main branches, including the coronary artery, the aortic valve, and the pulmonary artery. The early detection of mild stenotic and ectatic changes has been emphasized (Strachan, 1964; Ishikawa, 1978, 1981).

In recent years, a clinical classification of Takayasu's disease based on the presence and severity of the key complications attributed to the disease has been proposed as a basis for prognosis (Ishikawa, 1978, 1981). The following descriptive terms may also be identical to Takayasu's disease: Takayasu's arteritis, truncoarteritis productiva granulomatosa, Takayasu's arteriopathy, occlusive thromboaortopathy, aortitis syndrome, and nonspecific aortoarteritis.

ETIOLOGY

The cause of Takayasu's disease remains unknown. It has been theorized that an autoimmune mechanism may be one factor related to the pathogenesis because of similarities in clinical systemic symptoms and laboratory findings between the early phase of this disease and in systemic lupus erythematosus, and because of response to corticosteroid therapy during the inflammatory active stage. Concerning circulating antibodies against antigens of the arterial wall, however, results have been both confirmatory and negative, including a negative relation to circulating immune complexes. Group A streptococcal infection, tuberculosis, hormonal imbalance, ethnic susceptibility, and genetic predisposition have also been suggested as pathogenetic factors.

GEOGRAPHIC OCCURRENCE

Takayasu's disease has a worldwide distribution, and the incidence is much higher than earlier believed (Ask-Upmark, 1954; Domingo *et al.*, 1967; Lande *et al.*, 1976; Ishikawa and Matsuura, 1982). Geographic and ethnic influences on the incidence of the disease and the active general symptoms, age at occurrence, sex distribution, and the site of morphological changes of arterial lesions have been given attention (Joffe, 1965; Deutsch *et al.*, 1974; Lande and Rossi, 1975). Many series of ten cases or more have been reported from Japan, Korea, China, Hong Kong, the Philippines, India, Singapore, Iran, Israel, South Africa, France, Sweden, Finland, the USSR, and Mexico. A small series has been reported from Canada.

In the United States, the disease seems to be less common, but in New York City, particularly among Puerto Rican and black populations, the occurrence is more frequent (Lande *et al.*, 1976). The female-to-male ratio in patients with Takayasu's disease is 6 to 8 : 1 in Japan (Ishikawa, 1981; Nakao *et al.*, 1967). All patients reported from Sweden were females (Ask-Upmark, 1954; Waern *et al.*, 1983). The ratio of 2.2 to 5.3 : 1 is found in China, South Africa, Iran, the USSR, India, Korea, and Mexico. A report from France shows a ratio of 3.6 : 1; the Philippines and Finland show the ratio of 1.2 to 1.8 : 1. The average age at the time of the diagnosis or admission is 39 to 41, 30 to 32, and 21 to 25 years in reports from Finland and Sweden; Japan, Israel, and France; India, South Africa, and the Philippines; respectively (Paloheimo, 1967; Sen *et al.*, 1973; Ishikawa, 1981; Fiessinger *et al.*, 1982).

PATHOLOGY

On histologic examination, the lesions in Takayasu's disease show panarteritis of the aorta and its main branches and of the pulmonary artery. The lesions of the arterial wall begin with a mesoperiarteritis with subsequent fibrosis and are followed by fibrotic thickening of the adventitia and the vasa vasorum. These changes lead to an intimal fibrosis, which progresses usually into marked thickening, often with thrombi. The destruction of the arterial wall leads to both stenotic and ectatic changes of the lumen, particularly occlusion. The affected portions are clearly demarcated from the adjacent normal sites, and segmental "skipped" lesions have been observed (Nasu, 1982).

Inflammatory changes occur predominantly in the media and according to histological findings at the time of autopsy are broadly classified into three types: (1) granulomatous inflammation, (2) diffuse productive inflammation, and (3) fibrosis. The lesions in these three types are believed to progress in the sequence listed. In 65 of the 76 cases autopsied in Japan, 18 cases (28 percent) were Type 1, nine cases (14 percent) were Type 2, and 38 cases (58 percent) were Type 3 (Nasu, 1982).

CLASSIFICATIONS AND CLINICAL ASPECTS

Takayasu's disease shows protean clinical features, and there is a long interval between the onset of symptoms, which usually begins at a young age, and the established diagnosis, the average duration being eight or nine years (Ishikawa, 1978, 1981). The signs and symptoms may be dependent on the degree of the inflammatory activity, the site of involvement, and the main complications attributable to the disease. For a better understanding of the clinical profile in an individual patient with this disease, it is helpful to clarify to which group the patient belongs.

The erythrocyte sedimentation rate is a reliable index for the inflammatory activity of the disease (Lupi-Herrera *et al.*, 1977; Ishikawa, 1978). When the sedimentation rate (Westergren) is consistently 20 mm/hour or greater, particularly 40 mm/hour or more, the inflammatory activity may be defined as being in the active stage. During this period, most patients have general symptoms independent of the grade of the arterial luminal changes. The constitutional systemic complaints, which have various grades of severity, consist of easy fatigability, malaise, fever, stiffness of shoulders, nausea, dizziness, headache, neck pain, and arthralgia. The elevated sedimentation rate during the active period, which varies in duration with each patient, is generally followed by a gradual return to the normal range. A careful history taking is vital for the diagnosis, for often there is a stage during which there is a changing pattern of symptoms (Ishikawa, 1978).

When the narrowing of the involved arteries is severe, cardiovascular symptoms such as palpitation, dyspnea on exertion, syncopal attacks, intermittent claudication of the arms or legs, pulsus differens or pulselessness, bruits over the affected arteries, and high blood pressure are usually present. With a careful bedside examination a tentative classification of the type can be made (Inada *et al.*, 1962; Nakao *et al.*, 1967; Ueno *et al.*, 1967). Total aortography, however, is indispensable for confirmation and differential diagnosis. More than half the number of patients have the extensive type at the time of diagnosis or admission. This type is the combined aortic arch and descending aorta type.

Depending upon the presence and severity of the four principal complications attributed to the disease, Takayasu's disease can further be classified into four groups (Groups I, IIa, IIb, III):

Group I: Uncomplicated Takayasu's disease, with or without the involvement of the pulmonary artery.

Group II: Takayasu's disease characterized by presence of only one of the following complications: (1) Takayasu's hypotensive retinopathy, (2) secondary hypertension, (3) aortic regurgitation, or (4) aortic or arterial aneurysm. The entire group is subclassified according to the severity of these complications into group IIa (mild or moderate complication) and group IIb (severe complication).

Group III: Takayasu's disease with two or more complications.

At the time the diagnosis is established, about half the number of patients already belong to Group II and most have pulmonary arterial involvement (Ishikawa, 1978, 1981). Coronary arterial lesions are rarely associated with this disease. Plain roentgenograms will often show calcification of the affected aorta and a hyperlucency of the lung area in the occluded pulmonary arterial segments. Pulmonary arteriography or perfusion lung scanning aid in the diagnosis. Most patients in the very advanced stage have congestive heart failure or visual disturbances that may progress to blindness (Ishikawa, 1981; Ishikawa *et al.*, 1983).

CERVICAL ARTERIAL LESIONS

Characteristics

In over two thirds of all patients with Takayasu's disease there is an involvement of the aortic arch vessels at the time of the diagnosis or admission. Consequently, these patients usually have symptoms of aortic arch syndrome but seldom those of subclavian steal syndrome. However, attention should be directed to the other areas of the aorta and its main branches, for extensive lesions occur in more than half of all patients with the disease, particularly in cases of mild or moderate involvement of the arch vessels. In this disease, the proximal segments of the aortic arch vessels are affected, and the distal segments of the bifurcation of the common carotid arteries and those of the vertebral arteries are usually spared. Intra- and extracranial collateral circulations are generally developed in patients with considerable lesions of the cervical arteries in the disease (Ishikawa *et al.*, 1983; Sano *et al.*, 1970). Actually, severe cerebrovascular or ocular symptoms, such as recurrent syncopal attacks or blurred vision, often gradually subside (Ishikawa *et al.*, 1983).

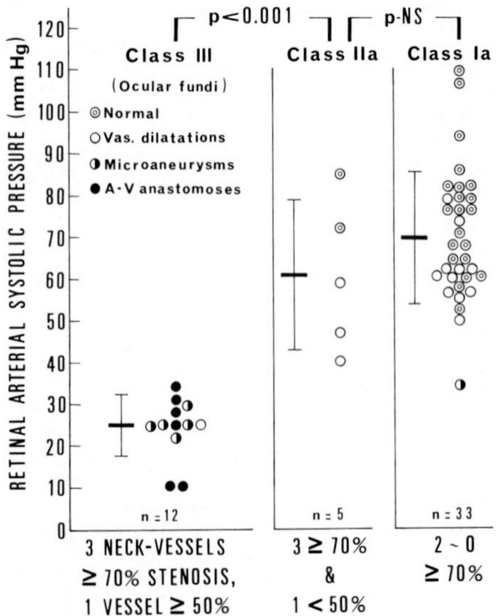

Figure 29–1. Relation of the degree and extent of diameter stenosis in the four cervical arterial systems to retinal arterial systolic pressure in 50 patients with Takayasu's disease. The vertical bars indicate the standard deviation (SD) of the mean. The average retinal arterial systolic pressure (± SD) was 70 ± 16, 61 ± 18, and 25 ± 8 mmHg in Classes Ia, IIa, and III, respectively. Vas. = vascular; *A-V* = arteriovenous; *p* = probability; *NS* = not significant. (From Ishikawa *et al.*: Occlusive thromboaortopathy (Takayasu's disease): cervical arterial stenoses, retinal arterial pressure, retinal microaneurysms and prognosis. *Stroke*, **14**:730–35, 1983. Reproduced by permission of the American Heart Association, Inc.)

Angiographic and Ophthalmological Findings

In patients with Takayasu's disease, a significant decrease in retinal arterial systolic pressure and definite changes in retinal vessels usually occur only after all the four cervical vessels become markedly narrowed. According to the degree and extent of diameter stenosis in the four proximal neck vessels in the disease, stenosis is classified into three groups (see Figure 29–1; Ishikawa *et al.*, 1983):

Class I: 70 percent or greater stenosis in less than three cervical arterial systems. Patients in Class Ia have no systemic hypertension.

Class II: 70 percent or greater stenosis in three-vessel systems and less than 50 percent stenosis in the remaining one. Patients in Class IIa have no systemic hypertension.

Class III: 70 percent or greater stenosis in three vessels and 50 percent or greater stenosis in one system (see Figure 29–2 left).

The ophthalmodynamometric systolic pressure in patients in Class III is significantly lower (under 40 mm Hg) than that in patients in Class IIa, but there is no significant difference between patients in Classes Ia and IIa. Microaneurysms (see Figure 29–3A; Ishikawa *et al.*, 1983) and/or arteriovenous anastomoses (see Figure 29–3B; Ishikawa, 1978) in the retinal vessels are usually observed in patients in Class III but seldom in those in combined Classes I and II. Significant differences in retinal arterial systolic pressure and in fundoscopic changes in both eyes are uncommon (Ishikawa *et al.*, 1983). The bilaterally reduced retinal arterial pressure associated with the severe hypoxic retinopathy is pathognostic because in patients with atherosclerotic occlusions the phenomenon of lowered retinal arterial pressure is usually unilateral (Paulson, 1976). The bilateral nature of the disease is also unlike the unilaterality of microaneurysms in patients with ipsilateral atheromatous obstruction of the internal carotid artery. Angiography is at present the most sensitive procedure for evaluating functional reserve capacity of the affected four vessels and the state of the collateral circulation (see Figure 29–2 right) in this disease as well as in transient ischemic attacks and carotid artery disease.

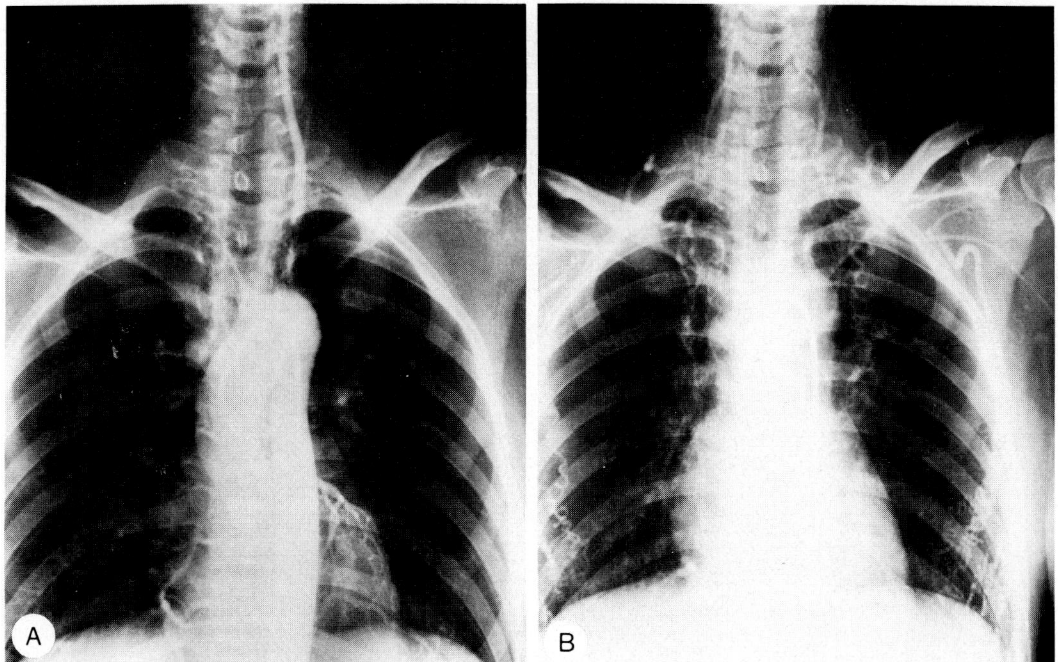

Figure 29–2. Serial thoracic aortograms of a 23-year-old Japanese female patient with Class III Takayasu's disease. **A:** Note there is no direct filling of the aortic arch vessels except the left vertebral artery following the ipsilateral markedly narrowed subclavian artery and the tapering brachiocephalic artery. **B:** (In the delayed phase) note very developed collateral channels in the neck and chest. The patient had no detectable blood pressure in either arm, but delivered a healthy baby at age 31 by elective cesarean section.

TREATMENT AND PROGNOSIS

Medical Therapy

In general, patients with Takayasu's disease in the inflammatory active stage respond well to corticosteroid therapy. Not only are their complaints reduced, but progression of arterial involvement during the active period of this disease may be retarded or even prevented (Nakao *et al.*, 1967; Fraga *et al.*, 1972; Ishikawa, 1981). The initial daily dose of corticosteroids is usually 30 to 50 mg of prednisolone, more often the latter, which is reduced to 10 to 20 mg. It is not uncommon for patients to be prescribed the drug for more than four years. To prevent thromboembolism, we often also prescribe aspirin or an oral anticoagulant independently of the presence of the inflammatory activity, particularly in patients receiving a large dosage of steroid therapy or in those with severe lesions of all the main cervical arteries. However, these treatment modalities are not completely established.

Clinical course and major treatments in 81 patients with this disease classified by angiographic severity of lesions of the four cervical arterial systems (Classes I, II, and III defined in the section on cervical arterial lesions) are presented in Table 29–1. Patients with the aortic arch type in Class II may be good candidates for medical treatment rather than reconstructive surgery of the affected aortic arch vessels, as are patients in Class I. In patients in Class III, the prognosis for life span and/or the eyes is not always good, despite medical treatment. In a recent large series, from which surgically treated patients were excluded, the ten-year overall survival rate after the diagnosis was established was 89 percent. The ten-year survival rate in patients in a "high-risk" group (Groups IIb and III) and those in a "low-risk" group (Groups I and IIa) is 74.2 and 100 percent, respectively (see Figure 29–4; Ishikawa, 1981). The most feared combinations of clinical features in this disease are multiple complications or a severe single complication attributed to the disease and severe disability.

Surgical Treatment

Surgical treatment mainly involves reconstructive surgery of the aorta and its main branches, but also includes endarterectomy,

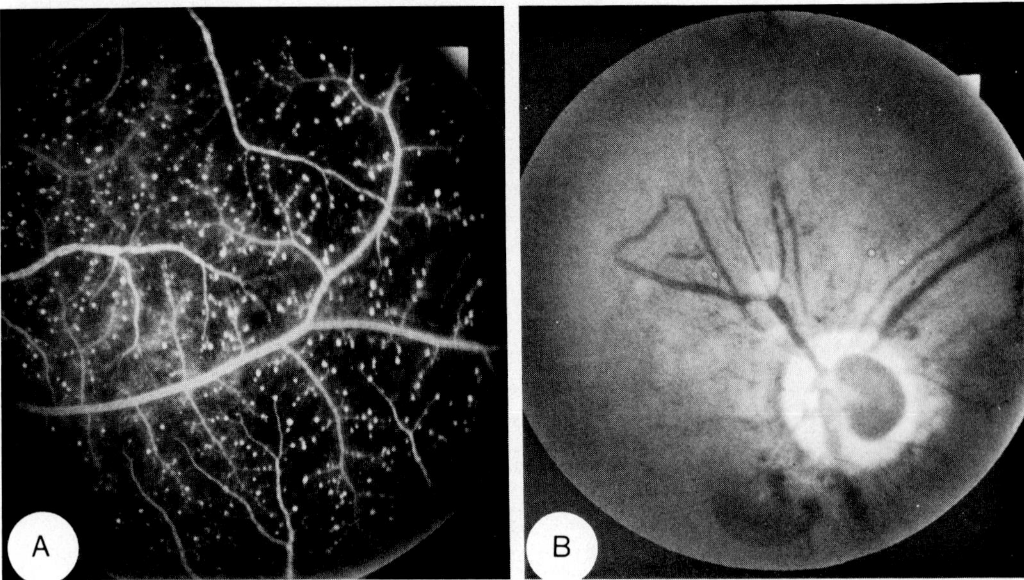

Figure 29-3. **A:** Fluorescein fundus angiogram of the left eye of a 32-year-old Japanese female patient with Class III Takayasu's disease showing numerous microaneurysms composed of saccular or fusiform dilatations of precapillary arterioles and postcapillary venules. (From Ishikawa *et al.*: Occlusive thromboaortopathy (Takayasu's disease): cervical arterial stenoses, retinal arterial pressure, retinal microaneurysms and prognosis. *Stroke,* **14**:730–35, 1983. Reproduced by permission of the American Heart Association, Inc.) **B:** Fundus photograph of the left eye taken approximately 11 months after the fundus angiogram. (*A*) Note arteriovenous anastomoses on and around the disc and preretinal hemorrhages. The patient died at age 34 from a cerebral embolism after blindness. (From Ishikawa, K.: Natural history and classification of occlusive thromboaortopathy (Takayasu's disease). *Circulation,* **57**:27–35, 1978. Reproduced by permission of the American Heart Association, Inc.)

Table 29-1. Clinical Course and Treatments in 81 Patients Classified by Angiographic Severity of Lesions of Four Cervical Arterial Systems

CLINICAL COURSE AND TREATMENTS	CLASS III (N = 12)	CLASS II (N = 6)	CLASS I (N = 63)
Onset to Diagnosis:			
Age at onset (mean ± SD)	25.4 ± 6.3 years	23.2 ± 10.1 years	21.4 ± 7.0 years
Age at diagnosis (mean ± SD)	34.8 ± 9.9 years	39.7 ± 15.2 years	30.0 ± 9.7 years
Cerebral infarction with sequelae	2 (17%)	0	0
Cerebral hemorrhage or SAH	0	0	0
After Diagnosis:			
Length of follow up (mean ± SD)	9.0 ± 5.1 years	4.0 ± 2.7 years	7.0 ± 4.9 years
Blindness (uni- or bilateral)	4 (33%)	0	0
Cerebral infarction	1 (8%)	0	2 (3%)
Cerebral hemorrhage or SAH	0	0	2 (3%)
Lethal heart failure	0	0	2 (3%)
Deaths related to operation	0	0	3 (5%)
Total number of patients who died from Takayasu's disease	2 (17%)	0	9 (14%)
Surgically treated patients	1 (8%)	0	10 (16%)
Corticosteroid therapy	5 (42%)	4 (67%)	31 (49%)
Oral anticoagulant therapy	11 (92%)	2 (33%)	29 (46%)

* SAH = subarachnoid hemorrhage; SD = standard deviation.

From: Ishikawa, K.; Uyama, M., and Asayama, K.: Occlusive thromboaortopathy (Takayasu's disease): cervical arterial stenoses, retinal arterial pressure, retinal microaneurysms and prognosis. *Stroke,* **14**:730–35, 1983. Reproduced by permission of the American Heart Association, Inc.

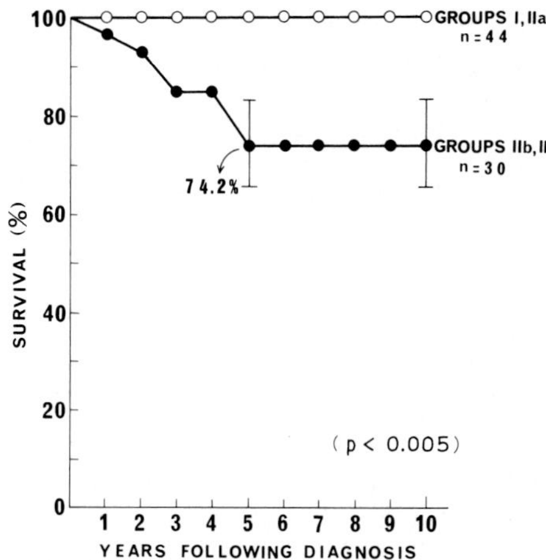

Figure 29-4. Comparison of survival rates after establishment of the diagnosis in patients with Takayasu's disease in Groups I and IIa and Groups IIb and III. The vertical bars indicate the standard error: p = probability. (From Ishikawa, K.: Survival and morbidity after diagnosis of occlusive thromboaortopathy (Takayasu's disease). *Am. J. Cardiol.*, **47**:1026-32, 1981. Reproduced with permission.)

aneurysmectomy, and aortic valve replacement. The surgical results seem to depend on the location, extent, and severity of the lesions in the aorta and its main branches. Of 67 patients who underwent surgical treatment, 18 (26.9 percent) died—11 (16.4 percent) were lost during surgery and 7 died later. Of these 67 patients, 18 had severe or moderate lesions in the four cervical arterial systems. Death occurred in three of these 18 and was attributed to intracerebral and subarachnoidal bleeding after the reconstruction of the aortic arch vessels. In one patient, retinal bleeding led to unilateral blindness (Kimoto, 1979). In a patient in Class III (see Table 29-1; Ishikawa *et al.*, 1983), retinal bleeding occurred after a bypass graft, and a subsequent occlusion of the graft led to bilateral blindness. Radical surgery of the cervical arterial lesions was performed in 29 patients with the disease. Three immediate postoperative deaths occurred in this group. In two patients, the cause of death was apoplexy (Pokrovsky and Tsyreshkin, 1975). In a report of 33 patients with the disease who underwent surgical therapy of the affected aortic arch vessels, no death related to the operation occurred, and 30 remained completely asymptomatic in the postoperative period (Kieffer and Natali, 1983). One patient died because of massive frontal hemorrhage five days after bilateral common carotid artery reconstruction. He also had microaneurysms in both eyes (Kusaba *et al.*, 1973).

Intracranial hemorrhage after cervical arterial reconstruction may develop not only in patients with acute stroke but also in those with severely affected aortic arch vessels from Takayasu's disease, despite no evidence of fresh cerebral infarction. Intrapartum cerebral hemorrhage (Ishikawa and Matsuura, 1982) occurs in some patients with extensive and severe occlusion and/or narrowing of the four cervical arteries. Such an intracranial hemorrhage, including retinal bleeding, under these conditions in patients with Takayasu's disease may be due in part to a combination of severity of rapid blood pressure elevation and some cerebral vasculopathy, the latter probably like a retinal vasculopathy in the disease owing to antecedent chronic cerebral ischemia (Ishikawa and Matsuura, 1982). In general, in patients with this disease who were selected for surgery, the markedly accelerated sedimentation rate should be treated with steroid therapy until the rate returns to normal before surgery is undertaken. A careful long-term follow up is required because of the surgical risks and because the activity of the disease may increase after operation (Ishikawa, 1981).

Patients with lesions of the cervical arteries, most of whom are good candidates for surgical treatment of the affected vessels, may also respond well to medical treatment or management, and some patients with a poor prognosis despite medical treatment may also have a poor prognosis despite surgical treatment.

REFERENCES

Ask-Upmark, E.: On the "pulseless disease" outside of Japan. *Acta Med. Scand.*, **149**:161-78, 1954.

Caccamise, W.C., and Whitman, J.F.: Pulseless disease: a preliminary case report. *Am. Heart. J.*, **44**:629-33, 1952.

Deutsch, V.; Wexler, L.; and Deutsch, H.: Takayasu's arteritis: an angiographic study with remarks on ethnic distribution in Israel. *A.J.R.*, **122**:13-28, 1974.

Domingo, R.T.; Maramba, T.P.; Torres, L.F.; and Wesolowski, S.A.: Acquired aorto-arteritis: a worldwide vascular entity. *Arch. Surg.*, **95**:780-90, 1967.

Fiessinger, J.N.; Tawfik-Taher, S.; Capron, L.; Laurian, C.; Cormier, J.M.; Camilleri, J.P.; and Housset, E.: Maladie de Takayasu: critères diagnostiques. *Nouv. Press. Med.*, **11**:583-86, 1982.

Fraga, A.; Mintz, G.; Valle, L.; and Flores-Izquierdo, G.: Takayasu's arteritis: frequency of systemic manifestations (study of 22 patients) and favorable response to maintenance steroid therapy with adrenocorticosteroids (12 patients). *Arthritis Rheum.*, **15**:617-24, 1972.

Frövig, A.G.: Bilateral obliteration of the common carotid artery: thromboangiitis obliterans? *Acta Psychiatr. Neurol. (Suppl.)*, **39**:1–79, 1946.

Inada, K.; Shimizu, H.; Ishiai, S.; Kobayashi, I., and Kawamoto, S.: Pulseless disease and atypical coarctation of the aorta. *Kokyu To Junkan.*, **9**:15–24, 1961 (in Japanese).

Inada, K.; Shimizu, H.; and Yokoyama, T.: Pulseless disease and atypical coarctation of the aorta with special reference to their genesis. *Surgery*, **52**:433–43, 1962.

Ishikawa, K.: Natural history and classification of occlusive thromboaortopathy (Takayasu's disease). *Circulation*, **57**:27–35, 1978.

Ishikawa, K.: Survival and morbidity after diagnosis of occlusive thromboaortopathy (Takayasu's disease). *Am. J. Cardiol.*, **47**:1026–32, 1981.

Ishikawa, K., and Matsuura, S.: Occlusive thromboaortopathy (Takayasu's disease) and pregnancy: clinical course and management of 33 pregnancies and deliveries. *Am. J. Cardiol.*, **50**:1293–1300, 1982.

Ishikawa, K.; Uyama, M.; and Asayama, K.: Occlusive thromboaortopathy (Takayasu's disease): cervical arterial stenoses, retinal arterial pressure, retinal microaneurysms and prognosis. *Stroke*, **14**:730–35, 1983.

Joffe, N.: Aortitis of obscure origin in the African. *Clin. Radiol.*, **16**:130–40, 1965.

Judge, R.D.; Currier, R.D.; Gracie, W.A.; and Figley, M.M.: Takayasu's arteritis and the aortic arch syndrome. *Am. J. Med.*, **32**:379–92, 1962.

Kieffer, E., and Natali, J.: Supraaortic trunk lesions in Takayasu's arteritis. In Bergan, J.J., and Yao, J.S.T. (eds.). *Cerebrovascular Insufficiency*. Grune & Stratton, New York, pages 395–415, 1983.

Kimoto, S.: The history and present status of aortic surgery in Japan: particularly for aortitis syndrome. *J. Cardiovasc. Surg.*, **20**:107–26, 1979.

Kusaba, A.; Inokuchi, K.; Kiyose, T.; and Oka, N.: Carotid reconstruction for Takayasu's (pulseless) disease using open thromboendarterectomy at aortocarotid junction. *Jpn. J. Surg.*, **3**:91–97, 1973.

Lande, A.; Bard, R.; Rossi, P.; Passariello, R.; and Castrucci, A.: Takayasu's arteritis: a worldwide entity. *N.Y. State J. Med.*, **76**:1477–82, 1976.

Lande, A., and Rossi, P.: The value of total aortography in the diagnosis of Takayasu's arteritis. *Radiology*, **114**:287–97, 1975.

Lupi-Herrera, E.; Sánchez-Torres, G.; Marcushamer, J.; Mispireta, J.; Horwitz, S.; and Vela, J.E.: Takayasu's arteritis: clinical study of 107 cases. *Am. Heart. J.*, **93**:94–103, 1977.

Nakao, K.; Ikeda, M.; Kimata, S.; Niitani, H.; Miyahara, M.; Ishimi, Z.; Hashiba, K.; Takeda, Y.; Ozawa, T.; Matsushita, S.; and Kuramochi, M.: Takayasu's arteritis: clinical report of eighty-four cases and immunological studies of seven cases. *Circulation*, **35**:1141–55, 1967.

Nasu, T.: Pathology of pulseless disease: a systematic study and critical review of twenty-one autopsy cases reported in Japan. *Angiology*, **14**:225–42, 1963.

Nasu, T.: Takayasu's truncoarteritis: pulseless disease or aortitis syndrome. *Acta Pathol. Jpn.*, **32**(Suppl. 1):117–31, 1982.

Niimi, Y.: A case of Takayasu's disease. *Sogo Ganka Zasshi*, **36**:1404–10, 1941 (in Japanese).

Oota, K.: Ein seltener Fall von beiderseitigem Carotis-Sublcaviaverschluss (Ein Beitrag zur Pathologie der Anastomosis peripapillaris des Auges mit fehlendem Radialpuls). *Trans. Soc. Pathol. Jpn.*, **30**:680–90, 1940 (in German in Japanese journal).

Paloheimo, J.A.: Obstructive arteritis of Takayasu's type: clinical, roentgenological and laboratory studies on 36 patients. *Acta Med. Scand. Suppl.*, **468**:7–45, 1967.

Paulson, O.B.: Ophthalmodynamometry in internal carotid artery occlusion. *Stroke*, **7**:564–66, 1976.

Pokrovsky, A.V., and Tsyreshkin, D.M.: Nonspecific aorto-arteritis. *J. Cardiovasc. Surg.*, **16**:181–91, 1975.

Ross, R.S., and McKusick, V.A.: Aortic arch syndromes: diminished or absent pulses in arteries arising from arch of aorta. *Arch. Intern. Med.*, **92**:701–40, 1953.

Sano, K.; Aiba, T.; and Saito, I.: Angiography in pulseless disease. *Radiology*, **94**:69–74, 1970.

Savory, W.S.: Case of a young woman in whom the main arteries of both upper extremities and of the left side of the neck were throughout completely obliterated. *Med. Chir. Trans. Lond.*, **39**:205–19, 1856.

Sen, P.K.; Kinare, S.G.; Kelkar, M.D.; and Parulkar, G.B.: *Non-Specific Aorto-Arteritis: A Monograph Based on a Study of 101 Cases.* Tata McGraw-Hill Publishing Company, Bombay, New Delhi, 1973.

Shimizu, K., and Sano, K.: Pulseless disease. *J. Neuropathol. Clin. Neurol.*, **1**:37–47, 1951.

Shimizu, K., and Sano, K.: Pulseless disease. *Rinsho Geka*, **3**:377–96, 1948 (in Japanese).

Strachan, R.W.: The natural history of Takayasu's arteriopathy. *Q. J. Med.*, **33**:57–69, 1964.

Takayasu, M.: A case with peculiar changes of the central retinal vessels. *Acta Soc. Ophthal. Jpn.*, **12**:554–55, 1908 (in Japanese).

Ueno, A.; Awane, Y.; Wakabayashi, A.; and Shimizu, K.: Successfully operated obliterative brachiocephalic arteritis (Takayasu) associated with the elongated coarctation. *Jpn. Heart J.*, **8**:538–44, 1967.

Waern, A.U.; Anderson, P.; and Hemmingsson, A.: Takayasu's arteritis: a hospital-region based study on occurrence, treatment and prognosis. *Angiology*, **34**:311–20, 1983.

30

Vertebral Artery Surgery: Pathology, Hemodynamics, and Technique

ANDREW L. CARNEY

In the past decade, vertebral artery surgery has been stimulated by many diagnostic and therapeutic developments. In 1976, the feasibility of vertebral artery anastomosis at the C1–C2 level was first demonstrated (Carney *et al.*, 1976). By 1978, reports of vein bypass to the vertebral artery at the skull base began to appear (Carney and Anderson, 1978).

The skull base has been called a neurovascular-neurosurgical no-man's land. The factors that combined to bring about the emergence of vascular surgery of the vertebral artery were multidisciplinary; neurosurgeons approached this region from above, and vascular surgeons from the neck. Neurotologic surgeons were already "at home" at the skull base but not yet active in neurovascular reconstruction.

The technical ability to reconstruct the vertebral artery at the skull base demolished the nihilistic attitude toward hindbrain ischemia. Radiological and clinical observations involving all age groups began to appear with greater frequency, treatment became more aggressive, and our perspective broadened. Thus, vertebral artery surgery has become more sophisticated over the past decade and has radically changed the way we treat vertebral artery disease. Brain function is now directly related to brain perfusion. New techniques for measuring brainstem perfusion with high resolution (see Figure 30–1) provide not only an objective hemodynamic basis for selecting patients for vertebral artery surgery and for evaluating its hemodynamic results, but also a method for calibrating neurofunctional testing as a reflection of brain perfusion. Thus, the electroencephalogram (EEG) has become the instrument of choice for monitoring cerebral perfusion in the operating room, and a tool for the measurement of brain perfusion as well as the standard with which other tests are compared.

The major roadblock to relying upon brain perfusion clinically was philosophical: the physiological standard would displace the anatomical "gold standard" of angiography, disability/dysfunction would become an indication for surgery, the measure of successful therapy would be not death or paralytic stroke but the relief of disability, and, finally, sensory and perceptive disorders could be evaluated for a hemodynamic etiology. Now it is accepted that brain function and perfusion, and not the angiogram, are the measures of adequate blood flow, and the disability, impairment of function, and focal ischemia are the measures of need. Congenital vascular patterns and trauma affect all ages; atherosclerosis is not the only disease that involves the vertebral artery.

The early misconceptions also created significant obstacles to the understanding of vertebral circulation. Hindbrain ischemia generally produces disability rather than death; but even when death occurs, the neck is usually not examined in the course of an autopsy, thus vascular pathology in that region goes undetected. Disequilibrium, the most sensitive manifestation of brain-stem dysfunction, can force a person to crawl or lie supine in order to improve brain perfusion and protect vital

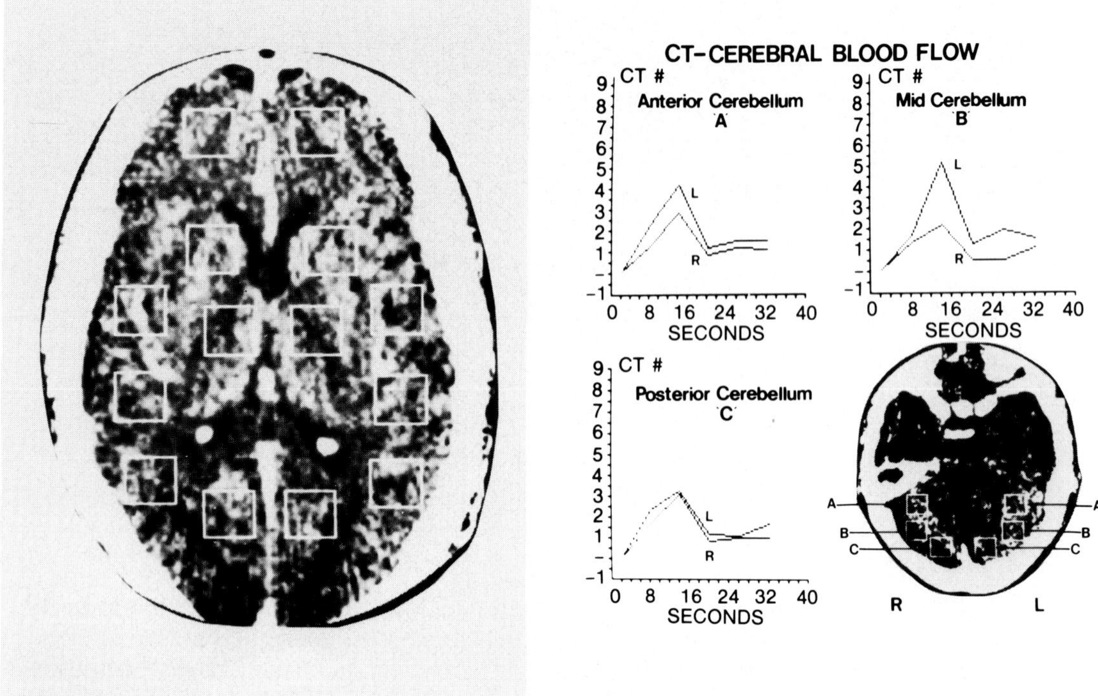

Figure 30–1. Dynamic computerized tomographic brain scan measures regional perfusion by contrast enhancement in the cerebral hemispheres and in the posterior fossa. The density change in the pixels are plotted against time following bolus injection. Mean transit time and amplitude of the curves are evaluated. The infratentorial study, performed in 1978 on a patient with right-sided trigeminal neuralgia revealed reduced perfusion on the right side.

functions, yet the episode leaves no "proof" of its passing. Furthermore, the manifestation of hindbrain ischemia often does not direct attention to the brain, like blindness directs attention to the eye, or deafness to the ear, or respiratory arrest to the lungs. Only a high degree of clinical astuteness prompts recognition of the true underlying pathology, i.e., abnormalities in the vertebral blood flow. This hemodynamic approach to the entire brain provides us with both a new nonneurologic language and with substantial useful tools for a sound approach to brain ischemia.

FUNCTIONAL ANATOMY OF THE VERTEBRAL ARTERY

The vertebral artery is characterized by its small diameter (0.5 to 5.5 mm) relative to its great length (15 to 35 cm). It is often asymmetrical and has many segmental branches before the paired arteries finally fuse into the basilar artery. The vertebral artery (see Figure 30–2) arises from the subclavian artery, courses within the bony canals of the cervical vertebrae anterior to the cervical nerve roots, and is surrounded by veins and nerve elements. It reverses direction on the atlas before piercing the dura mater to enter the cranium.

The volume of brain perfused by the vertebral artery varies individually from the region of a single end-artery to the entire brain. Compared with the carotid artery, it is a high-resistance vessel but vertebral revascularization, especially by a distal bypass, commonly results in dilatation of the vessels and extension of the vascular bed perfused.

The vertebral artery is best divided into segments according to the surgical exposure required. The anterior approach provides access to the vertebral artery within the neck. The proximal vertebral artery extends from its origin, which is variable, to the point of entry into the vertebral foramen, usually at C6. It is fixed in its course to the cervical spine by the vertebral nerve and by sympathetic fibers. It may be best aproached through a supraclavicular incision. The midvertebral segment of the artery may be approached by a longitudinal incision

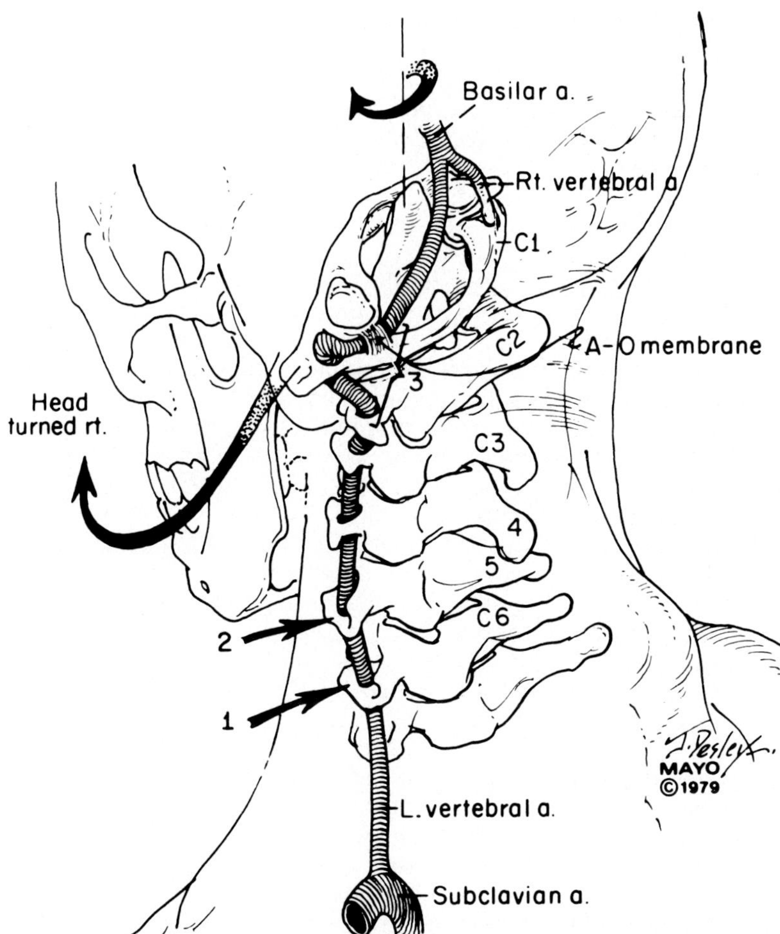

Figure 30–2. The effect of head rotation upon the vertebral artery. Head rotation, indicated by large curved arrows, carries the transverse process of the atlas forward which may stretch the artery, disrupt intima and cause thrombosis or dissection. The major contribution to head rotation occurs between C1 and C2 with a lesser contribution from the lower spine. See arrows 1 and 2 demonstrating the minimal rotation of C5 on C6. (From Krueger, B.R., and Okazaki, H.: Vertebral basilar infarction following chiropractic manipulation. *Mayo Clin. Proc.*, **555**:322–32, 1980.)

paralleling the course of the sternocleidomastoid muscle. The distal vertebral artery, the term designating the vessel at the level of the axis and the atlas, can be exposed through a high transverse cervical incision. Incisions from one section to the other may be continuous. The intracranial vertebral artery, which includes the suboccipital vertebral artery, must be approached posteriorly.

HEMODYNAMIC BASIS OF VERTEBRAL ARTERY SURGERY

All components that effect blood flow to the brain must be regarded as parts of a single system (Carney and Anderson, 1981; Carney *et al.*, 1981; Yates and Hutchinson, 1961). Evaluation of brain ischemia therefore involves the assessment of the hemodynamic levels, i.e., the system, the "precircle" arteries, the circle of Willis, and the end-arteries. Generalized brain ischemia may be due either to low cardiac output or to combined carotid and vertebral disease. About one third of patients presenting with symptoms of hindbrain perfusion deficit in reality suffer solely from a generalized brain ischemia due to low cardiac output.

The Precircle Level

Arterial obstruction proximal to the circle of Willis may produce ischemia either in the territory directly supplied or in a remote site. Ordinarily, the reserve flow from one carotid to the other will compensate, but this is less likely to occur between the carotid and vertebral systems, where such compensatory flow is dependent upon the posterior communicating arteries, the flow capacity of the patent vessels, and the resistance of the affected vascular bed. Normally, the pressure gradient between primary arteries and the circle is low but the flow capacity is high. In contrast, the gradient between the circle and the vascular bed of the end-arteries is high and the flow capacity is limited.

In a case of carotid obstruction, perfusion of the cerebral hemisphere may remain normal because of increased flow through the vertebral system, yet the brainstem itself may be ischemic (Bohmfalk *et al.,* 1979). This hindbrain ischemia may be relieved either by carotid endarterectomy to improve carotid flow or by vertebral artery reconstruction to increase vertebral artery flow. Vein bypass to the vertebral artery at the skull base results in maximal increase in blood flow and flow capacity of the vertebral basilar system.

The Circle of Willis

The circle of Willis is incomplete when any of the carotid or vertebral arteries have poor or no communication with it or whenever there is no connection between the segments of the circle itself. A hypoplastic vertebral artery ending in a posterior inferior cerebellar artery is an example of such an incomplete circle. It is also a true end-artery, and its occlusion may result in focal infarction of the brain stem and cerebellum. A hypoplastic vertebral system is also incomplete because the basilar artery terminates in the superior cerebellar arteries and has no primary communication with the circle. A hypoplastic system is one of high resistance because its diameter is narrow but its length is unchanged. Hypoplastic systems are commonly found in patients with longstanding symptoms. The primary function of the circle of Willis is to maintain blood flow to the brain during the intermittent obstruction of the cervical vessels produced by head motion. In this process, the principle of competitive flow applies, i.e., large primary vessels communicate freely with one another and have the capability of bidirectional flow. The cardinal characteristic of the circle is the ability of the primary channels to alter flow rapidly in response to slight changes in pressure. The circulation through the circle is dynamically balanced at "dead points," which may rapidly change with alteration in flow. This capability to immediately increase flow through the primary limbs of the circle was designated as "cognate" by Green and associates (1944), as "primary" by Nornes *et al.* (1979) and as "reserve" by Carney and Anderson (1981). Collateral flow is blood flow delivered through secondary channels and usually it is not immediately available. An artery, carotid or vertebral, directly supplying the circle is a primary limb of a high-flow reciprocating system. Competitive flow within this system is characterized by a low-pressure gradient, high-flow capacity, and ability to rapidly equilibrate flow and pressure. Even in the presence of total occlusion of a major limb, e.g., carotid occlusion, the resultant resting pressure gradient between limbs may be small. Only under the stress of increased flow demand or contralateral carotid compression, can the hemodynamic impact of minor obstructions in primary vessels be demonstrated.

Blood flow within an end artery to the brain is determined by a significant pressure gradient, it tends to be unidirectional, and it has a low flow capacity. Competitive flow within the end arteries after microvascular reconstruction may cause thrombosis at the junction of the end-artery with the circle of Willis or at the site of proximal stenosis where the pressure and flow are balanced: the dead point. For any end-artery reconstruction to remain open, the graft inflow must sustain the pressure within the vessel grafted. To prevent occlusion of the proximal end-artery, end-artery pressure must exceed that in the circle of Willis.

In general, reconstruction of a large vessel results in a better hemodynamic response than does that of a small vessel, and proximal reconstruction is more beneficial than end-artery reconstruction. Small-vessel reconstruction fares better in the presence of a high gradient and in the absence of significant competitive flow. Small vertebral arteries occlude more often than do large ones. Marked improvement of flow in one vertebral artery may be followed by a reduction in flow and diameter of the contralateral vessel. In an asymmetrical vertebral system, reconstruction of the larger vessel results in the greatest improvement in brain perfusion.

The extracranial completion of an incomplete circle of Willis can be achieved by creating a wide open communication between the carotid and vertebral systems in the neck. An anastomosis in the neck base will work well providing that there is no distal obstruction. In the presence of carotid siphon stenosis, vein bypass from the common carotid to the vertebral artery at the skull base may result in such high bypass flow that the internal carotid flow becomes severely reduced and thrombosis occurs.

The Post-Circle End-Artery

An end-artery, as distinguished from other small vessels, arises from the circle of Willis, the basilar artery, or the vertebral artery, and supplies a defined territory of the brain. Its presence is constant and the blood flow through it is determined by a high-pressure gradient. End-artery occlusion often results in the infarction of a specific segment of the brain. Hypotension within an end-artery is commonly due to extracranial arterial obstructions, but could be also caused by obstruction within the end-artery itself. If an end-artery is small, the resistance to flow will be high. Although some end-arteries are accessible for microvascular reconstruction, others are not.

End-arteries that arise from the basilar artery and supply the brain stem differ from the major cerebral and cerebellar vessels in that they supply regions so small that their occlusion may produce an infarct of only 3 to 5 mm in diameter, an arrangement useful in protecting against extensive infarctions. In the presence of basilar artery disease, these vessels show increased vulnerability to reduced systemic pressure and to decreased arterial blood flow (Camp, 1984; Kistler *et al.*, 1984).

THE MECHANICS OF HEAD MOTION

An understanding of the mechanics of head motion and its hemodynamic consequences is essential to the appreciation of the pathology of the vertebral artery. The head has the widest range of motion at the skull base. Extension and flexion take place at the articulation of the occipital condyles with the atlas and have a transverse axis of motion. Head rotation occurs between the atlas and the axis at the atlantoaxial articulation. The odontoid process serves as the pin around which the atlas rotates. The lateral masses of the atlas and the axis stabilize this rotation.

The cervical apophysical joints restrict the motion of the lower cervical spine. Each vertebra, from C3 to C6, has an upward projection or aphophysis, which interlocks with a downward extension of the vertebra above. This articulation is posterior and medial to the course of the vertebral artery. Henry (1957) notes that these articulations were already studied in detail by Luschka in 1848 and Trolard in 1892. The one between the atlas and the axis is anterior and slightly medial to the vertebral artery and serves as a prominent landmark during operations in this area.

Vascular Obstruction by Head Motion

In extreme head positions, one or more arteries, carotid and/or vertebral, normally obstruct. If the cardiac output is normal and if the circle of Willis is intact, there will be sufficient blood flow in the remaining vessels to maintain brain perfusion and normal brain function. The vertebral artery is particularly vulnerable to obstruction by normal head rotation (see Figure 30–3). To accommodate for this vulnerability, the vertebral system has a feature unique in the body: two vessels fuse in the direction of flow to form one vessel, the basilar artery. Nowhere else in the body does this occur. By this mechanism, the contralateral vertebral artery, if it is patent, can rapidly compensate for the transient obstruction.

Pathology of Head Motion

Hyperextension of the head produces stress at the occipito-atlantoid articulation. This is true even in the normal person, but is a greater problem in patients with anomalies of the skull base, or variant vascular patterns. In some patients the posterior, inferior cerebellar artery will prolapse through the foramen magnum into the neck and become particularly vulnerable to trauma.

Hyperextension of the neck stretches the proximal vertebral artery and produces maximum stress at the point where the vessel is fixed to the spine by the vertebral nerve. This may result in shearing of the intima, dissection (Simeone and Goldberg, 1968), and thrombosis. Extension injuries could also produce soft-tissue injuries on the anterior aspect of the cervical spine whereas flexion trauma may cause compression fractures of the anterior aspects of the bodies of the lower cervical vertebrae (see Figure 30–4).

The greatest contribution to head rotation occurs at the C1–C2 articulation, lesser

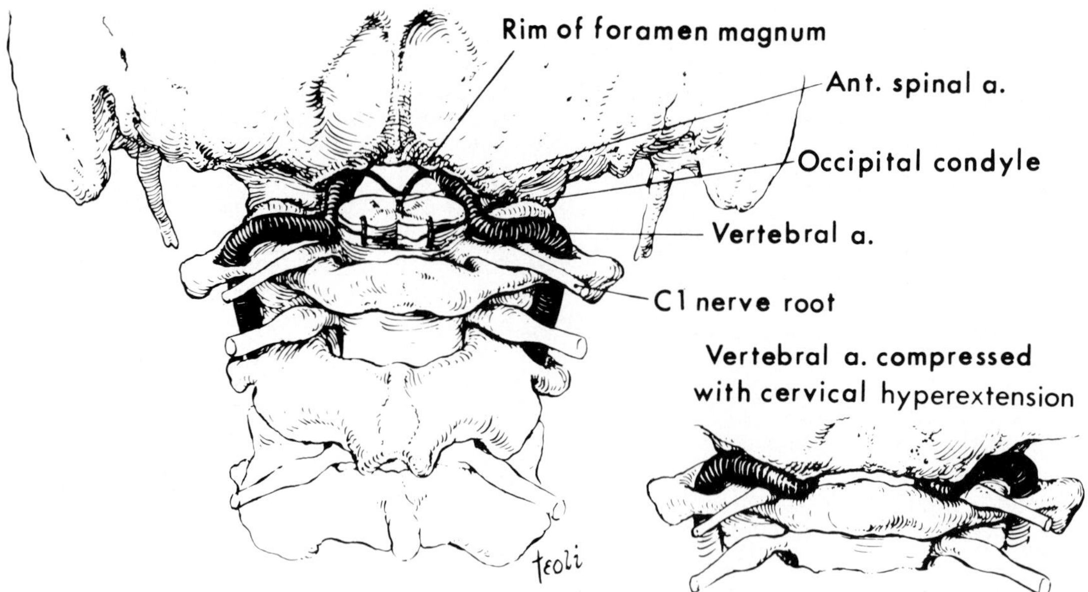

Figure 30–3. Cervical hyperextension can produce crushing injury to the vertebral arteries. Although the posterior-inferior cerebellar artery (PICA) usually projects off at right angles from the intracranial vertebral artery, occasionally an anomalous bifurcation will occur extracranially and project through the foramen magnum into the cervical spine, making it vulnerable to direct compression. (From Schneider, R.C.: *Head and Neck Injuries in Football.* Williams & Wilkins, Baltimore, MD, 1973.)

amounts take place in the lower cervical spine. Hypermobility which may predispose to vertebral artery injury, may occur with congenital deformities of the skull base, with traumatic disruption of ligaments in cases of rheumatoid arthritis. Congenital fusions, fractures or arthritis may restrict neck motion in one area, only to result in compensatory increase in motion in another region, resulting in arterial injury. Compression of the proximal vertebral artery by tendons of the scalenus anticus muscle may also cause obstruction whenever the head is turned extremely to the contralateral side. Kovacs (1955) pointed out that the posterior placement of the vertebral foramina in relation to the body of the vertebra increases vulnerability to compression of the vertebral artery by the subluxation of the apophyseal articulation. Brain (1963) emphasized the role these joints play in the production of symptoms. Studying the matter by cineangiography, he noted that whenever the head is rotated to the opposite side, the vertebral artery at the level of the atlas moves forward, angles acutely in relation to the transverse process of the axis, and is drawn up and out of the vertebral canal of the lower cervical vertebra. Trauma to the spine, which fixes the artery to the canal, eliminates this mobility. Norrell (1975) classified cervical spine trauma according to the mechanism of injury: extension, flexion, extension with rotation, and lateral flexion. These are normal mechanisms of motion made pathological by varying circumstances. Most head positions when stressed obstruct the vertebral artery and may produce symptoms of ischemia. When sufficient force is applied rapidly, the integrity of the arterial wall suffers and rupture or dissection can occur. A stressed head position can cause transient ischemic and arterial trauma, especially to the vertebral artery. This mechanism is primarily responsible for stroke in the young (Klein *et al.,* 1976; Latchaw *et al.,* 1974; Yates, 1959; Zimmerman *et al.,* 1978). Abnormalities of the occipital-atlantoid and atlantoid-axial articulations (Wackenheim, 1974), especially when combined with trauma, may contribute to vertebral artery injury and thrombosis. Computed tomographic scans can provide high quality pictures of the cross-sections of the spine for identifying skull base pathology. Conventional x-rays of this region are of limited value.

PATHOLOGY OF VERTEBRAL ARTERY DISEASE

Disease of the vertebral artery is neither confined to any one age group nor to a single

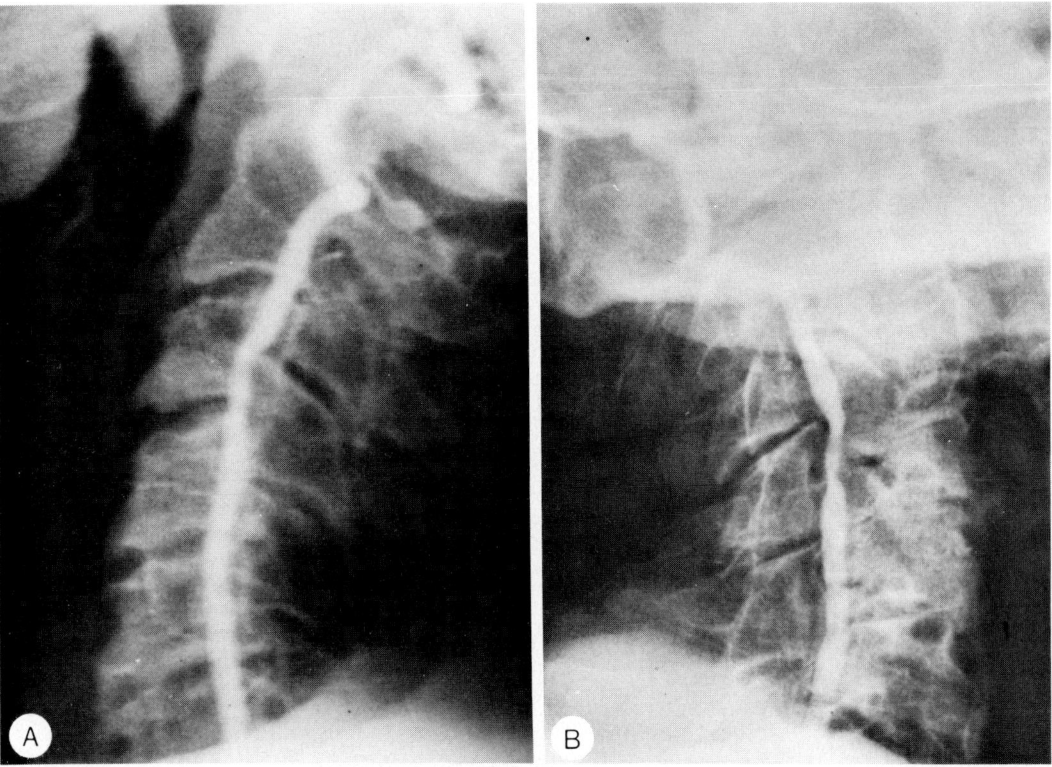

Figure 30-4. Angiogram of the vertebral artery in the lateral view in the neutral head position (*A*) and with the head rotated (*B*). Rotation of the head to the contralateral side in this patient caused syncope resulting from obstruction of the vertebral artery between C4 and C5 with dramatic changes in the EEG. The arterial diameter was reduced in the neutral position but was not associated with symptoms.

pathological process. The vertebral artery differs from the carotid artery by its variety, complexity, and subtlety. Because it is surrounded by bone, the motion of the bony canal can compress, injure, and occlude it. Dissection and acute thrombosis thus appear more frequently in the vertebral than in the carotid artery. The most provocative discoveries, however, are that head motion—even normal motion—could have pathological effects and that the major pathology of the skull base is mechanical trauma to its arteries.

The primary pathological mechanisms causing occlusion of the vertebral arteries are (1) trauma, (2) primary thrombosis, and (3) aneurysm. Arterial obstructions may be either static or dynamic. Static obstructions are caused by atherosclerosis, fibromuscular dysplasia, osteophytic compression, or thrombosis. Dynamic obstructions may be related to head position, entrapment, compression, or steal syndromes. Trauma may be penetrating or blunt or be the result of head motion. Thrombosis may be caused by dissection, disruption of the arterial wall, ulceration, or hypercoagulability, and may extend directly into intracranial vessels or embolize into the terminal portion of the basilar or posterior cerebral artery. Vertebral artery aneurysms are most often caused by trauma. The development of arteriovenous malformations may be either congenital or traumatic.

Static Obstruction

A significant number of patients with static obstructions have occlusive disease of more than a single vessel (see Figure 30-5). When the atherosclerotic obstruction is situated at the origin of the vertebral artery, the collaterals, especially the inferior thyroid artery, tend to be well developed. The inferior thyroid artery thus can be anastomosed end-to-end to the proximal vertebral artery. Atherosclerosis may make the subclavian artery friable and contribute to the development of subclavian steal. The atherosclerotic subclavian artery may also be more difficult to mobilize and ex-

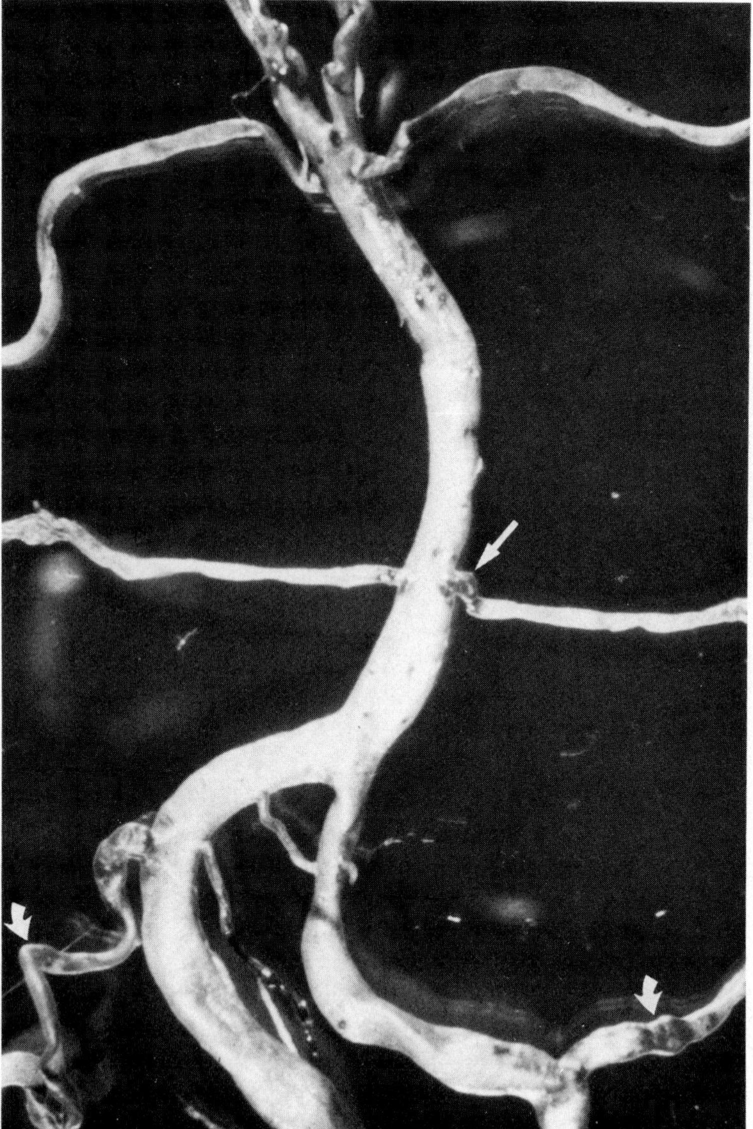

Figure 30–5. The primary branches of the vertebral system. The posterior inferior cerebellar branch arises from the vertebral artery. The anterior inferior and superior cerebellar branches arise from the basilar artery which terminates in the posterior cerebral branches to the occipital lobe. The penetrating branches supplying the brainstem have been removed. Scattered small vessel atherosclerosis can produce disabling symptoms but may not respond to large vessel reconstruction.

pose. Intracranial atherosclerosis is seldom localized enough to permit the performance of an endarterectomy, and extensive involvement of the basilar artery usually also prevents the performance of such a procedure.

Fibromuscular dysplasia occurs less frequently, but may involve any segment of the vertebral artery and could develop at any age. High quality selective angiography with magnification is necessary to identify this lesion.

Dynamic Obstruction

The loss of elasticity in the vascular wall results in dilation and elongation of the arterial system, which may give rise to recurrent obstruction aggravated by stressed head or arm positions. Because the obstruction is intermittent, collaterals do not develop. Extrinsic fixation, constriction, and entrapment of the proximal vertebral artery by sympathetic fibers, by the vertebral nerve, or by the ansa subclavia serve as a point of fixation of the artery to the spine. With advancing age, dilation and elongation of the arterial system elevate the aorta in the chest and the subclavian artery in the neck. The latter rotates as it rises because it is fixed to the first rib by the scalenus anticus muscle and it is tethered by the vertebral artery. The vertebral artery is, in turn, attached to the spine by nerve fibers. The dilated subclavian artery can be palpated and is often seen above the level of the clavicle so it can be readily delivered into the surgical field. The vertebral artery at C1-C2 is tightly secured by dense fibrous attachments. Nerves, veins, and/or small muscular arterial branches may cross the artery in an aberrant fashion, producing obstruction if the head is kept in a particular position. The artery may also penetrate a nerve and be caught in a snare that may tighten or loosen as the head is rotated. The turbulence thus created results in localized dilation of the involved artery segment which may cause platelet aggregation and embolism. Redundant loops below the atlantoaxial joint tend to have acute angulations which can lead to dynamic obstruction.

Mechanical head motion or trauma can result in the disintegration of the wall of the vertebral artery. The medial layer of the vertebral artery is elastic; the intima is not. The stress of stretch, distension, or direct compression may fracture the intima and leave the media intact. This traumatic etiology of dissecting aneurysm is well documented in the neurosurgical literature. Acute dissection and occlusion of the distal basilar and intracranial vertebral arteries during angiography have occurred (Takahaski, 1974), and were presumably caused by the rapid dilation of the arteries due to injection under pressure. The separation of intima from media is commonly seen during angiography. Furthermore, repeated trauma could compromise the integrity of the wall, making it friable and vulnerable to intimal separation. Acute dissection of the vertebral artery may be associated with delayed onset of symptoms caused by the extension of thrombosis into the posterior inferior cerebellar and basilar arteries. Fusion of the superior cervical ganglion with the anterior ramus of the second cervical nerve at the skull base may result in the *erosion of the anterior wall* of the vertebral artery. The damage to the arterial wall may make ligation the only possible course of action. Recurring occipital lobe *embolism* and severe disabling hindbrain ischemia can also be precipitated by minor accidents. If anticoagulants fail to prevent recurrence of emboli, ligation of the vertebral artery must be considered.

Dissection after reconstruction of a vertebral artery at skull base is associated with a state of predissection. In such cases, the artery is edematous and the flaky intima easily strips from the media with even minor surgical manipulation. The lack of adherence of the intima to the media is striking, and the inability to identify this problem preoperatively is frustrating. The operating microscope might be a most valuable asset in such a situation. One clinical finding is constant: pain localized over the artery. On angiography, close inspection may reveal loss of sharp wall definition.

Atherosclerotic stenosis with gradual progression will produce occlusion of the vertebral artery with reserved patency of the distal segment. *Thrombosis* arising out of ulceration, dissection, or trauma, however, will often propagate intracranially, but the onset of symptoms may be delayed. Although the principal source of embolism to the hindbrain is the vertebral artery itself, embolus to the forebrain often originates in the heart. Entrapment of the vertebral artery may also give rise to platelet aggregates at the site of stricture, which embolize to the occipital lobe causing acute visual field defects.

Although traumatic aneurysms of the vertebral artery are seemingly less common today than they were at the time of Matas (1893), they continue to occur. Whereas berry aneurysms are seldom seen on the vertebral artery, aneurysms and tortuosity of the vertebral artery may cause compression of the medulla or of a nerve root. *Aneurysms* of the subclavian artery may also encroach upon the vertebral artery and require vertebral reconstruction along with the repair of the subclavian artery. *Arteriovenous fistula* may be congenital or caused by fibromuscular dysplasia but more commonly by trauma. Congenital malformations of the head and neck may also be fed by branches of the vertebral artery.

The association of hindbrain ischemia with "whiplash" injury and with "thoracic outlet" symptoms is common. The onset of the thoracic outlet syndrome is often precipitated by whiplash injuries, and these patients have EEG findings that are frequently observed with hindbrain ischemia. Proximal vertebral artery obstruction caused by muscles and tendons were noted by Husni and associates (1966) and

Hardin (1965). The arterial pathology of the thoracic outlet syndrome is readily demonstrated by angiography (Bogousslavsky and Regli, 1985); however, compression of the brachial plexus and scalenus muscle is more difficult to appreciate because the outlines of soft tissues cannot be visualized by x-ray. In some cases thoracic outlet syndrome represents a hyperextension stretch injury to the brachial plexus. Stroke-associated thoracic outlet syndrome is an uncommon but a well-documented entity (DeVilliers, 1966).

SIGNS AND SYMPTOMS OF HINDBRAIN ISCHEMIA

Symptoms of hindbrain perfusion deficit are determined by the location and sensitivity of the ischemic area, as well as by the severity of the ischemia. In the presence of diffuse brain ischemia, symptoms are generated by the most sensitive site, often by the vestibular system. Diffuse ischemia with hindbrain symptoms must be differentiated from local ischemia with the same symptoms. Diffuse perfusion deficit must be approached with conservativism; focal ischemia must be dealt with aggressively. Often an associated second lesion of hemodynamic significance is present, usually obstruction of another vessel. Low-output syndromes, dehydration, or an unsuspected malignancy could also cause similar clinical pictures.

Focal Signs

Focal neurological signs neither identify nor localize vertebral artery obstructions. Although regional ischemia of the occipital lobe or the cochlear nucleus of the brain stem may be demonstrated, the site of arterial obstruction could well be the contralateral vertebral artery or even the carotid artery. Proximal obstruction can produce infarctions in the territory of end-arteries with discrete clinical manifestations, the Wallenberg's syndrome. Fisher and associates (1965) reported that of 16 fatal cases of lateral medullary infarction, the vertebral artery was occluded in 12 and the posterior inferior cerebellar artery supplying the region in two. Lateralizing signs of ischemia, especially in the territory of the basilar artery, are only randomly related to the side of vertebral obstruction (Hoobler, 1942). Williams and Wilson (1962) described the full scope of hindbrain symptoms and pointed out that one half of these patients have visual problems and two thirds have vertigo. They recognized that symptoms are primarily related to ischemia and not to infarction because the symptoms are generally reversible. Their clinical evaluation, however, involved speculation rather than proof about the immediate cause.

Disequilibrium

Central vestibular testing is directly concerned with brainstem and vestibular function and its modification by stressed head position and vestibular stimulation, which may be dependent upon blood flow within the vertebral artery. This technique has been found most useful in documenting brain-stem dysfunction. Brain-stem–evoked auditory responses have not been particularly helpful because the cochlea is less sensitive than the vestibular apparatus, and, to eliminate artifacts, the study must be done with a neutral head position and complete muscle relaxation. For us, brain-stem-evoked auditory potentials have not been useful in detecting vertebral artery obstruction produced by head position.

Loss of Hearing

Sudden deafness may be caused by reduced oxygenation of the perilymph. The level of oxygenation can be increased by artificially increasing the blood pressure (Fisch *et al.*, 1984). While use of mixtures of carbon dioxide and oxygen have also been helpful in reversing this type of neurological deficit (Buonanno *et al.*, 1984), they may also aggravate brain ischemia by increasing intracranial steals (Fisch *et al.*, 1984). The onset of sudden deafness commonly occurs during sleep, which suggests that the reduction of blood pressure and/or cardiac rate may be a contributing factor to decreased brain-stem perfusion.

Respiratory Arrest

Respiratory arrest, a common emergency, is rarely considered to be caused by a brain-stem ischemic attack. Angiographic evaluation of such patients and their aggressive management can be rewarding (Nenci *et al.*, 1983; Glenn *et al.*, 1980). Similarly, apnea and cardiac rhythm disturbances occurring during sleep, although studied extensively, have seldom been looked upon as manifestations of brain-stem ischemia.

Provoking Respiratory Dysrhythmia

Provocation of respiratory arrest or dysrhythmia by carotid compression is occasionally observed in the neurovascular laboratory. Kramer (1912) noted that injections of alcohol or chloroform into the carotid artery resulted in mild and transient manifestations, tachycardia and tachypnea; but injection into the vertebral artery resulted in hypotension, bradycardia, and respiratory arrest. Hardin (1965) presented four cases of patients presenting with acute respiratory arrest and paraplegia that recovered following emergency vertebral artery reconstruction. Thus, it appears that the control of respiration, heart rate, and blood pressure is mediated by the brain stem.

Nagashima (1970) evaluated the responses of the vestibular system during the temporary occlusion of the vertebral artery during surgery in the awake patient. He classified the resulting symptoms into three categories: (1) disorders of vision, (2) disorders of consciousness, and (3) visceral symptoms. His observations on abnormal ocular movements, amblyopia, alteration of visual fields, and disturbances of perception agreed with those of Hauge (1954). The level of consciousness acutely fell in five of the 25 patients studied but returned to normal after the occlusion was removed. In five patients, hypotension and bradycardia were preceded by nausea and vomiting. In one case, the vision suddenly blurred when the right vertebral artery was occluded for 30 seconds, after which nausea and vomiting occurred.

Neurovascular Stress Testing

The cardiovascular system in general and the cerebral circulation in particular have great reserve capacities. Both systems must function well to achieve effective brain perfusion, and both systems need to be tested under stress. The value of stress testing of the cardiovascular system has long been recognized (see Figure 30–6). The same is true of the blood supply to the brain. Common methods of stress testing of the cerebral circulation include the tilt table (Carney and Anderson, 1978; Furlan and Breuer, 1984), stressed head positions (Causse and Causse, 1979), inhalation of 5 percent carbon dioxide (Fisch *et al.,* 1984; Furlan and Brewer, 1984), the treadmill (Carney and Anderson, 1978), central vestibular testing (Kumar, 1981), and carotid compression (Eikelboom, 1981). Other forms of commonly occurring stress include the induction of anesthesia, surgical occlusion of a vessel, and hypotensive anesthesia with or without cardiopulmonary bypass and angiography.

Measurement of Brain Perfusion

Static and dynamic computed tomographic (CT) brain scans or their functional equivalent should be performed on patients considered for hindbrain revascularization. Diagnosis and localization of brain ischemia are based upon the objective findings of infarction, hypodensity, and focal atrophy seen on conventional CT scan and upon ischemia determined by dynamic contrast-enhanced CT studies. The newer techniques, like stable xenon-enhanced CT dynamic scanning, position emission scanning, and magnetic resonance imaging appear even more promising. It is important to remember that these studies are only performed when the patient is supine with the head in neutral position. If the patient is young and if symptoms occur only under stress, the dynamic CT studies may be normal. In this case, functional equivalent studies, such as central vestibular studies under stress, will often be diagnostic.

Selective Angiography with Magnification

Selective angiography of the carotid and subclavian arteries is employed with rotational views of the vertebral artery using magnification. We seldom use digital subtraction angiography because of the necessity of high resolution of the vessel at the skull base. The anatomical findings on angiography should be correlated with the results of general and topical hemodynamic evaluation.

TREATMENT ALTERNATIVES TO VERTEBRAL ARTERY SURGERY

Treatment for annoying and disabling hindbrain ischemia should begin by discontinuing or reducing the dose of antihypertensive medication, minimizing postural hypotension, and regulating diet. For some patients, pressure gradient supports are beneficial. Surgical intervention and treatment performed either

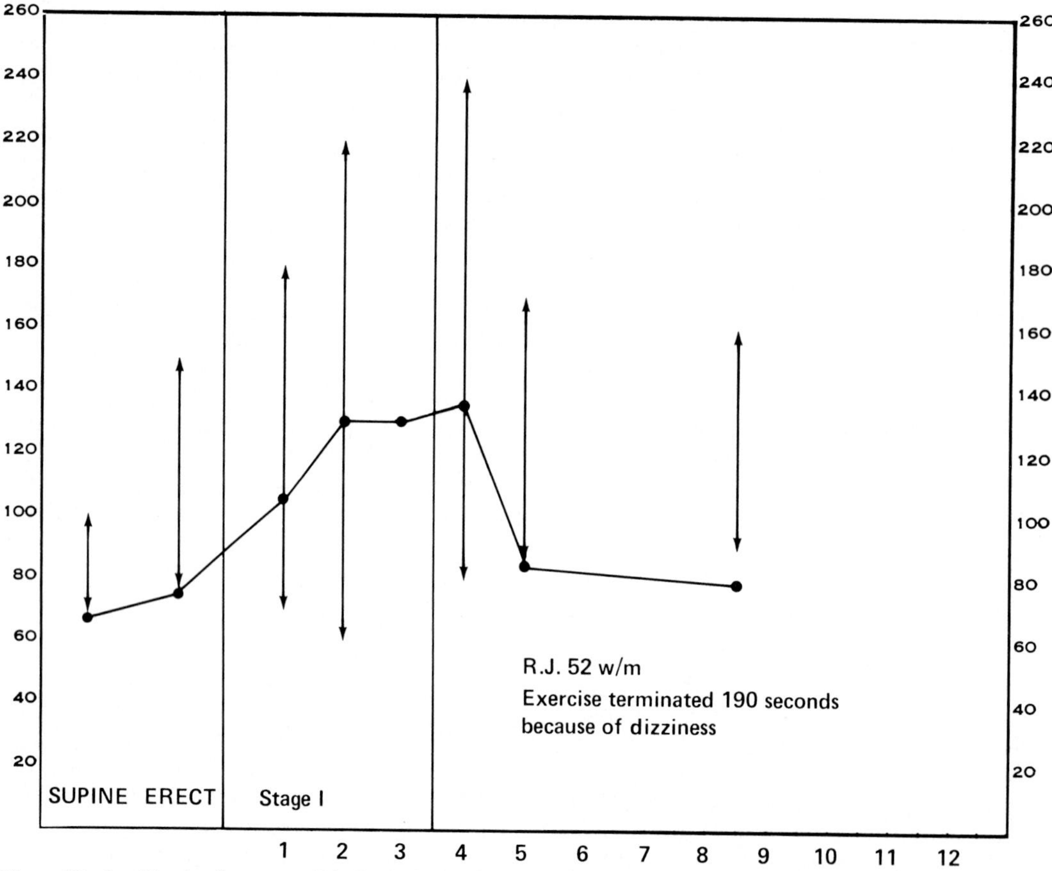

Figure 30–6. The development of hindbrain ischemia under stress may be demonstrated with the treadmill but not the bicycle ergometer. In this patient with dynamic obstructions of the carotid arteries, symptoms were related to the elevation of blood pressure.

electively or during crisis requires detailed neurovascular workup.

Hypervolemic Hemodilution

Plasma volume expansion, bed rest, and neck support are usually effective in controlling acute crises where respiratory arrest is not a threat. Hypervolemic hemodilution is the single most effective nonsurgical therapy available for episodes of acute brain ischemia (Carney and Anderson, 1981b). Cardiac dysrhythmia must be controlled, and if necessary physiologic pacing is used.

Carotid Surgery

In the presence of large posterior communicating arteries, endarterectomy of a stenosed carotid artery may be effective in relieving hindbrain ischemia. The same may be true when the obstruction of the internal carotid artery is dynamic rather than static. Relief of hypoglossal carotid entrapment with obstruction may substitute for vertebral artery reconstruction (Carney and Anderson, 1981a).

Thrombolysis

Thrombolytic therapy has been used for acute carotid and vertebral artery thrombosis in selected cases. Nenci and associates (1983) reported four cases of acute brain-stem stroke treated with streptokinase and urokinase. Three of the patients whose embolism to the distal end of the basilar artery or stenosis of the basilar artery were confirmed by angiography responded well to therapy. The fourth patient, who had bilateral cerebral artery occlusion, died. This therapeutic approach may be useful in the early treatment of respiratory failure caused by acute brain-stem injury. It may also have a place in treating delayed and late thrombosis at the site of surgical reconstruction.

Balloon Occlusion and Embolization

Interventional radiologists have used balloon catheters (DeBrun *et al.*, 1978), both for trial occlusion of the subclavian and vertebral arteries (George and Laurian, 1979) before surgery and also for permanent occlusion as definitive treatment of arteriovenous fistulas in the neck after bypass to the distal vertebral artery. In the latter case, the vertebral artery is occluded at a site proximal to the bypass but distal to the fistula. Both embolization and balloon inflation, distal and proximal, can then be performed. Additional bypass to the vertebral artery distal to the arteriovenous communication permits occlusion without compromising brain perfusion.

Balloon Angioplasty

Percutaneous balloon dilatation of lesions in the proximal vertebral artery has recently been reported (Motarjeme *et al.*, 1982). Percutaneous angioplasty of the basilar artery has not been reported. Intraoperative angioplasty of the basilar artery has unsatisfactory results. Disruption of the arterial media by the sharp edge of a calcified plaque, however, can result in intracranial aneurysm and hemorrhage (Sundt *et al.*, 1980). Postoperative balloon dilatation of the stenosed bypass to the distal vertebral artery, however, may be considered in the future. The presence of the distal vertebral artery bypass permits access by catheter to the intracranial artery for balloon placement, angioplasty, embolization, or chemotherapy.

Spinal Fusion, Decompression

In some patients with impaired vertebral artery flow, operating on the vertebra may be preferable to direct surgery of the vertebral artery. Persons with congenital or acquired hypermobility at the skull base of the atlantoaxial articulation should be evaluated for treatment to restrict this abnormal mobility. Bypass to the distal vertebral artery can be occluded by the mechanical rotation of the head. The unstable spine is better served by stabilization and cervical spinal stenosis by decompression. However, posterior decompression may change the relative position of the neck and aggravate head hyperextension. Hindbrain ischemia due primarily to vertebral artery obstruction distal to C-1 will not be benefitted by surgery proximal to C1.

Surgical fusion of the atlas and axis has been considered in lieu of or in combination with vascular reconstruction. Verbiest (1969) was of the opinion that fusion with unilateral distal vertebral artery reconstruction is not necessary. Extensive resection of the transverse process of C1 may result in symptomatic instability of this joint. Further experience is needed in this area.

VERTEBRAL ARTERY SURGERY: GENERAL CONSIDERATIONS

Indications

The general indication for vertebral artery reconstruction is underperfusion of the brain caused by a hemodynamically significant obstruction of the vertebral artery (see Table 30–1). Reconstruction is thereby expected to relieve disability, enhance function, and prevent brain damage. Pain caused by bone erosion, pressure on neural tissue, or ischemia owing to arteriovenous malformation is also a valid indication for surgery. The specific hemodynamic objective of vertebral artery surgery is to enhance perfusion to a particular area of the hindbrain as a whole or to the forebrain by increasing collateral flow through the circle of Willis. Advanced cortical atrophy, hydrocephalus, brain tumor, and intracranial aneurysm are some of the principal contraindications to reconstruction of the vertebral artery. Other conditions that may compromise results include cervical spinal stenosis, abnormalities of the skull base or cervical vertebrae, spinal cord pathology, left ventricular dysfunction, cardiac dysrhythmia, and systemic hypotension. Overlooked obstruction of the carotid artery (Carney, 1981) and vertebral artery stenosis distal to the site of reconstruction could also cause unsatisfactory results after technically successful vertebral surgery.

Preparation for Surgery

For elective surgery the patient should be neurologically stable, i.e., with absent or controlled symptoms when provoked by passive tilt. For the acute case of hindbrain ischemia, hypervolemic hemodilution combined with

Table 30-1. Potential Indications for Reconstruction of the Distal Vertebral Artery at the Base of the Skull

- Obstructive pathology at the C1-C2 level
- Obstruction of the vertebral artery proximal to C2
- Acute thrombosis of the proximal vertebral artery with patent distal segment
- Chronic occlusion of the proximal vertebral artery with patent distal segment
- Failure of proximal reconstruction
- Ligation of proximal vertebral artery
- Aneurysm of the vertebral artery
- Arteriovenous fistula involving the midvertebral artery
- Irradiation of the lower neck
- Previous carotid subclavian bypass
- Increased hazard of proximal reconstruction: the anterior spinal artery arising from the subclavian artery
- Inoperable carotid lesions: to increase collateral flow to the forebrain as an alternate to extracranial-intracranial bypass
- Hypoplastic systems with incomplete circle of Willis
- Interventional access to the posterior fossa: for balloon placement, angioplasty, embolization
- Safeguard against neurological damage under cardiopulmonary bypass, hypotensive anesthesia, general anesthesia
- Reestablishment of vascular continuity disrupted by tumor and/or resection
- Preservation as a conduit when the internal carotid artery is occluded or likely to become occluded by ligation or thrombosis.
- Completion of the circle of Willis—extracranial: when there is no effective posterior communication between isolated and hypoplastic systems and other vessels
- Control of recurrent occipital lobe embolism from the vertebral artery proximal to C2: anticoagulant failure

bed rest is the treatment of choice. In a patient with severe and longstanding hindbrain ischemia, intolerance to the erect position may be severe. Although the relief of symptoms can usually be achieved preoperatively when the patient is supine, this group is extremely sensitive to surgical manipulation. Vertebral artery surgery at the skull base requires sure hands and fine instruments to perform an anastomosis in a tight, deep hole. It must be done perfectly the first time. A high-intensity fiberoptic light source should illuminate precisely where it is needed. Magnification is necessary and the microscope desirable. Clamps, sutures, and forceps must be a combination of vascular, microvascular, and cardiovascular armamentaria because the anatomical regions of concern include the thorax, the neck, and the skull base.

Vertebral Artery Occlusion

Because it is necessary to temporarily clamp the vertebral artery during surgery, a brief review of clinical experience with vertebral artery ligation may be helpful. Dandy (1944) reported a case of sudden death after momentary pinching of a vertebral artery in the operating room. Bakay and Sweet (1953) measured the intraarterial pressures in the posterior inferior cerebellar artery and also in the exposed vertebral artery between the occiput and the atlas before and after intracranial ligation of the vertebral artery for aneurysm. They concluded that the ligation of one vertebral artery is unlikely to reduce distal pressure and proximal ligation is therefore probably of little benefit in treating an aneurysm arising from the basilar artery. Shintani and Zervas (1972) noted that in 100 cases of ligation reported in the literature, the overall mortality rate was 12 percent.

Rainer and associates (1970) reported two deaths in 54 cases of vertebral artery surgery owing to brain damage. One patient died in surgery and the other was lost postoperatively. They therefore recommended the use of temporary shunting while the vertebral flow is interrupted during surgery.

Cormier and Laurian (1976) observed a 1.5 percent mortality rate in a total of 172 patients, in whom 119 vertebral arteries were reconstructed. No further details were given. Edwards and Mulherin (1980) reported neither mortality nor stroke in 204 reconstructions of the vertebral artery. Use of shunts was abandoned early in their series. Senter and Long (1983) reported use of a shunt during the reconstruction of the midvertebral artery. I have not employed shunts for either carotid or vertebral reconstruction for a decade, and others have taken similar positions. On the other hand, I give careful attention to plasma volume expansion and monitoring in the operating room. If a patient is very high risk, intolerance to the induction of anesthesia warrants cancellation of surgery.

Selection of Procedures

The procedure used is determined by the site of pathology, the nature of the pathology, the findings at surgery and the ability of the surgeon. The principal decision relates to the level at which the artery is to be approached. There is no one standard procedure and combinations of techniques are applied in various circumstances (Carney *et al.*, 1981). Just as coronary bypass and carotid procedures have been performed simultaneously, reconstruction of the proximal vertebral artery at the time of coronary bypass is also possible (Moran, 1980). Reconstruction of the vertebral artery at the skull base, however, is too complex to combine with cardiac surgery.

RECONSTRUCTION OF THE PROXIMAL VERTEBRAL ARTERY

Exposure

The proximal vertebral artery is most conveniently exposed through a transverse supraclavicular incision extending from the midline over the lateral edge of the clavicular head of the sternocleidomastoid muscle. The clavicular head can be divided or retracted medially. If only retracted, then the lateral edge must be mobilized widely. The scalene fat pad is incised medially and retracted laterally. The scalenus anticus muscle with the overlying phrenic nerve is exposed high to permit radical excision (see Figure 30–7). Attention is then directed caudally toward the first rib for completion of the resection. Muscle bands extending between the cords of the brachial plexus or other encroaching bands are excised.

The subclavian artery is mobilized first laterally, then medially. The thoracic duct, if injured, is ligated. An attempt is made to preserve the branches of the subclavian artery. Commonly, the arch of this artery rides high in the neck, far above the entrance of the vertebral artery into the foramen of C6. The overlying nerve fibers are frequently divided. The vertebral artery is mobilized to the vertebral foramen. Occasionally, tendinous attachments of the scalenus muscles encroach upon the vertebral artery and are resected. If the nature of the procedure requires ligation of the vertebral artery, this should be carried out near its origin from the subclavian artery to gain maximal length. The vertebral vein is ligated when encountered. If the subclavian artery appears to be friable or lies deep and the operative plan does not call for its exposure, then it should be avoided because minor injury may lead to further damage, requiring complex repair or even replacement by prosthesis. Unusual situations may require extension of the

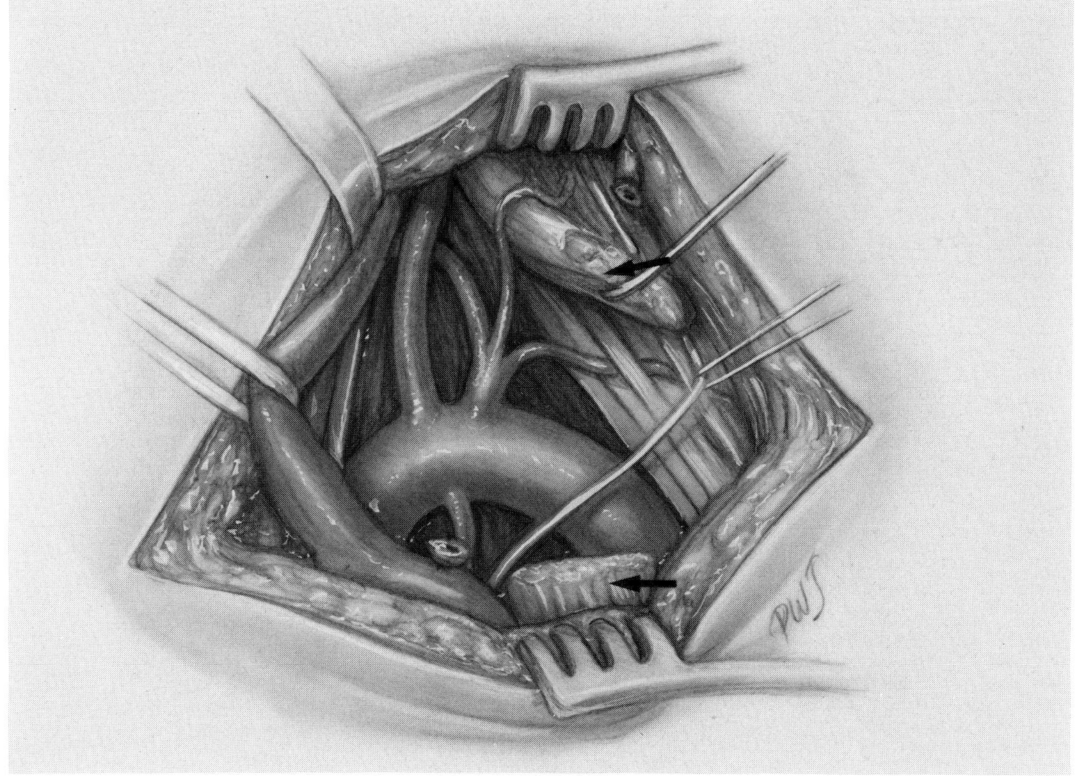

Figure 30–7. The normal anatomy of the proximal vertebral artery is illustrated, showing the basic relationships of soft tissues. The cisterna chyli and vertebral nerve are not shown.

incision into the thorax or mobilization of the vertebral artery above the C6 level.

Transsubclavian Endarterectomy

Cate and Scott (1959) described an endarterectomy of the origin of the vertebral artery through the subclavian artery (see Figure 30–8). No incision was made in the vertebral artery.

Endarterectomy with Patch Angioplasty

Vein patch angioplasty (see Figure 30–8B) is greatly facilitated by the use of fine monofilament suture. If the origin of the vertebral artery is very low in the thoracic inlet, the site of planned arteriotomy may be difficult to reach. Transthoracic vertebral patch angioplasty (see Figure 28–9) has recently been recommended concomitantly with replacement of the proximal subclavian artery (Robicsek, 1985).

Bypass to the Proximal Vertebral Artery

Berguer and associates (1976) reported on a bypass to the proximal vertebral artery from the subclavian artery. Autogenous vein is generally used as the graft, but the use of prosthetic material has also been reported (Bohl *et al.*, 1977). The distal anastomosis is usually per-

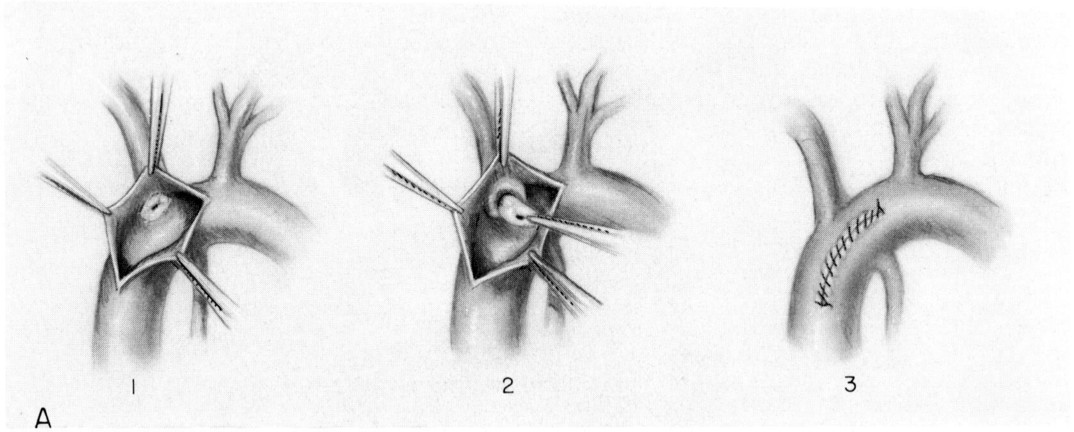

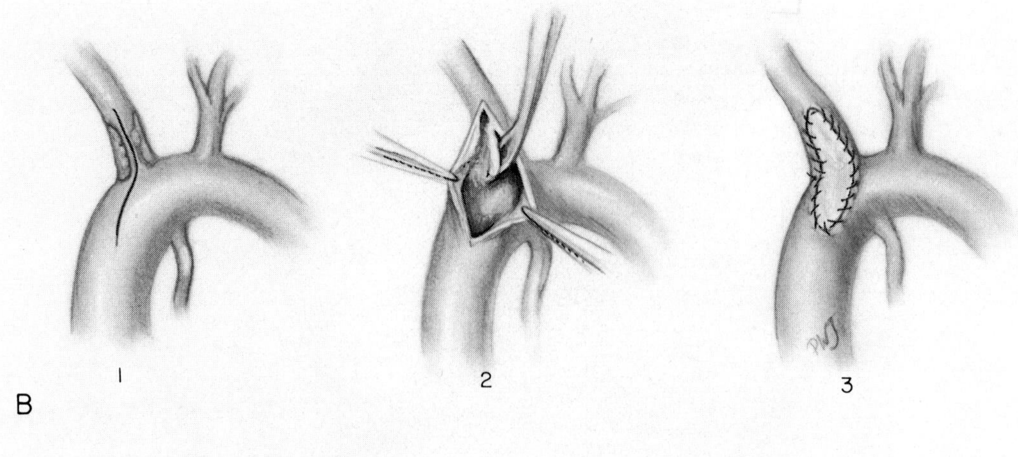

Figure 30–8. Vertebral endarterectomy performed through the interior of the subclavian artery (*A*) and by the direct route combined with patch arterioplasty (*B*).

formed end-to-side to leave the course of the vertebral artery undisturbed. In my experience, bypass to the proximal vertebral artery has rarely been necessary. However, its use permits bypass to the vertebral artery within the cervical spine when the proximal segment is not suitable for use.

Decompression

When only one vertebral is patent or if there is marked sensitivity to intermittent dynamic occlusion, decompression may be the procedure of choice. The proximal vertebral artery is mobilized from its origin to the foramen transversarium at C6. If the vertebral nerve fibers overlying the vertebral artery are divided, a mild Horner's syndrome will result but it usually disappears within a year. However, the vertebral nerve may be spared in cases where the artery is divided and primarily anastomosed. Radical excision of ganglia or fibers for microscopic confirmation of structure is not only unnecessary but worsens the sympathetic sequel. Bleeding from the vertebral vein near the vertebral foramen can be most troublesome. To assure long-lasting good results, all ligaments, muscles, and bands overlying the proximal vertebral artery are excised up to the foramen.

Segmental Resection

Segmental resection and end-to-end anastomosis may be applied in some cases of obstruction owing to entrapment. The artery should be of excess length and adequate diameter and the conditions for the performance of a convenient and unencumbered anastomosis should be present. If this is not the case, an alternative technique should be employed.

Subclavian-to-Proximal Vertebral Arterial Anastomosis

Obstruction of the proximal vertebral artery is often associated with an elongated and high-lying subclavian artery. Ligation and division of the vertebral artery near its origin permit moving the vessel anterolaterally to a more easily accessible surgical field (see Figure 30–9). If needed, shortening of the vertebral artery is accomplished by resection (see Figure 30–10). The origin of the thyrocervical trunk may be incorporated in the reconstruction, and used as the proximal site for the anastomosis.

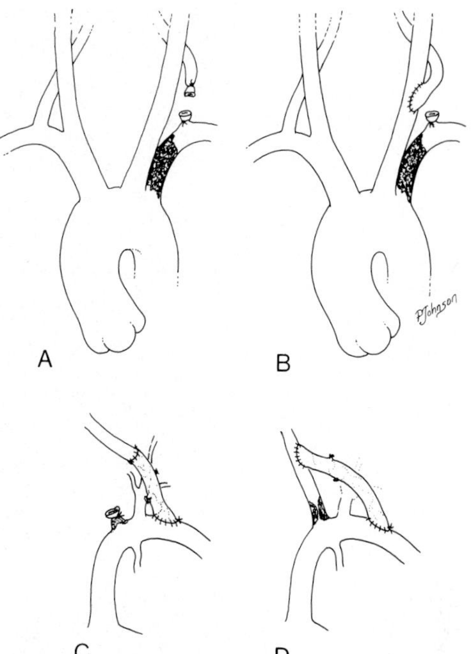

Figure 30–9. Ligation of the vertebral artery (*A*), implantation of the vertebral artery into the proximal common carotid (*B*), and end-to-end (*C*) and end-to-side (*D*) subclavian vertebral bypass grafts.

Common Carotid-to-Proximal Vertebral Arterial Anastomosis

This procedure does not require the resection of the scalenus anticus muscle because the vertebral artery may be approached medial to the muscle. Introduced by Wylie in 1970, it has received enthusiastic support from Edwards (Edwards and Mulherin, 1980) and has gained in popularity over the years. The procedure also has the limitation that its use requires simultaneous occlusion of both the carotid and the vertebral arteries. Edwards and Mulherin (1980), though, reporting on 204 cases, did not observe any neurological sequelae due to this maneuver.

Inferior Thyroid-to-Vertebral Arterial Anastomosis

If there is a high-grade atherosclerotic obstruction of the proximal vertebral artery, the interior thyroid artery is usually well developed because it serves as a collateral channel. It can be anastomosed end-to-end to the proximal vertebral artery (Carney *et al.*, 1981).

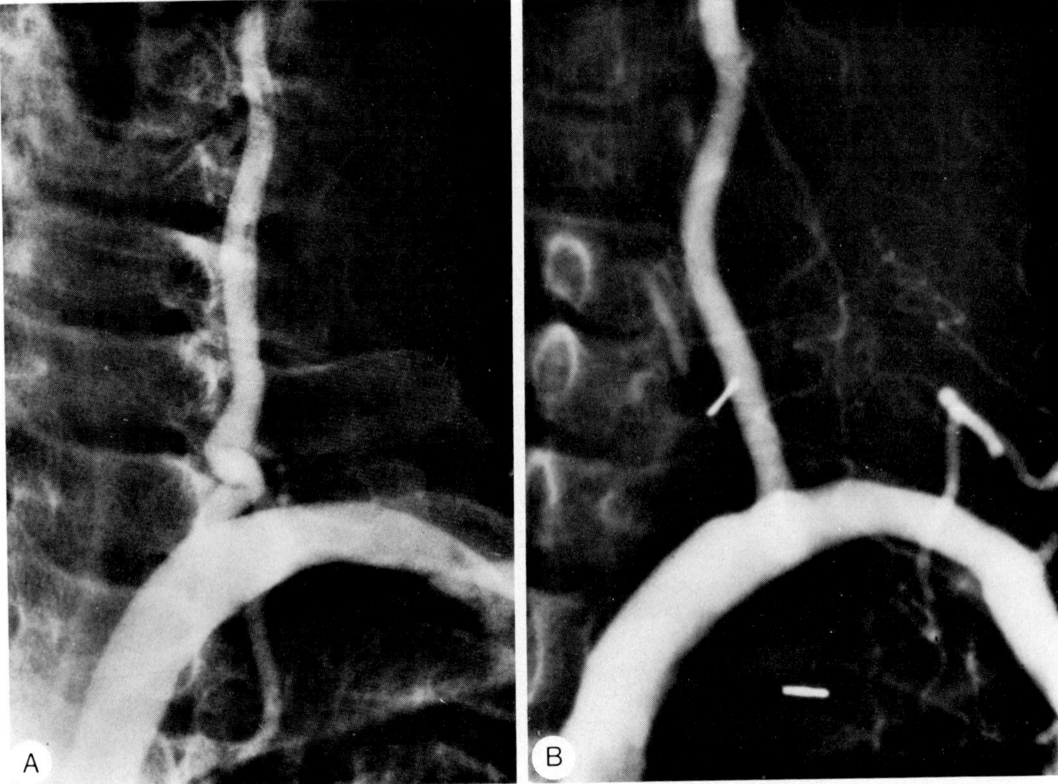

Figure 30–10. Vertebral artery obstruction due to entrapment by the vertebral nerve. Implantation onto the subclavian artery is performed distally for technical ease. Angiograms: **A**: Preoperative. **B**: Postoperative.

External Carotid-to-Midvertebral Arterial Anastomosis

Corkill and associates (1977) reported the anastomosis between the external carotid artery and the midvertebral artery for proximal disease. This technique is an alternative to distal vertebral artery bypass.

Superior Thyroid-to-Vertebral Anastomosis

Kojimi and associates (1983) reported microvascular anastomosis of the superior thyroid artery to the midvertebral artery in order to bypass atherosclerotic obstruction of the origin of the vertebral artery.

Ligation of the Proximal Vertebral Artery

Ligation of the vertebral artery may be required incidentally to procedures upon the subclavian artery or to control recurring hindbrain embolism (see Figure 30–9A). Confirmation of a patent contralateral vertebral artery is highly desirable. The use of heparin may decrease the likelihood of delayed thrombosis, and reconstruction at the skull base can be performed at the later date.

Replacement of the Subclavian Artery

Replacement of the subclavian artery with a prosthesis may be necessary if the performance of an anastomosis to it is part of the operative plan and the subclavian artery is of poor quality. Replacement of the vertebral artery with a Dacron prosthetis can be performed too, with patency persisting more than three years.

Contraindications

Contraindications particular to reconstruction of the proximal vertebral artery include (1) obstruction distal to the site of reconstruction, (2) opacification of the anterior spinal artery by a radiculomedullary branch arising from the subclavian artery (Carney *et al.*, 1981), and (3) presence of a carotid-subclavian bypass. Ligation of the anterior spinal artery should be avoided because it may result in paraplegia. The patient with borderline pulmonary function may be severely compromised by phrenic nerve injury or the loss of the scalenus muscle as an accessory muscle of respiration.

RECONSTRUCTION OF THE MIDVERTEBRAL ARTERY

Hutchinson and Yates (1957) first reported compression and obstruction of vertebral arteries by osteoarthritic spurs which resulted in death from stroke. Vascular reconstruction of the proximal artery was recommended by Crawford *et al.* (1958), whereas others pursued the issue by decompressing the vertebral artery within the cervical spine high at the skull base (Hardin, 1965).

Decompression

In the 1960s, Creighton Hardin, general and vascular surgeon, noted the filling of the basilar artery by right carotid injection in one case that sparked his interest in the vertebral system. In this case, the left vertebral artery was hypoplastic and the right vertebral artery was severely compressed by osteophytic spurs. The dominant right vertebral artery was decompressed on January 15, 1959, and the site was marked with silver clips. Postoperative films of the cervical spine revealed the clips at the incorrect vertebral level, and the larger spur was removed one week later. The bony mass reduced the arterial diameter by one half and was densely adherent to the arterial wall. Hardin in 1963 reported 15 additional cases using an incision paralleling the posterior edge of the sternocleidomastoid muscle. Bakay and Leslie (1965) also reported three similar cases and added interbody fusion of the vertebrae to the procedure. In Nagashima's (1970) experience with 20 additional patients, metal needle markers were used to localize the vertebral level by x-ray before injecting a small amount of dye to mark the tissue. He made a transverse cervical incision and carried dissection to the spine. The longus colli muscle was then resected and the osteophytes were excised with a dental burr, Hall air drill, or curette, but fusion was not performed. Head rotation during surgery resulted in near-total occlusion of the vertebral artery in seven of these patients and severe compression in the remaining 13. Verbiest (1969) combined decompression and mobilization of the vertebral artery during anterior decompression of nerve roots, removal of cervical disk, or fusion. He noted that in some cases scalenus anticus syndrome, if present, also cleared after the decompression of the nerve roots or the brachial plexus.

An argument against vertebral artery decompression is that the structural changes in the arterial wall are permanent. Gortvai (1964) noted that even after straightening the course of the artery, a crease remained in the adventitia where compression had been the most severe. He speculated that this crease may have represented either an atheromatous plaque or local fibrosis. Nagashima (1970), using the operating microscope, also noted that even after removal of bone and cartilage the vertebral artery still remained kinked because of a marked perivascular fibrosis.

The vertebral artery can erode bone and, in turn, osteophytes can erode the arterial wall. Such erosion by bony compression may necessitate ligation of the vertebral artery and may also be the source of thombosis and embolism (Verbiest, 1969). The primary pathology of the midvertebral artery has been the compromise of vertebral artery blood flow with stressed head positions, but other neurological lesions, such as tumors of nervous origin and aneurysms, are also occasionally encountered. Aneurysms may be either small or extensive with venous communications. In the 1960s, the primary reason for utilizing decompression of the anterior aspect of the midvertebral artery was that it was the sole therapy a surgeon could offer. Two criticisms of the procedure included (1) the changes noted in the arterial wall extended through its entire thickness and could not be relieved by decompression, and (2) the arterial lumen was not explored and the state of the lumen not determined.

With the development of bypass procedures to the vertebral artery at the skull base, the need for arterial decompression within the cervical spine has diminished while decompression of cervical nerves impinged by bone remained a mainstay of neurological and orthopedic surgery.

RECONSTRUCTION OF THE DISTAL VERTEBRAL ARTERY

Exposure

An anterolateral or anterior approach may be used to reach the vertebral artery at the skull base. The former is designed to expose the vertebral artery between the C1 and C2 segments by a route anterior to the internal jugular vein. The incision for the anterolateral approach, as described by Henry (1957) and also used by Verbiest (1969), can be extended first posteriorly toward the occiput, then medially and caudally. It permits wide access to the anterolateral structures of the neck.

The incision for the anterior approach (Nanson, 1966) mobilizes the earlobe and extends anterior to the ear. The dissection can then be extended to the base of the skull. This incision also provides good access to the parotid gland and facial nerve. Displacing the mandible forward improves access to the vertebral artery, the anterior cervical spine, and the high carotid. Both approaches work well, but the anterolateral one seems less cumbersome. In general, the less the experience of the operator, the wider the field that needs to be exposed. After the incision is made, the superior flap is carefully mobilized from the sternocleidomastoid muscle to avoid the deep lobe of the parotid gland and facial nerve. The greater auricular nerve is usually sacrificed and rarely reconstructed. The mastoid process is mobilized so that it can be divided with an osteotomy. Once the mastoid process is divided, the deep ligamentous attachment of the mastoid can be sectioned. This maneuver leads directly to the mastoid attachment of the posterior belly of the digastric muscle whose caudal edge is then mobilized to the hyoid before being elevated off the prevertebral fascia. The spinal accessory nerve lies posterior and lateral to the internal jugular vein. The superior cervical ganglion which sits astride the prevertebral fascia and medial to the jugular vein is not visualized unless it is fused with the anterior ramus of the second cervical nerve. The latter surrounds the vertebral artery and attaches it to the spine at the level of the atlantoaxial articulation. It is a sensory branch that can be divided with impunity. In a lean patient, aggressive superior traction may be followed by palsy of the mandibular branch of the facial nerve. Aberrant nerve fibers will often ensnare the vertebral artery, resulting in convolutions appreciated only at surgery.

In the course of the operation the transverse process of the atlas can be easily seen and palpated in the field. The caudal attachments include the levator scapulae, the scalenus medius, and the anterior intertransversalis muscles. Some of these muscle attachments must be divided. The atlantoaxial articulation can be palpated through the prevertebral fascia, which is then incised. The superior cervical ganglion lies medial to the anterior ramus of the second cervical nerve, which embraces the vertebral artery and holds it close to the vertebra. This ramus is divided and retracted. The venous plexus, if present, must also be controlled. The encircling sheath is incised, and the artery is mobilized to permit application of vascular clamps after exposing 1.5 cm of its length.

In some patients, the anterior capsule of the atlantoaxial articulation is worn thin by prominent flaring of the bony surfaces; in others, adhesions surround the artery. Entry into the capsule in such cases may reveal sharp edges of dense bone, which should be ground smooth. Occasionally, the bone overlying the foramen transversarium of C2 and C3 needs to be removed to gain access to the medial bight of the vertebral artery. Resection of the transverse process of C1 is well tolerated. Access to the artery high at C1 is much more readily secured than at the medial bight. Resection of extensive posttraumatic dystrophis calcification compromises joint stability.

TECHNICAL CONSIDERATIONS

When the lateral bight of the vertebral artery at C2 forms a free loop, mobilization can be accomplished with a minimum of dissection. The medial angle of the vertebral artery at the level of the axis, however, is more often the site of significant pathology. The bight of the vertebral artery may be buried deep in a bony cavern lined by veins or bony lakes. When the fibrous sheath extends to this area, it may be covered by Batson's venous plexus, and could cause severe blood loss if injured.

Bypass Grafts

The best substitute for artery is *artery*. The stress applied to a graft at the skull base is three-dimensional, and the position of the graft is important. The more posteriorly it is located, the less severe are the stresses involved. The more anterior is the position, the greater are the arcs cut by flexion and rotation. It is doubtful that the compound motion at the skull base would be tolerated by a synthetic prosthesis.

The *vein* is far from being a perfect graft material. Intimal hyperplasia can occlude a well-constructed vein graft. Thin-walled veins tend to dilate excessively, tear easily, and are prone to kinking. Generally, thick-walled veins work best and are easiest to gauge for 4 to 6 mm vertebral arteries. Discrepancy in size is more of a problem if the arteries are hypoplastic. A smaller diameter arterial anastomosis with the use of a microvascular technique may be preferred in such situations. Many neurosurgeons have anastomosed the external carotid directly to the vertebral artery; even the superior thyroid artery has been used for this purpose.

Clark and Perry (1966) mobilized the vertebral artery from C6 to C1 to gain a long enough segment to anastomose the vertebral artery to the external carotid artery at the level of the bifurcation. That reconstruction remained patent for more than a decade (Perry, personal communication, 1985). Shorter lengths of the vertebral artery have been used by others (Carney *et al.*, 1981; Diaz *et al.*, 1983).

The use of *artificial prostheses* has been unrewarding. Occlusion often occurred with Dacron prostheses and with reconstructions originating from the external carotid artery.

PROCEDURES AT THE SKULL BASE

Decompression and Mobilization

An occasional patient may have severe local obstruction of the vertebral artery caused by compression by arterial branches or neighboring nerves. Division of the obstructive tissues and arterial mobilization may be curative. If there is prominent flaring and spurring of the C1-C2 joint surfaces, it is recommended that the articulation be ground smooth.

Carotid-to-Vertebral Arterial Anastomosis

In 1966, Clark and Perry mobilized the proximal vertebral artery to the skull base to obtain a segment sufficient to anastomose the vertebral to the external carotid artery at the level of the bifurcation (see Figure 30–11). When direct anastomosis is planned between these vessels, the vertebral artery can be passed deep to the internal jugular vein to shorten the distance to the carotid.

Segmental Resection

Acute angulation or constriction may compromise blood flow at a specific point. In such cases, mobilization alone may not be enough and segmental resection and end-to-end repair may be applicable. Redundancy of the vertebral artery may facilitate the performance of such an operation. The medial angle of the vertebral artery at C2 is mobilized and the segmental branches are ligated and divided. Unroofing the foramen transversarium at C3 usually permits the surgeon to obtain an ade-

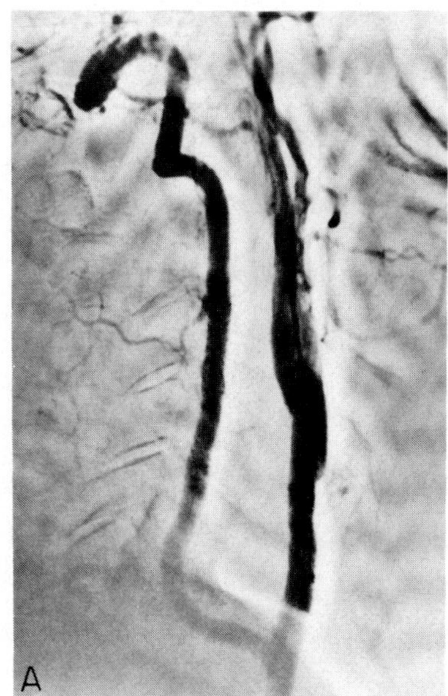

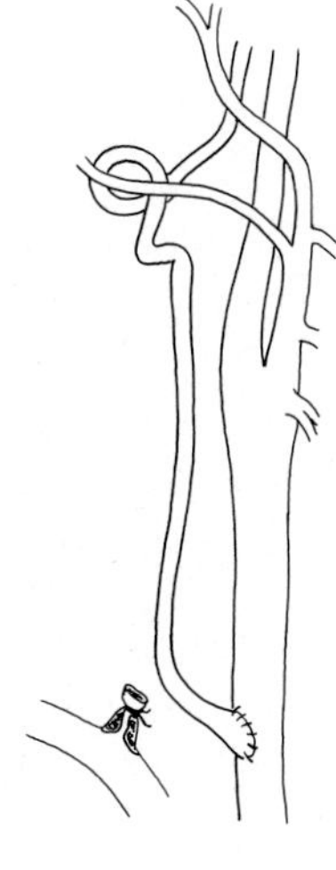

Figure 30–11. Anastomosis of the common carotid-to-distal vertebral artery: postoperative angiogram (*A*) and illustration of the surgical technique (*B*).

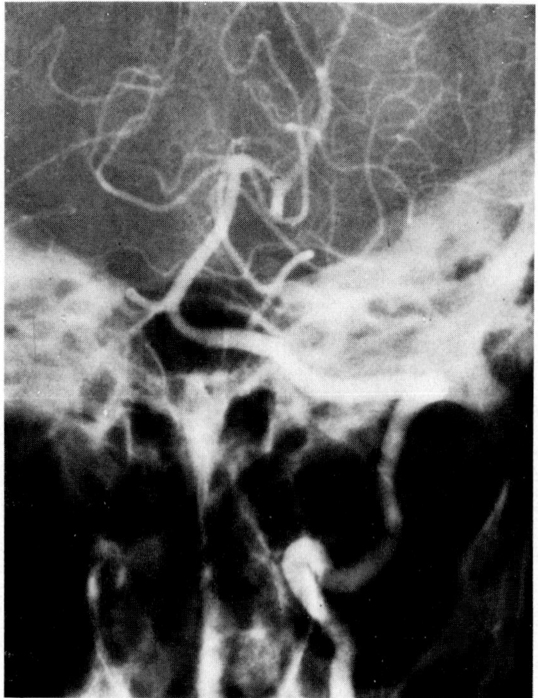

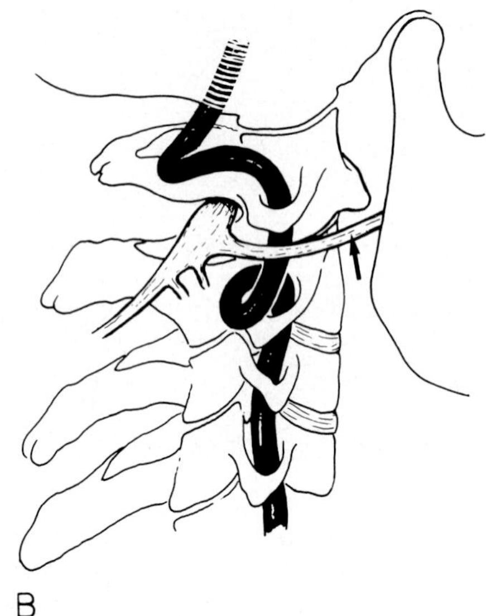

Figure 30 – 12. **A:** An intraosseous (C2) bight of the vertebral artery. **B:** Dynamic obstruction of the vertebral artery at C2.

quate length of the artery. Segmental resection allows restoration of flow without a graft, which is desirable in the younger patient. A three-year follow up with angiography has revealed good patency and excellent configuration of the anastomosis (see Figures 30 – 12 and 30 – 13).

Bypass to the Vertebral Artery at the Skull Base

When the proximal vertebral artery is patent and obstruction due to redundancy occurs at the C2 level, segmental resection is often adequate to restore normal flow. However, if vertebral artery obstruction exists proximal to C2 and cannot be corrected by reconstruction of the proximal segment, then reconstruction at the skull base by vein bypass is the procedure of choice (Carney *et al.,* 1977).

Distal Anastomosis

End-to-End Anastomosis. Because this technique requires ligation and division of the proximal end of the vertebral artery, it is easier technically to perform the anastomosis if the distal end of the artery is delivered out of the depth of the wound and into the surgical field. Hemodynamically, this type of anastomosis is less likely to lend itself to the occlusion because it eliminates competitive flow and provides better laminar flow within the vertebral artery, which should diminish the chance of failure. It is the procedure of choice when the proximal vertebral artery is to be excluded, as is the case with arteriovenous malformations. Its disadvantage is that the vertebral blood flow is interrupted during the performance of both the distal and the proximal anastomoses (see Figure 30 – 14).

Side-to-Side Anastomosis. The proximal vertebral artery is preserved with this technique. Also, if the bypass occludes later on, the postoperative status is not worse than it was preoperatively. The major advantages to vein bypass are that only a short length of artery needs to be mobilized for reconstruction, the dissection of the medial angle is avoided, and vertebral blood flow is only briefly interrupted. Vascular clamps can be applied and anastomosis accomplished in a mobilized arterial segment not more than 1.5 cm long. Ideally,

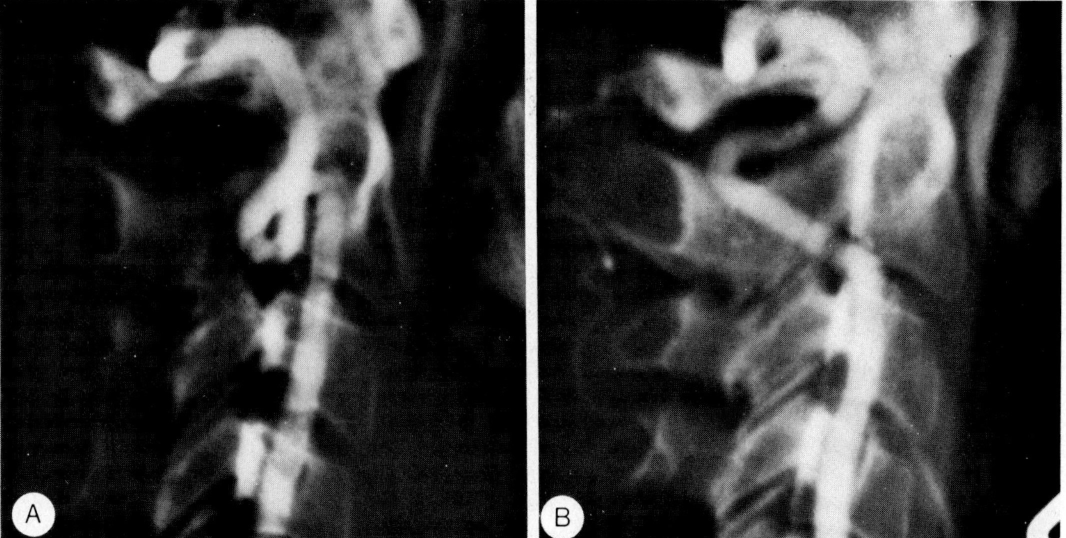

Figure 30–13. Angiograms: **A:** Preoperative. **B:** Postoperative 42 months. The principal indication for surgery in this patient was recurrent syncope resulting from head hyperextension.

this anastomosis should not compromise the lumen of the vertebral artery or the objective of the operation, i.e., preservation of the "native" vertebral artery, is lost.

The Proximal Anastomosis

Common Carotid Artery. The bypass to the vertebral artery should originate from a source that is adequate and will not be compromised by the position of the head, and does not jeopardize future surgery. The common carotid-to-distal vertebral arterial bypass which originates well below the carotid bifurcation fulfills these criteria. In the case of very low-lying bifurcation, bypass from the subclavian artery or from the internal carotid artery should be considered.

Subclavian Artery. This artery is a good site of origin for a bypass, because with the distal anastomosis at the skull base, it tends to place the graft posteriorly in the neck where it is less vulnerable to rotation. Another practical advantage to this procedure is that the contribution of the bypass to brain perfusion can be measured readily by compressing the graft. However, its use requires a second incision. One must also be careful because the subclavian artery is positioned lower than the vertebral artery so that air can be trapped in the vein graft. Backflow will not occur if the venous valves have not been removed, and passage of a probe is very difficult.

Internal Carotid Artery. After endarterectomy of an occluded internal carotid artery, its proximal segment offers an excellent takeoff site for a vein graft. Similarly, if the internal carotid is to be ligated for some reason, it should be made high at the skull base so that the proximal segment provides a satisfactory conduit to the vertebral artery (see Figure 30–15).

External Carotid Artery. The external carotid artery bypass to the C1-C2 vertebral artery fared poorly, with occlusions occurring in four of the first six reconstructions (Carney and Anderson, 1978). This type of reconstruction exposes the anastomosis to tension when the head is rotated to the opposite side. The bypasses that have remained open have shown considerable slack, and have taken on a "lazy-S" configuration as they cross superficial to the internal jugular vein without producing tension. Direct anastomosis of the external carotid to the midvertebral artery has also been reported (Bladin and Merory, 1975; Corkill *et al.*, 1977; Pritz *et al.*, 1981; see Figures 30–16, 30–17, and 30–18).

Occipital Artery. The occipital artery is a small-diameter vessel which approaches the vertebral artery at a right angle. Size discrepancy may make flow competition great. Attempts to use the occipital artery are often abandoned because of friability of the vessel. Mechanical motion at the skull base could also compromise the quality of vessel wall. Anasto-

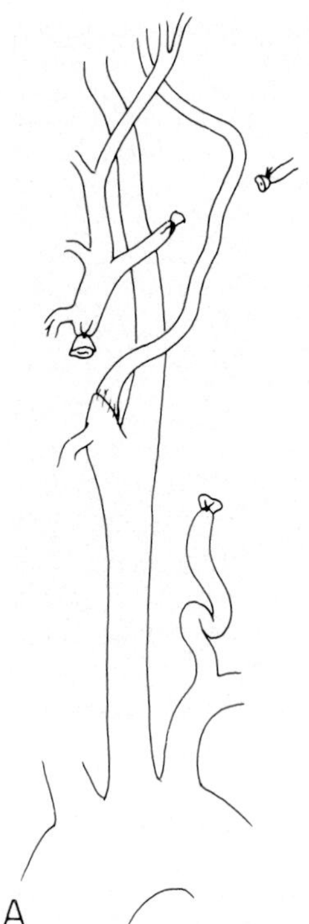

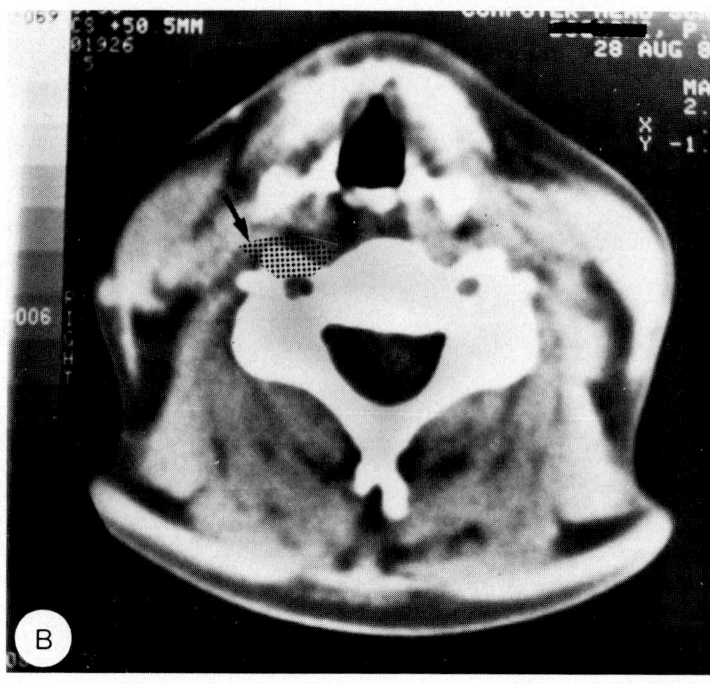

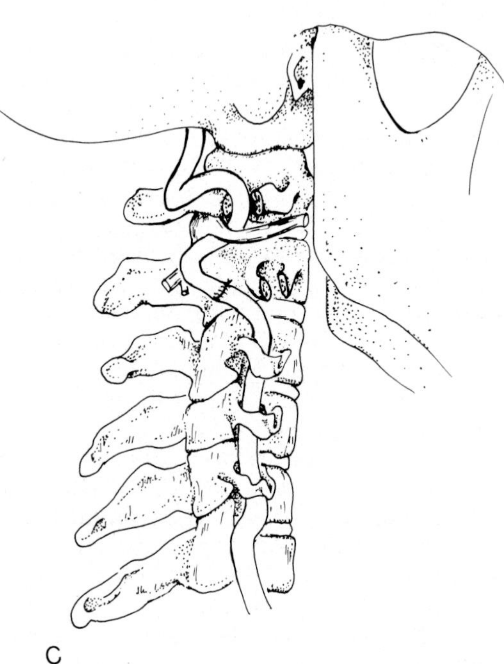

Figure 30–14. Mobilization of the entire vertebral artery to gain enough length to perform an end-to-end external carotid to proximal vertebral anastomosis at level of the carotid bifurcation. The principle of directly anastomosing the vertebral artery to the carotid artery involves the exclusion of the subclavian-vertebral artery inflow. When two large size vertebral arteries are present, this technique can be used (*A*). Cross section of a cervical vertebra on CT-scan. The shaded area of the cross-section of the bony vertebra indicates the limited amount of bone that must be removed to unroof and mobilize the vertebral artery (*B*). Segmental resection and anastomosis of the vertebral artery at the skull base (*C*).

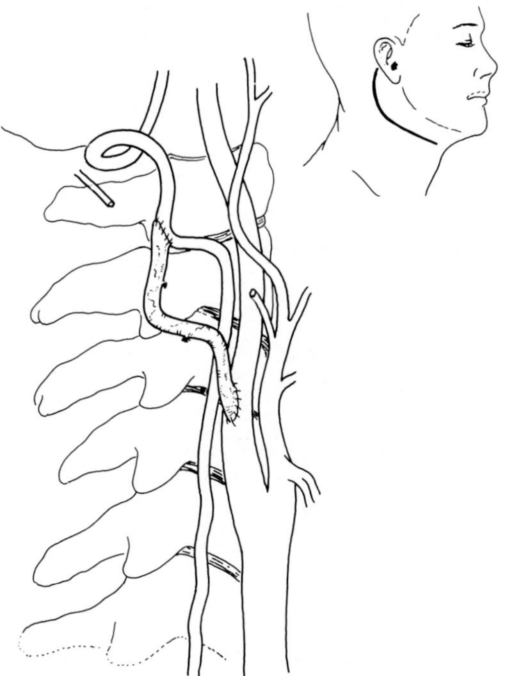

Figure 30–15. Internal carotid-to-distal vertebral artery bypass.

mosis of the occipital artery to a vessel of smaller diameter may have greater potential to remain open because of the lack of competitive flow.

COMPLICATIONS

Disruption of Reconstruction

In one of my patients, a thin-walled vein used as bypass graft disrupted on the fourth postoperative day at the site of segmental resection and anastomosis. In two other patients, vein patches utilized for angioplasty of the carotid artery ruptured, one from straining on the operating table, and the other during violent coughing on the fourth postoperative day.

Thrombosis Caused by Head Position

Head motion could cause graft failure even after a flawless reconstruction. The longitudinal axis of head rotation is posterior so that grafts so positioned are less subject to stress. Torsion and improper length of the bypass are also constant concerns to the surgeon. The course of the graft may be on either side of the jugular vein, but excess tension may compress the vein and also occlude the graft, whereas excess length can easily result in kinking. Grafts with a longitudinal axis fare much better than those with a horizontal axis. In one series, all bypasses from the occipital artery and all bypasses except two from the external carotid failed, irrespective of the level of the carotid bifurcation.

Neurological Deficit

There were no immediate operative deaths in this series. Of the two neurological deficits noted in the region supplied by the carotid artery, one was temporary and the other was permanent. The former patient had a tight stenosis of the carotid siphon and had a transient ischemic episode after surgery. The second patient had a low-lying carotid bifurcation and his vein bypass from the external carotid artery occluded asymptomatically in the postoperative period. Exploration failed to reveal any responsible mechanism for the occlusion. The situation was corrected by leaving the venous anastomosis intact, and placing a 4 mm Dacron prosthesis from the vein segment to the external carotid artery utilizing interrupted suture.

THE TRIGEMINAL ARTERY MODEL

The vein bypass to the distal vertebral artery has many similarities to the trigeminal artery, which connects the carotid to the basilar artery (see Figure 9–8). Complications may appear during the long-term follow-up of the bypass procedures. While the trigeminal artery is not subject to the stress of head motion and its wall is arterial not venous, the quality of the individual vein, its diameter, wall thickness and intima may affect long-term results.

Complications include embolism, thrombosis, and aneurysm (Carney, 1981; Kojimi *et al.*, 1983; McCormick and Greene, 1967) which may be manifested by brainstem transient ischemic attacks, visual symptoms, and even cortical blindness. Clinicians should watch for these complications in patients undergoing bypass to the distal vertebral artery. The effects of alterations in perfusion pressure and volume flow on the arterial system and on neurological functions require further observation.

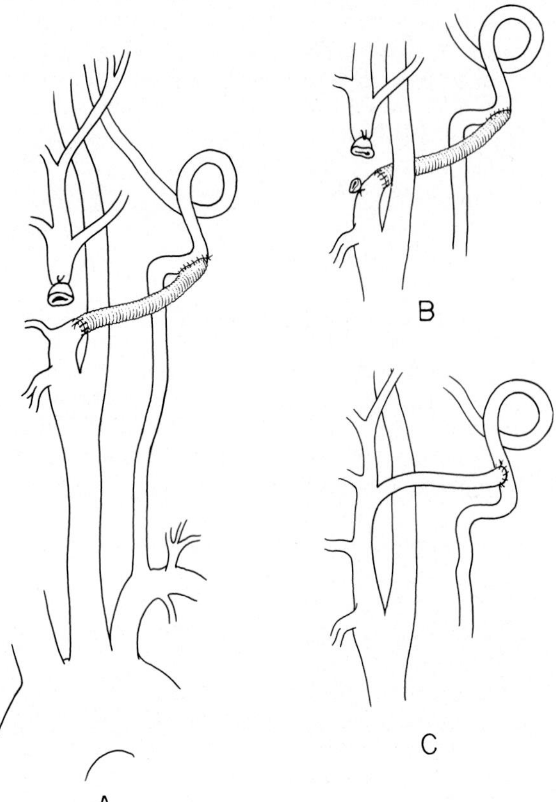

Figure 30–16. Different varieties of external carotid-to-distal vertebral artery bypass: superficial to the internal carotid artery (*A*), deep to the internal carotid artery (*B*), and occipital artery-to-distal vertebral artery bypass (*C*).

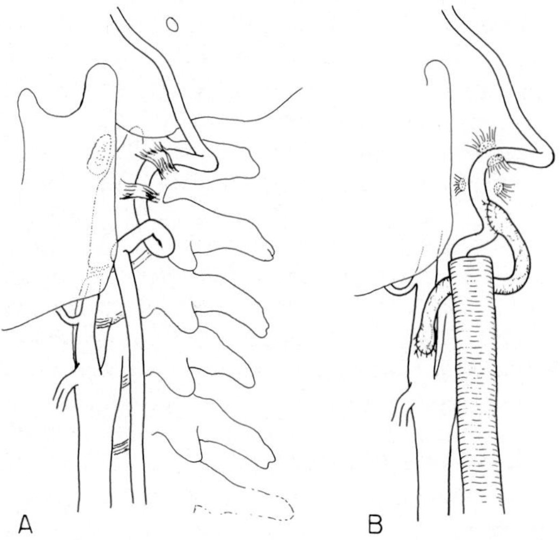

Figure 30–17. Schematic representation of the procedure used in a patient in whom vertebral flow was impeded by a combination of buckling and fibrous obstruction at the skull base (*A*) Surgical reconstruction consisted of releasing the fibrous compression and performing an external carotid-to-distal vertebral artery bypass using an autogenous saphenous vein graft (*B*).

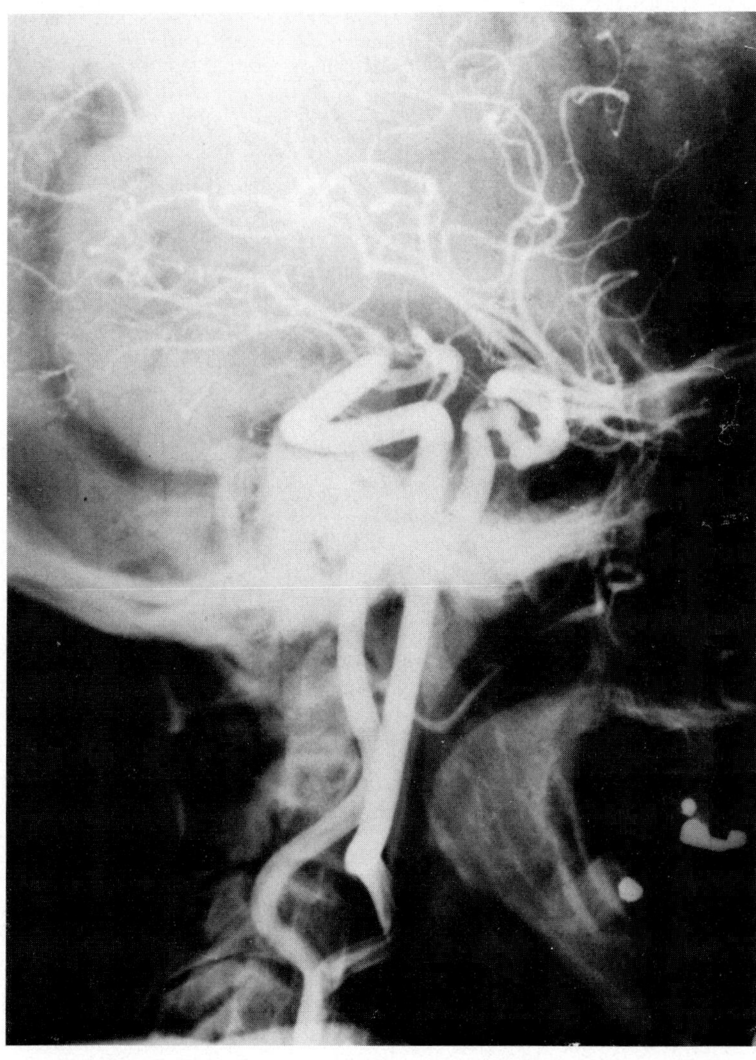

Figure 30-18. Extracranial-intracranial bypass to the posterior cerebral artery in a patient with basilar artery occlusion. The vein bypass arose from the external carotid artery.

Recovery

The patient usually feels better immediately after surgery. Within two to three weeks there is usually a relapse, but improvement is gradual thereafter. Being forewarned of this seems to benefit patients greatly. However, an occasional patient may require repeated hospitalization and administration of plasma volume expanders for relief. The use of a cervical pillow at night and a soft cervical collar is desirable in the early postoperative period.

In general, the time required to obtain relief of symptoms is directly related to their duration. Patients with symptoms of short duration obtain maximal improvement in about 12 weeks after surgery, which corresponds to the time when induration of the tissues of the neck subsides. If symptoms are longstanding, improvement continues more slowly over 24 months.

Although some patients will not experience anesthesia of the area supplied after division of the greater auricular nerve, most will retain some permanent numbness that is aggravated by cold weather. Patients should be informed of that in advance. Injury to the spinal accessory nerve will weaken shoulder stability, which requires six to 12 month to resolve.

THE INTRACRANIAL VERTEBRAL ARTERY

The history of ligation of the vertebral artery through the suboccipital approach goes back to 1888 (Matas, 1893). Before microvascular surgery was developed, this was the only operative procedure utilized on the intracranial vertebral artery. The objective was, naturally, not revascularization, but rather control of bleeding, obliteration of an arteriovenous fistula, or exclusion of a cervical aneurysm. Waga and associates (1978) controlled a dissecting aneurysm that extended to the posterior inferior cerebellar artery by clipping the intracranial vertebral artery proximal to the aneurysm.

CONCLUSION

In summary, vertebral artery surgery is more complex than that in the carotid artery. Revascularization is now possible at all levels of the head and neck. I have performed a total of 115 reconstructions of the vertebral artery at the skull base with minimal morbidity and mortality rates and have attained good relief of symptoms and the disappearance of disability. Long-term patency appears to be adequate, but the technical considerations of providing a suitable conduit and supply of blood and the biomechanics of head motion must continue to receive careful clinical and experimental trials.

Finally, the carotid-vertebral communication constitutes an extracranial limb of the circle of Willis, a revolutionary concept. The bypass to the vertebral artery at skull base is not simple, and its construction requires meticulous technique and understanding of the biomechanics of head motion. The reality of this procedure has necessitated a diagnostic approach which has integrated diverse specialties, extended the focus from the cerebral hemispheres to the entire brain and extended the realm of technical possibility. The system approach to brain blood flow integrates brain perfusion with neurological function.

REFERENCES

Bakay, L., and Leslie, E.V.: Surgical treatment of vertebral artery insufficiency caused by cervical spondylosis. *J. Neurosurg.*, **23**:596–601, 1965.

Bakay, L., and Sweet, W.H.: Intra-arterial pressures in the neck and brain: late changes after carotid closure, acute measurements after vertebral closure. *J. Neurosurg.*, **10**:353–59, 1953.

Berguer, R.; Andaya, L.V.; and Bauer, R.B.: Vertebral artery bypass. *Arch. Surg.*, **111**:976–79, 1976.

Bladin, P.F., and Merory, J.: Mechanisms in cerebral lesions in trauma to high cervical portion of the vertebral artery-rotation injury. *Proc. Aust. Assoc. Neurol.* **12**:35–41, 1975.

Bogousslavsky, J., and Regli, G.: Vertebrobasilar transient ischemic attacks in internal carotid artery occlusion or tight stenosis. *Arch. Neurol.*, **42**:64–68, 1985.

Bohl, J.; Fenshke, A.; Reuten, H.J.; and Schindler, E.: Giant aneurysm of the vertebral artery causing compression of the lower medulla oblongata. *J. Neurol.*, **214**:289–93, 1977.

Bohmfalk, G.L.; Story, J.L.; Brown, W.E., Jr.; and Marlin, A.E.: Subclavian steal syndrome. Part I: Proximal vertebral to common carotid transposition in three patients, and historical review. *J. Neurosurg.*, **51**:628–40, 1979.

Brain, L.: Some unsolved problems of cervical spondylosis. *Br. Med. J.*, **1**:771–77, 1963.

Buonanno, G.S.; DeWitt, L.S.; Kistler, J.P.; and Davis, K.R.: Proton nuclear magnetic resonance imaging in posterior circulation stroke. In Berguer, R., and Bauer, R.B. (eds.): *Vertebral Basilar Arterial Occlusive Disease.* Raven Press, New York, pages 149–61, 1984.

Camp, P.E.: Carotid to distal vertebral artery bypass for vertebrobasilar ischemia. *J. Neurosurg.*, **60**:187–89, 1984.

Carney, A.L.: Vertebral artery surgery: historical development, basic concepts of brain hemodynamics, and clinical experience of 102 cases. *Adv. Neurol.*, **30**:249–82, 1981.

Carney, A.L., and Anderson, E.M.: Carotid distal vertebral artery bypass for carotid artery occlusion. *Clin. Electroencephalogr.*, **9**:105–9, 1978.

Carney, A.L., and Anderson, E.M.: Hypoglossal carotid entrapment syndrome. *Adv. Neurol.*, **30**:223–47, 1981a.

Carney, A.L., and Anderson, E.M.: The system approach to brain ischemia. *Adv. Neurol.*, **30**:1–30, 1981b.

Carney, A.L.; Anderson, E.M.; and Burns, E.: Cerebral hemodynamic evaluation. *Adv. Neurol.*, **30**:335–60, 1981.

Carney, A.L.; Emanuele, R.; and Anderson, E.M.: *Carotid Distal Vertebral Artery Bypass.* Medicom A-V Productions, Chicago, 1977.

Carney, A.L.; Emanuele, R.; and Anderson, E.M.: *Surgery of the Vertebral Artery.* Medicom A-V Productions, Chicago, 1976.

Cate, W.R., Jr., and Scott, H.W., Jr.: Cerebral ischemia of central origin: relief by subclavian-vertebral artery thromboendarterectomy. *Surgery*, **45**:19–31, 1959.

Causse, J.B., and Causse, J.: A new nystagmographic test for the elicitation of sub-clinical vertebro-basilar insufficiency and poor cochleo-vestibular vascularization. *J. Laryngol. Otol.*, **93**:969–74, 1979.

Clark, K., and Perry, M.O.: Carotid vertebral anastomosis: an alternate technique for repair of the subclavian steal syndrome. *Ann. Surg.*, **163**:414–16, 1966.

Corkill, G.; French, B.N.; Michas, C.; Cobb, C.A.; and Mims, T.J.: External carotid-vertebral artery anastomosis for vertebrobasilar insufficiency. *Surg. Neurol.*, **7**:109–15, 1977.

Cormier, J.M., and Laurian, C.: Surgical management of vertebral-basilar insufficiency. *J. Cardiovasc. Surg.*, **17**:205–23, 1976.

Crawford, E.S.; Debakey, M.E.; and Fields, W.S.: Roentgenographic diagnosis and surgical treatment of basilar artery insufficiency. *J.A.M.A.*, **168**:509–14, 1958.

Dandy, W.E.: *Intracranial Arterial Aneurysms.* Comstock, Ithaca, New York, 1944.

DeBrun, G.; Lacour, P.; Caron, J.P.; Hurth, M.; Comoy, J.; and Keravel, Y.: Detachable balloon and calibrated-leak balloon techniques in the treatment of cerebrovascular spasm. *J. Neurosurg.*, **49**:635–49, 1978.

DeVilliers, J.C.: A brachiocephalic vascular syndrome associated with rib. *Br. Med. J.*, **2**:140–44, 1966.

Diaz, F.G.; Ausman, J.I.; de los Reyes, R.A.; Pearce, J.; Shrontx, C.; Mehta, B.; Patel, S., and Dujovny, M.: Combined reconstruction of the vertebral and carotid artery in one single procedure. *Neurosurgery*, **12**:629–35, 1983.

Edwards, W.L., and Mulherin, J.L., Jr.: The surgical management of the vertebral and subclavian arteries. *Surgery*, **87**:20–8, 1980.

Eikelboom, B.C.: *Evaluation of Carotid Artery Disease and Potential Collateral Circulation by Ocular Pneumoplethysmography.* Uitgeversmaatschappij Huisartsenpers B.V., Utrecht, 1981.

Fisch, U.; Nagahara, K.; and Pollak, A.: Sudden hearing loss: circulatory. *Am. J. Otolaryngol.*, **5**:488–91, 1984.

Fisher, C.M.; Gore, I.; Okabe, N., and White, P.D.: Atherosclerosis of the carotid and vertebral arteries: extracranial and intracranial. *J. Neurolpathol. Exp. Neurol.*, **24**:455–76, 1965.

Furlan, A.J., and Breuer, A.C.: Central nervous system complications of open heart surgery. *Stroke*, **15**:912–15, 1984.

George, B., and Laurian, C.: Surgical possibilities in the third portion of the vertebral artery (above C2). *Acta. Neurochir.*, Suppl. **28**:263–69, 1979.

Glenn, W.L.; Haak, B.; Sasaki, C.; and Kitchner, J.: Characteristics and surgical management of respiratory complications accompanying pathological lesions of the brain stem. *Ann. Surg.*, **191**:655–63, 1980.

Gortvai, P.: Insufficiency of vertebral artery treated by decompression of its cervical part. *Br. Med. J.*, **2**:233–34, 1964.

Green, H.D.; Cosby, R.S.; and Radzow, K.H.: Dynamics of the collateral circulation. *Am. J. Physiol.*, **140**:726–36, 1944.

Hardin, C.A.: Vertebral artery insufficiency produced by cervical osteroarthritic spurs. *Arch. Surg.*, **90**:629–33, 1965.

Hauge, T.: Catheter vertebral angiography. *Acta. Radiol.*, Suppl. **109**:1–219, 1954.

Henry, A.K.: *Extensile Exposure.* Williams & Wilkins, Baltimore, Maryland, 1957.

Hoobler, S.W.: Syndrome of cervical rib with subclavian arterial thrombosis and hemiplegia due to cerebral embolism. *N. Engl. J. Med.*, **226**:942–44, 1942.

Husni, E.A.; Bell, H.S.; and Storer, J.: Mechanical occlusion of the vertebral artery. *J.A.M.A.*, **196**:475–78, 1966.

Hutchinson, E.C., and Yates, P.O.: Carotico-vertebral stenosis. *Lancet*, **1**:2–8, 1957.

Kistler, J.P.; Buonanno, F.S.; DeWitt, L.D.; Davis, K.R.; Brady, T.K.; and Fisher, C.M.: Vertebral-basilar posterior cerebral territory stroke delineation by proton nuclear magnetic resonance imaging. *Stroke*, **15**:417–26, 1984.

Klein, R.A.; Snyder, R.D.; and Schwarz, H.J.: Lateral medullary syndrome in a child: arteriographic confirmation of vertebral artery occlusion. *J.A.M.A.*, **235**:940–41, 1976.

Kojimi, T.; Waga, S.; and Kanemaur, K.: Anastomosis of the superior thyroid artery to the vertebral artery for vertebrobasilar insufficiency. *Surg. Neurol.*, **20**:481–86, 1983.

Kovacs, A.: Subluxation and deformation of the cervical apophyseal joints: a contribution to the etiology of headache. *Acta Radiol.*, **43**:1–16, 1955.

Kramer, S.P.: Function of the circle of Willis. *J. Exp. Med.*, **15**:348–63, 1912.

Krueger, B.R., and Okazaki, H.: Vertebral basilar infarction following chiropractic manipulation. *Mayo Clin. Proc.* **555**:322–32, 1980.

Kumar, A.: Reliability of central vestibular testing in the identification of posterior fossa pathology. *Adv. Neurol.*, **30**:291–99, 1981.

Latchaw, R.E.; Seeger, J.F.; and Gabrielson, T.O.: Vertebrobasilar arterial obstruction in childhood. *Neuroradiology*, **8**:141–47, 1974.

Matas, R.: Aneurysms and wounds of the vertebral arteries. *Ann. Surg.*, **18**:477–516, 1893.

Moran, J.: Discussion. In Edwards, W.J., and Mulherin, J.L., Jr.: The surgical management of the vertebral and subclavian arteries. *Surgery*, **87**:20–8, 1980.

Motarjeme, A.; Keifer, J.W.; and Zuska, A.J.: Percutaneous transluminal angioplasty of the brachiocephalic arteries. *A.J.R.*, **138**:457–62, 1982.

McCormick, W.F., and Greene, J.: Carotid-basilar anastomoses. *J. Iowa Med. Soc.*, **57**:551–56, 1967.

Nagashima, C.: Surgical treatment of vertebral artery insufficiency caused by cervical spondylosis. *J. Neurosurg.*, **32**:512–21, 1970.

Nanson, E.M.: The surgery of the deep lobe of the parotid salivary gland. *Surg. Gynecol. Obstet.*, **122**:811–6, 1966.

Nenci, G.G.; Gresele, P.; Taramelli, M.; Agnelli, G.; and Signornini, E.: Thrombolytic therapy for thromboembolism of vertebrobasilar artery. *Angiology*, **34**:561–71, 1983.

Nornes, H.: The role of the circle of Willis in graded occlusion of the internal carotid artery in man. *Acta Neurochir.*, **28**:165–77, 1973.

Norrell, H.A.: Fractures and dislocations of the spine. In Rothman R.H., and Simeone, F.A. (eds.): *The Spine.* W.B. Saunders, Philadelphia, Pennsylvania, pages 529–66, 1975.

Pritz, M.B.; Chandler, W.F.; and Kindt, G.W.: Vertebral artery disease: radiological evaluation, medical management, and microsurgical treatment. *Neurosurgery*, **9**:524–30, 1981.

Rainer, W.G.; Quianzon, E.P.; Liggett, M.S.; Newby, J.P.; and Bloomquist, C.D.: Surgical considerations in the treatment of vertebrobasilar arterial insufficiency. *Am. J. Surg.*, **120**:594–97, 1970.

Robicsek, F., and Selle, J.G.: Transthoracic approach to the left subclavian and vertebral arteries. *J. Thorac. Cardiovasc. Surg.* **89**:144–46, 1985.

Senter, H.G., and Long, E.T.: Subclavian to distal vertebral artery bypass. *J. Neurosurg.*, **58**:607–10, 1983.

Shintani, A., and Zervas, N.T.: Consequence of ligation of the vertebral artery. *J. Neurosurg.*, **36**:447–50, 1972.

Simeone, F.A., and Goldberg, H.I.: Thrombosis of the vertebral artery from hyperextension injury to the neck. *J. Neurosurg.*, **29**:540–44, 1968.

Sundt, T.M.; Smith, H.C.; Campbell, J.K.; Vlietstra, R.E.; Cucchiara, R.F.; and Stanson, A.W.: Transluminal angioplasty for basilar artery stenosis. *Mayo Clin. Proc.*, **55**:673–80, 1980.

Takahaski, M.: *Atlas of Vertebral Angiography.* University Park Press, Baltimore, Maryland, 1974.

Verbiest, H.: Anterolateral operations for fractures and dislocations in the middle and lower parts of the cervical spine. *J. Bone Joint Surg.*, **51A**:1489–1530, 1969.

Wackenheim, A.: *Roentgen Diagnosis of the Cranioverte-bral Region.* Springer-Verlag, New York, 1974.

Waga, S.; Fugimoto, K.; and Morooka, Y.: Dissecting an-eurysm of the vertebral artery. *Surg. Neurol.*, **10**:237–39, 1978.

Williams, D., and Wilson, T.G.: The diagnosis of the major and minor syndromes of basilar insufficiency. *Brain*, **85**:741–74, 1962.

Yates, P.O.: Birth trauma to the vertebral arteries. *Arch. Dis. Child.*, **34**:436–41, 1959.

Yates, P.I., and Hutchinson, E.C.: *Cerebral Infarction: The Role of Stenosis of the Extracranial Arteries.* Medical Research Council, Special Report Series, No. 300. H.M. Stationery Office, London, 1961.

Zimmerman, A.W.; Kumar, A.J.; Gadoth, N.I.; and Hodges, G.J.: Traumatic vertebrobasilar occlusive dis-ease in childhood. *Neurology*, **28**:185–88, 1978.

Index

A

B

C

F

G

H

I

J

K

L

M

N

O

P

Q

R

S

T

U

V

W

X